Dictionary and Handbook
of
Nuclear Medicine
and
Clinical Imaging

Mario P. Iturralde, M.D., D.M.C., D.M.
Chief Specialist and Head
Department of Nuclear Medicine
H. F. Verwoerd Hospital, Pretoria

and

Professor and Chairman
Department of Nuclear Medicine
University of Pretoria
Pretoria, Republic of South Africa

CRC Press
Boca Raton   Ann Arbor   Boston

Library of Congress Cataloging-in-Publication Data

Iturralde, Mario P., 1933-
Dictionary and handbook of nuclear medicine and clinical imaging
Mario P. Iturralde.
p. cm.
Includes bibliographies and index.
ISBN 0-8493-3233-8
1. Diagnostic imaging—Handbooks, manuals, etc. 2. Nuclear
medicine—Handbooks, manuals, etc. I. Title.
[DNLM: 1. Diagnostic Imaging—dictionaries. 2. Nuclear Medicine-
-dictionaries. 3. Radiation Dosage—handbooks. 4. Radioisotopes-
-handbooks. WN 13 I91d]
RC78.7.D53I88 1990
616.07'54—dc20
DNLM/DLC
for Library of Congress
89-10006
CIP

Direct all inquiries to CRC Press, Inc., 2000 Corporate Blvd., N.W., Boca Raton, Florida 33431.

© 1990 by CRC Press, Inc.

International Standard Book Number 0-8493-3233-8

Library of Congress Card Number 89-10006
Printed in the United States

FOREWORD

This Dictionary and Handbook of Basic Nuclear Medical Science and Clinical Imaging was urgently needed. It bridges the gap between those highly sophisticated papers and publications dealing with specialized problems in clinical diagnostic imaging on the one hand, and on the other hand, the large volumes dealing with basic sciences generally.

General medical practitioners as well as specialists frequently find themselves being trapped in a multidisciplinary network which is characterized by crossroads of various scientific worlds: physics, chemistry, informatics, biology, medicine, etc. This means a vocabulary of variant origin and changing definition corresponding to the multidisciplinatory nature of the field.

The foreseeable merits of this Dictionary and Handbook are

1. The fast overview information to those readers who are still unfamiliar with the field of basic nuclear medical science and clinical imaging.
2. The more in-depth information for the postgraduate reader who wants to take the board examination in Nuclear Medicine or Radiology. This reference book may serve as a concise directory for the studies and as a source of key words to check the acquired pretest level of knowledge.
3. The realization of an abundant source of related data for the specialist.
4. The clear definition of terms which sometimes have an aura of indeterminacy and/or of double meaning.

In conclusion, these merits with regard to the present situation of nuclear medicine and clinical imaging literature seem to provide a bright future for this Dictionary and Handbook. However, not being a professional fortune-teller, the acceptance of this publication within the next years will decide whether my colleagues share the favorable opinion I have of this informative publication.

Prof. Dr. med. W. E. Adam, M.D.
Director, Department of Nuclear Medicine
University of Ulm Medical Center
Ulm/Donau
Federal Republic of Germany

NOTICE

Procedures and guidelines for the administration of radiopharmaceuticals as well as pharmacological interventions, are described in this Dictionary and Handbook. While every effort has been made to ensure that the suggested pharmacological dosage schedules comply with the standards accepted at the time of publication, new research and clinical experience may require changes in the recommended procedures and doses.

The author and publishers of this book suggest that readers consult the current literature and check the product information sheet included in the package of radiopharmaceuticals to make sure that changes have not been introduced in the dosage schedules, procedures, and/or special precautions for the administration of these products. This suggestion is of particular importance when trying new products or when using them for pregnant women and children.

Since the general recommendation provides for individual variations, the final decision regarding this matter is the responsibility of the attending physician.

PREFACE

Impressive advances in medicine and biology have been made recently by medical scientists who have used great ingenuity in adapting the tools and techniques of the physical, chemical, and mathematical sciences to their complex medical and biological problems. Perhaps no field in the life sciences so typifies this revolution as the field of nuclear medicine, which in the past 40 years has emerged as an integrated medical discipline. In so doing, this young and fast growing medical speciality has significantly expanded the physician's armamentarium, improving the quality of patient management.

Nuclear medicine has developed with the help of many disciplines from which it has borrowed and into which it has grown, reaching far beyond the field of medicine. Its vocabulary is therefore a complex and rich collection of terms and definitions contributed by each of the multiple disciplinary components that make up the field.

As expected with advances in knowledge, changes in terminology are logical and desirable developments. New discoveries, new concepts, new theories — all must have, it seems, new words or new groupings of words to describe and define them in speech and print. Proper terms are highly important for communication in any subject. They are powerful tools for directing thought, and if properly chosen can be a great aid in teaching the subject to those interested, but unfamiliar with it.

A need has become apparent for a compact, easy-to-use reference textbook which will interpret this new world of nuclear medical science to its readers. The present volume is designed to meet this need by supplying both a dictionary of the most commonly encountered words in nuclear medicine and a comprehensive handbook of the background material necessary for understanding their use in a wider context. The assembly of related data in tables serves the additional purpose of grouping information under broad headings of reference, thereby sparing the reader much searching in the literature.

The dictionary is certainly not original, because the author refrained from creating or inventing new terms which would form a further burden for existing medical terminology. The vocabulary in this dictionary is therefore a collection of widely used terms and definitions that appear in many of the textbooks, treatises, monographs and well-known periodicals dealing with the basic science of nuclear medicine and clinical imaging. This includes some slang words and other made-up terms which technical people use when talking to each other. Medical terms as such have been limited, as most of them can be easily found in any medical dictionary.

The topicality of the Dictionary and Handbook is, of course, an important consideration, and I have therefore included terms defining techniques which have recently blossomed in importance. These include theoretical and practical aspects of clinical imaging in all its modes: computerized axial tomography (CAT), digital subtraction angiography (DSA), ultrasound scanning (US), nuclear magnetic resonance imaging (NMRI), positron emission tomography (PET), single photon emission computerized tomography (SPECT), and radionuclide imaging in general.

In writing such a volume of diversified scientific information, it is possible that many errors of both commission and omission have been made. I would appeal to interested users finding any such errors to bring them to my attention.

The essence of knowledge is, having it, to apply it.
Confucius (551—479 B.C.)

Mario P. Iturralde

THE AUTHOR

Mario P. Iturralde, M.D., D.M.C., D.M., is Chief Specialist and Head of the Department of Nuclear Medicine, H. F. Verwoerd Hospital, Pretoria, and Professor and Chairman of the Department of Nuclear Medicine, University of Pretoria, Republic of South Africa.

Professor Iturralde graduated in 1960 with an M.D. degree from the Faculty of Medicine, Universidad Mayor de San Andres, La Paz, Bolivia. In 1963 he obtained the D.M.C. degree from the Universidad Mayor Real y Pontificia de San Francisco Xavier, Sucre, Bolivia, and in 1975, the degree of Doctor of Medicine (D.M.) from the University of the Orange Free State, Bloemfontein, Republic of South Africa. Professor Iturralde received intensive training in Nuclear Medicine in Brazil, Puerto Rico, and the United States with a grant from the World Health Organization.

Professor Iturralde is a member of the Society of Nuclear Medicine (U.S.), South African Society of Nuclear Medicine (charter member and first president), South African Institute of International Affairs, University of South Africa (UNISA) Centre for Latin American Studies, South African Association for Medical Education, and the South African Transplantation Society. He has served as scientific advisor to the Presidency of the Republic of Bolivia, as member of the Life Sciences Committee of the South African Atomic Energy Board, as member of the Biological Sciences Advisory Panel of the National Accelerator Centre of the South African Council for Scientific and Industrial Research, and as member of the Working Group for Nuclear Medicine for the implementation of SI Units for ionizing radiation and the Committee on Medical Use of Ionizing Radiation of the South African Bureau of Standards. In 1988, Professor Iturralde was invited to the Republic of China, Taiwan, as visiting professor of Nuclear Medicine, and he is an active correspondent member from South Africa and International Advisor to the World Federation of Nuclear Medicine and Biology. He is also a member of the Life Sciences Institute of the University of Pretoria, as well as a member of the editorial board of *Latin American Report* of the UNISA Centre for Latin American Studies. He has been awarded the decoration of the Order of Merit of the Republic of Egypt, the First Chris Jansen Memorial Lecture Medal by the South African Society of Nuclear Medicine, and Plaques of Honour by the Veterans General Hospital, Taipei, and the 4th Asia and Oceania Congress of Nuclear Medicine.

Professor Iturralde has presented 95 lectures at international and national meetings as well as 25 guest lectures at universities and institutes. He has published more than 100 research papers as well as 5 book chapters. His current major interests include radionuclide diagnostic imaging in organ transplantation, neuroendocrine disorders, and reproductive physiology.

ACKNOWLEDGMENTS

I am indebted to friends and colleagues who have helped me in the task of writing, compiling and reviewing this volume.

Special gratitude is extended to Professor Emeritus Bernard J. Meyer of the University of Pretoria, to whom I owe a great deal for his invaluable suggestions and friendly encouragement. Thanks are due to Dr. Aldo Serafini of the University of Miami, and Mrs. Naomi Eliovson, editor of *Nuclear Active*, for their comments on the contents of the book, and to Mrs. Marietjie Dowling of the Bureau of Computer Services at the University of Pretoria, for her technical assistance.

Cooperation and assistance in numerous ways from members of the Department of Nuclear Medicine and Medical Library at the University of Pretoria is greatly appreciated.

Finally, I am ever grateful and thankful to Mrs. Susan Wilbers, for her excellence and patient typing of the manuscript, while the assistance of the publisher, CRC Press, Inc., deserves my gratitude and recognition.

Dedicated to:

THE MEMORY OF MY MOTHER
for her selfless devotion to her family

MY WIFE
for her support and understanding without which this task would never have been accomplished

MY CHILDREN
for making everything worthwhile

DICTIONARY

DATA HANDBOOK

International System (SI) Units for the Measurement of Radioactivity and Ionizing Radiation

DICTIONARY

FUNDAMENTALS OF ENGLISH MEDICAL ETYMOLOGY

ENGLISH, THE LINGUA FRANCA OF MEDICINE

There was a time when no civilized person would have thought of writing about medicine in any language other than Latin, which was the Esperanto of the educated world, and its last traces probably disappeared when those responsible for the membership examination of the Royal College of Physicians of London some decades back decided to omit questions on Latin and Greek from the papers.

During the 40 years since World War II there has been a gradual takeover of medical communication by the English language. However, some familiarity with Greek and Latin, which contribute so largely to English medical terminology must obviously simplify the task of learning a basic vocabulary and understanding new words as they are encountered.

Even today, at least 50% of the modern general English vocabulary is of Greek or Latin origin, and it is a conservative guess that as much as 75% of the scientific component is of such origin (most of it in the form of anatomical nomenclature, as original Latin and not derivative). Greek words have come into English through Latin, in which they have undergone some change, or through a second intermediary language, such as French, with still further change.

Latin, in fact, borrowed heavily from Greek over the centuries. The Latin alphabet as we use it is derived with slight modifications from the Greek alphabet, which is almost completely phonetic. The most constant change, however, in the transition of Greek and Latin words to English is the loss of termination which produces the combining form.

In general, most words derived from Greek or Latin consist of a root or base which is modified by a prefix or a suffix, or both. The root is often abbreviated when the prefix or suffix is added. A prefix, commonly a preposition or adverb, consists of one or two syllables placed before a word to modify the meaning of it. A suffix, which constitutes the third element in the formation of compounds, is a syllable or syllables added to the end of a word or root in order to modify its meaning.

ANALYTICAL AND ETYMOLOGICAL WORD LIST OF GREEK AND LATIN COMBINED FORMS, PREFIXES AND SUFFIXES

a-	a- (n is added before words beginning with a vowel) negative prefix: asexual, anoxia
ab-	away from: abductor
abdomin-	abdomen: abdominal
acet-	vinegar: acetate
acid-	sour: aciduric
acou-	hear: acoustics
acr-	extremity, peak: acromegaly
act-	do, drive: interaction
actin-	ray, radius: actinomicosis
ad-	ad (d changes to c, f, g, p, s, or t before words beginning with those consonants) to toward: adrenal
aden-	gland: adenoma
adip-	fat: adiposity
aer-	air: aerobic
-agogue	leading, inducing: galactagogue
-agra	catching, seizure: podagral
alb-	white: albicans

alg-	pain: neuralgia
all-	other, different: allergen
alve-	through, channel, cavity: alveolar
amphi-	(i is dropped before words beginning with a vowel) both, doubly: amphibious
amyl-	starch: amyloidosis
ana-	(final a is dropped before words beginning with a vowel) up, positive: anaphylactic
andr-	man: androgen
angi-	vessel: angiology
ankyl-	crooked: ankylosis
ante-	before: antecubital
anti-	(i is dropped before words beginning with a vowel) against, counter: antigen, antagonist
antr-	cavern: antronasal
-aph-	touch: dysaphia
apo-	(o is dropped before words beginning with a vowel) away from, detached: apophysis
arachn-	spider arachnoid
arch-	beginning, origin: archetype
arter(i)-	artery, arteriosclerosis
arthr-	joint: arthritis
articul-	joint: articulation
aur-	ear: auricle
aux-	increase: auxanology
ax-	axis: axis
axon-	axis: axoneurone
bacill-	small staff, rod: lactobacillus
bacter-	small staff, rod: bacteriology
ball-	throw: ballistics
bar-	weight: barometer
bi-	life: aerobic
bi-	two, double: biarticular
bil-	bile: biliary
blast-	bud, a growing thing in its early stages: blastoma
blephar-	eyelid: blepharoptosis
brachi-	arm: brachialgia
brachy-	short: brachydactylia
brady-	slow: bradycardia
brom-	stench: podobromidrosis
bronch-	windpipe: bronchitis
bry-	full of life: embryonic
bucc-	cheek: buccal
cac-	bad, abnormal: cacosmia
calc-	stone, limestone, lime: calcification
calc-	heel: calcaneodynia
calor-	heat: calorimeter
cancr-	crab, cancer: cancroid
capit-	head: capitate
caps-	container: encapsulated
carbo(n)-	coal, charcoal: carbohydrate

carcin-	crab, cancer: carcinoma
cardi-	heart: cardiomegaly
cata-	(final a is dropped before words beginning with a vowel) down, negative: catabolism
caud-	tail: caudal
cav-	hollow: concavity
cec-	blind: cecum
-cele	tumor, hernia: varicocele
cell-	room cell: cellular
cen-	common: cenosite
cent-	hundred: fractions of units in the metric system, centimeter, centipede
cente-	puncture: centesis
centr-	center: neurocentral
cephal-	head: cephalic
cept-	take, receive: receptor
cer-	wax: cerumen
cerebr-	cerebrum: cerebrospinal
cervic-	cervix, neck: cervicitis
cheil-	lip: cheilitis
cheir-	(also spelled chir-) hand: chirurgical
chlor-	green: chlorophyll
chol-	bile: cholangiography
chondr-	cartilage: chondromucoid
chord-	string, cord: chordoma
chori-	protective fetal membrane: choriocarcinoma
chro-	color: monochromatic
chron-	time: chronology
chy-	pour: ecchymosis
-cid(e)	cut, kill: germicidal
cili-	eyelid: superciliary
circum-	around: circumferential
-cis-	cut, kill: excision
clas-	break: osteoclast
clin-	bend: incline, clinocephaly
clus-	shut: malocclusion
cocc-	seed, pill: streptococcus
coel-	or cel-, hollow: celiac
colon-	large intestine: colonic
colp-	hollow, vagina: colpitis
con-	con- (becomes co- before vowels or h; col- before l; com- before b, m, or p; cor- before r) with: conduction
contra-	against, counter: contraindication
copr-	dung: coproma
cor-	doll, little image, pupil: corectopia
corpor-	body: incorporation
cortic-	cortex, bark, rind: cortical
cost-	rib: costochondral
crani-	skull: craniotomy
creat-	meat, flesh: creatinin
cret-	distinguish, separate off; discrete

crin-	distinguish, separate off: endocrinology
crur-	leg: crural
cry-	cold: cryoagglutinin
crypt-	hide, conceal: cryptorchidia
cult-	tend: cultivate, culture
cune-	wedge: cuneiform
cut-	skin: cutaneous
cyan-	blue: cyancobalamin
cycl-	circle: cycle, cyclopentane
cyst-	bladder: cystitis
cyt-	cell: cytology
dacry-	tear: dacryocystitis
dactyl-	finger, toe: polydactylia
de-	down, from: decomposition
dec-[1]	ten, indicates multiple in metric system: decade
dec-[2]	ten, indicates fraction in metric system: decimeter
dendr-	tree: neurodendrite
dent-	tooth: dentist
derm(at)-	skin: dermatitis
desm-	ligament: desmopathy
dextr-	right-hand: ambidextrous
di-	two: diplopia
dia-	(a is dropped before words beginning with a vowel) through, apart: diagnosis
didym-	twin: epididymitis
digit-	finger, toe: digitalis
diplo-	double: diplopia
dis-	dis- (s may be dropped before a word beginning with a consonant) apart, away from: disability
disc-	disk: discotomy
dors-	back: dorsal
duct-	lead: conduct, oviduct
dur-	hard: induration
dynam(i)-	power: neurodynamic
dys-	bad, improper: dysfunction
e-	out from: ebonation
ec-	out of: eccentric
-echo-	have, hold, be: synechiotomy
ect-	outside: ectoderm
ede-	swell: edematous
electr-	amber: electrocardiography
-em-	blood: anemia
en-	(n changes to m before b, p, or ph) in, on: encephalitis
end-	inside: endocardium
enter-	intestine: gastroenterology
epi-	(i is dropped before words beginning with a vowel) upon, after, in addition: epiglottis
erg-	work, deed: ergometer
erythr-	red: erythrocyte
eso-	inside: esophagus
esthe-	perceive, feel: paresthesia

eu-	good, normal: euthyroid
ex-	out of: exfoliation
exo-	outside: exogenous
extra-	outside of, beyond: extracellular
faci-	face: facial
-facient	make: rubrefacient
fasci-	band: fascicular
febr-	fever: febrifuge
-ferent	carry: efferent
ferr-	iron: ferrokinetics
fibr-	fiber: fibrinogen
fil-	thread: filament
fiss-	split: fission
flagell-	whip: flagellation
flav-	yellow: riboflavin
-flect-	bend, divert: deflection
flu-	flow: fluid
for-	door, opening: foramen
-from	shape: archiform
fract-	break: refractory
front-	forehead: front, frontoparietal
-fug(e)	flee, avoid: vermifuge
funct-	perform, serve: function, malfunction
fund-	pour: infundibulum
galact-	milk: galactorrhea
gam-	marriage, reproductive, union: gametocyte
gangli-	swelling, plexus: ganglioma
gastr-	stomach: gastroscopy
gelat-	freeze, congeal: gelatin
gemin-	twin, double: quadrigeminal
gen-	become, be produced, originate: genetics
germ-	bud, a growth in its early stage: germinal
gest-	bear, carry: gestation
gland-	acorn: glandular
-glia	glue: neuroglia
gloss-	tongue, glossitis
glott-	tongue, language: epiglottis
glutin-	gluten, glue: agglutination
glyc(y)-	sweet: glycemia
gnath-	jaw: gnathoplasty
gno-	know, discern: prognosis
grad-	walk, take steps: gradient
-gram	scratch, write, record: electrocardiogram
gran-	grain, particle: granuloma
graph-	scratch, write, record: encephalography
grav-	heavy: multigravida
gyn(ec)-	woman, wife: gynecology
gyr-	ring, circle: gyrate
hapt-	touch: haptodysphoria
hect-	hundred, multiple in metric system: hectometer
helc-	sore, ulcer: helcoplasty

hem(at)	blood: hematology
hemi-	half: hemiplegia
hepat-	liver: hepatology
hept(a)	seven: heptavalent
hered-	heir: hereditary
hex-	six. An a is added in some combinations: hexagon
hex-	have, hold, be: cachexia
hidr-	sweat: hidronephrosis
hist-	web, tissue: histology
hod-	road, path: hodophobia
hom-	common, same: homogenous
horm-	impetus, impulse: hormone
hydat-	water: hydatiform
hydr-	water: hydrology
hyper-	above, beyond, extreme: hypertrophy
hpyn-	sleep: hypnotic
hypo-	(o is dropped before words beginning with a vowel) under, below: hypothyroidism
hyster-	womb: hysterectomy
iatr-	physician: iatrogenic
idi-	peculiar, separate, distinct: idiosyncrasy
ili-	ilium (ileum) lower abdomen, intestines (ili- is commonly used to refer to the ilium part of the pelvis): iliosacral
in-	fiber: inophragma
in-	in (n changes to l, m, or r before words beginning with those consonants): in, on insertion
in-	in- (n changes to l, m, or r before words beginning with those consonants) negative prefix: invalid
infra-	beneath: infraorbital
insul-	island: insulin
inter-	among, between: interdigital
intra-	inside: intramuscular
irid-	rainbow, colored circle: iridectomy
is-	equal: isotope
ischi-	hip, haunch: ischiopubic
jact-	throw: jactitation
ject-	throw: rejection
jejun-	hungry, not partaking of food: jejunoileostomy
jug-	yoke: conjugal
junct-	yoke, join: conjunctiva
kary-	(also spelled cary-) nut, kernel, nucleus: megakaryocyte
kerat-	(also spelled cerat-) horn: keratitis
kil-	thousand, multiple in metric system: kilogram
kine-	(also spelled cine-) move: hypokinetic
labi-	lip: dentilabial
lact-	milk: lactose
lal-	talk, babble: glossolalia
lapar-	flank: laparoscopy
laryng-	windpipe: laryngoscope
lat-	bear, carry: translation
later-	side: inferolateral

lent-	lens, lentil: lenticular
lep-	take, seize: analeptic
leuk-	(also spelled leuc-) white: leukocyte
lien-	spleen: hepatolienal
lig-	tie, bind: ligament
lingu-	tongue: lingula
lip-	fat: lipoprotein
lith-	stone: lithotome
loc-	place: locomotor
log-	speak, given an account: gynecology
lumb-	loin: lumbosacral
lute-	yellow: luteoma
ly-	loose, dissolve: fibrinolysis
lymph-	water: lymphoma
macr-	long, large: macroaggregate
mal-	bad, abnormal: malfunction
malac-	soft: osteomalacia
mamm-	breast: mammary
man-	hand: manual
mani-	mental aberration: maniac
mast-	breast: mastitis
medi-	middle: medial
mega-	great, large, also multiple in metric system (1,000,000): megaureter
megal-	great, large: megalomania
mel-	limb: melalgia
melan-	black: melanine
men-	month: menstruation
mening-	membrane: meningitis
ment-	mind: dementia
mer-	part: meromicrosomia
mes-	middle: mesoderm
meta-	(a is dropped before words beginning with a vowel) after, beyond, accompanying: metatarsal
metr-	measure: metrication
metr-	womb: endometriosis
micr-	small: microscope
mill-	one thousand, indicates fraction in metric system: milliliter
-mittent	send: intermittent
mnem-	remember: mnemonics
mon-	only, sole: monaster
morph-	form, shape: morphology
mot-	move: motility
myo-	muscle: myocardium
-myces	fungus: myelomyces
myel-	marrow: myeloma
myx-	mucus: myxedema
narc-	numbness: narcosis
nas-	nose: nasolabial
neo-	new, young: neonate
necr-	corpse: necrosis

nephr-	kidney: nephrology
neur-	nerve: neurology
nod-	knot: nodular
nom-	law, custom: nomogram
non-	nine: nona
non-	not: nonsecretory
nos-	disease: nosocomium
nucle-	kernel: nuclear
nutri-	nourisch: malnutrition
ob-	ob (b changes to c before words beginning with that consonant) against, toward: obturator
ocul-	eye: oculofacial
-ode	road, path: cathode
odont-	tooth: odontology
-odyn-	pain, distress: otodynia
-oid	form: sphenoid
ode-	oil: oleocranon
olig-	few, small: oligophrenia
omphal-	navel: omphalomesenteric
onc-	bulk, mass: oncology
onych-	claw, nail: onychiomycosis
oo-	egg: oopherectomy
op-	see: optometry
ophthalm-	eye: ophthalmology
or-	mouth: intraoral
orb-	circle: suborbital
orchi-	testicle: orchipexia
organ-	implement, tool: organ, organogenesis
orth-	straight, right, normal: orthopedics
oss-	bone: ossification
ost(e)-	bone: osteology
ot-	ear: otology
ov-	egg, synovia: ovulation
oxy-	sharp keen: oxyopia
pachy(n)-	thick: pachyderma
pag-	fix, fast together: thoracopagus
par-	bear, give birth to: multiparous
para-	(final a is dropped before words beginning with a vowel) beside, beyond: parasternal
part-	bear, give birth to: parturition
path-	abnormal, disease, sickness: pathology
ped-	child: pediatrics
pell-	skin, hide: pellagra
-pellent	drive: repellent
pen-	need, lack: leukopenia
pend-	hang down: appendix
pent(a)-	five: pentose, pentaploid, pentadactyle
peps-	digest: dyspepsia
pept-	digest: peptic
per-	through: peraxillary
peri-	around: perinasal

pet-	seek, tend toward: centripetal
pex-	fix, made fast: nephropexia
pha-	say, speak: aphasia
phac-	(also spelled phak-) lentil, lens: phacocele
phag-	eat: phagocytosis
pharmac-	drug: pharmacology
pharyng-	throat: nasopharyngeal
phen-	show, to appear: phenotype
pher-	bear, support: peripheric
phil-	like, have affinity for: eosinophilia
phleb-	vein: thrombophlebitis
phleg-	burn, inflame: phlegmon
phob-	fear, dread: claustrophobia
phon-	sound: telephone
phot-	light: photography
phrag-	fence, wall off, stop up: diaphragm
phren-	mind, diaphragm: phrenogastric
phthi-	decay, waste away: phthisis
phy-	bring forth, produce, be by nature: osteophyte
phyl-	tribe, kind: phylology
-phyll	leaf: chlorophyll
phylac-	guard: anaphylactic
physe-	blow, inflate: emphysema
pil-	hair: depilation
pituit-	phlegm, rheum: pituitary
placent-	cake: placenta
plas-	mold, shape: dysplasia
platy-	broad, flat: platycephallic
pleg-	strike: apoplegia
plet-	fill: complete
pleur-	rib, side: pleuritis
plex-	strike: apoplexy
plic-	fold: complication
pne-	breathing: apnea
pneum(at)-	breath, air: pneumatic
pneumo(n)-	lung: pneumocentesis, pneumonology
pod-	foot: podiatry
poie-	make, produce: hematopoiesis
pol-	axis of a sphere: poligonal
poly-	much, many: polyuria
pont-	bridge: pontocerebellar
por-	passage: porencephalic
por-	callus: porosis
posit-	put, place: reposition
post-	after, behind in time or place: postnatal, postnasal
pre-	before in time or place: prenatal, prerenal
press-	press: vasopressor
pro-	before in time or place: prodrome
proct-	anus: proctology
prosop-	face: prosopalgia
pseud-	false: pseudoarthrosis

pysch-	soul, mind: psychology
pto-	fall: nephroptosis
pub-	adult: ischiopubic
puber-	adult: puberty
pulmo(n)-	lung: pulmonology
puls-	drive: expulsion
punct-	prick, pierce, point: puncture
pur-	pus: suppuration
py-	pus, nephropyosis: pyogenic
pyel-	basin, pelvis: pyelonephritis
pyl-	door, orifice, gate: pylorus
pyr-	fire: pyrophosphate
quadr-	four: quadrigeminal
rachi-	spine: rachidian
radi-	ray: radiation
re-	back, again: repetition
ren-	kidneys: renal
ret-	net: reticuloendotothelial
retro-	backwards: retrograde
rhag-	break, burst: hemorrhagic
rhaph-	suture: gastrorrhaphy
rhe-	flow: rinorrhea
rhex-	break, burst: metrorrhexis
rhin-	nose: rhinitis
rot-	wheel: rotator
rub(r)-	red: bilirubin
salping-	tube, trumpet: salpingitis
sanguin-	blood: sanguineous
sarc-	flesh: osteosarcoma
schis-	split: schistoglossia
scler-	hard: sclerosis
scop-	look at, observe: gastroscope
sect-	cut: dissect
semi-	half: semiconcious
sens-	perceive, feel: sensation
sep-	rot, decay: septicemia
sept-	fence, wall: of nasoseptal
sept-	seven: septipara
ser-	watery substance: serosynovitis
sex-	six: sexdigitate, sexivalent
sial-	saliva: asialia
sin-	hollow, fold: sinusitis
sit-	food: parasitology
solut-	loose, set free: dissolution
somat-	body: psychosomatic
spas-	draw, pull: antispasmodic
spectr-	appearance, what is seen: spectroscope
sperm(at)-	seed: spermatogenesis
spers-	scatter: dispersion
sphen-	wedge: sphenoidal
spher-	ball: microsphere

sphygm-	pulsation: sphygmomanometer
spin-	spine: cerebrospinal
spirat-	breathe: inspiratory, respiratory
splanchn-	entrails, viscera: splanchnic
splen-	spleen: splenectomy
spor-	seed: sporophyte
squam-	scale: desquamation
sta-	make stand, stop: stasis
stal-	send: peristalsis
staphyl-	bunch of grapes: staphylococcus
stear-	fat: stearrhea (steatorrhea)
sten-	narrow, compressed: stenosis
ster-	solid: cholesterol
sterc-	dung: stercobilin
sthen-	strength: myasthenia
stol-	send: systole
stom(at)-	mouth, orifice: stomatitis
strep(h)-	twist: streptococus
strict-	draw tight, compress, cause, pain: constriction
stroph-	twist: strophocephalus
struct-	pile up: obstruction
sub-	sub (b changes to f or p before words beginning with those consonants) under, below: subphrenic
super-	above, beyond, extreme: superactivity
syn-	(n disappears before s, changes to l before l, and changes to m before b, m, p, and ph) with, together: synarthrosis
tact-	touch: contact
tax-	order, arrange: ataxia
teg-	cover: tegument
tel-	end, distant: telencephalon
tele-	at a distance: telephone
tempor-	time, timely: temporary
ten-	tight stretched band: tendon, tendonitis
tens-	stretch: extensor
test-	testicle: testicular
tetra-	four: tetralogy
the-	put, place: synthesis
thec-	box, case: thecodont
thel-	teat, nipple: thelalgia
therap-	treatment: radiotherapy
therm-	heat: thermometer
thi-	sulfur: thiemia
thorac-	chest: thoracotomy
thromb-	lump, clot: thrombophlebitis
thym-	spirit: dysthymia
thyr-	shield: thyroid
toc-	childbirth: tocology
tom-	cut: thyroidectomy
ton-	stretch, put under tension: peritoneum
top-	place: topalgia
tors-	twist: torsion

tox-	arrow, poison: toxic
trache-	windpipe: tracheotomy, endotracheal
trachel-	neck: trachelomyitis
tract-	draw, drag: traction
traumat-	wound: traumatic
tri-	three: tricuspid
trich-	hair: trichiasis
trop-	turn, react: chromotropic
troph-	nurture: trophoblast
tuber-	swelling, node: tuberculosis
typ-	type: typical
typh-	fog, stupor: typhoid
typhl-	blind, cecum: typhlomegaly
ultra-	beyond: ultrafiltration
uni-	one: unilateral
ur-	urine: nicturia
vacc-	cow: vaccine
vagin-	sheath: invaginated
vas-	vessel: vascular
vert-	turn: diverticulum
vesic-	bladder: vesicoureteric
vit-	life: vitamin
vuls-	pull, twitch: avulsion
xanth-	yellow, blond: xanthochromatic
zoo-	animal life: zoology
zyg-	yoke, union: zygomatic

REFERENCES

- *Dorland's Illustrated Medical Dictionary,* 26th Edition, W. B. Saunders Company, Philadelphia, 1981.
- *Illustrated Stedman's Medical Dictionary,* 24th Edition, Williams & Wilkins, Baltimore, 1962.
- International Dictionary of Medicine and Biology, John Wiley & Sons, New York, 1986.

COMMON PREFIXES, SUFFIXES, AND ROOTS

Prefixes

a, an	Without, negative, absence of
ab	From, away from
ad	Adherence, increase, near, toward
ante, antero	Before, forward, front
anti	Against
auto, aut	Self
bi, bis	Twice, double
brady	Slow
cata	Lower, down, negative
co, com, con	Together, with
contra	Against, counter, opposite
de	Down from
di	Double, twice
dia	Through, apart
dis, dys	Apart, away from; painful, difficult
ec	Out of
ecto	Outside
em, en	In, into
end, endo	Within
entero	Intestine
epi	Upon, at, in addition to
eu	Well, good
ex, exo	Out, away from, over, outside
gastro	Stomach
hemi	Half
hemo	Blood
hyper	Above, excessive, beyond
hypo	Decreased, under
infra	Beneath, below
inter	Among, between
intra, intro	Into, within
macro	Large
mal	Bad
medio	Middle
mes	Middle
meta	Beyond, over
micro	Small
multi	Many
myo	Muscle
neuro	Nerve
ortho	Straight, normal
pan	All, every
para	Around, beside, by, beyond, abnormal near
patho	Disease
per	Through
peri	Around
poly	Many
post	After, behind

pre	Before, in front of
pro	In front of, forward
pseudo	False
py	Pus
quadri	Fourfold
re	Again, back
retro	Back, backward
semi	Half
steno	Narrow, contracted
sub	Under, below, beneath
super, supra	Above, beyond, superior
sym, syn	With, along, together, beside
tachy	Fast
tendo	Tendon
trans	Across, over, through
tri	Three
ultra	Excess, beyond
uni	Single, one

Suffixes

algia	Pain
cente	Puncture
dynia	Pain
ectomy	Surgical removal of
ede	Swelling
genic	Origin, producing
genous	Kind
gram	Picture, tracing
lysis	Dissolution, breaking down
oid	Resembling, like
ology	Science of, study of
oscopy	Diagnostic examination
ostomy	Opening
otomy	Incision
penia	Lack, decrease
plegia	Paralysis
scler	Hardening
trophy	Nutrition
uria	Urine

Roots

aden	Gland
arteria	Artery
arthros	Joint
auris	Ear
brachion	Arm
bronchus	Windpipe
cardium	Heart
cephalos	Brain
cholecyst	Gallbladder
colon	Intestine

costa	Rib
cranium	Head
derma	Skin
enteron	Intestine
epithelium	Skin
esophagus	Gullet
gaster	Stomach
hemo	Blood
hepar	Liver
hydro	Water
hystera	Womb
kystis (cysto)	Bladder
larynx	Throat
myelos	Marrow
nasus	Nose
nephros	Kidney
neuron	Neuron
odons	Tooth
odynia	Pain
optikas	Eye
osteon	Bone
ostium	Mouth, orifice
otis	Ear
pes	Foot
pyretos	Fever
ren	Kidney
rin	Nose

BRITISH AND AMERICAN SPELLINGS

This dictionary uses the American spelling in preference to the British, in the cases where the two differ. The main differences are ae and oe, both of which have been retained in British spelling but contracted to e in American spelling. Other differences include the British -our for -or, ph for f and the word endings -tre for ter, or re for er and ise for ize.

The following are a few examples of British — American spellings:

	British	**American**
ae for e	aetiology	etiology
	naevus	nevus
	gynaecology	gynecology
	hyperaemia	hyperemia
	haematoma	hematoma
c for k	leucocyte	leukocyte
	ECG	EKG
ei for i	cleidocostal	clidocostal
	cheilosis chilosis	
	cheiroplasty	chiroplasty
ise for ize	ionise ionize	
	digitise digitize	
	standarise standarize	
oe for e	myxoedema myxedema	
	amoeba ameba	

	diarrhoea	diarrhea	
-our for -or	colour	color	
	tumour	tumor	
ph for f	sulphur	sulfur	
	sulphadiazine		sulfadiazine
re for er	centre	center	
	fibre	fiber	
tre for ter	metre	meter	
	litre	liter	

TERMS USED TO DESCRIBE ANATOMICAL POSITIONS AND PLANES

Terms of directional anatomical position come in pairs. Thus we have:

anterior or ventral	front of, toward the front of the body
posterior or dorsal	back of, toward the back of the body
superior	situated above, upper
inferior	situated beneath, lower
lateral	away from midline, to the side
medial	toward the midline, middle
cranial, cephalic	toward the head
caudal	away from the head, toward the feet
distal	away, further from
proximal	near, closer to
internal, inner	inside a body cavity
external, outer	outside a body cavity

Additional Terms

abduction	movement away from the middle line
adduction	movement drawing toward the middle line
afferent	bringing toward a center
efferent	conducting away from the center
bilateral	relating to both sides
unilateral	relating to one side only
deep	beneath the surface depth
superficial	situated near the surface
eversion	turning outward
inversion	turning inward
extension	movement to place a limb in a straight position
flexion	movement to bend a limb
plantar	referring to the sole of the foot
palmar	referring to the palm of the hand
prone	lying face downward
supine	lying face upward

The human body can be divided along imaginary flat fields or planes to identify the position of parts of the body. These are

median or sagittal	plane that passes vertically through the body from front to back and divides it into right and left halves
transverse	plane that passes horizontally through the body at right

angles to the sagittal plane and divides the body into upper and lower portions

coronal or frontal   plane that passes longitudinally through the body from side to side, at right angles to the median plane and divides the body into anterior and posterior portions

Abdominal Anatomical Regions

umbilical	region around the umbilicus
epigastric	region directly above the umbilical region
hypogastric	region directly below the umbilical region
hypochondriac	region to the right and left of the epigastric region
lumbar	region to the right and left of the umbilical region
iliac	region to the right and left of the hypogastric region

PLURAL ENDINGS FOR MEDICAL TERMS

In the English language, most plural endings are formed by simply adding s or es to the singular word. Besides these, in the language of medicine there are still other plural endings. These are examples of some of the most common plural endings for medical terms.

Singular ending	Plural ending	Examples	
		Singular	Plural
-a	-ae	aorta	aortae
-ax	-aces	thorax	thoraces
-(x)	-(es)	phalanx	phalanges
-ex	-ices	apex	apices
-is	-es	pubis	pubes
-ix	-es	cervix	cervices
-ma	-mata	fibroma	fibromata
-on	-a	ganglion	ganglia
-s	-es	pars	partes
-um	-a	antrum	antra
-us	-i	acinus	acini
-y	-ies	necropsy	necropsies

ABBREVIATIONS, ACRONYMS, SYMBOLS, DENOTATIONS, AND SIGNS COMMONLY USED OR DEFINED IN THE DICTIONARY

ABBREVIATIONS AND ACRONYMS

Ab	Antibody
ABNM	American Board of Nuclear Medicine
AC	Alternating current
ACC	Anticoincidence circuit
ACD	Annihilation coincidence detection
ACD	Acid citrate dextrose
ACTH	Adrenocorticotropic hormone
ADC	Analog to digital converter
ADH	Antidiuretic hormone
ADP	Adenosine diphosphate
AFC	Antibody forming cells

AFP	Alpha feto protein
AFP	Adiabatic first passage
Ag	Antigen
AIDS	Acquired immunodeficiency syndrome
AIUM	American Institute for Ultrasound in Medicine
ALARA	As low as reasonably achievable
ALGOL	Algorithmic language
ALU	Arithemetic logic unit
AMA	American Medical Association
AMP	Adenosine monophosphate
AMU	Atomic mass unit
ANOVA	Analysis of variance
ART	Algebraic reconstruction technique
ASCII	American Standard Code for Information Interchange
ASO	Antistreptolysin O (titer)
ATP	Adenosine triphosphate
AVM	Arteriovenous malformation
AVN	Atrioventricular Node
BASIC	Beginners all-purpose symbolic instruction code
BBB	Blood brain barrier
BBB	Bundle branch block
BCD	Binary coded decimal
BE	Barium enema
BGO	Bismuth germinate
BIDA	Parabutyliminodiacetic acid
BIT	Binary digit
BLEDTA	1-(p-bromoacetamidiophenyl) ethylenedinitrilotetracetic acid
BMR	Basal metabolic rate
BP	British pharmacopeia
BP	Blood pressure
BSA	Body surface area
BSP	Sulfobromophthalein
BSR	Basal skin resistance
BUN	Blood urea nitrogen
cAMP	Cyclic adenosine monophosphate
CABG	Coronary artery bypass graft
CAD	Coronary artery disease
CAI	Computed aided instruction
CAT	Computerized axial tomography
CBA	Competitive binding assay
CBC	Complete blood count
CBF	Cerebral blood flow
CBV	Cerebral blood volume
CCK	Cholecystokinen
CEA	Carcinoembryonic antigen
CERN	Conseil Europeen de Recherche Nucleaire
CF	Complement fixation, fixating
CFR	Code of Federal Regulations
CMI	Cell mediated immunity
CMOS	Complementary metal oxide semiconductor
$CMRO_2$	Cerebral metabolic rate for oxygen

CMRR	Common mode rejection ratio (amplifiers)
CNS	Central nervous system
CO	Carbon monoxide
CO	Cardiac output
CO_2	Carbon dioxide
COAD	Chronic obstructive airways disease
COBOL	Common business oriented language
CPB	Competitive protein binding
CPK	Creatine phosphokinase
CPM	Counts per minute
CPS	Counts per second
CPU	Central processing unit
CRAG	Cerebral radionuclide angiography
CR	Count rate
CRM	Counting rate meter
CRT	Cathode-ray tube
CSF	Cerebrospinal fluid
CT	Computed tomography
CVA	Cerebrovascular accident
CVP	Central venous pressure
CVS	Cardiovascular system
CW	Continuous wave (e.g. of doppler ultrasound)
DAA	Data access arrangement
DAC	Digital to analog converter
DADS	N, N' bis (mercaptoacetyl)-ethylenediamine
DASP	Double antibody solid phase
DBMS	Data base management system
DC	Direct current
D&C	Dilation and curettage
DDC	Diethyldithiocarbamate
DDL	Data definition language
DEIDA	Diethyliminodiacetic acid
DEL	Dose equivalent limit
DF	Duty factor
DFP	Diisopropyl flurorophosphate
DHF	Delta host functions
DHTA	Dihydrothioctic acid
DIDA	Diethyliminodiacetic acid
DIP	Dual in line package
DISIDA	Diisopropyliminodiacetic acid
DIT	Diiodotyrosine
DMA	Direct memory access
DML	Data Management Language
DMSA	Dimercaptosuccinic acid
DNA	Deoxyribonucleic acid
DOE	Department of Energy (USA)
DOS	Disk operating system
DPM	Disintegrations per minute
DPS	Disintegrations per second
DSA	Digital subtraction angiography
DTA	Diethylenetriamine

DTPA	Diethylenetriaminepentaacetic acid
DVT	Deep venous thrombosis
D/W	Dextrose in water
EC	Electron capture
ECF	Eosinophil chemotactic factor
ECT	Emission computerized tomography
EDTA	Ethylenediaminetetraacetic acid
EDV	End diastolic volume
EEG	Electroencephalogram, electroencephalograhy
EHDP	Ethane-1-hydroxy-1, 1-diphosphonate
EIDA	Diethyliminodiacetic acid
EKG (ECG)	Electrocardiogram, electrocardiography
ELISA	Enzyme-linked immunosorbent assay
EMF	Electromotive force
EMG	Electromyogram
EPROM	Erasable programmable read only memory
ERA	Electric response audiometry
ERCP	Endoscopic retrograde cholangiopancreatography
ERD	Estimated radiation dose
ERD	Equivalent residual dose
ERPF	Effective renal plasma flow
ERV	Expiratory reserve volume
ESC	Escape key (Computer)
ESR	Erythrocyte sedimentation rate
ESU	Electrostatic unit of charge
ESV	End systolic volume
EURATOM	European Atomic Energy Community
Fab	Antigen-binding fragment
FDA	Food and Drug Administration (USA)
FDG	2-fluror-2-deoxy-D-glucose
FEF	Forced expiratory flow
FEV	Forced expiratory volume
FFT	Fast fourier transformation
FET	Field effect transistor
FID	Free induction decay
FIFO	First in/first out (Computer)
FM	Frequency modulation (radio and tape recorders)
FN	False negative
FNF	False negative fraction
FORTRAN	Formula translation
FP	False positive
FPF	False positive fraction
FPR	False positive rate
FRC	Functional residual capacity
FSH	Follicle stimulating hormone
FT	Fourier transform
FTA	Fourier transform analysis
FTI	Free thyroxine index
FUO	Fever of unknown origin
FWHM	Full width at half maximum
Ge (li)	Germanium-lithium (drifted detector)

GFR	Glomerular filtration rate
GHP	Glucoheptonate
GI	Gastrointestinal
GM	Geiger-Müller
GMW	Gram molecular weight
G6PD	Glucose-6-phosphate dehydrogenase
GR	Grid ratio
GSD	Genetically significant dose
GSR	Galvanic skin response
GU	Genitourinary
HA	Hemagglutination, hemagglutinating
HAA	Human Australian antigen
HAM	Human albumin microspheres
Hb	Hemoglobin
HCAT	Homotaurocholate
HCG	Human chlorionic gonadotropin
HCL	Hydrochloric acid; Hydrochloride
HCO_3	Bicarbonate
Hct	Hematocrit
HEDP	Hydroxyethylidene diphosphonate
HEDSPA	1-Hydroxy-ethylidene-1, 1-disodium phosphonate
HEDTA	N-hydroxyethylethylenediamine-tetraacetic acid
HGH	Human growth hormone
HIDA	Dimethyliminodiacetic acid
HIPDM	2-Hydroxyl-3-methyl-5-iodobenzyl-1, 3-propanediamine
HM-PAO	Hexamethyl propilene amine oxime
HMDP	Hydroxymethylene diphosphonate
HPLC	High performance liquid chromatography
HSA	Human serum albumin
HU	Heat units
HVG	Host vs. graft
HVL	Half-value layer
IAEA	International Atomic Energy Agency
IC	Immune complex
IC	Integrated circuit
ICRP	International Commission on Radiological Protection
ICRUM	International Commission on Radiological Units and Measurements
ID	Information density
IDA	Iminodiacetic acid
IEC	International Electrotechnical Commission
IEP	Immunoelectrophoresis
I:E ratio	Inspiratory to expiratory ratio (Lung ventilator)
IF	Intrinsic factor
IgA, E, etc.	Immunoglobulin A, E, etc.
IMP	Iodoamphetamine
IMV	Intermittent mandatory ventilation
IND	Investigational new drug
I/O	Input/Output
IPPB	Inspiratory positive pressure breathing
IPPV	Intermittent positive pressure ventilation

IR	Inversion recovery
IRMA	Immunoradiometric analysis
ISO	International Organization for Standarization
IT	Isomeric transition
ITLC	Instant thin-layer chromatography
IU	International unit(s)
IVP	Intravenous pyelogram
JND	Just noticeable difference
KTS	Kethoxal-bis (thiosemicarbazone)
kV	Kilovoltage (X-rays)
LAN	Local area network
LATS	Long-acting thyroid stimulator
LCD	Liquid crystal display
LCMRG1e	Local cerebral metabolic rate of glucose
LD_{50}	Lethal dose
LDH	Lactic dehydrogenase
LED	Light-emitting diode
LET	Linear energy transfer
LFC	Loss free counting
LFOV	Large field of view
LIFO	Last in first out (Computer)
LSB	Least significant bit
LSF	Line spread function
LVEF	Left ventricular ejection fraction
MAA	Macroaggregated albumin
MAG_3	Mercaptoacetylglycyl-glycyl-glycine (Mercaptoacetyltriglycine)
MCA	Multichannel analyzer
MCH	Mean corpuscular hemoglobin
MCHC	Mean corpuscular hemoglobin concentration
MCV	Mean corpuscular volume
MDP	Methylenediphosphonate
MEK	Methylethyl ketone
MHC	Major histocompatibility complex
MI	Myocardial infarction
MIBG	Metaiodobenzylguanidine
MIF	Migration inhibitory factor
MIRD	Medical Internal Radiation Dose (Committee)
MIT	Monoiodotyrosine
MLC	Mixed leukocyte culture
MLD	Median lethal dose
MLT	Median lethal time
MLSI	Multiple line scan imaging
MOS	Metal oxide semiconductor
MODEM	Modular/demodulator
MPBB	Maximum permissible body burden
MPC	Maximum permissible concentration
MPD	Maximum permissible dose
MR	Magnetic resonance
MRI	Magnetic resonance imaging
mRNA	Messenger ribonucleic acid
MSB	Most significant bit

MTF	Modulation transfer function
MTT	Mean transit time
MUGA	Multiple gated acquisition
MVO_2	Myocardial oxygen consumption
MW	Molecular weight
MWPC	Multiwire proportional counter
NAND	Not-and
NBS	National Bureau of Standards (USA)
NCRP	National Council on Radiation Protection (USA)
NDA	New drug application
NEEP	Negative end-expiratory pressure
NEMA	National Electrical Manufacturers Association (USA)
NF	National Formulary (USA)
NIH	National Institutes of Health (USA)
NMR	Nuclear magnetic resonance
NOR	Nor-or
NRC	Nuclear Regulatory Commission (USA)
NSB	Nonspecific binding
NTA	Nitrilotriacetic acid
OD	Optical density
OER	Oxygen extraction ratio
OID	Object image distance
OIH	Orthoiodohippurate
PAC	Penicillamine-acetazolamide complex
PAO_2	Arterial oxygen pressure
PaO_2	Alveolar oxygen pressure
PAP	Pulmonary arterial pressure
PAWP	Pulmonary arterial wedge pressure
PBI	Protein-bound iodine
PBNAA	Partial body neutron activation analysis
PCO_2	Carbon dioxide pressure (or tension)
PO_2	Oxygen pressure (or tension)
$PaCO_2$	Arterial carbon dioxide pressure
PaO_2	Arterial oxygen pressure
PAO_2	Alveolar oxygen pressure
PCB	Printed circuit board
pCO_2	Partial pressure of carbon dioxide
PCT	Positron computed tomography
PCWP	Pulmonary capillary wedge pressure
PD	Pulse duration
PEEP	Positive end-expiratory pressure
PEFR	Peak expiratory flow rate
PET	Positron emission tomography
PETT	Positron-emission transaxial tomography
PG	Pyridoxylidene glutamate
PGNAA	Prompt gamma neutron activation analysis
pH	Hydrogen-ion concentration
PHA	Pulse height analyzer
PIPIDA	N-(para-isopropyl) iminodiaceitc acid
PIXE	Proton induced X-ray emission
PL	Permitted radiation exposure level

PLES	Parallel line equal space (phantom)
PMT	Photomultiplier tube
pO$_2$	Partial pressure of oxygen
Poly	Polyphosphate
POP	2,5-Diphenyloxazole
POPOP	1.4-Bis(5-phenoxazole)benzene
PPi	pyrophosphate
ppm	Parts per million
PPx	Polyphosphate
PRF	Pulse repetition frequency
PRFT	Partially relaxed fourier transform
PRO	Peer review organizations
PROM	Programmable read only memory
PS	Partial saturation
PSF	Point spread function
PSP	Phenosulfonphthalein
PTCA	Percutaneous transmural coronary angioplasty
PTH	Parathyroid hormone
PTU	Porpylthiouracil
PVP	Polyvinyl pyrrolidone
PYP	Pyrophosphate
PZT	Lead zirconate titanate (ultrasonic transducers)
QA	Quality assurance
QC	Quality control
QF	Quality factor
RAD	Radiation absorbed dose
RAI	Radioactive iodine
RAM	Random access memory
RAST	Radioallergosorbent test
RBA	Radiobinding assay
RBC	Red blood cell
RBE	Relative biologic effectiveness
rCBF	Regional cerebral blood flow
RCP	Radiochemical purity
RDP	Radiopharmaceutical drug product
REM	Roentgen equivalent man
RES	Reticuloendothelial system
RF	Radiofrequency
RF	Rheumatoid factor
RIA	Radioimmunoassay
RIS	Radioimmunoscintigraphy
RIT	Radioimmunotherapy
RNA	Ribonucleic acid
RNA	Radionuclide angiography
RNP	Radionuclide purity
RNV	Radionuclide venography
RNV	Radionuclide ventriculography
ROC	Receiver operating curve, characteristic
ROI	Region of interest
ROM	Read-only memory
RT	Total resolution

RV	Residual volume (lung)
SA$_{O2}$	Arterial oxygen saturation
SBE	Subacute bacterial endocarditis
SC	Sulfur colloid
SGOT	Serum glutamic oxaloacetic transaminase
SGPT	Serum glutamic pyruvic transaminase
SI	Système International (Units)
SNR	Signal-to-noise ratio
SOD	Source to object distance
SPECT	Single photon emission computerized tomography
SSKI	Saturated solution of potassium iodide
SV	Stroke volume
TAA	Tumor-associated antigens
T3	Triiodothyronine
T4	Thyroxine, levothyroxine
TAC	Time-activity curve
TB	Tuberculosis
TBG	Thyroxine-binding globulin
TBI	t-Butylisonitrile
TBNAA	Total body neutron activation analysis
TBPA	Thyroxine binding prealbumin
TC	Total count
TCA	Trichloracetic acid
TE	Echo time
TGC	Time-gain compensation (ultrasonic scanners)
TGC	Time gain compensation
THC	Transhepatic cholangiography
TI	Inversion time
TLC	Thin-layer chromatography
TLD	Thermoluminescent detector
TM	Time-motion (ultrasonic scanner)
TN	True negative
TNF	True negative fraction
TP	True positive
TPF	True positive fraction
TPO	Thyroid peroxidase
TPR	True positive rate
TRH	Thyrotropin-releasing hormone
TSA	Tumor-specific antigen
TSH	Thyroid-stimulating hormone
TVG	Time varied gain
UMU	Universal mass unit
USP	United States Pharmacopeia
USPHS	United States Public Health Service
VC	Vital capacity (lung function)
VCG	Vectorcardiogram
VDU	Visual display unit
VT	Minute ventilation
VT	Tidal volume (lung function)
VER	Visual evoked response (of sight)
VEP	Visual evoked potential (of sight)

WAN   Wide area network
WBC   White blood cell

SYMBOLS AND DENOTATIONS

a	Activity
A	Amplitude
A	Disintegration rate (= dN/dt)
A	Mass number (Atomic weight)
Å	Angstrom (10^{-10} m)
$\tilde{A}$	Cumulative activity
A_o	Original activity
a	Radius of Bohr orbit
b	Nuclear binding energy
B	Background count rate
B	Barrier factor
B	Buildup factor (from Compton scattering)
B	Bucky factor
B	Magnetic field
B	Blood
B_o	Unit of magnetic induction (NMR)
B_1	Radiofrequency magnetic induction field
B_x	Gradient magnetic field in x direction
Bq	Becquerel
b	Barn
b.p.	Boiling point
C	Concentration
C	Celcius
C	Centi
C	Contrast
C	Coulomb
CD	Contrast detail
CL	Confidence limits (statistics)
Ci	Curie
c	Velocity of light
cd	Candela
c/kg	Coulomb/kilogram
cm	Centimeter
c/s	Cycles per second
d	Density
D	Diameter
D	Average absorbed dose
$D_\beta D_\gamma$	Total beta dose; total gamma dose
d	Day
d	Distance
d	Deuteron, H^2
db	Decibel
df	Degrees of freedom (statistics)
D_m	Minimum separation
E	Erythrocyte
E	Kinetic energy of a particle
E	Exposure

ED_{50}	Median effective dose
E_b	Binding energy
E_γ	Gamma-ray energy
E_e	Electron energy
E_α	Kinetic energy of an alpha particle
E_{max}	Maximum energy of a beta spectrum
$\tilde{E}$	Average beta energy
e	Base of Naperian (natural) logarithms (= 2.71828)
e	Elementary charge (= 4.803×10^{-10} esu)
e	Electronic charge (= 4.803×10^{-10} esu)
emu	Electromagnetic unit
esu	Electrostatic unit
eV	Electron Volt
e^+	Electron positron
e^-	Electron negatron
F	Feces
F	Fahrenheit
F	Faraday
f	f-factor, rad to Roentgen ratio
f	f-Number of lens
f	Frame
f	Frequency
f	Packing fraction
f/s	Frames per second
ft	Foot
f_A, f_B, f_H, f_S, f_W	Counting geometry factors or coefficients for air-scattering, back-scattering, side-scattering, self-absorption, and window- and air-absorption, respectively
G	Gross count rate
G	Number of gray levels
G	Physical geometry factor
G_m	Magnification gain
G_n	Gaussian probability of obtaining a count of n
G_y	Gray
g	Gram
Hz	Hertz
h	Hour
h	Planck's constant
$h\nu$	Energy of a photon
I	Intensity of radiation
I	Current
IP	Ion product
I.P.	Ion pairs
IT	Internal transition
I_p	Current in transformer primary circuit
I_s	Current in transformer secondary circuit
$I^2 F$	Power loss due to current in a resistor
$I\gamma$	Specific gamma-ray emission or specific gamma-ray output
j	Joule
K	Contrast improvement factor
K	Linear pair production attenuation coefficient

K	Kelvin
KeV	Kilo-electron Volt
K_{sp}	Solubility product constant
k	Reaction rate constant
kg	Kilogram
LD_{50}	Median lethal dose
lb	Pound
ln	Naperian logarithm
ln	Natural logarithm
log	Base 10 logarithm
M	Magnetization
M	Magnification
M	Isotope mass of neutral atom, amu
MeV	Mega-electron Volt
M_H	Isotopic mass of neutral hydrogen atom, amu
M_{He}	Isotopic mass of neutral helium atom, amu
M_p	Proton mass, amu
M_n	Neutron mass, amu
M_t	Total mass
M	Momentum
m	Meter
m	Relativistic mass of a particle with a rest mass of m_o, g
m	Mass of a substance, g or mg
meq	Milliequivalents
min	Minute
ml	Milliliter
mm	Millimeter
mol	Mole
N	Newton
N	Number of counts
N	Number of turns in a transformer winding
N	Neutron number
N	Atoms/cm^3 in a target
N	Avogadro number
N	Number of atoms
N	Normality, equiv/liter
N	Number of observations (statistics)
N_p	Number of turns in the transformer primary
N_s	Number of turns in the transformer secondary
n	Neutron
n	Observed number of random events (statistics)
$\bar{n}, \bar{N}$	Mean value of n for a number of observations (statistics)
n	Principal quantum number
ni	Fraction of times a disintegration produces in ith radiation
P	Probable error (statistics)
P	Probability
P	Plasma
Pt	Patient
P_n	Poisson probability of obtaining a count of n
P	Proton, H^1 nucleus
P	Proportion (statistics)

P	Momentum
P	Probability of occurrence of a random event
P_Φ	Angular momentum
Q	Energy change in a nuclear reaction
Q	Q factor, ratio of resonant frequency to band width
Q_1	25th percentage value = first quartile
Q_2	50th percentage value (median) = second quartile
Q_3	75th percentage value = third quartile
R	Corrected counting rate
R	Nuclear radius
R	Dose rate
R	Range of a particle
R	Reflection coefficient
R	Resistance
R	Resolution
RC	Time constant of a circuit with resistance R and capacitance C
R_c	Collimator resolution
R_{eq}	Equivalent resistance
R_i	Intrinsic resolution
R_m	Maximum range of a beta particle
R_b, R_s, R_t	Count rate of backgrounds, sample and total activities
r	Number of rows in a table
r	Roentgen
r	Observed count rate (= n/t)
r	Radius
rad	Radiation absorbed dose
r_b, r_s, r_t	Observed backgrounds, sample and total count rates
S	Mean dose per cumulative activity
S	Area
S	Specific activity
S	Stopping power
S	Separation energy for an alpha particle
Sf	Cerebrospinal fluid
Sv	Sievert
S_a, S_n	Apparent specific activity
S_a, S_n	Normalized specific activity
s	Sample deviation (statistics)
s	Sample standard deviation
s	Second
s	Serum
sr	Steradian
s^2	Sample variance (statistics)
s^2	Sample variance
T	Kinetic energy
T	Resolving time of a nuclear particle detector
T	Tesla
T	Occupancy factor
T	Period
T	Time
T	Transmission
T_l	Spin lattice or longitudinal relaxation time

T_2	Spin-spin or transverse relaxation time
T_{Avg}	Average half time
T_d	Daughter half life
T_p	Parent half life
t	Variate or critical ratio
t	Time
t_b, t_r, t_e	Biological, radiological and effective half-lives
$t^1/_2$	Half-life
$t^1/_2$	Reaction half-time
U	Use factor
U	Potential energy
U	Urine
u	Apparent absorption coefficient for a Beta particle cm^2/mg
V	Volts
V	Volume
v	Velocity
W	Energy of a gamma transition
W	Total energy (kinetic + potential)
W	Watt
W	Work
X	Thickness of an absorber, cm
X	Sample mean
$X^1/_2$	Half-value thickness of half-value layer, cm
x	Thickness of absorber, mg/cm^2
yr	Year(s)
Z	Atomic number
Z	Acoustic impedence
Ze	Nuclear charge

GREEK ALPHABET-CODED SYMBOLS

α	Alpha particle
β	Velocity relative to velocity of light (= v/c)
β, β^-, β^+	Beta ray or particle negatron and positron
Γ	Radioisotope gamma factor
Γ	Slope of film characteristic curve
γ	Gamma ray or other photon
γ	Gyromagnetic ratio
Δ	Small increment
Δ	Mean energy of radiation per nuclear transformation (dosimetry)
Δ	Mass defect
ΔI	Change in intensity
ΔX	Change in thickness
Δ^V	Change in voltage
$\Delta \lambda$	Change in wavelength
Δ_i	Equilibrium absorbed dose constant for the ith radiation
ε	Efficiency
θ	Symbol for angle
θ_i	Angle of incidence
θ_r	Angle of reflection
θ_t	Angle of transmission
λ	Wavelength of electromagnetic radiation

λ	Decay constant
λ_c	Compton wavelength (= h/m c)
λ_{min}	Minimum wavelength
μ	Actual or true mean count
μ	Total linear absorption coefficient, cm^{-1} (Coefficient of attenuation)
μ	Permeability
μ	Micro-, micron(s)
μm	Mass attenuation coefficient
ν	Frequency of electromagnetic radiation
ν	Neutrino
$\nu*$	Antineutrino
σ	Standard deviation
σ	True standard deviation (statistics)
σ	Cross section of a target, cm^2/target particle
σ	Standard deviation of the difference
σ^z	Variance of a normal distribution
$\sigma, \sigma_s, \sigma_a$	Linear coefficients for Compton collision, Compton scattering and Compton absorption
$\sigma_x, (SE_x)$	Standard Error of the Mean
σ_q	Quantum noise
$\%\sigma$	Percent standard deviation
π	Ratio of circumference of a circle to its diameter (= 3.14159)
ρ	Density, g/cm^3
ρ	Proton density
ρ	Physical density gm/cm^3
Σ	Sigma, symbol for summation
Σ	Macroscopic cross section, cm^{-1}
τ	Mean life (= $1/\lambda$)
τ	Relative error or parameter of the counting error (= number of standard deviations)
τ	Photoelectric linear absorption coefficient
τ	Symbol for angle
τ	Dead time
τe	Effective mean life
	Absorbed fraction (dosimetry)
Φ	Neutron flux
Φ_β	Magnetic flux
O	Specific absorbed fraction (dosimetry)
ϕ	Absorbed fraction for the ith radiation
χ	Magnetic susceptibility
χ^2	Pearson's chi-square function
χ^2	Chi Square + $\Sigma^{(0-E)^2}$
ψ	Specific activity
Ω	Ohm
ω	Larmor precessional frequency
ω	Angular frequency
ω	Overvoltage
ω_o	Larmor frequency
δ	Chemical shift

COMMON BASIC SIGNS

+	plus, addition, positive, acid reaction
−	minus, subraction, negative, alkaline reaction
±	plus or minus, positive or negative, indefinite
$T^{\pm}$	minus or plus, negative or positive, indefinite
/	per
÷, /, −	division
×, ·, ( )	multiplication; in microscopy, magnification
( ) [ ]	collection
(a,b]	left open, right closed interval
$\lceil r \rceil$	smallest integer k with k≥ r
$\lfloor r \rfloor$	largest integer k with k ≤ r
$\lvert r \rvert$, $\lvert \beta \rvert$	absolute value of number r or vector β
=	is equal to
:=	equal per definition
≠	is not equal to
≡	is identical to
≃	equals approximately, congruent
>	greater than; whence, from which is derived
≯	not greater than
≥	greater than or equal to
<	less than; from, derived from
	not less than
≤	less than or equal to
Δ	corresponds to
::	proportional to; "as"
:	ratio; "is to"
~	similar to
∝	varies as, proportional to
→	approaches
∞	infinity
∴	therefore
⇌	if and only if
$\sqrt{\ }$	square root
$\sqrt[v]{\ }$	nth root
a^{n}	nth power of a
log, $\log_{10}$	common logarithm
ln, $\log_{e}$	natural logarithm
e or ε	base of natural logs, 2.718
π	pi, 3.1416
∠	angle
⊥	perpendicular to
‖	parallel to
n	any number
$\lvert n \rvert$	absolute value of n
$\bar{n}$	average value of n
a^{-n}	reciprocal of nth power of a = $[1/a^{n}]$
n°	n degrees
n′	n minutes, n feet
n″	n seconds, n inches
f(x)	function of x

Δx	increment of x
dx	differential of x
Σ	summation of
sin	sine
cos	cosine
tan	tangent
*	birth
†	death
♀	female
o	female
♂	male
□	male
%	percent
℞	recipe, take
'	foot; minute; univalent
"	inch; second; bivalent
‴	line; trivalent

OTHER USEFUL INFORMATION

PHONETIC ALPHABET

A	Alpha	N	November
B	Bravo	O	Oscar
C	Charlie	P	Papa
D	Delta	Q	Quebec
E	Echo	R	Romeo
F	Foxtrot	S	Sierra
G	Golf	T	Tango
H	Hotel	U	Uniform
I	India	V	Victor
J	Juliet	W	Whisky
K	Kilo	X	X-Ray
L	Lima	Y	Yankee
M	Mike	Z	Zulu

GREEK ALPHABET

Capital letter	Small letter	Sound	Name	Transliteration
A	α	a (draft)	alpha	a
B	β	b (bet)	beta	b
Γ	γ	g (get)	gamma	g
Δ	δ	d (do)	delta	d
E	ε	e (egg)	epsilon	e
Z	ζ	z (gaze)	zeta	z
H	η	e (late)	eta	e
Θ	θ	th (thin)	theta	th
I	ι	i (it)	jota/iota	i
K	κ	k (key)	kappa	k
Λ	λ	l (let)	lambda	l
M	μ	m (met)	my/mu	m

N	ν	n (net)	ny/nu	n
Ξ	ξ	x (axis)	xi	x
O	o	o (cod)	omicron	o
Π	π	p (pet)	pi	p
P	ρ	rh red (trilled)	rho	r, rh
Σ	σ	s (set)	sigma	s
T	τ	t (tell)	tau	t
Υ	υ	y (ü German)	upsilon	y; u after vowel
Φ	φ	ph (photo)	phi	ph
X	χ	ch (nach German)	chi	ch
Ψ	ψ	ps (tips)	psi	ps
Ω	ω	o (clover)	omega	o

EUROPEAN AND AMERICAN NOTATIONS FOR LARGE NUMBERS

Numbers expressed as a power of		European name	American name
10	1,000,000		
10^6	$1,000,000^1$	million	million
10^9		milliard	billion
10^{12}	$1,000,000^2$	billion	trillion
10^{15}			quartrillion
10^{18}	$1,000,000^3$	trillion	quintillon
10^{33}			decillion
10^{60}	$1,000,000^{10}$	decillion	
10^{303}			centillion
10^{600}	$1,000,000^{100}$	centillion	

BIBLIOGRAPHY

BOOKS

- *Amersham Nuclear Medicine Catalogue.* Amersham International, Plc., Amersham. 1986.
- *Basic and Clinical Immunology.* 3rd Edition. H. Hugh Fundenberg, Daniel P. Sites, Joseph L. Cladwell, J. Vivian Wells. Lange Medical Publications. Los Altos, California. 1980.
- *Basic Clinical Ultrasound.* Hylton B. Meire, Pat Farrant. Bir Teaching Series.
- *Basic Medical Statistics.* Anita K. Bahn. Grune and Stratton, New York. 1972.
- *Basics of Radiopharmacy.* Buck A. Rhodes and Barbara Y. Croft. The C. V. Mosby Company, Saint Louis. 1978.
- *Biomedical Instrumentation and Measurements.* 2nd Edition. Leslie Cromwell, Fred J. Weibell, and Erich A. Pfeiffer. Prentice-Hall, Englewood Cliffs, New Jersey. 1980.
- *Computer-Assisted Medical Decision Making.* Homer R. Warner. Academic Press, New York. 1979.
- *Computers and The General Practitioner.* Alastair Malcolm and John Poyser. Pergamon Press, New York. 1982.
- *Computers in Radiology.* George B. Greenfield and Lincoln B. Hubbard. Churchill Livingstone, New York. 1984.
- *Computers in the Practice of Medicine.* Vol 1. *Introduction to Computing Concepts.* H. Dominic Covvey and Neil Harding McAlister. Addison-Wesley Publishing Company. Menlo Park, CA. 1980.
- *CRC Handbook of Chemistry and Physics.* 67th Edition (Definitions. Robert C. Weast, Editor-in-Chief. CRC Press, Boca Raton, FL. 1986–1987.
- *CRC Handbook of Management of Radiation Protection Programs.* K. L. Miller, and W. A. Weidner, Editors. CRC Press, Boca Raton, FL. 1986.
- *CRC Handbook Series in Clinical Laboratory Science.* Section A: Nuclear Medicine, Volume II. David Selingson, Editor-in-Chief, Richard P. Spencer, Section Editor. CRC Press, Boca Raton, FL. 1982.
- *CRC Handbook of Medical Physics.* Vol III. Robert G. Waggener, James G. Kereiakes and Robert J. Shalek. CRC Press, Boca Raton, FL.
- *Diagnostic Ultrasound, Text and Cases.* Dennis A. Sarti and W. Frederick Sample. Martinus Nijhoff Publishers. The Hague. 1980.
- *Dictionary of Medical Equipment.* Malcolm Brown, Paul Hammond, and Tony Johnson. Chapman and Hall. London. 1986.
- *Dictionary of Radiation Protection, Radiobiology and Nuclear Medicine* (in four languages). Compiled by Rald Sube. Elsevier, Amsterdam. 1986.
- *Fundamentals of Immunology.* 2nd Edition. Quentin N. Myrvik and Russell S. Weiser. Lae and Febiger, Philadelphia. 1984.
- *Fundamentals of Nuclear Medicine.* Naomi P. Alazraki and Fred S. Mishkin. The Society of Nuclear Medicine, New York. 1984.
- *Fundamentals of Nuclear Pharmacy.* 2nd Edition. Copal B. Saha. Springer-Verlag, New York. 1984.
- *Glossary of Atomic Terms.* Public Relations Branch, Atomic Energy Authority United Kingdom. London. 1974.
- *Glossary of NMR Terms.* Leon Axel, Alexander R. Margulis, Thomas F. Meaney American College of Radiology, Chicago, IL, 1983.
- *Glossary of Terms in Nuclear Medicine and Technology.* American Nuclear Society Standard Subcommittee on Nuclear Terminology and Units. La Grange Park, IL, 1976.
- *Golden's Diagnostic Radiology.* Section 17: Tomography: Physical Principles and Clinical Applications. J. T. Littleton, M. L. Durizch, E. H. Crosby, and J. C. Geary. The Williams & Wilkins, Baltimore.
- *Health Physics Handbook.* General Dynamics. Fort Worth, Texas. 1963.
- *Introduction to Radiological Physics and Radiation Dosimetry.* Frank Herbert Attix. John Wiley & Sons, New York. 1986.
- *MR Imaging Compendium.* W. Koops. Philips Medical Systems. W. Koops, Rotterdam. 1986.
- *NEMA Standards for Performance Measurements of Scintillation Cameras.* The NEMA Standards Publication No. NU1-1980, Washington, D. C. 1980.
- *Newnes Concise Encyclopaedia of Nuclear Energy.* D. E. Barnes, R. Batchelor, A. G. Maddock, J. A. Smedley, and Denis Taylor. George Newnes, London. 1962.
- *NMR Data Handbook for Biomedical Applications.* Paula T. Beal, Sharad R. Amtey, and Sitapati R. Kasturi. Pergamon Press, New York. 1984.
- *Nuclear Magnetic Resonance, NMR Imaging.* C. Leon Partain, A. Everette James, F. David Rollo, and Ronald R. Price. W. B. Saunders, Philadelphia. 1983.
- *Nuclear Medicine Technology and Techniques.* Donal R. Bernier, James K. Langan, and L. David Wells. The C. V. Mosby Company. St. Louis. 1981.

- *Physics in Medicine and Biology Encyclopedia.* T. F. McAinsh. Pergamon Press, New York. 1986.
- *Physics in Nuclear Medicine.* 2nd Edition. James A. Sorenson, Michael E. Phelps. Grune and Stratton. Harcourt Brace Jovanovich, Orlando, 1987.
- *Practical Abdominal Ultrasound.* Constantine Metreweli. William Heinemann Medical Books, London. 1978.
- *Principles and Practice of Nuclear Medicine.* Paul J. Early, D. Bruce Sodee. The C. V. Mosby Company, St. Louis. 1985.
- *Principles of Radioisotope Methodology.* Grafton D. Chase, Joseph L. Rabinowitz. Burgess Publishing, Minneapolis, MN 1963.
- *Positron Emission Tomography.* Martin Reivich and Abass Alavi, Editors. Alan R. Liss, Inc. New York. 1985.
- *Quality Assurance in Nuclear Medicine.* World Health Organization, Geneva. 1982.
- *Quality Assurance of Radiopharmaceuticals.* M. Frier and S. R. Hesslewood, Editors. Special Issue of *Nuclear Medicine Communications.* The British Nuclear Medicine Society. Chapman and Hall, London. 1980.
- *Radiation Protection.* Carl B. Braestrup, and Harold O. Wyckoff, Charles C. Thomas, Springfield, IL. 1958.
- *Radiation Protection. Recommendations of the International Commission on Radiological Protection.* ICRP Publication 3. Pergamon Press, Oxford. 1960.
- *Radiological Health Handbook.* Division of Radiological Health. U.S. Department of Health, Education and Welfare. Bureau of State Services. Washington. 1960.
- *Scientific Table.* 7th Edition. K. Diem and C. Leintner. Ciba-Geigy, Basle, Switzerland. 1970.
- *Siemens. Computer Terms and Definitions.* Siemens Gassasonics, B. V. Uithoorn, The Netherlands. 1986.
- South African Bureau of Standards. *South African Standard Code of Practice for the Industrial Use of Ionising Radiation.* SABS 0203. Part 1. Pretoria. 1985.
- *The Radiochemical Manual.* 2nd Edition. The Radiochemical Centre, Amersham. 1966.
- *Ultrasound. Environmental Health Criteria 22.* World Health Organization, Geneva. 1982.

PERIODICALS

- *American Journal of Cardiology*
- *American Journal of Physiologic Imaging*
- *British Journal of Radiology*
- *European Journal of Nuclear Medicine*
- *International Journal of Cancer*
- *Journal of Computer Assisted Tomography*
- *Journal of Nuclear Medicine*
- *Journal of Ultrasound and Medical Biology*
- *Nuclear Medicine Communications*
- *Radiology*
- *Seminars in Nuclear Medicine*

RECOGNITION OF COPYRIGHTS

Recognition is granted with appreciation for reprinting, with permission, definitions of the following words previously published (with amendments introduced by the author) in:

T. F. McAinsh, Ed., *Physics in Medicine and Biology Encyclopedia* (1986), Pergamon Press, Oxford, England.

Biophysics, Biostatistics. Cardiac output, Cyclotrons, Cyclotron principle, Ficks principle, Impedance plethysmography, Indicator dilution method, Moving detector devices, Neutron activation analysis in vivo, Nuclear magnetic resonance spectroscopy. Positron emission tomography. Pulse-echo imaging, Quality assurance of instrumentation. (Nuclear medicine), Quench corrections, Radionuclide generators, Radiosensitizers, Semiconductor detectors, Time-of-flight detection. Two-dimensional scanning.

Malcolm Brown, Paul Hammand and Tony Johnson, Eds., *Dictionary of Medical Equipment* (1986), Chapman and Hall, London.

Absorber, Applicator, A-scanner, Atomic absorption spectrometer, Atomizer, Auto-gamma counter, B-scanner, Cathode ray tube, Centrifuge, Chart recorder, Cineangiography, Cobalt-60 treatment unit, Collimator, Compound ultrasonic scanner, C-scanner, Coulter counter, Electrode, Faraday cage, Grey scale display, Heat camera, Image Intensifier, Ionization chamber, Ionizing radiation, Light pen, Linear array (ultrasound) scanner, Linear accelerator, Liquid scintillation counter, M-mode (ultrasonic) scanner, Motorized syringe, Multichannel analyzer, Oscilloscope, Phantom, Phased array (ultrasonic) scanner, Photomultiplier tube, Pulse height analyzer, Real time ultrasonic scanner, Scintillation camera, Section (ultrasonic) scanner, Stop-action (ultrasonic) scanner, Time compression analyzer, Time-motion (TM) scanner, Tourniquet, Transducer, Transmission-mode (ultrasonic) scanner, Treadmill, Well counter, X-ray tube.

Glossary of Terms in Nuclear Science and Technology (1986), American Nuclear Society, IL.

Ablator, Accident conditions, Accumulated occupational dose equivalent, Activation detector, Activation foil, Active component, Active failure, Airborne radioactive material, Airborne radioactivity area. Amplifier laser fusion, Anticipated operational occurrences, Barytes concrete, Beam hole, Beam profile, Branching fraction, Branching ratio, Breit-Wigner formula, Broad beam, By-product material, Cadmium cut-off effective, Cadmium ratio, Calandria (reactor technology), Calibration point, Can, Canal, Capture gamma radiation, Cask. Centrifugal process, Cell correction factor, Charge exchange, Charged particle equilibrium (CPE), Chemical radiation protector, Chemonuclear, Chemonuclear reaction, Cladding material, Clean (reactor theory), Coincidence (Count), Cold testing, Cold trap, Collective dose equivalent (S), Collectron, Committed dose equivalent, Common-mode failure, Confinement system, Continuous discharge, Controlled area, Coulomb barrier, Critical experiment, Critical volume, Criticality accident, Cross section, Cryogenic stabilization, Cyclotron (or gyro) frequency, Cyclotron radiation, Cyclotron resonance heating, Decay branching, Decommissioning, Decontamination factor, Depletion, Differential absorption rate, Displacement factor, Dose commitment, Dose threshold, Dose transit, Dose volume, Dual temperature exchange separation process, Dynamic stabilization, Electromagnetic separation process, Emergency shutdown, Emission rate, Energy imparted to matter, Enrichment factor, Equilibrium time, Equivalent square beam or equivalent field, Exchange distillation, Exclusion area, Exponential decay, Fail safe, Fermi age theory, Fertile, Fission products, Fixation (solids), Fractional rate of elimination, Fractionation (of dose), Fuel cooling installation, G-value, Gonadal dose, Grenz rays, Hard radiation, Hot cell, Hot trap, Integral experiment, Intrinsic tracer, Inverse bremsstrahlung, Isocenter, Isodose, Isomeric state, Isotopic power generator, Knocked-on atom, Larmor radius, Magnetic axis, Magnetic island, Manipulator, Mass coefficient of reactivity, Mass decrement, Mass excess, Mass ionization, Mass ionization conversion coefficient, Maximum credible accident, Maximum permissible concentration (MPC), Mean free path, Median Lethal time (MLT), Mossbauer effect, Multigroup model, Narrow beam, Neutron density, Neutron diffusion, Neutron Economy, Neutron energy group, Nondestructive measurement, Nuclear battery, Nuclear disintegration, Nuclear emulsion, Nuclear transformation, Nuclear transition, Orbital electron capture, Ordinary wave, Output, Parent, Photon propulsion, Photopronton, Population center distance, Proliferation, Radiation damage, Radiation detector, Radiation protection, Radiation sensor, Radioactive chain; decay chain, Radioactive equilibrium, Radioactive source, Radioactive waste, Radioactivity standard, Radioresistance (Radiation protection), Radiosensitivity (radiation protection), Range-energy relation, Reaction rate, Reactivity, Recoil, Remote maintenance, Resonance energy, Resonance region, Resonance scattering, Resonance width, Runaway (reactor), Scatter factor, Scavenging, Sealed source, Self-shielding, Self-shielding factor, Separation Energy (isotope separation), Shielding, Slowing-down area, Slowing-down density, Source-surface distance, Specific energy, Spent fuel, Stabilizer, Standardization, Streaming, Strontium unit, Thermal leakage factor, Threshold energy, Tissue-air ratio, Unrestricted area, Unsealed source, Workload, Xenon equilibrium, Yellowcake, Zero-area tissue-air ratio.

Robert C. Weast, Ed., *CRC Handbook of Chemistry and Physics,* 67th Edition, (1986-1987), CRC Press, FL.

Absolute units, Abvolt, Absolute zero, Absorption spectrum, Absorptive index, Absorptive power, Acceleration due to gravity, Acceptor, Actinic, Actinometer, Active mass, Allotropy, Albedo, Alfven speed, Alfven wave, Allobar, Ampere's rule, Ampere-turn, Amplitude modulation, Amplitude (of wave), Angle, Anhydride, Anistropic, Antiferromagnetic materials, Anti-matter, Aperture ratio, Apochromat, Atomic theory, Avogadro's law, Avogadro's principle, Bar, Beam splitter, Beat(s), Beat frequencies, Beating, Binary notation, Bohr's atomic theory, Bolometer, Boltzmann constant, Bremsstrahlung effect, Brightness, Centripetal force, Circulation, Computer-generated holograms, Conductors, Conservation of energy, Conservation of mass, Conservation of momentum, Constitutive property, Cryopumping, Cryotron, Curie's law, Curie point, Current (electric), Day, Debye length, Decomposition, Definite proportions law of, Degree, Degree of association, Degree of dissociation, Diabatic process, Diamagnetic materials, Dielectric, Diffraction, Diffuse reflection, Dipole, Dissociation-field effect, Distribution law, Donor, Doppler broadening, Dulong and Petit law, Effective neutron cycle time, Elasticity, Electric dipole, Electrolytic dissociation or ionization theory, Electromagnetic spectum, Electrophoretic effect, Electrostatic unit, Emission spectrum, Entropy, Extraterrestrial radiation, Farad, Faraday constant, Faraday effect, Ferrimagnetic Materials, Fresnel, Gas, Global radiation, Bram atom, Gram equivalent, Harmonic, Heat capacity, Helsenber's theory of atomic structure, Henry, Hologram, Holography, Hydrogen ion concentration, Hyperon, Hysteresis, Lattice energy, Line of force, Liquid, Longitudinal wave energy, Loudness, Magnetic Anisotropy, Magnetic Domains, Mass and weight, Mixtures, Molecular volume, Mosley's Law, Neel point, Normal solution, Nuclear isomers, Ohm, Osmotic-pressure effect, Paramagnetic materials, Periodic law, Phase angle, Planck's constant, Proton-proton reaction, Real image, Relative humidity, Salt, Scattering coefficient, Scattering cross section, Shell, Solid, Subshell, Unit, Valence electrons, Vapor, Vapor pressure, Virtual image, Volume velocity, Weber.

DICTIONARY OF NUCLEAR MEDICINE AND CLINICAL IMAGING

A

A. Symbol for mass number. The sum of Z (atomic number) and N (neutron number).

Abdomen. That portion of the trunk located between the chest and the pelvis; the upper portion of the abdominopelvic cavity.

Aberrant. Deviated from normal structure.

Abiotic. Characterized by an absence of life.

Ablation. Separation or detachment; destruction, that is, by radiation.

Ablator. A layer of pellet material that, due to absorption of beam energy, is changed into a plasma that accelerates radially outward. This momentum creates a reaction force that drives an implosion of the remaining interior pellet material.

Abney effect. The change in the apparent hue of a light of given wavelength when the saturation of the light is decreased. The magnitude of the apparent shift in hue is wavelength dependent.

Abnormal. Contrary to the usual structure, position, condition, or rule.

Abscess. Localized pocket of pus caused by death of tissue.

Abscissa. The horizontal coordinate of a graph.

Abscopal effect. Refers to secondary effects of irradiation outside treated volumes due to abnormal factors.

Absolute disintegration rate. When carrying out a radioactive assay it is possible to write down a formula of the type

$$n = FaFbFcFdN$$

where n is the absolute disintegration rate (in dpm), N is the observed counting rate obtained experimentally, and Fa, Fb, Fc, and Fd are the degradation factors due to efficiency of the extraction process, self-absorption in the source, the geometry of the measurement arrangement, the detector efficiency, respectively.

Absolute refractory period. The portion of the depolarization-repolarization cycle during which myocardial fibers cannot respond to any stimulus, as opposed to relative refractory period.

Absolute sensitivity. The absolute plane sensitivity per unit detector area, S_a, is defined as the counting rate registered per unit detector area from an infinite plane source containing unit area activity of a given radionuclide, as expressed by:

$$S_a = cps/cm^2/MBq/cm^2$$

where cps/cm^2 expresses the mean count density averaged over the detector's field of view, and MBq/cm^2 refers to the specific activity of the radionuclide contained in the source. The resulting units are cps/MBq, and the observed counting rate is insensitive to the distance between the source and the face of the collimator when the source is considerably larger than the field of view of the instrument and when the source-to-collimator distance is small with respect to the source diameter.

Absolute units. A system of units based on the smallest possible number of independent units. Specifically, units of force, work, energy, power not derived from or dependent on gravitation.

Absolute zero. The theoretical temperature at which molecular motion vanishes and a body would have no heat energy; the zero point of the Kelvin and Rankine temperature scales.

Absolute zero may be interpreted as the temperature at which the volume of a perfect gas vanishes, or, more generally, as the temperature of the cold source which would render a Carnot cycle 100% efficient. The value of absolute zero is now estimated to be $-273.15°C$, $-459.67°F$, $0°K$, and $0°$ Rankine.

Absorbed dose. (D) Is the amount of energy imparted by ionizing radiation to matter of a defined mass in a finite volume. Thus, the absorbed dose is the expectation value of the energy imparted to matter per unit mass at a point. The dimensions and units of absorbed dose are the same as those used for kerma: the gray (Gy) or the non-SI unit, the rad.

$$1 \text{ Gy} = 1 \text{ J kg}^{-1} = 100 \text{ rad}$$

Absorbed dose index. The absorbed dose index at a point in a field of ionizing radiation is defined as the maximum absorbed dose occurring within a 30-cm-diameter sphere (simulating the body) centered at the point, and consisting of material equivalent to soft tissue with a density of 1 g/cm^3 The preferred unit is the gray (Gy).

Absorbed dose rate. The dose absorbed in a given time interval, divided by that time interval. The SI unit of absorbed dose rate is the gray per second (Gy s^{-1}).

$$1 \text{ Gy s}^{-1} = 1 \text{ J kg}^{-1} \text{ s}^{-1} = 100 \text{ rad s}^{-1}$$

Absorbed fraction. (Φ) It is that fraction of the photon energy which is absorbed in a medium of a specified volume.

Absorbed-fraction method. A method for calculating absorbed dose, which includes the effects of scattered as well as direct radiation. The absorbed fraction is the ratio of the total energy absorbed by the target to the total energy emitted by the source.

Absorber. Any material used to absorb radiation for a specific purpose. A sheet or other body of material placed between a source of radiation and a detector for purposes such as: determining the nature or the energy of the radiation; reducing the intensity of the radiation at the detector; as a shielding; or giving the radiation some desired characteristic, as by preferential transmission of one component of the radiation. Such an absorber may function through a combination of processes of radiation attenuation—namely, true absorption and scattering. Calibrated absorbers are usually made in the form of metal disks. This term is also used to refer to a carbon dioxide absorber of the type used in rebreathing anesthetic circuits. It consists of a container filled with soda lime through which the patient's expired gases are passed. The soda lime absorbs carbon dioxide from the expired gases so that the remainder can be fed back to the patient.

Absorption. The process whereby some of all or part of the energy of incident radiation is transferred to the substance through which it passes. This process results in a reduction of the radiation intensity or a reduction in the number of particles emerging from the absorbing material. Common mechanisms, electromagnetic in nature, are Compton scattering, photoelectric effect, ionization, pair production, and bremsstrahlung.

Absorption coefficient. Rate of change in the intensity of a beam of X or γ radiation per unit thickness (linear absorption coefficient), per unit mass (mass absorption coefficient), or per atom (atomic absorption coefficient) of absorber, due to deposition of energy in the absorber. The total absorption coefficient is based on the sum of individual energy absorption processes (Compton effect, photoelectric effect, and pair production).

Absorption curve. All materials absorb or attenuate radiation to some extent, that is, they remove energy from a beam of radiation. Hence, all materials are absorbers. The manner in which different types of radiation are affected by the presence of absorbers is well illustrated by the absorption curves obtained for these radiations. An absorption curve is obtained using a system where a well-collimated detector measures the intensity of a beam of radiation. The intensity of the beam is then plotted as a function of the thickness of the absorber, and the curve obtained is the absorption curve of the radiation being examined with the particular absorber used.

Absorption discontinuity. A discontinuity in a graph of (photoelectric) absorption coefficient against photon energy.

Absorption line. A line observed in a nuclear magnetic resonance (NMR) spectrum corresponding to a single transition or a set of transitions arising from absorption of the incident radio-frequency radiation by the nuclear spins.

Absorption profile. A curve of detector readings from one angle (view, projection) of the scanning movement in computerized tomography.

Absorption spectrum. The array of absorption lines and absorption bands which results from the passage of radiant energy from a continuous source through a selectively absorbing medium cooler than the source. The absorption spectrum is a characteristic of the absorbing medium just as an emission spectrum is a characteristic of a radiator. When the absorbing medium is in the solid or liquid state the spectrum of the transmitted light shows broad, dark regions which are not resolvable into lines and have no sharp or distinct edges.

Absorptive index. The imaginary part of the complex index of refraction of a medium. It represents the energy loss by absorption and has a nonzero value for all media which are not dielectrics Also called index of absorption.

Absorptive power. For any body is measured by the fraction of the radiant energy falling upon the body which is absorbed or transformed into heat. This ratio varies with the character of the surface and the wavelength of the incident energy. It is the ratio of the radiation absorbed by any substance to that absorbed under the same conditions by a black body.

Abundance ratio. Usually the relative abundance of an isotope to the total content of an element. Often this is expressed as a percentage, e.g. 0.71% for ^{235}U in natural uranium.

Abvolt. The cgs electromagnetic unit of potential difference and electromotive force. It is the potential difference that must exist between two points in order that 1 erg of work be done when one abcoulomb of charge is moved from one point to the other. One abvolt is 10^{-6} V.

Accelerating tube. An evacuated chamber or tube containing electrodes down which the particles travel as they are accelerated from the high voltage terminal to ground.

Acceleration. Is the rate at which velocity is changing. It is the change in velocity (change in speed or direction or both) divided by the time over which the change occurs.

$$\text{acceleration (m/s}^2) = \text{velocity change (m/s)/time (s)}$$

Acceleration due to gravity. The acceleration of a body freely falling in a vacuum. The International Committee on Weights and Measures has adopted as a standard or accepted value, 980.665 cm/s^2.

Accelerator. A device to increase the velocity, and therefore the energy, of atomic particles, linearly or in circular paths by means of an electromagnetic field. The accelerated particles can thus cause nuclear reactions in target atoms by irradiation. Common types of accelerators are the cyclotron, synchroton, synchrocyclotron, betatron, linear accelerator, van de Graaf accelerator, etc.

Acceptance inspection. (Acceptance test) Inspection to determine whether an item delivered or offered for delivery is acceptable. Such inspection may include tests carried out following the installation of equipment to determine whether it has been manufactured and installed in accordance with the agreed technical specifications; the results of these tests provide reference values against which the future performance of the equipment may be assessed when routine testing is undertaken.

Acceptance region. 1-α region of the null hypothesis curve.

Acceptor. In transistors, the P-type semiconductor, the electrode containing trivalent impurities (boron, gallium, or indium) to increase the number of holes which can accept electrons. Contrast with donor.

Access. To retrieve information from some computer storage device such as internal memory, disk, or tape.

Accessory cells. Lymphoid cells predominantly of the monocyte and macrophage lineage that cooperate with T and B lymphocytes in the formation of antibody and in other immune reactions.

Access time. The time required by a computer to locate and retrieve information from a specified location. In the case of memory, this is related to the electronic speed of the address register and read/write circuits. In the case of disks, the access time is the sum of the time taken of the read/write head to locate a particular track plus the time required for information to rotate into the read/write position. Thus, access time is the sum of the waiting time and transfer time.

Accident conditions. Substantial deviations from operational states that are expected to be infrequent and that may lead to release of significant quantities of radioactive materials if appropriate engineered safety features or administrative controls were not provided.

Accumulated occupational dose equivalent. The sum of all dose equivalents to an individual resulting from occupational exposures to ionizing radiations, including measured dose equivalents for monitored periods and calculated values of dose equivalents for periods for which no monitoring records are available.

Accumulator. Any computer storage where mathematical operations such as addition, subtraction, division, and multiplication take place. The accumulator stores a number, receives another number, and then holds the result of any mathematical operation carried out on those two numbers.

Accuracy. A term used to indicate how close a measurement of a quantity is to its true value, In diagnostic tests, the number of the tests results (i.e. the number of true positives and true negatives in relation to the total number of tests performed).

Acellular. Not made up of cells or containing no cells.

Acetabulum. The rounded (cotyloid) cavity on the external surface of the innominate bone that receives the head of the femur.

Acetylcholine. A reversible acetic acid ester of choline having important physiological functions, such as the transmission of a nerve impulse across a synapse.

Acid. Any chemical compound that can either donate a proton or accept a pair of electrons in chemical reaction.

Acidic. Having the characteristics of an acid, that is, a substance which gives hydrogen ion in solution or which neutralizes bases, yielding water.

Acidophilic. Stains easily with acid dyes; grows best on acid media.

Acidosis. Accumulation of acid in, or loss of base from, the body, causing decrease in blood pH.

Acinus. Saccular terminal division of a compound gland having a narrow lumen, as contrasted with an alveolus. Several acini combine to form a lobule.

Acoustic admittance. The reciprocal of acoustic impedance, the complex ratio of sound pressure to volume velocity. Acoustic admittance is measured in m^3 Pa^{-1} s^{-1} or cgs acoustic ohms.

Acoustic coupler. A device for changing a sequential train of pulses. corresponding to a binary number, into sounds of a given frequency, which are piped into the mouthpiece of a standard telephone set for transmission to a remote telephone receiver. The reverse process is achieved by changing the received sounds back into a train of pulses.

Acoustic enhancement. Overamplification of echoes lying behind fluid-filled structures.

Acoustic impedance. Ratio of the acoustic pressure to particle velocity in a medium. Measured in $Pasm^{-3}$ or cgs acoustical ohms. Its change at a surface causes sound to be reflected to an extent at that surface (the basis of distance ranging by means of echoes—sonar and ultrasound imaging).

Acoustic intensity. The intensity of a sound beam represents the average rate of energy flowing through a unit area and is usually expressed in W/cm^2. The intensity of a plane wave can be related to pressure amplitude, particle displacement amplitude, the velocity of sound, and the undisturbed density of the medium by various formulas. The intensity of a sound beam can also be related to the voltage applied to the transducer generating the sound energy. Sound intensities are difficult to measure directly.

Acoustic lens. Used to focus the ultrasound beam when placed in front of a flat crystal.

Acoustic pressure. The pressure inside a medium is alternately raised and lowered as a pulse of ultrasound passes through.

Acoustic propagation properties. Characteristics of a medium that affect the propagation of sound through it.

Acoustics. Having to do with sound.

Acoustic shadowing. The loss of acoustic power (illumination) of structures lying behind an attenuating or reflecting target. It is important to distinguish between acoustic shadows and regions of low reflectivity. The shadowing may be partial or complete.

Acoustic variables. Pressure, density, temperature, and particle motion—things that are functions of space and time in a sound wave.

Acoustic window. An area of a patient, which is free from bone or gas, through which ultrasound can be passed to study deeper structures.

Acoustic-optics. Interaction of light and sound.

Acquired immunity. Immunity acquired during life: may be either specific or nonspecific.

Acquired immunodeficiency syndrome. (AIDS) A recently described, severe, debilitating, and commonly fatal disease occurring in humans. The causative agent, a retrovirus (human immunodeficiency virus—HIV), is transmitted by sexual intercourse. blood and blood products, and vertically from mother to child. In some people, infection with the virus produces profound damage to the cell-mediated immune system resulting in the occurrence of opportunistic diseases—infections and certain cancers—with a high mortality rate.

Acquisition. Intake of data to the computer; process of measuring and storing image data.

Acquisition delay time. The time between the end of the radiofrequency pulse and the beginning of data acquisition in an NMR experiment.

Acquisition rate. The number of data points acquired per second. Also known as sampling rate or digitizing rate.

Acquisition time. The time during an NMR experiment in which data are acquired and digitized. Comprising only the imaging procedure data acquisition time. In comparing sequential plane imaging and volume imaging techniques, the equivalent image acquisition time per slice must be considered, as well as the actual image acquisition time.

Acromegaly. Enlargement of head and other symptoms associated with tumors of the pituitary gland.

Actin. A muscle protein which combines with myosin to form actomyosin.

Actinic. Pertaining to electromagnetic radiation capable of initiating photochemical reactions, as in photography or the fading of pigments. Because of the particularly strong action of ultraviolet radiation on photochemical processes, the term has come to be almost synonymous with ultraviolet, as in actinic rays.

Actinides. This term is used to denote the series of heavy elements of atomic number 89 and upwards. The name is taken from actinium, the first member of the series. All these elements may have had at least a transient natural existence at the first creation of the universe, but all above uranium are now regarded as synthetic elements, produced by nuclear processes in nuclear reactors, cyclotrons, etc.

Actinium. Element symbol Ac, atomic number 89, atomic weight 227.028.

Actinometer. The general name for any instrument used to measure the intensity of radiant energy, particularly that of the sun. Actinometers may be classified, according to the quantities which they measure, in the following manner: (1) pyrheliometer, which measures the intensity of direct solar radiation; (2) pyranometer, which measures global radiation (the combined intensity of direct solar radiation and diffuse sky radiation); and (3) pyrgeometer, which measures the effective terrestrial radiation.

Action potential. The electrical activity developed in muscle and nerve cells during activity—such as conduction of electrical impulses or contraction. The action potential may be elicited by electrical, chemical, or mechanical stimulation, and is characterized by definite phases that return the cell again to the membrane resting potential.

Activated charcoal. Carbon obtained from vegetable matter by carbonization in the absence of air, preferably in a vacuum. This material has the property of absorbing large quantities of gases. It has important applications in chemistry and technology, e.g., absorption of solvent vapors, clarifying liquids, and others.

Activated lymphocytes. Lymphocytes that have been stimulated by specific antigen or nonspecific mitogen.

Activated sludge. Term sometimes used with reference to radioactive effluent treatment processes employing biological slimes and sludges, to concentrate the radioactive materials.

Activated water. A transient, chemically reactive state created in water by absorbed ionizing radiations.

Activation. The process of inducing radioactivity. The majority of artificially produced radioactive substances are produced by neutron-capture reactions of the (n,γ) type in a nuclear reactor. It is also possible to use deuteron-induced reactions in a cyclotron. A process in which the members of the complement sequence are altered enzymatically to become functionally active.

Activation analysis. An analytical method of chemical analysis permitting the detection and measurement of trace quantities of elements that become radioactive following their bombardment with neutrons. These artificially made nuclides decay in a way similar to the naturally occurring radioactive elements.

Activation cross section. The activation cross section is the cross section for the formation of a radionuclide by a specified interaction. In computing it, one uses the total number of nuclei of the element being irradiated or that of the isotope which forms the nuclide in question.

Activation detector. A radiation detector in which the induced radioactivity produced by exposure in a radiation field is used to determine particle flux density or particle fluence.

Activation energy. The energy necessary to cause a particular reaction to begin. Nuclear: The amount of outside energy which must be added to a nucleus before a particular nuclear reaction will begin. Chemical: The amount of outside energy necessary to activate an atom or molecule so as to cause it to react chemically.

Activation foil. An activation detector in the form of a foil.

Active component. A component that has moving parts or that is designed to perform its functions by a change of configuration or properties.

Active deposit. The radioactive deposit produced by the disintegration of radioactive emanation: radium-active deposit comprises the solid decay products of radon.

Active failure. A malfunction or unintentional operation of an active component.

Active immunity. Immunity acquired following exposure to harmful agents such as toxins or microbes or their products; the effectors of active immunity may be specific, e.g., due to antibodies, or nonspecific, e.g., due to interferon or other nonspecific agents.

Active lattice. The core of a heterogenous reactor in which the fuel and moderator are arranged in a regular manner. The part of a nuclear reactor where the fuel is distributed in a regular manner throughout the moderator.

Active mass. Of a substance is the number of

gram molecular weights per liter in solution, or in gaseous form.

Active product. The product of a nuclear reaction or nuclear disintegration which is itself radioactive.

Active section. That portion of a reactor in which the infinite multiplication constant k is greater than unity. Thus, the section if large enough is capable of sustaining a chain reaction.

Active transport. A mechanism whereby a substance is concentrated against an electrochemical gradient. Example: the quantitative clearance of iminodiacetic acid (IDA) from the bloodstream by hepatic polygonal cells.

Activity. The average number of spontaneous nuclear transitions from a particular energy state occurring in an amount of radionuclide in a small time interval, divided by that time interval. The SI unit of activity is the becquerel (Bq); the non-SI unit is the curie (Ci).

$$1 \text{ Bq} = 2.7 \times 10^{-11} \text{ Ci}$$

$$1 \text{ Ci} = 3.7 \times 10^{10} \text{ Bq}$$

Activity coefficient. Defined as the ratio of the thermodynamic activity to the true concentration of the substance.

Activity concentration. The activity concentration of a radioactive material (liquid or gaseous, at a given temperature and pressure) is the ratio of the activity of the contained radionuclide to the volume of the material. The commonly used unit is the becquerel per liter (Bq l^{-1}) or a multiple of it.

Activity curve. Since the activity is the number of disintegrations per unit time taking place in a radioactive specimen, the activity curve is one showing the variation of activity of the specimen with time. It is therefore the decay curve.

Activity-mass formula. A formula for computing the activity of a given mass of a radioisotope. It is

$$M = 130000 \text{ G/A T}$$

where T is the half-life in days, M is the activity in megabecquerels (MBq), A is the atomic mass of the radioisotope, and G is the mass in micrograms.

Actomyosin. The system of actin and myosin protein filaments responsible for muscle contraction.

Acute dose response. A response occurring either during or shortly after completion of treatment or acute exposure to radiation.

Acute exposure. An exposure in which a significant dose of radiation is received in a short space of time. The time may be as short as a fraction of a second or might extend to a day or even several days. If the dose is large enough it will give rise to acute effects such as erythema, radiation sickness, or death.

Adaptation. Spoken of in radiology as dark adaptation of the eyes, that is, remaining in a darkened room or using red-tinted goggles until it is possible for the eyes to distinguish a low intensity of illumination.

Adapter card. A printed circuit card that gives a computer more memory, enables it to control a new device, or gives it some other new capability. It is plugged into one of the system expansion slots in the system unit or system expansion unit.

Additivity. Refers to doses of different types of radiation (e.g., γ-rays and neutrons) or radiation from different sources (e.g., an external source and material deposited in an organ) which are received by the same volume of tissue. All such doses must be added together to determine the total dose or the fraction of permissible dose which has been received by the body or by any part of it.

Address. Address refers to a specific location in the computer's memory. Each location in memory contains a different piece of information. A computer address can be identified with either a number code or letters of the alphabet, depending on whether using machine language or a high-level language.

Addressing modes. The ways a computer can refer to a memory address, for example: direct, indirect, absolute, relative, implied, and indexed.

Address register. Memory location where an address is stored.

Adenitis. Inflammation of a gland or lymph nodes.

Adenocarcinoma. A type of malignant tumor in which the cells are arranged in the form characteristic of glands.

Adenoma. A benign epithelial tumor derived from glandular tissue. The numerous types are prefixed by cell or origin, e.g., papillary adenoma, fibroadenoma, tubular adenoma.

Adenosine deaminase. An enzyme that catalyzes the conversion of adenosine to inosine and is deficient in some patients with combined immunodeficiency syndrome.

Adenosine monophosphate. (AMP) Nucleotide containing adenine, a pentose sugar, and one phosphoric acid; product of metabolism.

Adenosine triphosphatase. (ATPASE) An enzyme that degrades ATP to ADP (adenosine diphosphate) and Pi (inorganic phosphate).

Adenosine triphosphate. (ATP) High-energy molecule that provides the energy for muscle contraction.

Adenosine 5′-diphosphate. (ADP) An energy-rich phosphate compound.

Adenosis. Any disease of a gland.

Adenylate cyclase. Enzyme found in the liver and muscle cell membranes.

Adhesion. The property of remaining in close approximation owing to molecular attraction between contiguous surfaces of adjacent bodies.

Adiabatic. A body is said to undergo an adiabatic change when its condition is altered without gain or loss of heat. The line on the pressure volume diagram representing the above change is called an adiabatic line.

Adiabatic fast passage. (AFP) A method of conducting an NMR experiment in which either the static field or the radio-frequency field is swept while the other is held constant. This sweeping can be done either slowly or quickly, compared with the spin-lattice proton relaxation time (T1). If the sweep is done quickly, it is adiabatic. (An adiabatic process is an irreversible thermodynamical process carried out with no charge or entropy, i.e., without any change in the magnetization, in this case of fast passage). This method can be used to invert the spins in a continuous-wave NMR experiment (it is similar to the 180° pulse in pulsed NMR).

Adiabatic process. A thermodynamic change of state of a system in which there is no transfer of heat or mass across the boundaries of the system. In an adiabatic process, compression always results in warming, expansion in cooling.

Adipose tissue. Consists of fat-filled cells supported by strands of collagen fibers. Tissue forms a protective padding around organs.It forms the insulating layer in the hypodermis and serves as a fat deposit for the body's reserves of "fuel".

Adjuvant. A substance which increases the formation and persistence of antibodies when injected together with antigens.

Adoptive immunity. Immunity due to immune lymphocytes provided by injection or allo-grafting; such immunity is temporary because of the host vs. graft (HVG) response expressed by allogeneic recipients.

Adoptive transfer. The transfer of immunity by immunocompetent cells from one animal to another.

Adoral. Toward or near the mouth.

Adrenal gland. Gland situated on top of kidney, produces epinephrine (adrenaline).

Adrenaline. A hormone produced at the medulla of the adrenal glands. Its effects include the stimulation of heart action, the constriction of blood vessels, and the relaxation of the bronchial muscle. Epinephrine.

Adrenergic receptors. Receptors for various adrenergic agents of either the α or the β class that are present on a variety of cells and from which the action of various adrenergic drugs can be predicted.

Adsorption. The condensation of gases, liquids, or dissolved substances on the surfaces of solids.

Adventitia. Loose connective tissue covering an organ.

Aerobic. A term used to indicate the growth of microorganisms in the presence of oxygen.

Aerobic activity or exercise. Exercise performed, using large muscle groups, at an intensity low enough so that all the energy (ATP) required for muscular work is produced from the complete metabolism of glucose and fatty acids with oxygen.

Aerobic capacity. The amount of oxygen required or used by the body during peak or maximal work; a measure of cardiovascular fitness.

Aerobic power. The degree of physiological capacity to obtain and transport oxygen necessary for biological oxidation and provide the energy requirements of physical activity.

Aerosol. A dispersion of fine particles as dust or droplets in the air.

Aerosol scan. Use of a nebulized radioactive mist deposited in the lung airways to form an image.

Afferent pathway. A pathway conveying inwards toward the center of organs of other structures or areas, e.g., one which conveys sensory nerve impulses toward the central nervous system.

Affinity. Related to the energy of reaction and most often used synonymously with avidity. The simple difference between these two terms is that avidity specifically refers to the quality of the antibody, whereas affinity reflects the quality of the antigen. Both avidity and affinity affect the overall binding in antigen/antibody complex formation.

Affinity chromatography. A technique in which a substance with a selective binding affinity is coupled to an insoluble matrix such as dextran and binds its complementary substances from a mixture in solution of suspension. Separation of compounds based on differences in their affinities for a given species.

Affinity constant. (K) For the reaction A + BR, $K_a = A - BR$ between the total analyte [A] and binding regent [BR], then

$$K_a = [A - BR] / [A][BR]$$

at equilibrium under defined conditions where [ ] indicates molar concentrations.

After heat. Heat generated in a reactor after it has been shut down, which comes from the radioactive decay of fission products formed in the fuel elements.

After image. The image seen after the retina, or a portion of it, has been fatigued by exposure to intense light or a continued fixed-light stimulus.

Afterload. The load or resistance against which the left ventricle must eject blood. One index of afterload is aortic pressure (i.e., the force resisting the ejection of blood from the left ventricle). Another is aortic impedance.

Afterloading technique. A technique used in radiotherapy, Empty containers are first placed in position on or in the patient and are then filled with sealed radioactive sources which are passed rapidly along guide tubes from a protected safe. The technique reduces the risk of radiation exposure for the personnel who manipulate the sealed radiation sources used in brachytherapy.

After pulse. Some photomultiplier tubes give rise to a train of subsidiary pulses immediately following the main pulse. The subsidiary pulses are called after pulses or satellite pulses and occur for an interval of a few microseconds after the main pulse.

After repair test. A procedure carried out following the repair of defective equipment in order to determine whether the repairs have been properly affected and whether the instrument is functioning according to specifications.

Agar. Dried mucilaginous polymer extracted from algae, used as a gel for growth of microorganisms.

Agenesis. Failure of development of an organ.

Agglutination. Mass formed by the joining together or aggregation of suspended particles, sticking together to form a clump. An antigen-antibody reaction in which a solid or particulate antigen forms a lattice with a soluble antibody. In reverse agglutination, the antibody is attached to a solid particle and is agglutinated by insoluble antigen.

Agglutinin. An antibody which produces agglutination (clumping) of a particulate or insoluble antigen.

Aggregated albumin. Conglomerates of human serum albumin in a suspension. Careful heating and controlled pH adjustment produce radioaggregates not more than 1 μm in diameter (microaggregated albumin) for liver and spleen imaging and from 10 to 50 μm in diameter (macroaggregated albumin) for lung imaging.

Aggregate recoil. An atom of the source material which is ejected from the surface of a radioactive source. This occurs principally in α-particle disintegrations. Kinetic energy from the α particle and recoiling daughter nucleus is transferred to atoms of the parent element as a result of collisions, and, occasionally, sufficient energy is donated to a single parent atom to eject it from the surface of the source.

Airborne radioactive material. Radioactive material dispersed in the air in the form of dusts, fumes, mists, vapors, or gases.

Airborne radioactivity area. An area in which airborne radioactive materials exist in concentrations exceeding the maximum permissible concentration.

Air condition. The process whereby atmospheric air is cleaned and brought to a suitable condition of temperature and humidity prior to admission to buildings, laboratories.

Air coolers. Air since it is readily available, is an obvious fluid to consider for cooling in a reactor plant. It is, however, not a good heat-transfer material, and has the disadvantage in common with most other gases, of consuming large amounts of power to pump it through the cooling system.

Air count. A measurement in which the amount of radioactivity in a standard volume of air is determined; measurement can be made by using a vacuum cleaner to draw a standard volume of air through a filter paper on which the radioactive solids are deposited.

Air dose. Radiation dose at a point in free air. It consists only of the radiation of the primary beam and of that scattered from the surrounding air.

Air equivalent. Of a given absorber, the thickness of a layer of air at standard temperature and pressure which causes the same absorption, attenuation, or energy loss.

Air equivalent material. A substance that can be used for the walls of an ionization chamber without introducing appreciable energy-dependence effects. It will be composed of elements of low atomic number so that photoelectric effects are avoided. Such materials as graphite, paper, and certain plastics are satisfactory.

Air monitor. A detecting device, used for control and warning purposes, to measure the amount of radioactivity present in the air.

Air wall ionization chamber. Ionization chamber in which the materials of the wall and electrodes are so selected as to produce ionization essentially equivalent to that in a free-air ionization chamber. This is possible only over limited ranges of photon energies. Such a chamber is more appropriately termed an air-equivalent ionization chamber.

Airway resistance. Resistance to flow in the airways.

Akinesia. Absence of motor function or activity.

Alara concept. National Regulatory Council (NRC) recommendation stating that radiation safety practices should not only be to keep radiation levels within the legal limits, but, in addition, *As Low As Reasonably Achievable.*

Albedo. The ratio of the amount of electromagnetic radiation reflected by a body to the amount incident upon it, often expressed as a percentage, e.g., the albedo of the earth is 34%. The concept defined above is identical with reflectance. However, albedo is more commonly used in astronomy and meteorology and reflectance in physics. The albedo is to be distinguished from the spectral reflectance, which refers to one specific wavelength (monochromatic radiation). Usage varies somewhat with regard to the exact wavelength interval implied in albedo figures; sometimes just the visible portion of the spectrum is considered, sometimes the totality of wavelengths in the solar spectrum.

Albumin. One of the important proteins of the body, most of which circulates in the bloodstream. It is of importance in controlling water exchange between the blood and the tissue fluids.

Albumin microspheres. Microspheres of albumin 40 to 60 μm in diameter, produced under specific conditions of heat and pH, in oil. Used for temporary arteriolar capillary blockade.

Alcohol. Organic molecule containing the func-

tion –OH group.

Aldosterone. A steroid hormone produced by the adrenal cortex whose principal action is to facilitate potassium exchange for sodium in the kidney. Excessive secretion leads to sodium and water retention, and increase in blood volume.

Alfvén speed. The speed at which Alfvén waves are propagated along the magnetic field. For a perfectly conducting fluid with a mass density of 1 kg/m³ in a magnetic field of 10,000 G, the Alfvén speed is about 1000 m/s, while the speed of sound in air is about 300 m/s.

Alfvén wave. A transverse in a magneto-hydrodynamic field in which the driving force is the tension introduced by the magnetic field along the lines of force. Also called magneto-hydrodynamic wave. The dynamics of such waves are analogous to those in a vibrating string, the phase speed C being given by

$$C^2 = \mu H^2/4\pi\rho$$

where μ is the permeability, H is the magnitude of the magnetic field, and ρ is the fluid density. Dissipative effects due to fluid viscosity and electrical resistance may also be present.

Algae. Unicellular plants accounting for 90% of the earth's photosynthetic production of oxygen.

Algol. (Algorithmic language) High-level compiler language particularly well suited to arithmetic and string manipulations.

Algorithm. An explicitly defined process made up of a number of discrete steps or instructions designed to solve a particular problem; these instructions are frequently coded using computer languages.

Aliasing. Ambiguous plotting of velocities which are too high to be determined with certainty due to pulse repetition frequency (PRF) (Nyquist) sampling limitation in pulsed or range-gated Doppler. Aliasing is a form of loss of information in the processing of radionuclide-generated images acquired by a planar or tomographic imaging instrument. A common example of aliasing is the way the spokes of wagon wheels in old westerns on television appear to rotate backward while the wagon is going forward. This occurs because the sampling rate of video (around 30 frames per second) is not fast enough to show a true representation of the wheel going forward. The positions of spokes of the wheels change more rapidly than the sampling rate. In the same way, if the image source has changes in intensity over a distance shorter than two pixels (at a higher frequency than the Nyquist frequency) the result will be an image that does not accurately reflect the radioactive source distribution.

Aliquot. A small but representative and reproducible part of something, such as part of solution or a sample of a volume of a liquid.

Alkali metals. Collective name of the group of electropositive metallic elements lithium, sodium, potassium rubidium, cesium, and francium.

Alkaline earths. Collective name of the group of divalent electropositive metallic elements and their earths or oxides, beryllium, magnesium calcium, strontium, barium, and radium.

Alkalosis. Condition characterized by an increase in blood pH above 7.4.

Allele. A pair of genes, each occupying the same relative position on homologous chromosomes, but carrying contrasting inheritance characteristics.

Allergy. An altered state of immune reactivity, usually denoting hypersensitivity to drugs and biological substances.

Allobar. A form of an element differing in isotopic composition from the naturally occurring form.

Allogeneic. Denotes the relationship that exists between genetically dissimilar members of the same species.

Allograft. A graft in which the donor and the recipient are of the same species but are genetically dissimilar. (Also called homograft.)

Allotropy. The property shown by certain elements of being capable of existence in more than one form, due to differences in the arrangement of atoms or molecules.

Allotype. The genetically determined antigenic difference in serum proteins, varying in different members of the same species.

Alpha (α) emission. Particulate radiation consisting of fast-moving helium nuclei (two protons, two neutrons) produced by the disintegration of heavy nuclei, atomic number >52.

Alpha chamber. An ionization or proportional counting tube for the detection and measurement of α-particles. Due to the small range of the α-particles, either the source must be placed inside the chamber or the α-particles must be introduced through a thin window.

Alpha counter. Any nuclear detector which is used to detect α particles as individual pulses is called an α counter. It is usually either a gas

(alpha chamber) or a scintillation counter.

Alpha decay. The radioactive transmutation of one element into another by the emission of an α-particle.

Alphanumeric. Alphanumeric code consists of characters that represent both the letters of the alphabet and the digits 0 to 9. Alphanumeric code also contains characters that represent various symbols, including punctuation marks and the signs for mathematical operations. Computer output may be represented as alphanumeric data (equations, symbols, and sentences) or as graphic data (pictures, graphs, and charts).

Alpha particle. Positively charged subatomic particle emitted spontaneously from some radioactive substances in their change from one element into another. It consists of two protons and two neutrons and ionizes heavily due to its relatively large charge and mass. α-particles are emitted with high energy, typically between 3 and 7 MeV. Due to their heavy mass and double electronic charge, they interact strongly with surrounding atoms giving a very high ionization density and linear energy transfer along their track. For example, a 5-MeV α-particle creates 7000 ion pairs per millimeter at the start of its track (in tissue) and has a linear energy transfer of 55 keV μm^{-1}. This rapid loss of energy results in a very short range, typically less than 0.1 mm. The rapid deposition of energy also results in considerable biological damage. For both these reasons, radionuclides emitting α-particles are not suitable for use in nuclear medicine.

Alpha-particle model of the nucleus. In view of the exceptional stability of the α-particle, it is reasonable to suppose that the system of two protons and two neutrons may retain the identity of an α-particle inside the nucleus. Thus, a nucleus such as carbon-12 may be considered as three α-particles bound together. On this simple model it is possible to explain some of the properties of some simple light nuclei.

Alpha-ray. A synonym for a stream of fast-moving α-particles; a strongly ionizing and weakly penetrating radiation.

Alpha spectrometer. A device which measures the energies of α-particles.

Alternating current. (AC) An electrical current in a circuit that reverses direction alternately, at regular intervals of time.

Alternating gradient accelerator. A high-energy cyclic accelerator in which the particles pass in succession through magnetic fields which increase rapidly with radius and which fall rapidly with radius. The system has the useful property of reducing the amplitude of vertical and horizontal oscillations, so allowing the use of a vacuum box with smaller cross-sectional area much smaller magnet pole pieces.

Alternative hypothesis. The hypothesis that is accepted when the null hypothesis is rejected.

Aluminum. Element symbol Al, atomic number 13, atomic weight 26.9815.

Aluminum filter. Various thicknesses of aluminum used as filtration in the X-ray beam to absorb the longer, ineffective rays. Usually 1 to 3 mm thick.

Alveolar ventilation. The volume of air entering the alveoli per minute, or the amount of alveolar air expired per minute.

Alveoli. Air sacs clustered along the aveolar ducts. Lined with epithelium and covered with surfactant, forming parts of the respiratory membrane through which gas exchange occurs in the lungs.

Alzheimer's disease. A presenile, diffuse, degenerative, organic brain disease with loss of memory.

Ambient background. Count rates of radiation levels arising from materials of low radioactivity in the local surroundings or from cosmic radiation.

Amelioration. Improvement of a disease.

Amenorrhea. An abnormal absence of menstruation.

Amentia. A congenital lack of mental ability.

American standard code for information interchange. (ASCII) A standard code consisting of eight-bit coded characters for letters, numbers, punctuation, and special communication control characters.

Americium. Element symbol Am, atomic number 95, atomic weight ~243.

Amino acid. A class of chemicals containing a carboxyl group (COOH) of an amino group (NH_2) plus a side chain, thus having both basic and acidic properties. Basic constituents of proteins.

Ammeter. An instrument for the measurement of the quantity of an electric current.

Amniocentesis. The transabdominal aspiration of amniotic fluid.

Amniotic fluid. The fluid which surrounds the fetus in utero.

A-mode scanning. An ultrasonic scanning method employing ultrasonic pulses in the megahertz range used to detect the depth of reflecting structures within the body. The dis-

tance into the body is displayed on the X-axis of a cathode ray tube (CRT) and the returning echoes are displayed as vertical movements on the Y-axis, the echo amplitude being shown by the extent of the vertical movement. A-scanners were first used to detect the correct position of the "midline echo" in the brain, which originates from the falx cerebri. Early A-scanners were converted industrial echo-sounders intended for detecting microcracks in metals. Now, medical A-scanners are intended purely for midline detection and incorporate "swept gain" correction circuits to compensate for the attenuation of ultrasound that occurs in human tissue.

Amorphous. Having no definite form, shapeless, not crystallized.

Ampere. (A) Is that constant current that, if maintained in two straight, parallel conductors of infinite length, of negligible circular cross section, and placed 1 m apart in vacuum, would produce between these conductors a force equal to 2×10^{-7} newton per meter of length.

Ampere's rule. A positive charge moving horizontally is deflected by a force to the right if it is moving in a region where the magnetic field is vertically upward. This may be generalized to currents in wires by recalling that a current in a certain direction is equivalent to the motion of positive charges in that direction. The force felt by a negative charge is opposite to that felt by a positive charge.

Ampere-turn. A measure of magnetomotive force, especially as developed by an electric current, defined as the magnetomotive force developed by a coil of one turn through which a current of one ampere flows, that is, 1.26 Gb.

Ampere's law. A vector equation relating current flow and magnetic fields. The law states that if a current (l) flows through an infinitesimal distance (dl) along a line at some point (P) a distance (r) away, there is produced an infinitesimal element of a magnetic field (dH) such that

$$dH = 1 \sin \theta \ d \ l/r^2$$

where θ is the angle between the direction of current flow and the line joining P and dl. More compactly,

$$dH = 1 \ d \ l \times r/r^3$$

Amplification. The process whereby signals derived from ionization are magnified to a degree suitable for measurement.

Amplifier. A device that accomplishes amplification.

Amplitude. Maximum variation of an acoustic variable or voltage.

Amplitude analysis. The image analysis technique for cyclical studies such as multigated blood pool. The maximum count rate change for each computer pixel during the cycle is presented as composite image.

Amplitude modulation. The variation of the amplitude of a wave in a way that corresponds to another wave. In general, the positive or negative envelope of the modulated wave (carrier wave) contains enough information to allow the modulating wave to be recovered, provided that the carrier wave has at least twice the frequency and twice the peak amplitude of the modulating signal.The modulated carrier C(t) is given by

$$C(t) = A_o \, [1 - k \, M(t)] \, \cos \omega_o t$$

where M(t) is the modulation.

Amplitude of wave. A measure of the maximum displacement of the wave crest from its undisturbed position (or the maximum electric or magnetic field strength of an electromagnetic wave).

Anabolism. A process by which cells convert simple substances into complex compounds; opposite of catabolism.

Anaerobic. A term used to indicate the growth of microorganisms in the absence of oxygen.

Anaerobic exercise. Muscular activity of an intensity that exercising muscle's energy requirement (ATP) cannot be met aerobically. The extra energy is obtained by the metabolism of glucose without oxygen to lactic acid (lactate), which is toxic to the muscles.

Analgesia. Diminished sense of pain.

Analgesic. An agent that relieves pain.

Analog. A physical quantity whose measurable magnitude may take on a continuum of values as opposed to digital quantities that can have only discrete values; any signal that is continuously variable (e.g. X send Y signals of a γ camera); structure with a similar function.

Analog computers. Computers that perform operations on continuous signals. Their output is in the form of continuous signals such as voltage fluctuations, waveforms, etc.; not as precise or accurate as a digital computer.

Analog data. Nondigital information that is continuously variable; film recording is an analog means of data storage.

Analog rate-meter system. A system of circuitry whereby a time-average frequency of radioactive events is converted into a proportional electrical signal and appropriately displayed.

Analog scan converter. A type of scan converter consisting of a vacuum tube in which the image is stored as electrical charge on a silicon target.

Analog-to-digital converter. (ADC, A/D) A device which converts analog quantities or signals to digital quantities. In digital scintigraphy the analog video signal is converted (digitized) to digital values and stored in a digital memory. It can also transform words and numbers into a binary value. A digital-to-analog converter does the opposite and has application in electronic and electromechanical output devices.

Analysis of variance. (ANOVA) A method of partitioning variance into its parts, such as between two or more treatment groups and within treatment groups so as to yield independent estimates of the population variance. The ratio of these independent estimates then can be tested using the F distribution. This provides a method of significance testing on the sample means.

Analyte. The substance in the specimen to be analyzed in an assay.

Analyzer. An instrument for discriminating energy levels of detected radiation.

Anaphase. The stage of cellular nuclear division at which the chromosomes separate into two groups which leave the equatorial plate in opposite directions and move to the poles of the spindle.

Anaphylactoid shock. Anaphylaxis-like shock that can be produced by injection of a variety of foreign agents such as colloids.

Anaphylaxis. A reaction of immediate hypersensitivity present in nearly all vertebrates which results from sensitization of tissue-fixed mast cells by cytotropic antibodies following exposure to antigen; shock mediated by IgE antibodies.

Anastomoses. To unite an end to another end; bridge between vessels, as between the smaller arteries that supply the heart muscle. Increase in their size and number provides a collateral circulation to regions of the myocardium threatened with ischemia by gradual narrowing of a larger artery.

Anatomy. Science of the structure of the human body and its parts.

And. A logical operation within a computer. For example, the statement "A and B are true" is correct only if each is individually true. If one is false, the statement is false. By applying such logic, a computer can make decisions.

And gate. An electronic logical circuit that produces an output only if all input signals are the same. For example, a "1" appears in the output if all inputs are a "1".

Androgen. Hormone or substance that possesses masculinizing activity.

Anemia. Decreased number of red blood cells or decrease amount hemoglobin in red blood cells.

Anergy. The inability to react to a battery of common skin test antigens.

Anesthesia. Partial or complete loss of sensation with or without loss of consciousness as a result of disease, injury, or administration of an anesthetic agent, usually by injection or inhalation.

Aneurysm. A circumscribed dilatation of an artery, vein, or the heart due to weakness of their walls.

Anger camera. Type of γ ray scintillation camera, named for its inventor Hal O. Anger. A detecting system (employing a single crystal 25 to 90 cm in diameter and 0.6 to 1.25 cm thick, and 37 to 91 photodetecting circuits) that views the entire field at once and is most effective in the 100- to 300-keV energy range.

Angina. Pressure, discomfort, or actual pain in the front of the chest (angina pectoris) or arms, usually provoked by effort or tension. Angina occurs because of an inadequate supply of blood to the heart muscle. Almost all cases of angina are caused by narrowing or blockage of the coronary arteries by atherosclerosis.

Angiocardiography. Angiocardiography is the radiologic or scintigraphic examination of the various cardiac chambers of the heart. In radiology this involves introduction of a catheter either into the right heart (through the vena cava) or the left heart (through the arterial side of the circulation). The chief indications for this investigation are the evaluation of pediatric congenital heart disease, ventricular aneurysm, and the well-known but rare occurrence of primary cardiac tumor.

Angiography. Radiologic or scintigraphic study of the blood vessels. Arteriography is a subheading of angiography and involves the evaluation of arteries, wheres venography is concerned with evaluation of veins. In radiologic angiography an iodinated contrast material is injected directly into the blood vessel to be examined through a flexible polyethylene tube (catheter) leading to the organ of interest outlining the anatomy of the vascular system in the region. (This direct introduction through a puncture without utilizing a surgical incision is termed "percutaneous" introduction.) Scintigraphic angiography with a radioisotope injected (mostly intravenously) is simpler, sensitive, but poorer in resolution.

Angioma. A tumor whose cells tend to form a blood vessel or related to blood vessels.

Angioplasty. Plastic surgical reconstruction of a diseased injured blood vessel. Percutaneous transluminal angioplasty is an invasive but nonsurgical technique for relieving regional ischemia due to artery disease.

Angiotensin. Vasoconstrictor substance present in blood.

Angle. The ratio between the arc and the radius of the arc. Units of angle, the radian, the angle subtended by an arc equal to the radius; the degree, 1/360 part of the total angle about a point.

Angle of incidence. The angle to the perpendicular made by the incident sound beam, which is equal to the angle of reflection.

Angle of reflection. The angle to the perpendicular made by the reflected sound beam.

Angstrom. (Å) One ten-thousandth of a micron (10^{-8} cm), unit of length used for measuring wavelengths in the visible, ultraviolet, and roentgen-ray spectra. A useful unit of distance in atomic and molecular physics since it is about equal to an atomic diameter.

Angular distribution and correlation. The relative number of particles emitted in different directions by the nuclei in a radioactive source or in a target which is being bombarded by a beam of particles.

Angular frequency. (ω) Rotational or oscillation frequency expressed in terms of radians per second. There are 2π radians in a circle; therefore, $\omega = 2\pi f$, where f is the frequency in terms of cycles per second or Hertz (Hz).

Angular momentum. A vector quantity expressing the momentum or intensity of rotational motion of a particle. In the absence of external forces, the angular momentum remains constant, with the result that any rotating body tends to maintain the same axis of rotation. When a torque is applied to a rotating body, the resulting change in angular momentum results in precession. Atomic nuclei possess an intrinsic angular momentum referred to as spin, measured in multiples of Planck's constant.

Angular variation of flood field uniformity and sensitivity. System stability with respect to rotation of the scintillation camera is measured for both uniformity and sensitivity. Use of the system for single photon emission computerized tomography (SPECT) requires a high degree of stability or nonvariability in intrinsic performance characteristics as a function of angular position.

Angular variation of spatial position. System stability with respect to rotation of the scintillation camera is measured for registration of spatial position.

Anhydride. (Of acid or base) An oxide, which when combined with water, gives an acid or base.

Anion. A negatively charged ion.

Anion exchange. An anion exchange material consists of solid polymeric polyvalent cations, which must always carry an equivalent amount of replaceable anions. Many anion exchange resins consist of a polystyrene or similar polymeric skeleton with attached cationic groups such as substituted ammonium ions. For example, resin, in the chloride form, will exchange chloride ions for other ions present in the solution into which it is introduced.

Anisotrophy. Change of a physical parameter with directions in a substance, e.g., variation of the self-diffusion coefficient of water and spin-spin relaxation time (T2) with the static magnetic field direction being along or perpendicular to muscle fiber orientation.

Anisotropic. Exhibiting different properties when tested along axes in different directions.

Anisotropic motion. Motion of an atomic or molecular species about one preferred axis, e.g., rotating about one axis in a molecule.

Ankylosis. Permanent consolidation, restriction of joint motion from abnormal fibrous or bony overgrowth.

Annihilation. (Radiation) The process that occurs when a positive electron (positron) interacts with a negative electron so that both of them disappear and their energy is transferred into electromagnetic radiation (usually as two photons, each of 511-KeV energy emitted in opposite directions).

Annular array. Array made up of ring-shaped elements arranged concentrically.

Anode. Positive electrode; electrode to which negative ions (anions) are attracted.

Anomaly. An unusual anatomical variation in the development of a structure or organ.

Anoxia. Oxygen deficiency; a condition that results from a diminished supply of oxygen to the tissues, and, therefore, threatening tissue death.

Antagonist. A substance that binds to a receptor but does not activate it, in the process of blocking the binding of the natural agonist and so preventing its action.

Antecubital. In front of the elbow; at the bend of the elbow.

Antegrade pyelography. Under local anesthetic and fluoroscopic visualization, a fine-gauge needle is introduced into the collecting system (pelvis) of the kidney. Contrast material is injected in an antegrade fashion to outline the collecting system, distal ureter, and the bladder. The most frequent indication for this examination is an obstructing lesion of the bladder or distal ureters.

Antenna. Device to send or receive electromagnetic radiation. Electromagnetic radiation per se is not relevant to NMR, as it is the magnetic vector alone that couples the spins and the coils, and the term coil should be used instead.

Anterior. Front or forward part of an organ.

Antiarrhythmic drug. An agent that prevents or alleviates cardiac arrhythmia.

Antibiotic. A chemical produced by a microorganism which can inhibit the growth of other microorganisms.

Antibody. (Ab) A protein which is produced as a result of the introduction of an antigen and which has the ability to combine with the antigen that stimulated its production.

Antibody affinity. The binding attraction of identical antibody (Ab) molecules for identical corresponding antigen (Ag) determinants.

Antibody avidity. The combined binding attraction of a population of antibodies (Abs) specific for various respective antigen (Ag) determinants on an Ag molecule. Avidity is used to designate the relative binding strength of an antiserum for an Ag.

Antibody-combining site. That configuration present on an antibody molecule which links with a corresponding antigenic determinant.

Antibody feedback. A regulatory mechanism whereby the production of antibodies (Ab) is finally slowed and halted by the immunosuppressive effects of the immunecomplexes (ICs) being formed.

Antibody-reacting sites. The two inverted surface sites at the ends of the antibody that react with the antigen-determinant sites on antigens.

Antibody response. Antibody production induced by antigen (Ag).

Anticipated operational occurrences. Events

expected to occur one or more times during the operating life of a nuclear power plant.

Anticoagulant. Substance which prevents the coagulation or clotting of blood.

Anticoincidence. The occurrence of a count in a specified detector unaccompanied simultaneously or within an assignable time interval by a count in one or more specified detectors.

Anticoincidence circuit. An electronic circuit with two input terminals that delivers an output pulse if one input terminal receives a pulse, but not if both input terminals receive a pulse simultaneously or within a predetermined time interval. A principle used in anticoincidence counting applied to pulse height analysis.

Antidepressant. Drug that results in behavioral and emotional stimulation; may belong to one or two classes, the nonamine oxidase inhibitors or the tricyclic antidepressants.

Antidiuretic hormone. (ADH) Also called vasopressin. Octapeptide that increases water retention through its action on kidney tubules.

Antiferromagnetic materials. Those in which the magnetic moments of atoms or ions tend to assume an ordered arrangement in zero applied field, such that the vector sum of the moments is zero, below a characteristic temperature called the Neel point. The permeability of antiferromagnetic materials is comparable to that of paramagnetic materials. Above the Neel point, these materials become paramagnetic.

Antigen. (Ag) A substance which can incite the formation of antibodies and which can react specifically with the antibodies formed, therefore eliciting an immune response.

Antigen/antibody complex. (Ag/Ab) The product of the joining of an antigen to an antibody. The complex has both chemical and physical properties different from either the antigen or the antibody.

Antigen-combining site. The binding site of the antibody (Ab) molecule that combines with antigen (Ag).

Antigen-determinant sites. Small three-dimensional everted surface sites on the antigen molecule which react with the antibody-reaction sites on the antibody molecules.

Antigenic. A term designating the capacity of a substance to serve as an antigen (Ag).

Antigenic competition. The suppression of the immune response to two closely related antigens when they are injected simultaneously.

Antigenicity. The ability of a substance to induce the immune response. Antigenicity of a substance depends on both its molecular size and its chemical composition. Certain sub-

stances, because of their small molecular size (for example, digoxin, angiotensin I, angiotensin II, triiodothyronine), will be able to induce the immune response only when they are coupled to large molecules.

Antigenic modulation. The spatial alteration of the arrangement of antigenic sites present on a cell surface brought about by the presence of bound antibody.

Antigen processing. The series of events that occurs following antigen administration and antibody production.

Antigen receptors. The receptors on a lymphocyte that bind antigen (Ag) determinants of a single configuration. Whereas the Ag receptors on B cells are intrinsic membrane immunoglobulins (Igs), the nature of the Ag receptors on T cells is controversial, albeit they appear to resemble the V regions of classical antibody (Ab) molecules.

Antigen trapping. The arrest of circulating antigens (Ags) (either particulate of soluble) in lymphoid organs.

Antiglobulin test. (Coombs test) A technique for detecting cell-bound immunoglobulin.

Antimatter. Matter consisting of antiparticles.

Antimony. Element symbol Sb (stibium), atomic number 51, atomic weight 121.75.

Antineutrino. Neutral nuclear particle emitted in either positron decay or electron capture.

Antinuclear antibodies (ANA). Antibodies that are directed against nuclear constituents, usually in nucleoprotein, and which are present in various rheumatoid diseases, particularly systemic lupus erythematosus.

Antiparticle. That particle (known or hypothetical) whose interaction with a given particle results in their mutual annihilation. Examples of particle-antiparticle pairs are electron-positron, proton-antiproton, and so on.

Any particle with a charge of opposite sign to the same particle in normal matters. Thus, the proton has a positive charge; the antiproton a negative charge. When a particle and its antiparticle collide, both may disappear with the creation of lighter particles; this process is called annihilation.

Antiproton. A particle possessing exactly the same properties of a proton except that its charge is negative.

Antiserum. Serum containing antibodies. In radioimmunoassay (RIA) the term often indicates an antibody solution that has not been subjected to purification steps.

Antitoxins. Protective antibodies that inactivate soluble toxic protein products of bacteria.

Antrum. A cavity or hollow, particularly a cavity surrounded by bone.

Anuria. Lack of urine excretion.

Aorta. The main and largest artery of the body, emerging directly from the left ventricle of the heart, which then branches, carrying arterial blood to all organs and tissues of the body systems.

Aortic stenosis. Narrowing of the aorta or its orifice because of lesions of the wall with scar formation; infection, as in rheumatic fever; or embryonic anomalies.

Aortic valve. Outlet valve from left ventricle to the aorta.

Aperture. An opening in an optical lens system. In digital radiography, the aperture opening is varied (f-stop setting) to control the amount of light from the output phosphor of the image intensifier to the video camera.

Aperture ratio. The ratio of the useful diameter of a lens to its focal length. It is the reciprocal of the f-number. In application to an optical instrument, rather than to a lens, numerical aperture is more commonly used. The aperture ratio is then twice the tangent of the angle whose sine is the numerical aperture.

Aperture time. The time interval during which the signal is received by the sampling device in signal processing, e.g., the aperture time of the boxcar integrator is the duration of the gate pulse during which the signal is allowed into the integrator.

Apex cardiogram. A measurement of the pressure variations at the point where the apex of the heart beats against the rib cage. Frequency response required: 0.1 to 50 Hz. Measured with special pressure-sensitive microphone or crystal transducer.

Apex of the heart. The rounded tip of the heart forming the left ventricle. The apical portion of the ventricular myocardium is thinner than other portions.

Aphasia. The loss of power of expression by speech, writing, etc., or of comprehending what is said or spoken as a result of brain disease or brain injury.

Aplasia. Developmental defect or congenital absence of an organ or tissue.

Apnea. A temporary absence, or cessation, of breathing.

Apochromat. A term applied to photographic and microscope objectives indicating the highest degree of color correction.

Apophysis. A projection, especially from a bone; an outgrowth without an independent center of ossification.

Application program. Computer program that performs a task specific to a particular user's needs. Application program can be any program that is not part of the basic operating system.

Applicator. A device fitted to teletherapy apparatus which fixes the spacing between the x-ray source and the patient. It mounts onto the x-ray or γ head and may have parallel steel walls or conical lead-lined walls, with or without a Perspex endpiece. The device will also define the width of the treatment beam.

Approach to criticality. The process in which neutron absorber is removed from (or fuel, moderator, or reflector is added to) a multiplying assembly or reactor either continuously or in several small increments to cause the effective multiplication factor to approach unity. At each increment, neutron subcritical multiplication is determined. As criticality is approached, the subcritical multiplication approaches infinity. Plotting the reciprocal of neutron multiplication vs. the parameter affecting reactivity and extrapolating to infinite multiplication predicts the point where criticality will occur.

Apraxia. Inability to perform useful movement correctly, notwithstanding the preservation of muscular power, sensibility, and coordination in general.

A priori. Condition prior to obtaining an item of data, i.e., *a priori* probability.

A programming language. (APL) A language for interactive terminals—the type of terminal where the user asks questions that are immediately answered by the computer. APL offers programmers many powerful mathematical functions, each represented by a special character. This concise notation makes programs written in APL shorter than programs written in other languages such as Pascal, BASIC, and FORTRAN, APL is especially useful for handling arrays.

Apyrogenicity. Pyrogens are defined as heat-stable substances which exist as a result of contamination by bacteria, viruses, yeasts, or molds and which when administered parenterally produce fever and hematological disorders; endotoxin, a component of the cell walls of Gram-negative bacteria, is a potent pyrogen; pyrogens are water soluble and they cannot be removed by autoclaving or by filtration; pyrogen tests have normally been carried out in rabbits by measuring rectal temperature under controlled environmental conditions; alternately, a Limulus test may be performed (gel formation of a lysate of the circulating amebocytes of the horseshoe crab); the Limulus test is sensitive and convenient.

Aquation. The replacement of coordination groups by water molecules.

Aqueous. Referring to anything dissolved in water; pertaining to water.

Arachnoid. The middle one of the three membranes surrounding the brain and spinal cord.

Architecture. Architecture refers to the design of a computer system. The goal of computer architecture is to organize the computer's components—processing units, memory, terminals, programs, etc.—in a way in which the different parts work together to achieve the objective of the design. Some computers may be designed to handle complex scientific calculations; others may be constructed to perform routine computations over and over again at very high speed.

Archival storage. Long-term storage, image filing.

Archived file. An archived file contains dated information, not needed to be retrieved quickly. An archived file is not stored in the main memory within the computer itself. Instead, it is kept outside the computer on some secondary storage medium: magnetic tape, microfilm, disk, paper ("hard copy").

Arc scan. A type of ultrasound scanning motion in which the transducer is moved over the subject in such a way as to describe a circumference around the object of interest.

Area. The unit of area is the square centimeter. The area of a square whose sides are 1 cm in length. Other units of area are similarly derived.

Area density. The method of expressing the thickness of a layer of absorbing material, as mass per unit surface area (mg/cm^2).

Area detector. In photoelectronic imaging, a video-image intensifier is an area X-ray detector. An entire area is digitized in a very short period of time.

Area monitoring. Routine monitoring of the level of radiation or of radioactive contamination of any particular area, building, room, or equipment. Usage in some laboratories or operation distinguished between routine monitoring and survey activities.

Arene. Hydrocarbon compound that contains any aromatic portion.

Argon. Element symbol Ar, atomic number 18, atomic weight 39.948.

Argument. (Legal) An effort to establish belief by a course of reasoning.

Arithmetic instruction. An instruction that tells the computer to perform an arithmetic operation such as addition, subtraction, multiplication, or division. These operations are performed upon numbers of variables called operands and yield a numerical result.

Arithmetic-logic unit (Alu). That part of the control processing unit that carries out arithmetic operations such as add, subtract, increment, decrement, etc.

Aromatic compound. Chemical compound containing a ring system that has $(4n + 2)$ n electrons.

Array. A way of organizing pieces of information. There are two types of arrays: the vector and the matrix.

The vector is a one-dimensional array, a list of items in a horizontal row. Each item is given in the vector a number corresponding to its place in the list, and the list itself is given a name, usually a letter of the alphabet.

The matrix is a two-dimensional array: it has horizontal rows and vertical columns. Each item in the matrix is assigned two numbers. The first corresponds to its row; the second, to its column.

Array phased. A type of real-time scanner where the ultrasound beam is electronically steered through a sector.

Array processor. Special hardware which is designed for high-speed processing of large volumes of digital information. Some systems have fixed programs while others can be reprogrammed as needed.

Arrhenius concept. Concept stating that an acid is a compound that acts as a proton donor.

Arrhythmia. Irregularity of the pulse; too slow or rapid beating of the heart; or abnormality in the conduction of the heart's impulse to the different parts of the heart.

Arsenic. Element symbol As, atomic number 33, atomic weight 74. 9216.

Arterial blood pressure. Pressure in the large arteries of the body; usually measured in the brachial artery because it is about the level of the arch of the aorta and therefore indicative of aortic pressure. Varies from 30 to 400 mm-Hg.

Arteriole. Minute terminal branch of the arteries that ends in capillaries.

Artery. A blood vessel that carries blood away from the heart to the rest of the body. All arteries, except the pulmonary artery and its branches, carry oxygen-rich red blood for use by the tissues.

Arthritis. Inflammation of joints owing to infections, metabolic or other constitutional causes.

Arthrography. Radiologic or scintigraphic study of the joints. Usually involves the administration of a contrast material, or a radionuclide and air to distend the interior of the joint. This is useful in evaluation of joint cartilage and articulating surface abnormalities following trauma.It is sometimes useful in the evaluation of some forms of arthritis.

Arthus phenomenon. A local necrotic lesion resulting from a local antigen-antibody reaction and produced by injecting antigen into a previously immunized animal.

Artifact. Unwanted, spurious false feature in the image produced by the imaging process. Artificial product or error in the reconstructed images.

Artificial intelligence. Artificial intelligence is a man-made intelligence—a machine designed to mimic human learning. It refers to the ability of a machine or program to reason, to learn, and to improve its performance as a result of the repeated experience of a given situation or set of problems.

Artificial isotopes. Certain nuclides have the property of emitting radiation spontaneously by the disintegration of their nuclei. Natural radioactivity is due to the nuclides which occur in nature. Artificial radioactivity is due to nuclides formed under bombardment with particles or photons. Artificial isotopes can therefore be prepared by submitting suitable specimens to bombardment in a cyclotron. They are now being produced in large numbers in nuclear reactors for use in research, industry, and medicine.

Artificial radioactivity. The property of radioactivity induced in certain elements under controlled conditions.

Ascites. Accumulation of serous fluid in the abdominal cavity.

A-scope display. An oscilloscope display in which ultrasound echoes (converted to amplified electrical signals) are presented as deflections (peaks) of the timebase of the oscilloscope. The distance between the peaks is proportional to the depth of the echoes along the ultrasound beam.

Aseptic. Free from infection or germs, antiseptic.

Assay. A procedure to measure the presence or amount of test substance (for example, hormone in blood), usually by comparing the reactive behavior of sample to that of a standard or series of standards in which the amount of substance is known.

Assay meter. An instrument used for the assay of radioactive material. It can comprise a radiation detector sensitive to the emissions from the radioactive material and a counting-rate meter or a scaler.

Assembler. A program that converts computer instructions into machine language (binary code).

Assembly language. Commands for the minicomputer system written in symbolic or mnemonic form. Typically, three-letter abbreviations, called mnemonics, are used to represent each instruction, and each mnemonic can usually be equaled to one machine-code or binary instruction. An assembly language program is translated to binary code by an assembler.

Assembly listing. A list, produced by an assembler, that shows the symbolic code written by a programmer next to a representation of the actual machine instructions generated.

Associated corpuscular emission. The full complement of secondary charged particles (usually limited to electrons) associated with an X-ray or γ-ray beam in its passage through air. The full complement of electrons is obtained after the radiation has traversed sufficient air to bring about equilibrium between the primary photons and secondary electrons. Electronic equilibrium with the secondary photons is intentionally excluded.

Association constant. (K value) The mathematical representation of the affinity of binding between antigen and antibody.

Astatine. Element symbol At, atomic number 85, atomic weight ~210.

Asthenia. Lack or loss of strength and energy; weakness.

Astigmatism. An irregularity of the cornea of the lens of the eye, causing the image to be out of focus and resulting in faulty vision. Imaging visual display cathode ray tubes may also present this irregularity due to electronic tuning problems.

Asynchronous. The completion of one instruction triggers the next instruction. The computer hardware operations are scheduled by "ready" and "done" signals rather than by fixed time intervals. In addition, it implies that a second operation can begin before the first operation is complete. Describes a type of data transmission used for communication between computer devices through modems.

Asynchronous serial communication. Transmission of packets of randomly timed data in the form of a start bit, 8 bits of data, a parity bit, and a stop bit from one system device to another.

Asynergy. Lack of coordination of groups of organs or muscles which usually act in unison.

Ataxia. Failure or irregularity of muscular coordination, especially that manifested when voluntary muscular movements are attempted.

Atelectasis. Collapse of the alveoli of all or part of a lung.

Atheroma. A fat-like cyst or growth: a yellowish plaque that may be deposited in an artery wall, decreasing the size of the lumen (or channel).

Atherosclerosis. Aging damage, degeneration, and often thickening and infiltration by fatty substance of the inner layers of the arteries. If the process is severe enough, partial or complete blockage of blood flow through the arteries may occur. Although the term "hardening of the arteries" and "arteriosclerosis" do not have precisely the same meaning as atherosclerosis, most people use the terms interchangeably.

Atherosclerotic plaque. Fibrous tissue, sometimes calcified, around a central core of lipid that locally replaces normal lining of an artery and protrudes out into the arterial lumen.

Atmospheric radiation. Infrared radiation emitted by or being propagated through the atmosphere. Atmospheric radiation, lying almost entirely within the wavelength interval of from 3 to 80 μm, provides one of the most important mechanisms by which the heat balance of the earth-atmosphere system is maintained. Infrared radiation emitted by the earth's surface (terrestrial radiation) is partially absorbed by the water vapor of the atmosphere which in turn reemits it—partly upward, partly downward. This secondarily emitted radiation is then, in general, repeatedly absorbed and reemitted as the radiant energy progresses through the atmosphere. The downward flux, or counter-radiation, is of basic importance in the greenhouse effect; the upward flux is essential to the radiative balance of the planet.

Atom. The smallest unit of an element consisting of a single nucleus surrounded by one or more orbital electrons. The number of electrons is normally sufficient to make the atom electrically neutral. Adding or removing one or more electrons turns the atom into a negative or positive ion, but this is regarded as a state of the same atom. The atom is characterized by its nucleus which can only be changed by a process that requires very much more energy than changing the state of the atom. The atom of a given element is identified by its atomic number, for example, the number of electrons about the nucleus, or protons in the nucleus.

Atomic absorption coefficient. The linear absorption coefficient of a nuclide divided by the number of atoms per unit volume of the nuclide. It is equivalent to the nuclide's total cross section for the given radiation.

Atomic absorption spectroscopy. This is a method of chemical analysis where a flame photometer measures the absorption of particular wavelengths of light when passing through a flame in which atoms from metal salts (e.g., sodium and potassium) are being ionized. Small samples of body fluids are aspirated into a nebulizer and injected into a flame of propane or natural gas, or into a flameless electrothermal arc (e.g., carbon rod furnaces). Light is passed through the flame generated by a hollow cathode lamp lined with a coating of the metal to be analyzed. The characteristic spectral lines of the metal in question are radiated from the lamp and partially absorbed in the flame. A photometer detecting the radiation passing out of the flame can measure the quantity absorbed. Light emitted in the flame is separated from that absorbed, by pulsing the light source.

Atomic beam. A stream of atoms, which may or may not be ionized, emitted from a furnace of an ion source.

Atomic clock. A device which utilizes the exceptional constancy of the frequencies associated with certain electron spin reversals (as in the cesium clock) or the inversion of ammonia molecules (the ammonia clock) to define an accurately reproducible time scale.

Atomic density. The number of atoms in a unit volume of a substance. For an isotope of density p g/c.c and atomic weight A,

$$\text{atomic density} = pN_o/A \text{ atoms/ml}$$

where $N_o = 6.023 \times 10^{23}$ atoms/grams-molecule is Avogadro's number.

Atomic energy. A misnomer for nuclear energy, but accepted because of common usage to denote the energy released in nuclear reactions.

Atomic interaction. Any force that occurs between atoms, e.g., the valency forces joining atoms in a molecule.

Atomic mass. Mass of a neutral atom usually expressed in atomic mass units.

Atomic mass unit. (amu) This unit, used commonly in chemistry, is equivalent to $1/16$ of the mass of one neutral atom of oxygen-16; equivalent to 1.66×10^{-24} g, 931 MeV, 1.49×10^{-3} erg, or 0.999728 atomic weight units.

Atomic number. A number assigned to an element in the periodic table of the elements depending upon the number of electrons revolving about the nucleus. According to present theory, the number of protons in the nucleus; hence the number of positive charges on the nucleus (symbol: Z).

Atomic pile. An obsolete synonym for nuclear reactor. The term was used because the earliest reactor was essentially a pile of moderator (graphite) and uranium.

Atomic ratio. The ratio of the number of atoms of different isotopes in a given material. For example, in natural uranium, the atomic ratio $^{235}U/^{238}U = 0.00717$.

Atomic structure. The whole of matter is made up of a limited number of chemically distinct substances called elements. There are 92 of these occurring in nature, and a small number have been made artificially. Any sample of an element is made up of atoms, the smallest particle of an element still preserving its chemical and physical properties. All atoms are made up of three fundamental particles: electrons, protons, and neutrons. The electrically neutral neutrons and the positively charged protons are contained in a small central nucleus around which the negatively charged electrons revolve, occupying a much larger volume.

Atomic theory. All elementary forms of matter are composed of very small unit quantities called atoms. The atoms of a given element all have the same size and weight. The atoms of different elements have different sizes and weights. Atoms of the same or different elements unite with each other to form very small unit quantities of compound substances called molecules.

Atomic weapons. On July 16, 1945 the first nuclear weapon was exploded at the top of a high steel tower which had been erected in the arid desert area of Alamagordo in New Mexico. The target center became a cratered zone of total destruction; the sand melted under the searing intensity of the mighty heat flash and many neighboring substances were irradiated by the colossal neutron flux generated to yield radioisotopes giving nuclear emissions of dangerous character and intensity. On August 6 and 9 of the same year, fission weapons having explosive yields equivalent to 20 000 tons of TNT were dropped on the Japanese cities of Hiroshima and Nagasaki. In the two cities a total of about 100,000 people were killed, and it is reported that many times this number suffered blast or radiation injury to a greater or lesser degree. At once it became apparent that a new military device of awe-inspiring power had been forged, and that a scientific discovery of the greatest importance was, for good or evil, within the grasp of mankind.

Atomic weight. For a given specimen of an element, the mean weight of its atoms, expressed in either atomic mass units (physical scale) or atomic weight units (chemical scale). All elements have several isotopes, which differ in the weights of their atoms. Therefore, the average mass of the atoms in a sample will depend on whether it is a mixture of isotopes (e.g., in their naturally occurring proportions) or a single isotope. It is possible for two different elements (with neighboring atomic numbers) to have the same atomic "weight": in that case they are called isobars. Since 1961 this standard has been provided by the Carbon isotope ^{12}C whose atomic mass is defined to be actually 12. On this scale atomic weights for the naturally occurring elements range from 1.008 (hydrogen) to 238.03 (uranium).

Atomism. The theory that all matter consists of atoms—minute, indestructible particles, homogeneous in substance but varied in shape. Developed in the 5th century B.C. by Leucippus and Democritus and adapted by Epicurus, it was expounded in detail by the Roman poet Lucretius.

Atomizer. A liquid may by broken up into small particles in a gas (an aerosol) by a variety of methods. One method used in medical nebulizers is to force the driving as (propellant) through a small nozzle close to a supply of the liquid to be atomized. Droplets of the liquid are drawn into the stream of propellant by the Bernoulli effect where they may join a stream of low-pressure gas for delivery to the lungs or for humidification of the air in a room.

Atom percent. The number of atoms of an element or isotope in a mixture expressed as a percentage of the total number of atoms present.

Atom smasher. Colloquial term for accelerator.

Atony. Lack of tension of a muscle.

Atopy. A genetically determined abnormal state of hypersensitivity as distinguished from hypersensitivity responses in normal individuals, which are not genetically determined.

Atresia. Closure or absence of a normal passage, orifice, or cavity.

Atrial fibrillation. An arrhythmia of the heart characterized by irregular, disordered beating of the atria (storage chambers) of the heart.

Atrioventricular node. (AV node) The specialized mass of tissue located just beneath the surface of the interventricular septum that forms the only normal conduction pathway from the atria to the ventricles.

Atrioventricular septum. The fibrous "skeleton" to which are attached atria and ventricles, the heart valves, and the trunks of the aorta and pulmonary artery.

Atrioventricular valves. The mitral and tricuspid valves.

Atrium. The upper chambers of the heart leading into the ventricles.

Atrophy. A wasting away or decrease in size of a part; the result of a failure or abnormality of nutrition.

Attenuated. Rendered less virulent, reduced.

Attenuation. The process by which a beam of radiation is reduced in intensity when passing through matter. It is the combination of absorption and scattering processes and leads to a decrease in flux density of the beam when projected through matter. A general term to denote a decrease in magnitude in transmission from one point to another. This can also refer to attenuation of sound in tissue, which is the physical process by which the intensity of the ultrasound beam diminishes through tissue by reflection, scatter, and absorption in that tissue.

Attenuation coefficient. Attenuation per unit length of wave travel.

Attenuation correction. Attenuation correction is the ability to compensate for photons which have been absorbed in the patient, never reaching the detector. Since activity located deeper in the body is attenuated more than activity near the surface, attenuation manifests itself in an emission tomographic transaxial slice by artifactually decreasing the counts near the center of the body. The relatively higher counts near the edges of the radionuclide distribution are known as a "hot rim" artifact. The two methods most commonly used to correct radionuclide distribution are the Sorenson preprocessing method and the Chang postprocessing method.

In Sorenson's method, the length of the attenuating tissue traversed by each projection ray is either assumed or determined from the patient's transaxial body contour. A hyperbolic sine function of this attenuating length is then multiplied by the mean count value of the 180° opposing projections.

In Chang's method, the patient's transaxial body contour is used to define the length of medium which attenuates each pixel in each projection. The inverse of the average attenuation from all of the projections is then multiplied by the pixel value in order to yield the corrected pixel value.

Attenuation factor. A measure of the opacity of a layer of material for radiation traversing it; the ratio of the incident intensity to the transmitted intensity. It is equal to I_o/I where I_o and I are the intensities of the incident and emergent radiation, respectively. In the usual sense of exponential absorption $(I = I_o e - \mu x)^1$ the attenuation factor is $e - \mu x_1$, where x is the thickness of the material and μ is the absorption coefficient. The attenuation of photons from a ^{99m}Tc source 10 cm deep in the body is calculated by:

$$I = I_o e^{-\mu D}$$

where D = 10 cm and μ = 0.15 cm^{-1}; I = e$^{-0.15(10)}$ = 0.223 I_o. That is, only 22.3% will leave the object without being scattered or absorbed.

Audit trail. An audit is a record of a specific transaction that takes place in a computer's system. The trial is stored as a file (collection of information) and is created during routine processing of information.

Auger effect. The nonradioactive transition of an atom from an excited electronic energy state to a lower state with the emission of an electron. It usually refers to the X-ray region of energy states. The electron ejected in the Auger effect is known as an Auger electron.

Auger electrons. Those electrons emitted from an atom due to the filling of a vacancy in an inner electron shell.

Auscultation. The act of listening to sounds within the body as aid to diagnosis or for evaluating the condition of such organs as the heart and lungs.

Authorized limits. Upper levels of radiation exposure and of dose-equivalent limits, laid down by the competent authority and not to be exceeded.

Autoantibody. Antibody to self-antigens.

Autoantigens. Self-antigens.

Autoclave. This is vessel, constructed of thick-walled steel, for carrying out chemical reactions under pressure and at high temperature.

Auto-gamma counter. This is an automated well counter for assessing the radioactive content of test samples. Several hundred samples may be moved along a conveyer and lowered one at a time into a scintilation counter, of which the scintillation crystal is shaped into a well to receive the sample. The result of the counting from each sample is often handled by computer and the preparation of the samples is simpler than that required for a liquid scintillation counter. The crystal is housed in a thin aluminum can to exclude light but allow γ-ray to pass through. γ–Ray energies above about 20 keV may be counted.

Autograft. A tissue graft between genetically identical members of the same species.

Autoimmune. Immunity directed against the body's own tissues.

Autoimmune disease. (Autoallergic disease) A self-generated disease that results from antibodies or immune cells against self-antigens.

Autologous. An immunologic term for "derived from self" (for example, skin graft, blood cells). Related terms are isologous (synonym, syngeneic), derived from identical twin (same genetic makeup); homologous, derived from the same species; and heterologous, derived from a different species. All may be related to immunochemical specificity.

Automaticity. The ability to initiate an impulse or stimulus. The cells of the cardiac conduction system—called pacemaker cells—have this inherent capacity. They spontaneously depolarize, without external stimulation.

Autonomic. Acting independently of volition; relating to, affecting or controlled by the autonomic nervous system.

Autonomic nervous system. The part of the nervous system that is not under voluntary control. Its two major components, the sympathetic and parasympathetic nervous systems, control such functions as breathing, heart rate and function, blood pressure, and intestinal activity.

Autonomous nodule. A thyroid nodule that functions independently of thyroid-stimulating hormone.

Autoradiograph. A photographic record of the distribution and concentration of radioactivity in a tissue or other substance made by placing a photographic emulsion on the surface of, or in close proximity to, the substance, followed by the usual developing process.

Availability. The percentage of time for which an installation or instrument is available and capable of rendering services.

Avalanche. The multiplicative process in which a single charged particle accelerated by a strong electric field produces additional charged particles through collision with neutral gas molecules. This cumulative increase of ions results in the production of an extremely large number of charged particles, also known as Townsend ionization or a Townsend avalanche.

Avascular. Lacking in blood vessels or having a poor blood supply, said of tissues such as cartilage.

Average life. (Mean life) The average of the individual lives of all the atoms of a particular radioactive substance. It is the reciprocal of the disintegration constant and is equal to 1.443 times the half-life ($T_{1/2}$).

Avidity. The tendency of a specific reactor substance to hold its ligands; an intense eagerness for.

Avogadro's law. Equal volumes of different gases at the same pressure and temperature contain the same number of molecules.

Avogradro's number. (6.025×10^{23} physical scale) Number of atoms in a gram atomic weight of any element; also, the number of molecules in the gram molecular weight of any substance.

Avulsion. A tearing away forcibly of a part or structure.

Axial resolution. The smallest distance that can be resolved along the length of the ultrasound beam. This resolution is limited by the transmitted pulse length.

Axon. A usually long and single nerve-cell process that, as a rule, conducts impulses away from the cell body of a neuron.

Axon reflex. A triple response of the skin to a simple stimulus, such as a scratch, caused by antidromic conduction along a branch of the stimulated sensory nerve axon, resulting in vasodilation of the blood vessels in the skin.

Azimuthal resolution. The separation required to distinguish adjacent reflectors at the same depth. This resolution is limited by beam width of the transducer at the depth of the targets.

B

Background counts. In any form of nuclear detector giving electrical pulses, unwanted background counts may be recorded due to radiations other than those arising from the process under observation.

Background cutoff. Adjustment of an organ scanner to eliminate (or progressively minimize) nontarget counts.

Background monitor. A monitor used to give an indication of prevailing level of background radiation. Such instruments are calibrated to measure dose rate from a fraction of a gray per hour upwards.

Background program. Pertaining to the computer, a program that runs at a low priority; that is, when a higher priority (foreground) program is not using system resources. Pertaining to the user, a program not requiring any user interaction.

Background radiation. Ionizing radiation arising from sources other than the one directly under consideration. Background radiation due to cosmic rays and natural radioactivity is always present, the latter being accentuated by the presence of radioactive substances in the materials used in the construction of buildings.

Backing store. Also known as bulk store. A backup to the computer's main memory. Backing store can hold more information, but it takes longer to get to the information in backing store. Examples of backing stores include floppy disks, magnetic tapes, and drums.

Backprojection reconstruction. Backprojection is the imaging process of distributing a projection back across the plane to be reconstructed. It is employed by nearly all emission tomography restruction methods. If this is the sole technique employed, then it is a crude form of reconstructing which is called simple backprojection. The image obtained by simple backprojection is badly blurred; its low-frequency cosine wave components have large amplitudes, while its high-frequency wave components have small amplitudes. The amplitude of the frequency space representation of the image falls rapidly with increasing distance from the origin. Comparing the frequency space representations of the original object and the image formed by simple backprojection, it will be found that simple backprojection suppresses the amplitudes of the cosine waves in proportion to their frequencies. This provides the basis for the filtered backprojection method.

Backscatter. The process of scattering or deflecting into the sensitive volume of a radiation measuring instrument that originally had no motion in that direction. The process is dependent on the nature of the mounting material, the nature of the sample, the type of energy of the radiation, and the particular geometric arrangement.

Backup. The process of creating a computer-compatible duplicate of information stored on a computer system. Also, the procedure for redundant recording of information. Backup hardware usually refers to a duplicate or equivalent of any peripheral device or of the computer itself. Backup procedure usually refers to a procedure for manually recording and managing information during a system failure.

Bacteria. In general, any microorganism of the order Eubacteriales; a nonsporeforming, rod-shaped or nonmotile, rod-shaped microorganism. A loosely used generic name for any rod-shaped microorganism, especially enteric bacilli and morphologically similar forms.

Bacteriolysis. The disintegration of bacteria induced by antibody and complement in the absence of cells.

Bacteriophage. A virus that destroys bacteria.

Bacteriostat. An agent that inhibits the growth of bacteria.

Ballistocardiogram. Slight movement of body due to forces exerted by beating of the heart and pumping of blood. Patient placed on special platform. Movement measured by accelerometer. Required frequency response: dc to 40 Hz. Used to detect certain heart abnormalities.

Balloon-tip catheter. An instrument that can be passed into the pulmonary artery for continuous hemodynamic monitoring in critically ill patients. With its balloon tip deflated, the catheter is passed through a peripheral vein to the right atrium. The balloon is then inflated, and as the catheter is pushed forward, the blood flow carries it through the right atrium and right ventricle, and into the pulmonary artery. The balloon is then deflated, permitting continuous measurement of pulmonary artery pressure. Transient reinflation of the balloon will occlude a segment of the pulmonary artery, so that pulmonary capillary wedge pressure can be recorded.

Bandwidth. Of an electrical device or circuit: the frequency range within which the device or circuit acceptably operates, in respect of a given characteristic, usually the gain of a device or circuit. The range of frequencies (lowest to highest) that a system can transmit. High-spatial-frequency objects (small objects or objects with sharp edges) within X-ray images require large bandwidths.

Bar. International unit of pressure 10^2. Unfortunately, some writers have used this term for 1 dyn/cm^2. 1 bar = 0.987 atm = 1000 mbar =

29.53 in. of mercury.

Bar code. One of a variety of schemes for representing numerical or alphanumerical (letters and number digits) sequences, typically as black strips of varied width and spacing. One variation of these appears on many consumer packages.

Barium. Element symbol Ba, atomic number 56, atomic weight 137.337.

Barium enema. (Air contrast) In this examination the colon or large bowel is half filled with barium and subsequently distended with large volumes of air. This allows excellent coating of the mucosal surface and is particularly helpful in looking for small, erosive or ulcerative abnormalities in addition to small polyps or early cancers.

Barium swallow. (Esophagus and pharynx) Barium is administered orally and the swallowing mechanism from the pharynx through the esophagus to the top of the stomach is examined both fluoroscopically and with selected spot radiographs. This is done principally to examine esophageal motility, detect esophageal cancers, evaluate the patient for the presence or absence of esophageal (hiatal) hernia and cardiac abnormalities that displace the esophagus.

Barn. (b) Area unit expressing the area of nuclear cross section; 1 barn = 10^{-24} cm^2.

Baroreceptor. Nerve receptors in the blood vessels, especially the carotid sinus, sensitive to blood pressure.

Barrel distortion. A nonlinearity in gamma camera images such that straight-line objects appear to bow outward. Pincushion distortion is an inward bowing.

Barrier. Barrier of radiation-absorbing material, such as lead, concrete, and plaster, that is used to reduce radiation hazards.

Barytes concrete. A type of heavy concrete containing barytes (a dense barium mineral) added to improve its shielding characteristics.

Basal cell. A cell in the deepest layer of a stratified epithelium.

Basal metabolic rate. (BMR) Rate of activity of the tissues at rest, measured under controlled conditions of temperature, food intake, and activity and adjusted for body surface area, age, and sex.

Basal metabolism. The minimum energy expenditure required to maintain life processes during a resting state.

Basal skin resistance. (BSR) Is a measure of the slow baseline changes instead of the variations caused by the autonomic system. Frequency-

response requirements; dc to 0.5 Hz.

Base. Any compound that either acts as a proton acceptor or an electron pair donor in a chemical process, or which neutralizes acids, yielding water.

BaseBand. Unmodulated, original frequency of a signal.

Base line. Refers to the discriminator setting that determines the lowest-energy photon that will be counted or recorded. Normal evaluation; evaluation before administration of a substance.

Base of the heart. The region formed by the atrium and roots of the great vessels; thus the "top" of the heart, located opposite the apex of the heart.

BASIC. (*B*eginners *A*ll-purpose *S*ymbolic *I*nstruction *C*ode) An easy-to-use programming language using simple English words, abbreviations, and the like, to instruct the computer to perform a set of predetermined operations. As a language, it is widely used by many hardware manufacturers. Unfortunately, programs written for one microcomputer cannot be used on others without considerable modification, because the differing computer designers have introduced into the language certain peculiarities to suit the operation of their machine. The different varieties of BASIC are called "dialects".

Basophil. Structure, cell, or histological element staining easily with basic dyes; immature erythrocytes staining blue or gray.

Batch. A group unit in assay processing comprising controls, standards, and a set of test samples.

Batch mode. A mode or method of processing data in which similar data are collected together for processing at one time using the same program. It is a mode that contrasts with real-time processing. A system using the batch mode is called a "batch system".

Batch table. In data processing by computer, a table defined by the user that lists parameters such as type, position, and number of replicates—in effect describing the makeup of an assay batch.

Baud. The data transmission rate between devices per second. In the case of a train of binary signals (ASCII) one baud equals one bit per second. In the case if image transfer composed of bytes or words, including control signals (start and stop bits) and parity bits, the actual data transfer rate is less than 1 b/s. For example, a 10-Bd specification might, in practice, translate effectively to a 3.5-Mb/s data transfer rate.

Bayes theorem. A theorem that is useful in

obtaining conditional probabilities. One application is determining the probability of a disease given a symptom complex (or positive test) P(D/S), which takes into account knowledge of the probability of the symptom complex (or positive test) given the disease P(S/D). A simplified expression is

$$P(D/S) = \frac{P(D) \cdot P(S/D)}{[P(D) \cdot P(S/D)] + [P(D) \cdot P(S/D)]}$$

B cell. (Also known as B lymphocyte) Strictly a bursa-derived cell in avian species and, by analogy, bursa-equivalent-derived cells in nonavian species. B cells are the precursors of plasma cells that produce antibody.

Bead. A bead is a small part of a program written to perform a specific job. Beads can be developed individually and then strung in "threads" to form a complete program.

Beam. A unidirectional or approximately unidirectional flow of electromagnetic radiation or of particles. The acoustic field produced by a transducer.

Beam area. Cross-sectional area of a sound beam.

Beam axis. A straight line (calculated according to regression rules) joining the points of maximum pressure amplitude in planes parallel to the surface of the transducer assembly in the far field of the acoustic beam.

Beam crossection. The surface in a plane perpendicular to the beam axis, consisting of all the points at which the intensity is greater than X% of the spatial maximum intensity in that plane. For beams from therapy equipment, X is usually 5%; for ultrasound fields from diagnostic equipment, X is usually 25%.

Beam hardening. A heterogeneous beam traversing an absorbing medium becomes richer in higher energy X-rays.

Beam hole. A hole through a reactor shield into the interior of the reactor for the passage of a beam of radiation for experiments outside the reactor.

Beam nonuniformity ratio. The ratio of the value of the temporal average intensity at the point in the ultrasonic field where the temporal average is a maximum (i.e., the spatial peak temporal average intensity) to the spatial average temporal average intensity in a specified plane.

Beam profile. The magnitude of radiation intensity as a function of position in a cross-sectional plane of a radiation beam.

Beam profiler. A device that plots three-dimensional reflection amplitude information.

Beam reactor. A reactor specially designed to produce external beams of neutrons for research.

Beam splitter. A device to produce two separate beams from one incident beam.

Beam/vessel angle. The angle between the Doppler ultrasound beam and the long axis of a vessel under examination. This has to be measured to enable blood flow computations to be performed.

Beamwidth. The sound beam has a definite width at specific distances from the transducer face. This depends on width of transducer face; degree of focusing; intensity of the sound.

Beamwidth effect. Essentially the loss of lateral resolution because of beamwidth.

Beat frequencies. The beat of two different frequencies of signals on a nonlinear circuit when they combine or beat together. It has a frequency equal to the difference of the two applied frequencies.

Beating. A wave phenomenon in which two or more periodic quantities of different frequencies produce a resultant having pulsations of amplitude. This process may be controlled to produce a desired beat frequency.

Beat(s). Two vibrations of slightly different frequencies f_1 and f_2 when added together, produce in a detector sensitive to both these frequencies a regularly varying response that rises and falls at the "beat" frequency $f_b = |f_1 - f_2|$. It is important to note that a resonator that is sharply tuned to f_b alone will not resound at all in the presence of these two beating frequencies.

Becquerel. The SI unit of radioactivity. One becquerel (Bq) is equivalent to one nuclear disintegration per second. The conventional unit for radioactivity is the curie. 1 Bq = 2.70 $\times 10^{-11}$ Ci.

Bel. This is a mathematical expression that compares the relative intensity of two signals by a logarithmic relationship and is used in order not to have to deal with large numbers.

Bence Jones proteins. Monoclonal light chains present in the urine of patients with paraproteinemic disorders.

Benign. Not malignant.

Bergonie-Tribondeau law. The radiosensitivity of a tissue is directly proportional to its reproductive capacity and inversely proportional to its degree of differentiation.

Berkelium. Element symbol Bk, atomic number 97, atomic weight ~ 247.

Bernoulli equation. Relationship between velocity change across an obstruction and the pressure gradient. Neglecting viscous and early phasic accelerational factors, it is commonly simplified to: gradient = 4 × maximal velocity.

Beryllium. Element symbol Be, atomic number 4, atomic weight 9. 0122.

Beta applicators. Are beta-ray sources used for the radiotherapy treatment of very superficial skin conditions. The beta-ray emitter, usually strontium 90 is spread in a very thin layer over an area of a few square centimeters, and sealed between two thin layers of silver.

Beta blockade. Beta blockade reduces contractility and, with it, oxygen consumption. The attendant bradycardia at the same time prolongs the duration of the diastole and increases the perfusion time of the coronary system. These two favorable effects contrast with a frequent increase in end-diastolic pressure, hence decrease in the pressure gradient between arterial pressure and capillary pressure in the subendocardial region during diastole. Beta blockers are particularly beneficial in cases of angina pectoris that are provoked or aggravated by the secretion of epinephrine in response to excitement or stress.

Beta decay. The transformation of nuclei either by the spontaneous emission of electrons or positrons, or by the capture of an orbital electron from the K-shell, is known as beta-decay. The rate of decay is proportional to the number of nuclei present, the constant of proportionality being known as the decay constant. For all three processes the mass number of the nucleus does not change. The reaction schemes for the three processes—electron emission, positron emission, and K-capture—are

$$Z^A \rightarrow (Z + 1)^A + \beta^- \text{ electron emission}$$

$$Z^A \rightarrow (Z - 1)^A + \beta^+ \text{ positron emission}$$

$$Z^A + \beta_k \rightarrow (Z - 1)^A \text{ K-capture}$$

where the symbol Z^A characterizes a nucleus of atomic number Z and mass number A.

Beta emitter. Any radioactive nuclide that decays by beta decay with the emission of a beta particle.

Beta-gamma emitter. Beta disintegrations are sometimes accompanied by the emission of γ-rays. In such cases the emission of a β particle leads to a product nucleus in an excited state, which subsequently de-excites by the emission of a γ-ray. If the nuclear spin change associated with the emission of the γ-ray is not too large,

the γ-ray and β-particle will be emitted at approximately the same time and the event can be observed as a beta-gamma coincidence.

Beta particle. In 1900 Becquerel showed that the β-rays behaved in exactly the same way as cathode rays and, hence, identified the constituent particles, called β particles, as electrons. Some of the artificially produced radioisotopes decay by emission of a positron or positive electron; the name of β particle is also applied.

In the case of negative β particle emission the product nucleus has the same mass number as the original nucleus, but its atomic number is one unit greater. The process can be described as a neutron in the original nucleus breaking up into a proton and electron. As expected, therefore, it takes place with nuclei which have too many neutrons for complete stability. Conversely, positive β-emission occurs with nuclei which contain too many protons; one of the protons breaks up into a neutron and positron, leaving a product nucleus with an atomic number one unit less than the original nucleus. The ionization produced by a β particle is much less intense than that produced by an α-particle, and so, for the same energy, it will travel much further. It can also lose some energy by radiation when it passes the electric field of a nucleus. This energy loss, which at low energy is only a small percentage of that lost by ionization, appears as a continuous X-ray spectrum, called bremsstrahlung.

β particles interact very weakly with nuclei and so they are not useful projectiles for inducing nuclear reactions. A positive β particle which has been slowed down sufficiently can, however, unite with an electron. The positron and electrons are then annihilated and the energy appears as two γ-rays, each of energy about 0.511 MeV, which are emitted in opposite directions.

Beta-ray. Synonym for a stream of beta particles.

Beta-ray spectrometer. This is an instrument for measuring the distribution in energy of the electrons (or positrons) emitted in a beta-decay process. Such instruments are also used for measuring the energy and intensity of internal conversion electron groups.

Betatron. This machine is used to accelerate electrons to high energies. The electrons may be used to produce very penetrating X-rays for use in radiotherapy work or the examination of industrial castings, welds, etc., and in research work. Unlike most other accelerators, the betatron uses an electromagnetic field to accelerate the particles.

Bevatron. The name given to the large 6000-MeV particle accelerator which was completed in 1954 at the University of California Radiation Laboratory. This machine works on the principle of the proton synchrotron and used four large magnets, of total weight 10 000 tons, to make protons move in an orbit of 16.4 m radius. A large AC generator and rectifier set supplies the magnet with the necessary current which is made to rise from a small value to a maximum of 8300 amp in about 1 s.

Bezold-brücke effect. The apparent change in hue of a spectral light as the brightness of the light is altered.

B_0. A conventional symbol for the constant magnetic (induction) field in an NMR system. (Although historically used, H_0 [units of magnetic field strength, ampere/meter] should be distinguished from the more appropriate B_0 [unit of magnetic induction, tesla]). In competitive binding analysis or other such assays using a standard curve, an index of the amount of tracer (for example, labeled antigen) reacting with binding reagent (for example, antibody) in the absence of any added test substance (unlabeled standard antigen).

B_1. A conventional symbol for the radiofrequency magnetic induction field used in an NMR system (another symbol historically used is H_1). It is useful to consider it as composed of two oppositely rotating vectors, usually in a plane transverse to B_0. At the Larmor frequency, the vector rotating in the same direction as the precessing spins will interact strongly with the spins.

Bias. A systematic difference between a population value and the corresponding value derived from samples taken from that population. Bias does not necessarily involve prejudice. An asymmetry in interpretation or function. Example: The potential applied to the grid of a vacuum tube or the base of a transistor to preferentially allow current in a particular direction.

Biconcave. Having two concave surfaces.

Bifunctional chelates. Complexing agent with two sites for complexation.

Bifunctional drug. Drug with ability to attack two types of symptoms or disease.

Bifurcation. Branching, as in blood vessels.

Bigeminy. Occurring in pairs; bigeminal pulse pair.

Bilateral. Having two sides; symmetrical procedure such as bilateral adrenalectomy—removal of both adrenal glands.

Bile. A fluid continuously manufactured by the liver, stored and concentrated in the gallbladder, and released into the duodenum. It helps to emulsify and absorb fats and alkalinize the intestine content.

Bile acid breath test. Test that measures the presence of gut bacteria deconjugating a bile acid; radioactive CO_2 in the breath is collected and measured after administration of a ^{14}C-radiolabeled bile acid.

Bile duct. The duct through which bile is transported from the gallbladder to the duodenum .

Bile salts. Fat-emulsifying substances that are present in bile.

Biliary system. System including liver serving both a digestive and an excretory function.

Bilirubin. Bile pigment; breakdown product of hemoglobin, causes yellow color in serum and tissues.

Bimodular cavity. A special type of microwave cavity used in electron spin resonance experiments. This type of cavity can be simultaneously subjected to two microwave frequencies.

Binary. Refers to number of the base 2. Such numbers can be composed of only the digits 0 and 1: numbers are thus strings of 0s and 1s, in which each digit position toward the left represents an increasing power of 2. Computers use binary numbers because such numbers are easy to represent on and off states in simple circuits and because they are easy to process, since rules for logical and arithmetic operations in the base 2 can be implemented in simple circuits.

Binary digit. One of the symbols 1 or 0; called a "bit".

Binary notation. A system of positional notation in which the digits are coefficients of powers of the base 2 in same way as the digits in the conventional decimal system are coefficients of powers of the base 10. Binary notation employs only two digits, 1 and 0; therefore, it is used extensively in computers where the on and off positions of a switch or storage device can represent the two digits. In decimal notation $111 = (1 \times 10^2) + (1 \times 10^1) + (1 \times 10^0) = 100 + 10 + 1 =$ one hundred and eleven. In binary notation $111 = (1 \times 2^2) + (1 \times 2^1) + (1 \times 2^0) = 4 + 2 + 1 =$ seven.

Binary scale. A numerical system based upon the number 2 (the normal decimal system is based upon 10). In this scale the numbers 1, 2, 3, 4, 5, 6, 7, 8, 9, 10, 11, etc. are represented by 1, 10, 11, 100, 101, 110, 111, 1000, 1001,

1010, 1011, etc. The use of the binary scale in nuclear counting techniques arose from the need for electronic circuits to speed up counting. A second use of the binary scale is in the employment of computer storage techniques.

Binary scaler. A counting device utilizing the binary system of numbers.

Binding. In competitive radioassay, the reactive forces between ligand and binding agent describable by the mass action law and measurable by the fraction of reagent tracer bound in the ligand-binding agent complex.

Binding agent. In competitive radioassay, the test reagent chosen, most commonly antibody, to react specifically with the substance under test via mass action, reversible reaction.

Binding assay. An *in vitro* test employing the principles of reversible reactions.

Binding capacity. The amount of specific binding sites available per quantity of binding reagent. The extrapolated point of the X-axis of a Scatchard plot performed under defined conditions.

Binding constant. The equilibrium constant for a reaction between an antibody or binding protein and its antigen or ligand.

Binding energy. For a particle in a system, the net energy required to remove it from the system; for a system, the net energy required to decompose it into its constituent particles. The energy with which a particle is held to an atom or nucleus. Electron binding energy is a synonym for ionization potential. Nuclear binding energy for a neutron, proton, or alpha particle is equal to the difference in mass between the original nucleus and the sum of the product particles.

Binding site. Site of specific attachment of macromolecules to one another. In immunoassay, antibody tends to be bivalent and antigen multivalent. Sites of a protein where they bind to radionuclides.

Binomial distribution. Frequency distribution (probability distribution) of all possible outcomes when sampling from a binomial population,

Binomial population. Population of two mutually exclusive categories, e.g., those with and without specified attribute a.

Bioassay. The estimation of the potency and other characteristics of a drug or other material by studying the reaction in living matter.

Biochemical. Referring to the chemistry of living organisms.

Biochemical analogs. Chemicals of the living system that resemble one another in function but not in structure.

Biocompatibility. The ability of a material, and a physiological environment into which the material has been introduced, to coexist, as evidenced by the presence or absence of any adverse effect on the material or the physiological environment as a result of their coexistence.

Biodistribution. The distribution of material in a biologic system, such as an experimental animal.

Bioeffects. Effects on the biologic system.

Bioelectricity. The electrical phenomena that appear in living tissues.

Biofeedback. Process by which information about subject's response (usually heart rate, blood pressure, or skin temperature) is relayed back to the subject as an auditory or visual signal. The subject can be taught to regulate these involuntary responses on the basis of the feedback leading to a beneficial change in that specific function.

Biogenesis. The origin of life; the theory that organisms can originate only from organisms already living.

Biological clock. An intrinsic mechanism believed to reside in the pineal or hypothalamus or both that is responsible for the periodicity of certain biological circadian rhythms.

Biological effects of radiation. The biological effects of radiation were noticed soon after the discovery of X-rays in 1895 and of radioactivity in 1896. It was not long before that evidence of biological damage—dermatitis, leukemia, and cancer—appeared among its practitioners.

A second source of interest stemmed from the discovery of the induction of gene mutation by X-rays. This process apparently begins with the interaction between the ionizing particles and the matter of which living organisms are composed; trace these effects to their influences on biochemistry and structure at the cellular level, then to the assemblages of cells in tissues and organs, and eventually to effects observable in the whole multicellular organism, such as carcinogenesis, aging, and killing in the experimental mammal and man. The direct ionization of biologically important molecules within the cell makes a contribution to the totality of damage resulting from a given dose, but since living substance consists very largely of water, it has been contended that the products of its interaction with radiation play a major role. The important products are the free radicals H and OH which, like all free radicals, are highly reactive. Experiments with inorganic aqueous systems have shown that the biologically damaging hydrogen peroxide (H_2O_2) is formed secondarily by the union of OH radicals; also, that in the presence of dissolved oxygen the strongly oxidizing radical HO_2 is produced, at least by α and γ radiation.

Biological half-life. (T_b) The time required for the body to eliminate one half of an administered dose of any substance by regular processes of elimination. This time is approximately the same for both stable and radioactive isotopes of a particular element.

Biological shield. A shield whose prime purpose is to reduce ionizing radiation to biologically permissible levels.

Biological target volume. The volume of discrete biological entities (i.e., chromosome strand, bacterium, gene, virus, etc.) primarily responsible for a given radiation effect.

Biologic effectiveness of radiation. Ratio of X- or γ-ray dose to that required to produce the same biologic effect by the radiation in question.

Biologic matrix. Basic materials of living systems.

Biology. The science that deals with the phenomena of life.

Biomedical irradiation reactor. A reactor employed for the primary purpose of affecting biological processes by utilization of the reactor-generated ionizing radiation. Examples of such utilization are cancer research, and determining the effects of varying radiation levels on living matter.

Biometry. The application of statistical techniques to analysis in biological research.

Biophysics. Biophysics is the study of the physics of biological systems. Individual contributions to this field may emphasize structure or function, may focus on any scale from ion to ecosystem, and may be theoretical or experimental in approach. Concern with physical ideas is, however, the essential feature. In contrast to the routine use of a physical instrument, its development in the biological context often requires penetration into the physics of the biological system concerned. For reasons of this kind, it is unfruitful to define the borders between biophysics and biological or medical physics, and between biophysics and bioengineering; these disciplines differ in mainstream emphasis, but not at their interfaces.

Biopsy. Removal and examination of a portion of an organism or tissue, used to establish a diagnosis; usually a small piece of tissue.

Biopsy transducer. A transducer with some form of guide to allow the passage of a biopsy needle into the tissue beneath the transducer.

Biostatistics. Biostatistics consists of that part of the theory and application of formal statistics that pertains to biological and medical problems. The range of subject matter is broad; techniques are drawn from data collection, sampling, experimental design, interval estimation, hypothesis testing, correlation and regression, probability theory, simulation, and stochastic modeling. Applications lie in the area of vital statistics, clinical trials, bioassay, growth and development, agriculture, genetics, ecology, and epidemiology. The simplest techniques, descriptive procedures such as tabular display, graphical display, and the calculation of averages and accompanying measures of dispersion are very widely employed. Their aim is to represent a set of more or less complex data in such a way that its salient features are readily recognizable. Studies of association that compute measures of association without attempting generalization beyond the observed data also fall in this category.

Biosynthesis. Formation of a compound from other compounds by living organisms.

Biplane imaging. A special Anger camera collimator allowing two simultaneous views, 60° apart, of an organ. Each view is presented on half of the crystal.

Bismuth. Element symbol Bi, atomic number 83, atomic weight 208.980.

Bistable. A method of displaying B-mode information, whereby echoes that fall above a particular threshold are displayed and those that fall below are not displayed.

Bistable circuit. An electronic circuit that is stable in either of two states.

Bistable display. Display in which all recorded image elements have the same brightness.

Bistable tube. A cathode ray oscilloscope showing only "black or white". This is a form of storage tube.

Bit. Constructed from the words *BInary* digi*T*, the term refers to a single digit of a binary number. Its value is either one or zero. For example, the binary number 101 is composed of three bits.

Bit map. Each bit in a string corresponds to a location (word, sector, or page) in memory which is occupied (1) or available (0).

Bit-slice processor. A microprocessor chip that comes in variable bit widths and can be cascaded in parallel with other bit slice processors to form a processor of almost any bit length. It is programmed in microcode (firmware) that can be downline loaded in to writable control store (RAM). It is capable of doing mathematical operations on a large volume of data very quickly.

Bits per second. (BPS) A unit used to measure the speed of transmission in a telecommunication channel.

Black. Of a body or medium effectively absorbing all of the radiation of some specified energy or range of energies. Allowing no transmission or reflection or radiation.

Bladder. Membranous sac or organ used to hold urine; sometimes other sacs such as gallbladder.

Blanket. Fertile material put around a reactor core to breed new fuel, e.g., uranium becomes plutonium by absorption of spare neutrons.

Blast. Immature stage of cell development; precursor of differential cell type, i.e., lymphoblast, fibroblast, neuroblast.

Blastula. A fertilized ovum in an early stage of development, consisting of a fluid-filled cavity surrounded by a layer of cells.

Bleomycin. An antibiotic substance having antineoplastic properties.

Bliss system of communication. A method of communication used by the vocally handicapped. Thoughts and emotions, as well as objects and their descriptions, are conveyed by pictorial symbols.

Bloch equations. Phenomenological "classical" equations of motion for the macroscopic magnetization vector. They include the effects of precession about the magnetic field (static and radiofrequency) and the T1 and T2 relaxation times (NMR). Nuclear magnetic resonance in hydrogenous materials such as water as first observed in 1946 independently by Professor Bloch at Stanford and Professor Purcell at Harvard. Bloch proposed phenomenologic equations of motion for the macroscopic magnetization.

Block. A block in a computer is a group of smaller pieces of information (words or records) treated as a single unit of information to be moved from place to place. The blocks in a computer may all be the same length, or they may be different lengths. Blocking is putting together blocks from individual words or records.

Block floating point. An array of floating point numbers with a common exponent. Used in simple array processors for easier computation.

Blocking antibodies. Antibodies that react with antigens (Ags) to preempt Ag determinants, thus denying other antibodies (Abs) and cells with greater effect of potential the opportunity to react effectively with Ag.

Blocking factors. Substances that are present in the serum of tumor-bearing animals and are capable of blocking the ability of immune lymphocytes to kill tumor cells.

Blood. Composed of a pale yellow fluid, called plasma, containing proteins and mineral salts, and, suspended in the plasma, the formed elements known as red cells (erythrocytes), white cells (leukocytes), and platelets (thrombocytes). In man the total amount of circulating blood ranges form about 250 ml in the newborn infant to 5 or 6 liters in the average adult. Blood circulating through the heart, arteries, capillaries, and veins carries nutrients and oxygen to body cells. Blood groups are defined by antigens on red cell surfaces.

Blood apheresis. The removal blood component from whole blood, commonly done with blood separators, e.g., plasmapheresis and leukopheresis.

Blood-brain barrier. (BBB) Typically described as the tight endothelial junctions at the capillary wall that restrict transport and diffusion from blood to brain or brain to blood of some natural body substances, drugs, and chemicals circulating in the blood.

Blood count. The estimated number of blood cells in a sample of blood. The normal values are ~5 × 10^{12}/l for red blood cells and 5 to 10 × 10^9/l for white blood cells.

Blood dyscrasia. Any persistent change from normal of one or more of the blood components.

Blood flow measurements. A measure of the velocity of blood in a major vessel. In a vessel of a known diameter, this can be calibrated as flow and is most successfully accomplished in arterial vessels. Range is from –0.5 to +1650 ml/s. Required frequency response: dc to 50 Hz. Used to estimate heart output and circulation. Requires exposure of the vessel. Flow transducer surrounds vessel. Methods of measurement include electromagnetic and ultrasonic principles.

Blood grouping. Placing the red blood cells of various individuals into major and minor blood groups depending on difference in the panels of antigens they possess, e.g., the human blood groups of the ABO system.

Blood pigments. Pigments normally found in blood, such as hemoglobin and bilirubin.

Blood plasma. All-liquid portion of the blood without cells.

Blood serum. Liquid portion of the blood plasma left after clotting of fibrinogen; has slightly lower protein concentration than plasma.

Blood urea nitrogen. (BUN) Nitrogen in the form of urea found normally in whole blood or serum. Elevated BUN values occur in many disorders, especially with reduction of cardiac and renal output following myocardial infarction.

Blood volume. Measure of total blood volume in the system. Measured by injection of an indicator such as dye or radioactive tracer and subsequent measurement of indicator concentration.

Blooming. Tendency of an overilluminated area on a cathode ray tube to spread and coalesce with neighboring area.

B-mode scanning. This is an ultrasonic method employing pulsed ultrasound in the megahertz (MHz) range which records the depth from which echoes arise and the position in an X-Y plane. Depth into the body is usually displayed on the Y-axis of a CRT, distance along the skin surface in the direction of the scan is displayed on the X-axis, and the echo amplitude is presented via the Z-modulation (brightness modulation on a time base). Thus, in its simplest (but less than usual) mode of presentation, a B-scan display is a single line, with brightness modulated along its length. B-scanners were first used for visualization of the fetus in utero, but have since been used for examining other organs within the body such as the heart, liver, kidneys, thyroid, bladder, spleen, and eyes.

Board. A rectangular sheet on which the circuits of a computer are mounted. The board, in turn, is mounted on a chassis. A circuit board contains the circuitry of a microprocessor. A number of circuit boards may be mounted on what is known as a mother board.

Body burden. Radioactive material may be absorbed by the body and retained. The total amount present at any time is said to be the body burden.

Bohr magneton. The unit of atomic magnetic moment denoted by β or $_\beta$. It is equal to $eh/4\pi m_e c$ where e is the electron charge, h is Planck's constant, m_e is the electron rest mass, and c is the speed of light. It is the magnetic moment of a single electron spin and its value is 0.927×10^{-20} erg/G (cgs units or 9.27×10^{-24}

[joules/tesla, SI units]).

Bohr radius. The orbital radius calculated from the Bohr equation,

$$a = n^2h^2/4\pi^2mZe^2$$

$$= (0.529 \times 10^{-8}) \, n^2cm$$

where n is the principal quantum number.

Bohr's atomic theory. The theory that atoms can exist for a duration solely in certain states, characterized by definite electronic orbits, i.e., by definite energy levels of their extranuclear electrons, and in these stationary states they do not emit radiation; the jump of an electron from orbit to another of a smaller radius is accompanied by monochromatic radiation.

Boiling water reactor. (BWR) A reactor in which water is used both as coolant and moderator and allowed to boil in core. Steam is produced directly in the reactor vessel, under pressure, and in this state can be supplied to a turbine.

Bolometer. An instrument which measures the intensity of radiant energy by employing a thermally sensitive electrical resistor; a type of actinometer. Also called actinic balance. Two identical, blackened, thermally sensitive electrical resistors are used in a Wheatstone bridge circuit. Radiation is allowed to fall on one of the elements, causing a change in its resistance. The change is a measure of the intensity of the radiation.

Boltzmann constant. (Symbol k) The ratio of the universal gas constant to Avogadro number; equal to 1.38054×10^{-14} erg/degree Kelvin. Sometimes called gas constant per molecule, Boltzmann universal conversion factor.

Boltzmann distribution. If a system of particles which are able to exchange energy in collisions is in thermal equilibrium, then the relative number of particles, N_1 and N_2, in two particular energy states with corresponding energies, E_1 and E_2 is given by

$$\frac{N_1}{N_2} = \exp[-(E_1 - E_2) / kT]$$

where k is Boltzmann's constant and T is absolute temperature. For example, in NMR of protons at room temperature in a magnetic field of 0.25 T, the difference in numbers of spins aligned with the magnetic field and against the field is about one part in a million; the small excess of nuclei in the lower energy state is the basis of the magnetization and the resonance phenomenon. Population distribution of a system of particles in thermal equilibrium. The number of particles in energy level E at absolute temperature T (degrees Kelvin) is proportional to $e^{-E/kT}$, where e is the base of the Napierian logarithms and k is Boltzmann constant. More specifically, in the case of nuclear spins, the number of nuclear spins in parallel (N_+) and antiparallel (N_-) orientations with respect to the magnetic field is given by $N = Ne^{-\mu H/kT}$, where μ is the magnetic moment, H is the magnetic field in gauss, and k is Boltzmann's constant. This small excess of nuclear spins in the lower energy state (orientation parallel to the static field) gives rise to the resonance phenomenon.

Bolus. A quantity of opaque medium or radiopharmaceutical introduced into an artery or vein at one time. In NMR method of blood flow measurement, the bolus consists of a certain volume of blood whose protons have been tipped by the radiofrequency (rf) pulse.

Bombarding voltage. A term used to describe the energy of ions produced by an accelerator. The voltage is that which would be required to accelerate the particles to the velocity attainable by the machine.

Bombardment. The impact of accelerated atomic particles on nuclei, usually in connection with the production of radioactive isotopes.

Bonding. May be of two types, mechanical or chemical. The former bonds involve the interlocking of particles and the penetration of one component into the pores and grain boundaries of the other. Chemical bonds involve a definite interaction between the components such as that which occurs in the formation of compounds or solid solution.

Bone. Bone consists of an organic component, the bone matrix, and a crystalline inorganic component, hydroxyapatite, It also contains an appreciable amount of water. The most important constituents of the matrix are the collagen fibers surrounded by amorphous ground substances of mucoproteins and mucopolysaccharides. Reticulin fibers are also present. Upon or within the collagen fibers are laid down the hydroxyapatite crystals that give to bone its characteristic hardness.

Bones grow rapidly throughout childhood and adolescence both in length and to some extent in thickness, but even in maturity small areas of bone are constantly being removed and replaced. Apposition and resorption are continuous throughout life. Apposition takes place through the activity of a cell, the osteoblast, which first of all appears to lay down the ground substance and collagen fibers which subsequently become calcified. Resorption takes place through the activity of another cell, the osteoclast, which removes both the apatite and the matrix, simultaneously releasing them to the bloodstream.

Bone is a tissue that has many functions: (1) it provides a rigid but jointed structure for the body; (2) It protects within its rigid walls the essential blood-forming tissue, the hemopoietic marrow which gives rise to the circulating red cells, the platelets, and the majority of types of white cells; (3) it serves as a reservoir of certain minerals, particularly calcium, that are essential to the body. (4) it serves to protect delicate organs within its cavities, e.g., the skull protecting the brain, the thoracic cage protecting the heart and lungs.

Bone marrow. Soft material that fills the cavity in most bones; it manufactures most of the formed elements of the blood.

Bone seeker. Any compound or ion which migrates in the body preferentially into bone because it is either chemically similar to calcium or takes part in bone-forming processes, e.g., strontium, radium, plutonium, or phosphonates.

Boolean algebra. System of logic followed by computer circuits to decide if statements are true or false; includes such operators as and, or, not, except, if, and then.

Boot. To start a computer's operation system. The term "boot" comes from the notion of a computer "pulling itself up by its bootstraps", because a small portion of the operating system that is stored in read-only memory (ROM) loads the rest of the operating system from disk.

Boron. Element symbol B, atomic number 5, atomic weight 10.811.

Boron chamber. An ionization chamber lined with boron or boron compounds or filled with boron triflouride gas, used for counting neutrons. The counting pulse results from particles emitted when neutrons react with the ^{10}B isotope. Also called boron counter.

Bose-Einstein statistics. The kind of statistics to be used with system of identical particles having the property that the wave function remains unchanged, if any two particles are interchanged.

Bouguer-Lambert law. The law governing the absorption of light in a homogeneous transparent medium such that $I = I_o \exp(-kx)$, where I is the intensity of light transmitted, I_o is the incident intensity, x is the thickness of the transmitting layer, and k is the absorption coefficient.

Bound. In competitive binging assay, the fraction of tracer test substance recovered in or calculated to be in the ligand-binding agent complex (for example, antigen/antibody) at reactive completion.

Bound-atom cross section. The cross section for a neutron scattered by an atom when it is rigidly bound in a molecule or crystal. It is related to the free atom cross section through

$$\sigma \text{ bound} = (M + m / M)^2$$

where M is the mass of the atom and m is the mass of the neutron

Bowman's capsule. (Glomerular capsule) The blind funnel-like end of a nephron that surrounds a glomerulus.

Boxcar integrator. A type of signal processing equipment used to improve the signal-to-noise ratio in pulsed NMR experiments. It is usually a single-channel or dual-channel averaging device.

Brachial. Relating to the arm or a comparable process.

Brachytherapy. Therapy at short distances; e.g., implantation or placement therapy with needles, inserts or other such applications containing sealed radioactive materials useful in the treatment of various disease entities.

Bradycardia. Slow heart rate; usually applied to rates below 60 beats per minute.

Bragg curve. When heavy ionizing particles pass through matter they gradually lose energy be collisions with molecules in their path, producing ion pairs. The plot of specific ionization against distance traveled along the path provides a characteristics shape called the Bragg curve.

Bragg-Gray theorem. The theorem underlying the use of cavity ionization chambers for the measurements of absorbed radiation dose. It states that the amount of ionization in a gas-filled cavity in an irradiated medium is proportional to the energy absorbed by the medium at the location of the cavity.

Bragg peak. A peak in a Bragg curve showing that the amount of ionization per millimeter of tissue traversed by charged particles increases sharply as the particles slow down near the ends of their tracks.

Brain. The portion of the central nervous system within the skull; also called encephalon, cerebrum; complex organ with many types of tissues.

Brain scan. The study of changes in cerebral perfusion in various neurological conditions using radioisotopic procedures. The term was initially coined when rectilinear scanners were used for brain scintigraphy. However, the term scan is now used generically for any of the recently developed brain-imaging techniques. There are mainly two types of brain scans: some focus on the structural aspects and include computer-assisted tomography (X-ray scanning), traditional scintigraphy, and nuclear magnetic resonance imaging. Others concentrate on the functional aspects and give a picture of the cerebral metabolism and cerebral blood flow, whether normal or pathological. These techniques include positron and single photon emission tomography.

Branch. A detour away from the normal sequence of instructions followed by a computer.

Branching. The phenomenon involving the radioactive decay of certain species of nuclei by a choice of modes, a given statistical fraction of the nuclei of a species undergoing decay by one process, the remainder by a different process. For example, ^{137}Cs may decay in either of two modes, a direct β-emission of energy 1.17 MeV to ^{137}Ba or a β-emission of energy 0.51 MeV to an excited state of ^{137}Ba followed by the decay of this to the ground state accompanied by the emission of a γ-ray of 0.66 MeV. The first process occurs in 8% of disintegrations, the second in 92%. The branching fraction is the fraction decaying by a particular mode and the branching ratio is the ratio of the two branching fractions.

Branching fraction. In branching decay, the fraction of nuclei that disintegrates in a specific way. It is usually expressed as a percentage.

Branching ratio. The ratio of the branching fractions for two specified modes of disintegration.

Branch instruction. An order that causes the computer to retrieve its next instruction from outside the next sequential location.

Brönsted-Lowry concept. Concept stating that an acid is a proton donor and a base is a proton acceptor in a chemical process.

Breeder reactor. A nuclear reactor so designed

that it produces more fuel than it consumes. This is accomplished by producing in the nuclear reaction more atoms of fissionable plutonium than the number of uranium atoms consumed.

Breeding. The process of generating nuclear fuel, e.g., plutonium from uranium, by absorption of neutrons.

Breeding gain. In a breeder reactor, the gain is the excess of fissile atoms created over those consumed per unit volume per unit time.

Breit-Wigner formula. A formula describing the cross section for nuclear reaction in the vicinity of one or more resonances. For a single resonance, the formula is

$$\sigma(x,y) = (2l + 1)\pi\lambda^2 \frac{\Gamma_x\Gamma_y}{(E - E_0)^2 + (\Gamma/2)^2}$$

where $\sigma(x.y)$ = cross section for particle x to enter and y to leave a nucleus; Γ_x = partial width of the energy level for reemission of x without energy loss; Γ_y = partial width of the energy level for emission of y; Γ = total width of the level $\lambda = \lambda/2\pi$ where λ is the de Broglie wavelength; 1 = orbital angular momentum quantum number of the incident particle; E = energy of the reactants; and E_0 = resonance energy.

Bremsstrahlung. The electromagnetic radiation produced when a charged particle is accelerated in the coulomb field of a charged body. The radiation means an energy loss of the electron and is produced, for example, when an electron passes near a nucleus and is deflected from its path, this deflection being an acceleration toward the nucleus, The name (braking radiation) originates in the radiation produced when electrons are stopped in an absorber.

A well-known example of bremsstrahlung is the continuous band of radiation produced by an X-ray tube due to the interaction between the electron beam and target nuclei. The radiation is important in beta shields since although the hazard due to beta radiation may be removed by absorption in a shield, a new hazard due to gamma radiation may be created. This may be minimized by using material of low atomic number for the shield. Bremsstrahlung produced by the coulomb interaction between a particle and a nucleus other than that from which the particle originated as described above is also known as outer (or external) bremsstrahlung. Inner bremsstrahlung originates within transpiring atoms and is attributed to the sudden change of nuclear charge which occurs when a β-ray is emitted or when an orbital electron is captured.

Bremsstrahlung effect. The emission of electromagnetic radiation as a consequence of the acceleration of charged elementary particles, such as electrons, under the influence of the attractive or repulsive force fields of atomic nuclei near which the charged particle moves. In cosmic-ray shower production, bremsstrahlung effects give rise to emission of γ-rays as electrons encounter atmospheric nuclei, The emission of radiation in the bremsstrahlung effect is merely one instance of the general rule that electromagnetic radiation is emitted only when electric charges undergo acceleration.

Bridgeware. Computer components and programs used to translate instructions and information written for one type of computer into a format that another type of computer can understand. This is necessary because computers made by different manufacturers often have different languages.

Briggsian logarithmic system. System of logarithms based on the decimal system, using the base 10.

Brightness. Is measured by the flux emitted per unit emissive area as projected on a plane normal to the line of sight. The unit of brightness is that of a perfectly diffusing surface giving out 1 lm/cm^2 of projected surface and is called the lambert. The millilambert (0.001 L) is a more convenient unit. Candle per square centimeter is the brightness of a surface which has, in the direction considered, a luminous intensity of 1 cd/cm^2.

Bright up. Alternative term for acoustic accentuation found behind fluid-filled structures.

Broadband. High bandwidth, modulated signal capable of supporting high data transmission rates.

Broadband decoupling. A technique used in high resolution NMR spectroscopy in which nuclei of the same isotope but possibly different chemical shifts are decoupled simultaneously from a heteronucleis; e.g., in ^{13}C NMR spectroscopy, the coupling of all protons to the ^{13}C nuclei is removed by broadband decoupling.

Broad beam. In beam attenuation measurements, a beam in which the unscattered radiation and some of the scattered radiation reach the detector.

Broad-beam attenuation. Attenuation obtained under such conditions that the maximum amount of scattered radiation is included in the transmitted beam.

Brodmann's areas. Forty-seven numbered regions of the cerebral cortex, each of which is assumed to have a specific function.

Brodmann's area 17. In the cortex of the brain, the receptive area for visual images; also known as the projection area.

Bromination. Chemical addition of bromine to a compound.

Bromine. Element symbol Br, atomic number 35, atomic weight 79.904.

Bronchiectasis. A chronic disorder in which there is loss of the normal elastic tissues and dilation of lung air passages; characterized by difficulty in breathing, coughing, expectoration of pus, and unpleasant breath.

Bronchiogenic carcinoma. A malignant tumor originating in the lungs.

Bronchiole. The smallest branch of the bronchial tree.

Bronchography. Local anesthetic is applied to the mucosa of the trachea and bronchial tree and an iodized contrast material is introduced into the trachea and bronchial tree through a small opaque catheter to the area of lung under investigation. The principal indication for this examination is to attempt to determine whether an abnormality is intrinsically within bronchus (endobronchial) or extrinsic to the bronchus in the surrounding lung. It is also possible to document the location and degree of residual inflammatory change in areas of the lung that have been subjected to repeated episodes of pneumonia (bronchiectasis).

Bronchus. Either of two primary divisions of the trachea that lead, respectively, into the right and left lung; broadly, bronchial tube.

Brownian movement. Motion of minute particle suspended in a colloidal solution caused by unbalanced impacts with molecules of the surrounding medium.

Bubble memory. A type of computer memory that stores information as microscopic magnetic bubbles on a thin wafer of garnet or other silicate material. Bubble memory can store a great deal of information in a very tiny space. A magnetic field shifts the position of the bubble on the wafer to alter the contents of the memory.

Bucket brigade device. Also known as a charged-coupled device. A type of storage technology that shifts stored information by transferring a charge of electric current from one capacitor in the device to the next. The capacitors in this device are high-density integrated circuits.

Bucky diaphragm. A device used in diagnostic radiography to minimize haziness (due to scattered X-rays) when radiographing thick body parts.

Buffer. Storage area used to temporarily hold information being transferred between two devices or between a device and memory; often a special register of a designated area of memory.

Buffer solution. Solution containing mixtures of weak acids and the corresponding sodium salts, or weak bases and the corresponding nitrate or chloride which change their pH much less on the addition of small amounts of other acids or bases than, for example, ordinary solutions of salts, acids, or bases.

Buffy coat. The thin upper layer of leukocytes on sedimented red blood cells.

Bug. An error, defect, or other problem that prevents computer from working properly. Software bugs are errors in programs; hardware bugs are malfunctions in equipment.

Build-up factor. In the passage of radiation through a medium, the ratio of the total value of a specified radiation quantity at any point to the contribution to that value from radiation reaching the point without having undergone a collision.

Bundle branches. The right and left cardiac conduction pathway continuing from the bundle of His and proceeding along both sides of the interventricular septum to the tips of the ventricles.

Bundled. Refers to the fact that the cost of the software is included in the overall price of a computer system. This often means that the software cannot be obtained separately.

Bundle of His. The band of cardiac nervelike fibers that originates at the atrioventricular node and propagates the impulse originating in the sinoatrial node through the right and left bundle branches to the terminal Purkinje fibers.

Burial ground. (Graveyard) A place for burying unwanted radioactive objects to prevent escape of their radiations, the earth acting as a shield. Such objects must be placed in watertight, noncorrodible containers so that the radioactive material cannot be leached out and get into an underground water supply.

Burner reactor. A reactor which consumes fissile material but is not designed to produce new fissile material.

Burn-up. Induced nuclear transformation of atoms during reactor operation. The term may be applied to fuel or other materials.

Bursa. Fluid-filled sacs generally located where tendons (the ends of muscles) run over bony prominences near the joints. They are designed to cushion the tendons and prevent irritation and damage.

Bursa of fabricius. A cloacal lymphoepithelial structure in birds that regulates the development of B cells and the production of antibodies.

Burst. A term used in describing the location of an atomic weapon at the moment of detonation, i.d., sea-burst, ground-burst, air-burst, etc.

Burst cartridge. A fuel element in which a leak — usually a very small crack or pinhole — has developed in the can, "burst" being somewhat of an exaggeration, but conventional by use.

Bus. In computing, a set of wires along which signals representing addresses or data travel between the units that comprise a computer.

Butterworth filter. A low-pass filter for emission tomographic imaging reconstruction. Two parameters are needed to define the Butterworth filter, the cutoff frequency and the order of the filter. The order of the filter is related to how fast the filter is cut off: the higher the order the sharper the cutoff. The Butterworth filter may be applied using a sharper cutoff than the Hann filter, retaining contrast at higher frequencies while still eliminating the Poisson noise.

Bypass. Auxiliary flow route; replacement of major blood vessels by synthetic tubes, or natural vessels.

By-product material. Any radioactive material (except special nuclear material) yielded in or made radioactive by exposure to the radiation incident to the process of producing or utilizing special nuclear material. The tailings or waste products produced by the extraction or concentration or uranium or thorium from any ore processed primarily for its source material content.

Byte. Eight consecutive bits treated and stored as a group. One byte, for example, may represent one letter or two numbers.

Byte mode. A method of storage used for images in which the value for one pixel is stored in one byte (8 bits = $^1/_2$ word) and has value between 0 and 255.

C

Cache memory. High-speed memory the central processing unit (CPU) has direct access to. Generally smaller than main memory.

Cachexia. A profound and marked state of con

stitutional disorder; general ill health and malnutrition.

Cadaver. A dead body; generally a dead human body.

Cadmium. Element symbol Cd, atomic number 48, atomic weight 112.411.

Cadmium cutoff effective. The energy value which, for a given experimental configuration, is determined by the condition that if a cadmium cover surrounding a detector were replaced by a fictitious cover back to neutrons below this value and transparent to neutrons with energy above this value, the observed detector response would be unchanged.

Cadmium ratio. The ratio of the response of a bare neutron detector to its response under the same conditions but when covered with cadmium of a specified thickness.

Calandria. (Reactor technology) A closed reactor vessel with interval tubes or channels arranged so as to keep the liquid moderator separate from the primary coolant, to provide irradiation facilities, or to contain pressure tubes.

Calcification. Process by which an organic tissue becomes hardened by a deposit of calcium salts.

Calcitonin. A polypeptide, occurring naturally in the body, which plays a part in the regulation of blood calcium level. The synthetic form can be used in the treatment of Paget's disease.

Calcium. Element symbol Ca, atomic number 20, atomic weight 40.08.

Calcium antagonists. The favorable therapeutic effect of this group of drugs rests on two factors: they cause a reduction of peripheral resistance and, consequently, a reduction of myocardial work. Further, they reduce oxygen consumption by inhibiting calcium influx. On occasion, they may, in addition, improve the oxygen status through antiarrhythmic action.

Calculus. Commonly called stone, any abnormal concretion within the body. A calculus is usually composed of mineral salts, which can occur in the kidneys, ureter, bladder, or urethra.

Calder Hall. The world's first full-scale commercial-size nuclear power station, which started operating in October 1956. Four gas-cooled, graphite-moderated, natural-uranium reactors are at the Calder site in Cumberland, U.K. and this set is duplicated at Chapelcross. The designed heat output of each reactor was 180 MW (Th) but operational experience has allowed the output to be raised to 270 MW (Th).

Calibration. Determination of variation from standard, or accuracy, of a measuring instrument to ascertain necessary correction factors. A procedure for standardizing radiation detection instruments for various parameters such as quantitation of the amount of radioactivity, uniformity of response, spatial resolution, etc.

Calibration point. (Radiation therapy) The location in a radiation field at which a calibration is conducted. In air, the distance and the depth below the surface are usually specified. The calibration point is used in air only for X-rays generated by potentials less than 400 keV. For higher energy photon beams, it is to be used only in a phantom.

Calibration velocity. The velocity of sound assumed during the setting up of an ultrasound scanner. Usually 1540 m/s, but some calipers are set for 1600 m/s. Also called caliper velocity.

Californium. Element symbol Cf, atomic number 98, atomic weight ~251.

Calipers. Two electronic cursors generated on a display that can be manipulated to coincide with echoes of interest. Indicators of distance between the cursors are calibrated so that they can be used to measure the dimensions of the structure of interest.

Calix. Cup-shaped organs or cavities, for example, funnel-shaped recesses of the kidney pelvis. The name derives form the sacramental calix where wine is consecrated during mass.

Call. A transfer from one part of a computer program to another with the ability to return to the original program at the point of the cell.

Callus. The thickening or overgrowth of the skin caused by chronic friction or irritation. The hard bone-like substance produced at the fracture line early in the healing phase of a fracture.

Calorie. A unit of quantity of heat. When the term is used to describe the human body, it defines the heat produced by the metabolism or burning of energy sources, carbohydrates, fats, and proteins in food or body tissues. The quantity of heat required to raise the temperature of 1 g of water 1°C. The SI unit for quantity of heat is the joule (J).

Calorimeter. A device that measures temperature rise due to energy absorbed in a liquid.

Calutron. An American term for an electromagnetic separator used for the separation of isotopes on a production basis.

Calvarium. The upper half of the skull.

Can. A sealed container enclosing nuclear fuel or other material to provide protection from a chemically reactive environment, to provide containment of radioactive products produced during the irradiation of the composite, or to provide structural support.

Canal. A water-filled channel leading to or serving as a fuel-cooling installation into which radioactive objects are discharged from a reactor.

Canaliculus. Small canal or channel.

Cancellous. Having a reticular, porous, or spongy structure description used mainly with reference to bone tissue.

Cancer. A cellular tumor or malignant neoplasm whose natural course is usually fatal. Cancer cells, unlike benign tumor cells, exhibit the properties of invasiveness and spread to other organs. There are two broad categories termed: carcinoma — meaning a malignant new growth of epithelial cells that infiltrate surrounding tissues, and sarcoma — referring to a tumor made up of embryonic connective tissue. For further definition these suffixes are preceded by the name of the tissue or organ they are associated with; i.e., adeno — carcinoma of a gland; melanotic — carcinoma (abbreviated melanoma) of the melanin pigment-producing cells; lympho — sarcoma of the lymphatic glands; osteo — sarcoma of the bone; fibro — sarcoma of the fibroblasts which are collagen-producing cells.

Candela. (cd) Is the luminous intensity, in a given direction, of a source that emits monochromatic radiation of frequency 540×10^{12} Hz and that has a radiant intensity in that direction of 1/683 W/sr.

Canning. In a heterogeneous reactor the fuel is canned separately from the coolant and moderator by means of a can. The can serves to prevent contamination of the coolant by gaseous fission products, and reaction between the coolant and the fuel; the can itself must not react with either fuel or coolant, i.e., it must be compatible; it may be used as a load-bearing member or as a plastic imperious container; it may be only in physical contact with the fuel or metallurgically bonded to it.

Cannula. A hollow tube which is inserted into a body passage or cavity and used to withdraw or introduce fluids. Also used to remove tissue core samples.

Canthi. The parts of the eye which form the outer and inner angles of the eyelids.

Capacitance. Ratio of the charge on a condenser to the voltage across the plates: $C = Q/e$ where C is the capacitance in farads, Q is the charge in coulombs, and E is the voltage.

Capacitor. Capacitor is an electrical device for storing electrical charge. Capacitance of the capacitor indicates the amount of charge stored in it when its potential is raised by 1 V.

Capillary. The smallest vessel of the vascular system that connects arterioles with venules, forming a network in almost all parts of the body for the exchange of nutrients and gases between blood and other tissue.

Capillary bed. The combined mass of capillaries within the body.

Capillary blockade. Blockage of a fraction of a capillary bed by metabolizable particles injected downstream towards the capillary bed, for diagnostic or therapeutic purposes. Lung scanning is accomplished by intravenously injecting macroaggregates, which are trapped in the pulmonary capillary bed and, thus, lung perfusion is visualized. Starch microspheres can be used to block the capillaries of a segment of a diseased organ, to enhance or retain within that segment a therapeutic agent.

Capping. The movement of cell surface antigens toward one pole of a cell after the antigens are cross-linked by specific antibody.

Capsula. A sheath or continuous enclosure around an organ or structure.

Capture. A process involving a collision between a particle and a nucleus resulting in the retention of the particle within the nucleus and the emission of electromagnetic radiation called capture γ-rays.

Capture cross section. The probability that a nucleus will capture an incident particle. The unit of cross section is commonly the barn (10^{-24} cm^2).

Capture efficiency. (Trapping efficiency) The fraction of injected particles actually captured into orbit in a circular particle accelerator.

Capture gamma radiation. The gamma radiation emitted in radiative capture.

Carbohydrate. Substances containing only the elements carbon, hydrogen, and oxygen, arranged to form compounds called sugars, which in turn may be joined together in various combinations. Simple carbohydrates; substances containing only one or two sugar molecules (e.g., table sugar or honey). Complex hydrates; substances composed of many sugars linked together (e.g., starches and grains).

Carbon. Element symbol C, atomic number 6, atomic weight 12.011.

Carbon cycle. A theory proposed by H. Bethe has been advanced to explain the heat of the sun by a cycle of thermonuclear reactions involving carbon, hydrogen, nitrogen, and oxygen, and leading ultimately to the production of helium. This cycle is often referred to as the carbon cycle and is now adequately confirmed by laboratory experiments.

Carbon dioxide. Gas formed by tissue respiration; constitutes about 0. 5% by volume of the atmosphere. Essential for stimulation of the respiratory centers. A relatively inert gas which is often used to extinguish fires. It is used as coolant in nuclear power stations.

Carbonic acid anhydrase. An enzyme that catalyzes reversibly the conversion of CO_2 and H_2O to carbonic acid.

Carbon monoxide. Metabolic poison that combines firmly with hemoglobin, preventing hemoglobin from picking up oxygen and transporting it to the tissues.

Carbon-11. A 20-min half-life positron-emitting radioactive carbon; used with CO or CO_2 to derive cardiopulmonary information and in other applications requiring carbon-labeled imaging agents.

Carbon-14. This important long-lived isotope of carbon (5730-year half-life) decays by the emission of soft beta particles. It is produced by the reaction ^{14}N (n,p) ^{14}C which, unlike most (n,p) reactions, takes place with thermal neutrons. ^{14}C is proving very useful in studies on the reaction mechanisms or organic compounds, and particularly in biochemical studies, For these purposes a large number of ^{14}C compounds have been synthesized. By using ^{14}C as a tracer it is possible to follow radiometrically the course taken by carbon compounds in complex reactions; this technique has been applied in particular in the elucidation of the processes which occur in the photosynthesis of carbon compounds by plants etc. Small amounts of ^{14}C are formed naturally as a secondary effect of the cosmic radiation. Measurement of this natural activity in carbonaceous remains can be used for the dating of such materials.

Carboxyhemoglobin. A stable compound of carbon and hemoglobin, the latter possessing 300 times greater affinity for carbon monoxide than for oxygen. Its formation in the blood reduces the amount of oxygen that can be carried.

Carboxylic acids. Organic molecules with the

$$O = C\text{–}OH$$

functional group, which have acidic properties because of this functional group.

Carcinoembryonic antigen. (CEA) An antigen that is present on fetal endodermal tissue and is reexpressed on the surface of neoplastic cells, particularly in carcinoma of the colon.

Carcinogen. Any cancer-producing substance; often referring to chemicals that cause changes in cell properties. Substance stimulating the formation of cancer.

Carcinoma. A malignant new growth of cells from the epithelial layer (lining of organs, vessels, cavities) that tends to invade surrounding tissues and gives rise to metastases; organ name precedes to indicate type.

Cardiac. Pertaining to the heart.

Cardiac arrest. Standstill of normal heartbeat.

Cardiac cycle. Period from the end of one heart contraction (systole) and relaxation (diastole) to the end of the next systole and diastole.

Cardiac output. Cardiac output is the volume of blood ejected from the left ventricle into the systemic circulation or from the right ventricle into the pulmonary circulation. It is conventionally measured in liters per minute, while in physiological studies the concept of cardiac index is employed. This permits a comparison of output measurements in individuals of different body weight and is defined as

$$\text{cardiac index} = \frac{\text{cardiac output}}{\text{body surface area (m}^2)}$$

the volume of blood ejected per heartbeat and

$$\text{stroke index} = \frac{\text{stroke volume}}{\text{body surface area (m}^2)}$$

Cardiac transverse diameter. A measurement made frequently in radiography, defined as

$$\frac{\text{maximum cardiac width}}{\text{transverse thoracic diameter}} \times 100\%$$

Its value should be less than 50%, except in young children.

Cardiogenic shock. Acute peripheral circulation failure due to severely diminished cardiac output.

Cardiology. The study of the heart, its action, and disease.

Cardiomegaly. Hypertrophy, or enlargement, of the heart, usually due to disease that increases the cardiac workload.

Cardiomyopathy. A term which usually refers to a disease of the heart muscle or myocardium.

Cardiotachometry. The technique of counting the total number of heartbeats of an active sub-ject over a long period of time.

Cardiovascular. Referring to the heart and blood vessels that carry blood to the tissues (arteries) and from the tissues back to the heart. (veins).

Cardiovascular efficiency. The adaptive response of the heart to exercise. It is related to the efficiency of oxygen taken into the lungs and into the bloodstream and the ability of the heart to pump oxygenated blood to muscles for energy production and activity.

Cardiovascular fitness. The capacity of the body to perform aerobic muscular exercise. Its level is defined by VO_2Max, the amount of oxygen consumed by the body at peak exercise. Cardiovascular fitness can be improved by the regular performance of aerobic exercise.

Cardioversion. The process of converting the heart rhythm from an abnormal rhythm to normal sinus rhythm, also called defibrillation.

Carditis. Inflammation of the heart, especially the endocardium, myocardium, or pericardium.

Card reader. Advice that reads information from holes in punched cards and loads it into the computer's memory.

Carina. A projection of the lowest tracheal cartilage, forming a prominent semilunar ridge running anteriorly-posteriorly between the orifices of the two bronchi.

Carotid arteries. The arteries originating at the innominate artery (right carotid) and the aortic arch (left carotid), respectively, each dividing at approximately the middle of the neck into two branches — the internal and external carotid arteries which provide blood flow to the tissues of the head.

Carrier. A substance in ponderable amount which when associated with a trace of another substance will carry the trace with it through a chemical or physical process, especially a precipitation process. If the added substance is a different element from the trace, the carrier is called a nonisotopic carrier. A transmission signal upon which other signals can be piggybacked (modulated) for transmission. A carrier signal is a continuous signal transmitted over some medium at a particular frequency that is capable of being amplitude or frequency modulated to carry other signals containing data or information. An immunogenic substance that, when coupled to a hapten, renders the hapten immunogenic. An individual who harbors and sheds pathogens but who lacks overt symptoms of disease.

Carrier free. A preparation of a radioisotope to which no carrier has been added, and for which precautions have been taken to minimize contamination with other isotopes. Material of high specific activity is often loosely referred to as "carrier free", but more correctly this should be termed material of high isotopic abundance. In the strict sense the term means that all atoms of a given element present in a product are radioactive.

Carrier proteins. Macroscopic amounts of nonlabeled proteins present with trace amounts of radiolabeled proteins.

Carrier tone. An audio signal generated by a modem. The modem transmits data by modulating the tone, much as a radio station transmits sound by modulating a radio signal.

Carr-Purcell-Meiboom-Gill sequence. A modification of the Carr-Purcell sequence designed to correct any inaccuracies in the setting of the 180° pulses. This method gives the most accurate T_2 value.

Carr-Purcell sequence. Sequence of 90° and 180° radiofrequency RF pulses used to measure T_2. This approach tends to reduce errors from molecular diffusion which are more apparent in simpler spin-echo experiments. (NMR.)

Carry. When the total of two numbers exceeds register space, the computer indicates this condition, or forwards the results for further processing.

Cartilage. Fibrous connective tissue; infiltration with calcium minerals leads to bone development.

Cartridge. A fuel element cartridge consists of a rod of atomic fuel hermetically sealed into a suitable metal container. The container, referred to as a can, serves to protect the fuel from attack by the coolant etc., and to retain the volatile fission products.

Cascade. An arrangement of isotope separation stages such that the small change in isotopic abundance effected by a single stage is multiplied to give the desired change in abundance. In a simple cascade the enriched fraction is fed to the succeeding stage and the impoverished fraction to the preceding stage. An ideal cascade is one in which the turnover of each stage is so chosen that the total turnover of all the stages required to produce a specified output of specified abundance is a minimum. This means that as the abundance increases the total flow of material containing the product diminishes, so that the ideal cascade is large at the feed point and tapers off towards the product end. A square cascade is one in which the turnover is the same in each stage. This is uneconomic on a large scale because of the large holdup of

desired isotope and as a consequence of this its long equilibrium time. A squared-off cascade is an approximation of an ideal cascade and comprises sections in each of which all the stages have the same turnover. The successive transition of electrons to orbits of lower energy states, resulting in a possible spectrum of x radiation. The successive γ-ray emission in nuclear radiation.

Cascade generator. A design of high voltage supply in which transformers are connected in series in such a way that the full output voltage is not across any one winding.

Cascade shower. By a sequence of bremsstrahlung and pair production interactions, a high energy electron, positron, or γ-ray can give rise to a large number (shower) of less energetic electrons, positrons, and γ-rays.

Cassette cart. A movable storage device designed to collect data generated for processing by a device like an electrocardiogram. At a later stage the data can be transmitted to a computer for processing. In this example the information from the EKG is stored on a cassette tape. Synonym: data acquisition trolley.

Cask. A shielded container used to store or transport radioactive material,

Catabolism. Destructive phase of metabolism in which complex compounds are broken down by the cells of the body often with the liberation of energy; the opposite of anabolism.

Catalyst. A substance which affects the speed at which a chemical reaction occurs without affecting the end point of the reaction and without being changed itself by the reaction.

Catastrophe theory. A mathematical theory which deals with systems which do not exhibit "smooth" behavior, but which are subject to sudden discontinuities (catastrophes).

Catecholamine. One of a group of compounds that produces effects similar to those of the sympathetic nervous system. Epinephrine (adrenaline), norepinephrine, and dopamine are examples.

Catheter. A rubber or plastic tube. The two most commonly used types are the hollow catheter and the electrode catheter. The hollow catheter has at least one lumen connecting a hole at or near the tip of the catheter to an external port through which fluid samples may be withdrawn, pressures may be measured, and fluids (drugs, radiopaque, radiopharmaceuticals) may be injected, or to keep a passage open. The electrode catheter usually has no lumen, and has one or more platinum electrodes on its surface near to the tip, through which the heart's electrical activity may be recorded and electrical stimuli transmitted.

Cathode. A negative electrode; the electrode to which positive ions are attracted or from which electrons are emitted.

Cathode rays. Electrons emitted by the cathode of a low pressure discharge tube and accelerated by the electric field.

Cathode ray tube. (CRT) The most common form of display device used for the presentation of high-speed or text data is the cathode ray tube. The device consists of a glass envelope containing a very high vacuum in which a narrow beam of electrons is directed toward a phosphorescent screen. The electron beam is steered by electrostatic or magnetic means to cause illumination of different parts of the screen. Its value lies in the extremely high speed by which the bright spot can be steered to different parts of the screen. There are also specialized types of CRT (storage CRTs) used to retain the track of the bright spot. These are used in some imaging devices to build up the picture. Other types of "nonfade" displays utilize computer memories to store the image. Most CRTs for monitoring EKG or pressure waveforms used to have hong-persistence phosphors so that the path of the spot could be seen the whole way across the screen as a "comet's tail". These have now been largely superseded by short-persistence tubes backed up by a relatively simple computer memory to retain the whole line. Thus several cycles of a waveform are viewed clearly and this can be "frozen" for closer examination.

Cation. A positively charged ion.

Cationic proteins. Antimicrobial substances present within granules of phagocytic cells.

Caulking compounds. Sometimes used to ensure a perfect seal between a replaceable filter and its housing. The effects of radiation on such compounds may have to be considered.

Cave. A heavily shielded compartment in which highly radioactive material can be handled, e.g., by remote control.

Cavitation. An activity (which may be simple, but is often very complex) produced by sound in liquids or any medium with liquid content, involving bubbles or cavities containing gas.

Cavity wavemeter. Device for measuring microwave frequency used in electron spin resonance spectroscopy. (NMR.)

Cecum. The blind pouch at the entry to the large intestine, to which the appendix is attached.

Cell. Fundamental unit of structure and function in living organisms. A small, usually microscopic mass of protoplasm bounded externally by a semipermeable membrane, usually including one or more nuclei, capable (alone or interacting with other cells) of performing all the fundamental functions of life, and of forming the least structural aggregate of living matter capable of functioning as an independent unit. (Nuclear reactor): In a reactor which may be considered as a set of similar regions, one such region is called a cell.

Cell-bound antibodies. Antibodies that are bound to cells, irrespective of the manner of binding: comprise cytophilic antibodies and antibodies bound to antigen receptors.

Cell correction factor. A correction factor to correct for the effects of discrepancies between the true reactor cell and its idealized calculational model, applied to the calculated value of any neutron-physics characteristic which is arrived at by use of the cell approximation.

Cell division. The splitting of a parent cell into two daughter cells. The two separate processes involved are cytokinesis (division of the cytoplasm) and mitosis (division of the nucleus).

Cell-mediated immunity. Immunity in which the participation of lymphocytes and macrophages is predominant.

Cell sequestration. The process by which damaged erythrocytes are removed from the circulation by the spleen. Example: Thermally or chemically damaged radiolabeled red blood cells are used for spleen imaging.

Cellulitis. Inflammation of cellular or connective tissue. An infection of soft tissue in or close to the skin is usually localized by the body defense mechanism.

Cellulose. Carbohydrate polymer forming the skeleton of plants that is largely indigestible; provides roughage in the diet.

Center frequency. The frequency determined by $(F_1 + F_2/2)$, where F_1 and F_2 are the frequencies defined in bandwidth. Generally, the frequency at which the amplitude spectrum is a maximum.

Central-axis depth-dose function. In radiotherapy, the variation of radiation dose with depth in tissue along the central axis of a beam of ionizing radiation.

Central limit theorem. The distribution of means of random samples from a nonnormal population approaches the normal distribution as the sample size (n) becomes sufficiently large.

Central lymphoid organs. Lymphoid organs that are essential to the development of the immune response, i.e., the thymus and the bursa of Fabricius.

Central nervous system (CNS). The portion of the nervous system consisting of the brain and spinal cord.

Central processing unit (CPU). The part or parts of computer hardware that carry out data manipulation (processing or moving data) and control the sequence of operations performed by the computer that interpret and execute instructions. One important part of the CPU is the arithmetic unit, which performs arithmetics. Another part is the control unit that supervises the sequencing of operations. The internal memory contains the instructions (programs) that determine what is to be done in what sequence.

Central venous pressure (CVP). The blood pressure at the level of the inferior and superior venae cavae and the right atrium of the heart. Raised CVP is indicative of hypervolemia (high blood volume), of tricuspid valve insufficiency, or of cardiac insufficiency and failure.

Centrifugal process. A process for the separation of gaseous or liquid mixtures of isotopes making use of a centrifuge.

Centrifuge. Different constituents of body fluids or body fluids mixed with reagents can be separated on the basis of their density by artificially increasing gravity in a centrifuge. The samples are mounted in tubes on a metal disk which is rotated at high speed so that the heavier components move toward the outside of the disk. Suspensions and emulsions such as blood are used so that the various component parts are separated into layers which may be identified by eye, or by a densitometer or colorimeter.

Centriole. Small granule situated just outside the nuclear membrane in cells, which divides just before mitosis.

Centripetal force. The force required to keep a moving mass in a circular path. Centrifugal force is the name given to the reaction against centripetal force.

Centronics interface. A kind of parallel interface used by many peripherals and computers including the PC. Properly called a "Centronics-compatible interface", since it is a de facto standard first used by the Centronics Corporation. The terms "Centronics interface" and "parallel interface" are often used interchangeably, although a Centronics interface is really a specific type of parallel interface.

Cerebellum. A large, dorsally projecting part of the brain especially concerned with the coordination of muscles and the maintenance of bodily equilibrium, and of movements.

Cerebral angiography. A direct percutaneous puncture of the carotid arteries or puncture of a femoral artery and subsequent insertion of a catheter are the most common methods used to study the vascular circulation of the brain. This is usually done under local anesthesia in the radiology department and is of great assistance particularly in the evaluation of vascular abnormalities. Now superseded by digital substraction angiography.

Cerebral blood flow (CBF). Strict definition is blood flow in units of ml/min.. by convertion CBF refers to ml/min/g tissue which is more correctly called perfusion (i.e., blood flow per mass of tissue). LCBF refers to local value.

Cerebral cortex. The outer layer or gray matter of the cerebral hemispheres.

Cerebral metabolic rate for oxygen ($CMRO_2$). $LCMRO_2$ refers to local value and units are μmol/min/g (units of ml/min/g are also commonly used).

Cerebral metabolic rate of glucose (CMRGle). LCMRGlc refers to local value, and units are μmol/min/g (units of mg/min/g are also commonly used).

Cerebral radionuclide angiogram (CRAG). Rapid sequential acquisition of a radionuclide passage through the blood vessels of the brain; display and analysis of regional cerebral blood flow.

Cerebrospinal fluid (CSF). The fluid secreted by the choroid plexuses fills the brain ventricles and subarachnoid space surrounding the brain and spinal cord, to be, after circulation, reabsorbed into the large venous sinuses, through special structures, the arachnoid villi (granulations).

Cerebrum. The part of the brain, consisting of two large hemispheres divided into lobes. It contains the motor and sensory nerve centers which control voluntary actions and give the sensations of sight, hearing, taste, smell, etc.

Cerenkov counter. A particle counter in which is observed the Cerenkov light emitted when a charged particle passes through a transparent medium. Such counters are extensively used for the detection of highly energetic particles, since only for these particles is the condition for the emission of Cerenkov light satisfied. (The velocity of the particle must be greater than the velocity of light in the medium.) The relationship between the velocity of the particle and the angle emission of the light makes it possible to design a counter which indicates the velocity of the particles detected.

Cerenkov radiation. In 1934 the Russian physicist P. A. Cerenkov discovered that water, glass, and other transparent substances emitted a weak light when exposed to gamma radiation. Three years later I. Frank and I. Tamm were able to show theoretically that such light was produced when the velocity of charged particles exceeded the velocity of light in the medium. In the case of Cerenkov's experiments, the charged particles were electrons knocked on by the γ-rays. The frequency spectrum of the emitted light is continuous over the region for which the particle velocity is greater than that of light.

Cerium. Element symbol Ce, atomic number 58, atomic weight 140.115.

Cern. Abbreviation of Conseill Europeen de Recherche Nucleaire which is based at a site near Geneva where several large accelerators have been built. Renamed Organisation Europeen pour la Recherche Nucleaire.

Cervical spine. The cervical spine is the most flexible portion of the entire spinal column. As a result of this extreme degree of mobility it is extremely common to have degenerative changes in the vertebral bodies. The degenerative change is usually manifest as some degree of increased bone production ("spur formation") which may ultimately result in narrowing of the neural foramina (exit pathway for cervical nerve roots). Additionally, the cervical spine is vulnerable to injury from all manner of athletic endeavors as well as being frequently involved in motor vehicle accidents.

Cervix. Term denoting connection of two parts of a functional organ; in female mammals the cervix connects the uterus and vagina.

Cesium. Element symbol Cs, atomic number 55, atomic weight 132.905.

Cesium-137. A fission product isotope (half-life of 37 years) valuable as a γ source emitting photons of moderate energy for medical and, especially, industrial radiography.

Chaining. Storing large programs that exceed the capacity of the computer's memory by breaking them down into shorter segments.

Chain reaction. Any chemical or nuclear process in which some of the products of the process or energy released by the process are instrumental in the continuation or magnification of the process or initiating further reactions of the same type.

Chang method for attenuation post correction. This method first computes a reconstructed scintigraphic image using a conventional filtered backprojection algorithm and the assumption of no attenuation. Based on independently measured body contour, a correction

matrix is computed, each element $C(x,y)$ of which is equal to the reciprocal of the average attenuation along all rays from the pixel (x,y) to the boundary of the attenuating medium. Typically, constant linear attenuation coefficient is assumed. To obtain a first-order compensated image, the original reconstructed image is multiplied by the correction matrix.

Channel. An energy or time discriminator used in the multichannel analyzer. The resolution of the discriminator is set by the number of channels in the multichannel analyzer's acquisition group. A connection between the computer and a terminal or other external device. The computer and the terminal transmit information over the channel. In radioassay, the discriminator setting for the energy range selected for an isotope counted in a γ or liquid scintillation counter.

Channeling. (For chromatography columns) During column chromatography, channeling is a process in which liquid flows through a few pathways instead of washing the whole column.

Channels ratio. A method of quench correction in liquid scintillation counting.

Character. Any letter, digit, symbol, or punctuation mark. Characters are usually represented by a binary code composed of eight or nine bits in length; is usually referred to as a byte,

Characteristic X-ray emission. When an electron is removed from one of the inner shells of an atom, an electron from outer shell promptly moves in to fill the vacancy, and energy is released in the process. The energy released when an electron drops from an outer to an inner shell is exactly equal to the difference in binding energies between the two shells. The energy may appear as a photon or electromagnetic radiation. Electron binding energy differences have exact characteristic values for different elements; therefore, the photon emissions are called characteristic radiation or characteristic X-ray emissions.

Charge. The fissionable material or fuel placed in a reactor to produce a chain reaction. To assemble the charge in a reactor.

Charged-particle accelerators. Device used to electronically accelerate any charged particle.

Charged particle equilibrium. (CPE) The condition existing at a point within a medium under irradiation when, for every charged particle leaving a volume element surrounding the point, another charged particle of the same kind and energy enters. (Health physics.)

Charge exchange. The exchange of an electron between a neutral atom (or molecule) and an ion.

Charge holes. A hole or tube in the charge face of the shield of a reactor through which fuel elements are fed into or withdrawn from fuel channels in the moderator block.

Charge particles. Most atomic particles carry an electrostatic charge, the exceptions being the neutron, and certain mesons. The charged particles may have either positive or negative charge which is always one or more units of the charge of the electron ($e = 1.6 \times 10^{-19}$ C). The positively charged particles comprise atomic nuclei, positive electrons (positrons), and positive mesons, while the negatively charged particles are electrons, antiprotons, and negative mesons.

Chart recorder. A permanent record of measurements may be required if several variables are being monitored simultaneously or the rate of change is very rapid. A chart recorder saves the information as a graph written by a pen. The chart may show the variables on the Y-axis and time on the X-axis (Y-T recorder) on a single sheet of graph paper (as opposed to a strip of paper). The paper strip may be driven by a motor and gearbox over a roller, sometimes with a choice of speeds. The pen(s) usually move along the vertical axis and the two main types are potentiometric and galvanometric. The pens may write using ink, or using special paper responding to pressure or heat of the pen.

Checksum. The added total of all bits in a byte of data used to determine whether data have been faithfully transferred. Necessary number used in performing a parity check.

Chelate. Ligand that has two or more potential bonding sites.

Chelate compounds and chelating agents. When a metal ion combines with a group containing an electron donor, a coordination compound is formed. If the substance which combine with the metal contains two or more donor groups, or if the metal is already combined with another atom in the molecule containing the donor atom so that one or more rings are formed, the resulting structure is said to be a chelate and the attached molecule a chelating agent. Although a large number of chelating agents are known, the donor atoms are commonly restricted to nitrogen, oxygen, and sulfur.

Chemical bond. The directed attractive force between two atoms in molecule. A common type of chemical bond arises when two atoms share a pair of electrons.

Chemical equation. Symbolic statement describing a process and showing the stoichiometric relationships between the individual species involved in the process.

Chemical equilibrium. State of lowest energy for a chemical system undergoing a chemical reaction.

Chemical exchange reactions. If two compounds containing a common element, but of different isotopic composition in the two compounds, are mixed together, the system generally undergoes an exchange reaction such that the isotopic composition of the element in the two chemical forms eventually becomes almost the same.

Chemical formula. A combination of symbols with their subscripts representing the constituents of a substance and their proportions by weight.

Chemical purity. Chemical purity is the fraction of the total mass present in the stated chemical form. Chemical impurities arise from the production process. In generator-produced radionuclides, the most probable contaminant is the column material, e.g., aluminum.

Chemical radiation protector. A chemical agent that reduces the intensity of a particular radiation effect when added to chemical or biological system. The agent may be added prior to exposure, as with potassium iodide for thyroid action blocking, or after exposure, as with chelating agents for metal excretion enhancement.

Chemical shift. (δ) The change in the Larmor frequency of a given nucleus when bound in different sites in a molecule, due to the magnetic shielding effects of the electron orbitals. Chemical shifts make possible the differentiation of different molecular compounds and different sites within the molecules in high-resolution NMR spectra. The amount of the shift is proportional to magnetic field strength and is usually specified in parts per million (ppm) of the resonance frequency relative to a standard.

Chemical tracers. A radioactive form of compound is often called a tracer since it permits the subsequent identification of the compound or element by means of the activity.

Chemiluminescence. The emission of light during a chemical reaction as a result of the direct transformation of chemical energy into light.

Chemistry. Study of matter and the changes that

matter undergoes.

Chemonuclear reaction. A chemical reaction induced by nuclear radiation or fission fragments.

Chemonuclear reactor. A reactor designed as a source of radiation for effecting chemical transformations on a industrial scale.

Chemoreceptor. A nerve ending which can detect and differentiate substances according to their chemical properties; a sensory receptor sensitive to some chemical change.

Chemotaxis. Movement of an organism toward a higher chemical concentration or in response to a chemical presence. A process whereby phagocytic cells are attracted to the vicinity of invading pathogens.

Chemotherapy. Treatment of malignancies with drugs which act on the entire system of the body; consequently, these drugs are called systemic treatment.

Chest fluoroscopy. This study enables a dynamic evaluation of the cardiac structures, major vessels, and also the range of diaphragmatic motion. Localization of various chest nodules, the presence or absence of calcium in coronary arteries or cardiac valves, and the evaluation of the esophageal swallowing mechanism are several common indications for chest fluoroscopy.

Chimera. Organism which develops from combined portions of different types of tissues.

Chip. Chips are tiny circuits. Thousands of microscopic electronic components are etched on the chip's surface, forming what is known as an integrated circuit. Each component on the chip can represent a single binary digit as an on or off voltage. Because there are so many components on the chip, the chip can process thousands of pieces of information per second. For protection, chips are enclosed in ceramic or plastic packages. These packages include connectors that let the chips be plugged into circuit boards in various configurations.

Chirp z transform. An algorithm which may be used to generate the discrete Fourier transform for spectral analysis. It is commonly used to implement spectrum analysis utilizing primarily analog electronics.

Chi-square (χ^2) contingency test. A chi square test of qualitative data in which two or more sample distributions are compared with each other (contingency table). Has $(r - 1) \times (c - 1)$ df.

Chi-square (χ^2) distribution. A distribution used in tests of significance on qualitative data. It can be used to compare sample distributions or a sample distribution with a theoretical distribution. The approximate formula for χ^2 is

$$\Sigma \frac{(\text{observed number} - \text{expected number})^2}{\text{expected number}}$$

or

$$\Sigma \frac{(O - E)^2}{E}$$

Shape of the distribution depends on the number of degrees of freedom (df).

Chi-squared (χ^2) test. One of a large class of statistical significance tests for determining whether variations in a measurement are random counting errors. Sometimes termed goodness-of-fit tests, based on a single test statistic, the distribution of which is of a particular type (the χ^2 type). The test is appropriate to a series of data which are quantitative only in that the number of different categories into which they fall is known.

Chloramine-t. *N*-Chloro-4-methylbenzenesulfonamide sodium salt; an oxidizing agent used in radioiodination of proteins.

Chlorine. Element symbol Cl, atomic number 17, atomic weight 35.453.

Cholangiography. (Intravenous study) An iodine-containing contrast material which is water soluble is injected through a peripheral vein, excreted by the liver, collects in the gallbladder, and is ultimately routed into the intestinal tract for excretion. The i.v. examination is not dependent on the small bowel for absorption (cf. oral cholecystogram), but is again dependent on normal liver metabolism to concentrate and deliver the material to the gallbladder.

(Percutaneous transhepatic) A fine-gauge needle (23 gauge) is inserted under local anesthesia directly through the skin into the biliary ductal system. The primary indication for this examination is the evaluation of obstructive jaundice. The two most common causes of obstructive jaundice are malignant neoplasm or gallstone obstructing the common bile duct.

Cholecystography. (Oral gallbladder study) An organic compound containing iodine in tablet form is administered by mouth the evening prior to examination. The material is absorbed through the mucosa of the small bowel, passed through to the liver where it is excreted onto the biliary system, and concentrated in the gallbladder by the extraction of water molecules. This examination is aimed at the evaluation of the gall bladder, but is inherently dependent on normal liver function. The most common clinical indication is suspected gallstones (cholelithiasis).

Cholecystokinin. Hormone secreted by the small intestine; stimulates contraction of the gallbladder.

Cholesterol. One of the major fats or lipids contained in both food and the body's cells and fluids. Its level can be measured in the blood. High levels of cholesterol are associated with an increased risk of atherosclerosis. Precursor of the steroid hormones of the adrenal cortex, the sex hormones, and the bile acids.

Chondroblasts. Embryonic tissue cells from which cartilage develops.

Chordae tendineae. Fibrous ligaments attaching the cusps of the mitral and tricuspid valves to the papillary muscles and the ventricular walls of the heart.

Chorionic gonadotropin. A hormone secreted by the chorion and later the placenta which stimulates the release of estrogen and progesterone during pregnancy.

Choroid. The vascular coat of the eye, between the retina and the sclera, that nourishes the retina and the lens, and darkens the eye.

Choroid plexus. A vascular fold of the pia mater in the third, fourth, and lateral ventricles of the brain that secretes cerebrospinal fluid.

Chromatid. The two halves of a chromosome that has divided longitudinally at mitosis and meiosis, and which are held together at the centromere.

Chromatin. The part of a cell nucleus which is readily stainable; composed of DNA and proteins.

Chromatoelectrophoresis. Method of separating bound from free based on differential migration in an electrical field (electrophoresis) in which the support medium exhibits a higher affinity for free ligand relative to bound complex.

Chromatography. This method of chemical analysis uses a group of methods for separating a mixture of substances into their component parts. Chromatography is a misnomer for the technique since the color of the components is not really used for identifying substances in modern techniques. There are four basic types of chromatography using one phase or substrate which may be liquid or solid through which the test substance (gas or liquid) moves. A common feature of these methods is that the difference in rate of movement of the components of the test sample (plus reagents) is used to identify the separate components. In the clinical laboratory these methods are used to detect complex substances such as drugs and hormones. Examples of chromatographs are the gas-liquid chromatograph (GLC) and the thin-layer chromatograph (TLC). Both of these are being superseded by high-performance liquid chromatography (HPLC), although some compounds can only be measured by GLC.

Chromium. Element symbol Cr, atomic number 24, atomic weight 51.996.

Chromophore. A characteristic group, such as $-NO_2$ or $-N=N-$, that gives rise to color in many organic compounds. In combination with proteins, chromophores form photopigments in the retina.

Chromosome. The thread-shaped bodies in the nucleus of a cell consisting of connected strands of DNA molecules (genes); involved in the transmission of genetic information during cell division; as the cell divides, one half goes to the nucleus of each of the daughter cells. The number of chromosomes per cell varies greatly from organism to organism; man has 46.

Chromosome deletion. Loss of part of a chromosome are usually lethal to the cell in which they occur. Some mutations are probably due to small deletions.

Chronic exposure. When the radiation dose received is spread more or less uniformly over a long period of time the exposure is said to be chronic as opposed to acute exposure. Such exposure will not give rise to the usual acute effects but may, if the total exposure greatly exceeds the permissible dose, cause such long-term effects as leukemia or cancer.

Chronotron. An instrument used for the measurement of very short time intervals.

Chronotropic. Affecting time or rate, applies especially to nerves whose stimulation or agents whose administration affects the rate of heart contraction. Interventions that increase heart rate have a positive chronotropic effect, whereas those that decrease heart rate have a negative chronotropic effect.

Chylomicrons. Lipid-protein particles of very small size that pass from the epithlial cells of the small intestine into the lymphatics after a meal.

Chyme. The semifluid liquid material produced during the digestion of food.

Cilia. Fine threads found on the surfaces of many cells. Their motion causes movement of the surrounding fluid.

Cineangiography. This is an X-ray system or gamma camera producing a cine or video view of the movement of an X-ray contrast medium or a radioisotope through the cardiovascular system. Such techniques are used to investigate arterial disease and also to provide information about the function and hemodynamics of the heart and valves. Injection of the contrast medium into the coronary artery (cinecoronary arteriograms) may reveal the location and severity of plaque buildup. Injection just downstream to a heart valve gives an indication of the amount of regurgitation through the valve. Calculation may be made of ventricular volumes and ejection fraction. Cine is normally produced on high-resolution video and digital (computer-aided) image enhancement.

Cine display. Playing back a sequence of computer images in a dynamic display, much like a movie.

Cinefluorographic. (Cinefluorography) Utilization of a moving picture camera in conjunction with an image intensifier to record on motion pictures the fluoroscopic observations.

Cipher text. The result of converting "plaintext" (or English should it be the case) into text can be read by decoding, Synonym: scrambled text.

Circulating-fuel reactor. A reactor whose fuel (fluid or fluidized) circulates through the core.

Circulation. The flow or motion of a fluid in or through a given area of volume. A precise measure of the average flow of fluid along a given closed curve. Mathematically, circulation is the line integral.

$$\oint v \cdot dr$$

About the closed curve, where v is the fluid velocity and dr is a vector element of the curve. By Stokes theorem, the circulation about a plane curve is equal to the total velocity of the fluid enclosed by the curve. The given curve may be fixed in space or may be defined by moving fluid parcels.

Circumflex coronary artery. The branch of the left coronary artery that normally supplies the posterior wall and a portion of the inferior and lateral walls of the left ventricle.

Cirrhosis. Chronic, progressive disease of the liver, essentially inflammatory; characterized by proliferation of connective tissue, degeneration of parenchymal cells, and distortion of architectural pattern. The liver may be either enlarged or reduced in size.

Cistern. Fluid reservoir; enclosed space.

Cisternography. Delineation of the cerebrospinal fluid flow and spaces surrounding the brain after intrathecal instillation of a suitable radiopharmaceutical.

Cladding material. An external layer of material applied directly to nuclear fuel or other material that provides protection from a chemically reactive environment and containment of radioactive products produced during the irradiation of the composite. It may also provide structural support.

Class interval. Arbitrary unit into which raw data are grouped.

Clastic. Causing or undergoing a division into parts.

Clean. (Reactor theory) Refers to a reactor having no induced radioactivity and no poisons other than those present when it was constructed.

Cleanup. In radioassay, any preliminary treatment of test sample to remove interfering or competing substances.

Clearing field. A small electric field applied in a cloud chamber to remove unwanted ions formed by background radiation such as cosmic rays.

Clinical. Pertaining to the observed symptoms and cause of disease. The care of patients.

Clinical staging. A method for describing the extent of a primary tumor, the condition of the regional lymph nodes, and the absence or presence of distant metastases determined by history, clinical examination, radiography, scans, laboratory reports, and initial biopsy report.

Clipping time. The time-constant which characterizes the rate of decay of the output pulse from a counter amplifier.

Cloaca. A common term of fecal, urinary, or reproductive discharge.

Clock. A device within a computer system that keeps time, counts pulses, or generates regular periodic signals for synchronization.

Clonal selection theory. The theory of antibody synthesis proposed by Burnet that predicts that the individual carries a complement of clones of lymphoid cells that are capable of reacting with all possible antigenic determinants. During fetal life, clones reacted against self-antigens are eliminated on contact with antigen.

Clone. A group of cells all of which are the progeny of a single cell.

Closed cycle. Usually refers to reactor coolant circuits where the gas or liquid travels in a completely enclosed path.

Closed loop. A loop is a sequence of instructions that computers repeats until a certain condition is satisfied. When the condition is met, a computer moves on to the nest step in the program. A closed loop is a continuous loop from which there is no escape; the computer performs the sequence of steps over and until the operator intervenes.

Closed transport vehicle. A vehicle equipped with a securely attached exterior enclosure that during normal transportation restricts the access of authorized persons to the cargo space containing the radioactive materials. The enclosure may be either temporary or permanent, and in the case of the packaged materials may be of the "see-through" type, and must limit access from top, sides, and ends.

Closed water bath. A bag of polythene or other suitable material used in ultrasound examination which rests on a layer of contact gel over the area of interest and which contains water to the required depth.

Closing down. Refers to the procedure to be followed by a computer operator to ensure that the data which have been processed will be saved and not lost when the memory of the computer is cleared by switching off the electric power.

Clot. A semisolid mass of blood or lymph; coagulate of blood.

Clot retraction. Contraction or shrinkage of a blood clot resulting in the extrusion of serum.

Cloud chamber. An early type of nuclear radiation detector, by which the track of an ionizing particle may be observed and recorded photographically. Its operation depends on the formation of a supersaturated region in a gas containing a condensible vapor. The saturated vapor pressure near a drop increases with the curvature of the surface, and thus a vapor pressure which is saturated for a large drop or flat surface is below saturation for a small drop. For a given supersaturation, therefore, there exists a critical drop size below which the drop will evaporate and above which it will grow. The nuclei upon which drops will tend to form and grow include dust particles and positive and negative ions; the latter allow growth because their electrostatic charge reduces the saturation vapor pressure in their vicinity. The result is that the track of an ionizing particle appears as a line of small droplets. There are two types of cloud chamber, expansion and diffusion.

C-mode scanning. This is an ultrasonic scanning method which builds an image of a plane in the tissue which is perpendicular to the ultrasonic beam. This was originally done by time gating the returning echoes to correspond only to the chosen depth into the tissue. However, modern computerized tomography makes reconstruction of any plane of the tissue feasi-ble. C-scanning, though theoretically useful, has not gained wide acceptance in clinical ultrasound practice.

Coagulation. The transformation of a soluble protein into an insoluble protein.

Coarctation. The compression, narrowing, or stricture of the walls of a vessel, such as the aorta.

Coated tube. A form of solid-phase radioimmunoassay involving the attachment of antibody to a solid structure such as a test tube wall or plastic bead to facilitate separation.

Cobalamin (vitamin B$_{12}$). Vitamin and coenzyme essential for normal maturation of erythrocytes; contains cobalt and is the extrinsic factor that can be absorbed only in the presence of the intrinsic factor, a glycoprotein in the parietal cells of the stomach. Absence of cobalamin generally results in pernicious anemia.

Cobalt. Element symbol Co, Atomic number 27, Atomic weight 58.933.

Cobalt-60. The most important gamma source for medical and industrial radiography. The gamma radiation has similar characteristics to radium, but the cost of ^{60}Co source is but a fraction of that of radium. ^{60}Co can be produced at high specific activities and fabracated into wire, rods, or foil before activation.^{60}Co produces gamma radiation at 1.17 and 1.33 MeV which is useful in the treatment of deep-seated tumors. ^{60}Co has a half-life of 5.26 years and thus a sealed unit containing the cobalt will last for a few years. The source is fitted into a treatment head that contains massive shielding and a mechanism for exposing or closing the source by rotating it away from the collimator. The γ-ray beam is directed at the tumor to be treated via a set of collimators and moved during the treatment so that maximum radiation dose is delivered to the focal point at the center of rotation, other parts being irradiated less.It is also used as a source of penetrating ionizing radiation for industry (sterilization, γ radiography).

COBOL. *Common Business-Oriented Language;* a programming designed for business application. Its statements are close to English.

Cockcroft-Walton accelerator. Is of particular historical importance since, in 1930, it was the first to accelerate nuclear particles and so cause an artificially induced transmutation of the elements. Like the van de Graaf machine it produces a high voltage which is applied to an accelerator tube. If a voltage is applied between electrodes in an evacuated tube, and positive ions are introduced near the anodes, they will be accelerated away from the anode and will reach the cathode with an energy proportional to the voltage applied. The difficulties associated with the production of potential differences of more than 100 kV using a simple transformer-rectifier arrangement led to the introduction by Cockcroft and Walton of the voltage multiplier circuit.

Cocktail. In liquid scintillation counting, a mixture of organic solvents and fluors into which the sample is dispensed for counting. Radioactive cocktail, term applied for an oral dose of ^{131}I.

Code. A system of symbols used to represent data or instructions that are executed by a computer.

Code-operature imaging. System for obtaining series of tomographic images. A pattern of holes in a thin lead sheet (coded aperture) is used to form a source pattern on a detector. Light passed through a transparency of the image and aperture produces images in focus at different planes.

Co-deposition process. There are two main processes by which co-deposition can take place. These are by (1) co-precipitation, in which ions of the radionuclide to be carried can replace ions of the precipitate, i.e., isomorphous incorporation. This might be termed syncrystallization since the compound of the carrier element and the radionuclide, for example, barium and radium, have the same crystal forms; (2) adsorption of the radionuclide onto the surface of the precipitate.

Coding. The process of representing information in some other form. To encode data involves changing it from one form such as decimal to another form such as binary. To "decode" data means to change it back from encoded to original form. When referring to a program, "coding" refers to the action of writing the programs in a given programming language.

Codon. A sequence of three consecutive bases on messenger RNA that specifies a particular amino acid in the cellular synthesis of proteins.

Coefficient. Constant by which a variable or other quantity is multiplied in an equation.

Coefficient of determination. r^2, the square of the sample correlation coefficient. Like r, a measure of the degree of association between two variables. It indicates the proportion of variance in y associated with or explained by the variance in x. (Statistics.)

Coefficient of variation. The size of the standard deviation relative to the size of the mean (in percentage).

Coenzyme. A compound required for some particular enzymatic reaction to occur. It is loosely bound to the enzyme and usually acts as a carrier of an intermediate product of the reaction; e.g., coenzyme A.

Coffin. A large, heavily shielded box used for transporting or storing highly radioactive objects. Coffins are employed on reactor sites for storing materials, components, and so on, irradiated in the reactor, until such time as the induced radioactivity has decayed sufficiently for the items to be handled and buried.

Coherence. Maintenance of a constant-phase relationship between rotating or oscillating waves or signals of the same frequency. Loss of phase coherence of the spins results in a decrease in the NMR signal.

Coherent scattering. Scattering of photons or particles in which there are definite phase relationships between the incoming and the scattered waves. Coherence manifests itself in the inference between the waves scattered by two or more scattering centers. Examples are the Bragg scattering of X-rays and of neutrons by the regularly spaced atoms in a crystal, for which constructive interference occurs only at definite angles, called Bragg angles.

Coil. Single or multiple loops of wire (or other electrical conductor, such as tubing etc.) designed either to produce a magnetic field from current flowing through the wire, or to detect a changing magnetic field by voltage induced in the wire.

Coincidence. The occurrence of counts in two or more detectors simultaneously or within an assignable time interval: a true coincidence is one that is due to the incidence of a single particle or of several genetically related particles. An accidental, chance, or random coincidence is one that is due to the fortuitous occurrence of unrelated counts in the separate detectors. An anticoincidence is the occurrence of count in one or more other specified detectors. A delayed coincidence is the occurrence of a count in one detector at a short, but measurable, time later than a count in another detector, the two counts being due to a genetically related occurrence such as successive events in the same nucleus.

Coincidence counter. A circuit with two input terminals, or counters, which produces an output pulse only when a coincidence occurs, i.e., when each of two or more particles or photons is detected by different counters within the resolving time of the system and is therefore assumed to have its origin in the same event. A principle used in the detection of positron emitters.

Coincidence imaging. Any method or organ imaging, principally employing positron emitters, that suppresses background or possibly nonfocal counts by recording only simultaneous events.

Coincidence loss. The loss or register of events caused by their occuring within a span of time too short to be resolved by the electronic circuit. Also referred to as dead time loss, counting loss, or resolving time loss. The correction applied is termed the coincidence correction.

Cold testing. Testing of method, process, apparatus, or instrumentation with highly radioactive materials replaced by inactive materials or materials that may contain radioactive tracers.

Cold trap. A device for removing impurities from fluid systems by lowering the temperature to the point at which the impurities precipitate.

Colitis. Inflammation of the colon.

Collagen. The main fibrous protein of skin, tendon, bone, cartilage, and connective tissue; collagenase — an enzyme which breaks up collagen.

Collateral. Secondary or accessory; alternate passage.

Collateral chain. A chain of radioactive isotopes beginning with an isotope produced by a nuclear transmutation, and ending in one of the four radioactive series. For example,

$$^{242}_{96}Cm \rightarrow\ ^{238}_{94}Pu \rightarrow\ ^{234}_{92}U\ \rightarrow$$

(Uranium Series)

Collection time. The time taken for either positive or negative ions to arrive at the appropriate electrode of a pulse ionization chamber, proportional counter or Geiger counter after being formed inside the counter. These times depend upon ion mobilities, electric field strengths, and distances traveled.

Collective dose equivalent. (S) The dose equivalent to the entire exposed population. It is defined as

$$S\ =\ \sum_i H_i P_i$$

where H_i is the per capita dose equivalent in the whole body or any specified organ tissue of the P_i members of subgroup i of the exposed populations.

Collectron. A neutron detector in which an electric current is produced without the application of an external power source through the emission of β particles by a short-lived radionuclide. This radionuclide is produced by neutron activation in the part of the detector called the "emitter".

Colligative. A property of matter numerically the same for a group of substances, independent of their chemical nature.

Collimate. To restrict or define the cross section of a beam of radiation to the required dimensions.

Collimator. A collimator is a device for restricting and directing X-rays or other radiation by simply passing the rays through a tube (or set of parallel or divergent tubes), a cone, diaphragm, or grid made of metal which strongly absorbs the rays. In nuclear medicine collimators are described as a metal (usually lead) attachment to the crystal in a gamma camera. γ-Rays are directed through holes are absorbed in the metal. A crude focusing can be effected by arranging tapered holes so that only rays from a single point can reach the crystal. The effect is enhanced by having a larger number of small holes arranged in rings (e.g., 7, 19, 37, etc.) although the sensitivity may be reduced if the total surface area of hole is reduced as well. Collimation is more effective at lower energies of rays, since high-energy rays are less absorbed in the metal. Collimators are also used in radiotherapy to confine the treatment beam to the area to be irradiated. In this case they are single-hole collimators which may also form part of an applicator to define the distance from the source to the skin. In diagnostic radiology the X-ray unit is fitted with a collimator to limit the maximum field size, and diaphragms are fitted to allow the operator to select the field size and position.

Collision. Encounter between two subatomic particles (including photons) which changes the existing momentum and energy conditions. The products of the collision need not be same as the initial systems.

Collision density. In neutron transport theory, the number of collisions per cm^3/s undergone by a neutron with energy E, equal to the neutron flux divided by the scattering mean free path, is called the collision density.

Collision reactions. Any reaction produced when a neutron strikes a nucleus, including elastic scattering, inelastic scattering, radioactive capture, and fission.

Colloid. An intimate mixture of two substances, one of which, called the dispersed phase (or colloid), is uniformly distributed in a finely divided state through the second substance, called the dispersion medium (or dispersing medium), The dispersion medium may be a gas, a liquid, or a solid, and the dispersed phase may also be of these, with the exception that one does not speak of a colloidal system of one gas in another. Also called colloidal dispersion, colloidal suspension.

A system of liquid or solid particles colloidally dispersed in a gas is called an aerosol. A system of solid substance or water-insoluble liquid colloidally dispersed in liquid water is called a hydrosol. There is no sharp line of demarcation between true solutions and colloidal systems, on the one hand, or between mere suspensions and colloidal systems on the other. When the particles of the dispersed phase are smaller than about 1 nm in diameter, the system begins to assume the properties of a true solution; when the particles dispersed are much greater than 1 μm, separation of the dispersed phase from the dispersing medium becomes so rapid that the system is best regarded as a suspension. Colloids such ^{99m}Tc-tin colloid are phagocyted by the reticuloendothelial system when given intravenously, allowing liver, spleen, and bone marrow imaging.

Colon. Part of the large intestine between the cecum and the rectum.

Color flow imaging Doppler. In color flow imaging, the blood flow is superimposed on a two-dimensional image and displayed in real time. Flow towards the transducer is depicted as shades of red and flow away as shades of blue.Turbulent flow is depicted by the addition of green giving a mosaic pattern. This relatively new technique shows great promise as a means for assessing regurgitant valvular lesions and demonstrating shunt flow in congenital heart disease.

Colorimetry. Measurement of color.

Colposcope. An instrument used for examination of the vagina and cervix of the uterus.

Colposcopy. Examination of the vagina and cervix by means of the colposcope.

Colpostat. An appliance for retaining something, such as a radium applicator in the vagina.

Columnar recombination. The random recombination of positive and negative ions in the path of an ionizing particle through a gas.

Column generator. Column device of a generator using a parent radionuclide absorbed to a medium on the column; the daughter radionuclide is usually obtained by elution of the column with a solution that washes the daughter but not the parent off the column.

Coma. A state of unconsciousness from which the individual cannot be aroused by external stimuli.

Combination. A selection of terms (objects) arranged in any order.

Command. A keystroke or a line of input that enters to make an operating system or application program work. A word processing program would accept commands that did things like delete a word, insert a block of text, or start a new page.

Committed dose equivalent. The dose equivalent in a given organ or tissue that will be accumulated over 50 years (representing a working life), following a single intake of radioactive material.

Common-mode failure. Multiple failures attributable to a common cause.

Compartmental localization. The distribution of an injected radiopharmaceutical in a specific body space or compartment. Example: Labeled human serum albumin remains in the intravascular compartment for a sufficient time to allow blood pool imaging.

Compensation. Equalizing received ultrasound reflection amplitude difference due to reflector depth.

Competitive binding. The underlying principle of radioimmunoassay (RIA), namely, the competition between labeled (tracer) and unlabeled test substance molecules for binding sites on test reagent molecules during a reversible reaction.

Competitive binding assay. An *in vitro* test procedure using the principles of competitive binding, commonly employing but not limited to the use of radioactive isotopes as a tracer, antigen as ligand, and antibody as binding agent.

Competitive protein binding assay. A competitive binding assay that uses for binding agent some protein other than antibody, commonly a serum or plasma protein. A synonym for saturation analysis.

Compile. To produce a binary-code program from a program written in source (symbolic) language, by selection of appropriate subroutines from a subroutine library, as directed by the instructions or other symbols of the source program; the linkage is supplied for combining the subroutines into a workable program, and the subroutines and linkage are translated into binary code.

Compiler. A master program which translates a user's program, written in a high-level language such as FORTRAN, into a low-level language or into machine language object code.

Complement. A system of serum proteins that is the primary humoral mediator of antigen-antibody reactions.

Complementary metal oxide semiconductor. (CMOS) An integrated circuit widely used in computers because of its low power consumption.

Complement fixation. A standard serologic assay used for the detection of an antigen-antibody reaction in which complement is fixed as a result of the formation of an immune complex. The subsequent failure of lysis of sensitized red blood cells by complement that has been fixed indicates the degree of antigen-antibody reaction.

Complex. A compound of two or more parts, in which the constituents are more intimately associated than in a simple mixture.

Complex constants. Two real physical constants which it is convenient to unite together as a single complex number for mathematical analysis; for example, the complex index of refraction, of which the "imaginary" part is proportional to the coefficient of absorption.

Complex decay schemes. Many radionuclides have complex decay schemes. These may be due to the emitted particle having several possible maximum enerties, leading to different energy levels in the daughter nucleus and to a number of gamma radiations of different energies. For example, ^{132}I has 6 different beta energies and 11 gamma energies with abundance of 4% or more. A combination of electron capture and positron emission is quite common, for example, in ^{58}Co where 85% of transitions are by way of electron capture and 15% by positron emission.

Complex ion. The charged product of the association of two or more simple ions, or an ion and one or more neutral molecules. The ability to form complex ions increases with increasing charge and decreasing hydrated radius of the components.

Compliance. Term used to describe the passive or diastolic stiffness properties of the left ventricle. A hypertrophied or fibrosed heart with a stiff wall, for example, has decreased compliance; the expansibility of the lungs and/or thorax expressed as the volume change per unit pressure change.

Composite video. The standard form of a television signal containing both image brightness and synchronization information.

Composite video interface. A kind of interface used between a computer and monitor that combines all of the image and color information in a single signal.

Compound. Distinct substance formed by a union of two or more elements in definite proportions by weight.

Compounding. To form by combining parts, to form a whole, to put together. A pharmacy term describing the making of a drug or radiopharmaceutical.

Compound nucleus. A term, introduced by N. Bohr in 1936, describing a nucleus which has absorbed a nuclear particle. Bohr described nuclear reaction as a two-stage process: A + a → C → B + b. In the first stage, the target nucleus A absorbs an incident particle a to form the compound nucleus C. In the second stage, C disintegrates in one of a number of alternative ways to form a residual nucleus B with the emission of a particle b.

Compound scanning. Ultrasonic B-scanners may provide simple or compound scanning. A simple scan provides an image which is made up of a series of parallel or diverging scan lines such that each point in the tissue is interrogated from a single direction. Most real-time scanners produce these simple scans. This has a theoretical disadvantage in that a reflecting surface which is oblique to the ultrasound beam produces an echo which is reflected away from the receiving transducer such that some reflecting surfaces may not appear on the scan image. Compound scanners produce linear (parallel line) and sector (divergent) scans during the scanning process which are overlaid on the resulting image so that echoes are received irrespective of the orientation of the surfaces being represented. Hand-operated static B-scanners produce a compound scan, which is why they are sometimes preferred to real-time scanners.

Compression. Decreasing differences between small and large amplitudes.

Compton attenuation coefficient. The fractional number of photons removed from a beam of radiation per unit thickness of a material through which it is passing as a result of Compton effect interactions.

Compton effect. Absorption or attenuation effect observed for X- and γ- radiation in which the incident photon interacts with an orbital electron on the absorber atom to produce a recoil electron and a photon of energy less than the incident photon. When γ-rays fall on an organic crystal scintillation spectrometer, they generally interact in this manner and the pulse height spectrum observed for a monoenergetic γ-ray line corresponds to the energy distribution of the Compton electron. This is generally called the Compton spectrum of the γ-rays.

Compton recoil particle. The accelerated electron resulting from the process of Compton scattering. Also known as Compton electron or recoil electron.

Compton scattering coefficient. That fractional decrease in the energy of a beam of X- or γ-radiation in an absorber due to the energy carried off by scattered photons in the Compton effect.

Compton shift. The Compton shift is the difference between the wavelengths of the scattered and incident photons in the Compton effect.

Compton wavelength. For the electron the compton wavelength λ_o is defined as $\lambda_o = h/m_ec = 2.43 \times 10^{-10}$ cm.

Computed tomography. Use of a computer and data processing from X-rays, radionuclides, or nuclear magnetic resonance to produce body section images. These calculated images represent the following: X-ray (CT): tissue densities from absorption coefficients when X-rays are transmitted; radionuclide emission computed tomography (ECT): origin of emitted photons when radionuclides are administered and photons emitted; nuclear magnetic resonance (NMR): tissue T_1 and T_2 values, as well as quantities of magnetically polar nuclei such as hydrogen, which emit a characteristic resonant frequency in a uniform, graded magnetic field when excited by radiofrequency.

Computer. A data processing system or device able to accept and manipulate data in a prescribed and meaningful way. It consists, in most cases, of input and output devices, storage devices, and arithmetic and control unit. The main types of computer may be classified as follows:

Mainframe computers.—These are large digital computers usually remote from the sites of input and output. They usually handle many jobs simultaneously, often in different languages. They are used for financial information (salaries, sales and purchase ledgers, budgets) and for personnel and patient records.

Minicomputers.— Usually these are in a single cabinet at the site of use. Typical applications are calculating and presenting the results of dynamic isotope studies in the nuclear medicine department and for controlling process control apparatus such as the energy usage in a large hospital. Minicomputers often do the jobs which used to be performed on mainframe machines, but the smaller jobs are now commonly performed on microcomputers.

Microcomputers.— The central processor (arithmetic and logic unit) on these machines is contained on a single integrated circuit (microprocessor chip), and the whole computer (including memories, peripheral interface units, and disk controllers) may be contained on a single printed circuit board. Some of these are extremely powerful and fast computers, while their low cost permits them to be used on a single and often relatively trivial application such as converting the results of a single machine into a more useful form. They have an increasingly important application in the handling of text information (word processors) and at the other end of the scale may be used within medical equipment to control the operation of the equipment and manage the display of results.

Calculators.— It is not easy to draw a distinction between an electronic calculator and a microcomputer, but, in general, a calculator is not fully programmable in that the range of functions is limited by the internal program and design, whereas a microcomputer is normally taken to mean a device which can be programmed to a variety of tasks and usually can deal with different computer languages if these are fed into it by an external device (keyboard, tape cassette, or disk drive).

Analog computer.— High-speed mathematical computation can be performed without converting the signals into digital code. Instead, the mathematical functions (e.g., addition, subtraction, multiplication, differentiation, and integration) are performed by a series of operational amplifiers.

Computer-aided design/computer-aided manufacturing. (CAD/CAM) The technique of employing computers to assist in the design of electronic circuits, ,mechanical systems, and manufacture of a wide range of items.

Computer-aided instruction. (CAI) The use of a computer system in education. In medical training, computers have been used to provide multiple-choice quizzes or even to simulate patients or physiological systems. The computer engages in a dialogue with the student, informs him of mistakes, goes over new material, or conducts a review, depending on his responses.

Computer-generated holograms. A hologram made synthetically and based on computer calculations of amplitude and/or phase.

Computer graphics. Pictures created by a computer on a video display screen, printer, or other output device. Today computers are capable of producing very sophisticated graphics including movies, color illustrations, and three-dimensional drawings.

Computerized axial tomography. (CAT or CT) A radiographic technique in which X-ray images representing slices through a patient are reconstructed by means of computer programs. This produces an image on a cathode ray tube (CRT) screen of a section through the body, with each point on the image having a brightness corresponding to the X-ray absorption properties of the point represented. The scanner comprises one or more X-ray sources collimated to produce very thin X-ray beams which pass through the patient to a scintillation detector. The overall attenuation of the X-ray beam as it passes through the body is calculated from the intensity reaching the detector. Similar attenuation measurements are made thousands of times as the position and direction of the X-ray beam are changed. A computer with suitable programs calculates the attenuation occurring at each point within the section being scanned, which would be necessary to account for the measured overall attenuations. A variety of different scanning methods and arrangements of single or multiple heads and/or detectors are in use. Earlier systems used a complex movement called rotate-translate in order to economize on the number of detectors needed, but they have been mainly superceded because of their slower scan times and patient throughput.

Computer languages. Rather than operating in tedious machine language (the binary code of "0" and "1"), a programmer can talk to the computer in assembly language (symbolic names) or high-level language (which is close to English).

Computer-limited spectral resolution. It is the spectral width divided by the number of data points.

Computer output microfilm. (COM) A device for producing photographic film output directly from a computer. Such devices are very high speed, often using an electron beam on a cathode ray tube to produce light patterns that can be recorded on film.

Computer program. A series of coded instructions for solving a problem by means of a computer.

Computer system. This always refers to the entire hardware package and would most properly include all software as well. The emphasis here is on a working system.

Concatenation. The joining of two or more strings of characters to produce a single string.

Concentration. The amount of a substance in weight or moles present in unit volume of a solution. Strength of substance in a solution.

Concentration gradient. The continuous variation in concentration of a dissolved substance, such as potassium, along some dimension of a confined solution; used to describe the difference in concentration of positive potassium and sodium ions across the myocardial cell membrane.

Concentrations of radioactivity. Amount of radioactivity per volume unit, e.g., 1 MBq/ml.

Concomitant immunity. The ability of a tumor-bearing animal to reject a test inoculum of its tumor at a site different from the primary site of tumor growth.

Concurrent centrifuge. The centrifuge is often employed for the separation of both liquid and gaseous mixtures of isotopes. In the concurrent centrifuge one or more streams of gas enter at one end, the partially separated isotopes are removed in two or more streams at the other end.

Condenser ionization chamber. An ionization chamber which, having been charged to a certain potential, can be irradiated and subsequently attached to an electrometer to measure the residual charge, whereby the dose received is ascertained.

Condenser R-meter. An instrument consisting of an "air-wall" ionization chamber together with auxiliary equipment for charging and measuring its voltage; it is used as an integrating instrument for measuring the quantity of X or γ radiation in roentgen or c/kg.

Conditional probability. Probability of event "b" given that "a" occurred.

Conditioned reflex. Reflex response to a stimulus that has replaced the physiological stimulus.

Conductance. Reciprocal of the nonelastic resistance.

Conductivity. The ability to transmit impulses to other areas. Both the cells of the conduction system and the myocardial muscle fibers have this property.

Conductors. A class of bodies which are incapable of supporting electric strain. A charge given to a conductor spread to all parts of the body

Condyle. A rounded protuberance at the end of bone, forming an articulation.

Cone of radiation. (Treatment cone) In the medical use of γ-rays and X-ray beam is frequently restricted to a narrow cone by the use of diaphragms in in order to avoid unnecessary exposure of those parts of the patient's body which are not being treated or radiographed.

Confidence interval estimation. Determination of the interval within which a true value (population parameter) lies with a stated degree of confidence (e.g., 95 or 99 out of 100 times).

Confidence limits. In statistics, the two limits within which a given parameter or characteristic has a specified probability of being found.

Confinement system. A barrier and its associated systems, including ventilation, that are placed around an area containing radioactive materials to prevent the uncontrolled release of those materials.

Confinement time. Average lifetime of a particle in a plasma confinement system.

Conformation. It is the three-dimensional structure of a molecule. The angles of rotation about the different chemical bonds with molecules make up the conformation of the molecule. More than one conformation of the molecule can be allowed.

Conformational change. This is the change of the conformation of a molecule. This conformational change can be either gross or small. An example of a gross change is the unfolding of a protein or uncoiling of a DNA molecule, etc. Small changes in the conformation of big molecules can occur in the binding of a ligand, such as the binding of a substrate to an enzyme.

Congenic. (Originally called congenic resistant) Denotes a line of mice identical or nearly identical with other inbred strains except for the substitution at one histocompatibility locus of a foreign allele introduced by appropriate crosses with a second inbred strain.

Congenital. A condition present at birth, not necessarily inheritable.

Conjugate acid. Remainder of a basic compound after it has either accepted a proton or donated an electron pair in a chemical process.

Conjugate base. Remainder of an acidic compound after it has either donated its acidic proton or accepted an electron pair in a chemical process.

Conjunctiva. The thin, delicate membrane that lines the eyelids and is reflected over the front of the eyeball.

Conservation of energy. The principle that the total energy of an isolated system remains constant if no interconversion of mass and energy takes place. The principle takes into account all forms of energy in the system; it therefore provides a constraint on the conversions from one form to another. The law of

conservation of energy states that energy can neither be created nor destroyed and therefore the total amount of energy in the universe remains constant.

Conservation of mass. In all ordinary chemical changes, the total of the reactants is always equal to the total mass of the products.

Conservation of mass-energy. Energy and mass are interchangeable, as evidenced by the equation $E = mc^2$, where E is energy, m is mass, and c is velocity of light.

Conservation of momentum. For any collision, the vector sum of the momenta of the colliding bodies after collision equals the vector sum of their momenta before collision. If two bodies of masses m_1 and m_2 have, before impact velocities v_1 and v_2 and after impact velocities u_1 and u_2

$$m_1u_1 + m_2u_2 = m_1v_1 + m_2v_2$$

Console. A portion of a computer that is used for communication between operators and the computer, usually by means of displays, manual controls, and instruction execution commands.

Conspicuity. The ability of a structure to stand out from its surroundings. In digital radiology bones and other anatomy are removed so that the opacified vessels can be more conspicuous.

Constitutive property. A property which depends on the constitution or structure of the molecule.

Contact medium. A substance such as oil or gel that is placed on the skin to minimize the amount of air between the transducer and the skin and thereby achieve good acoustic coupling.

Contact radiation therapy. X-ray therapy with specially constructed tubes in which the target-skin distance is very short (less than 2 cm). The voltage is usually between 40 and 60 kV.

Contact scan. A scan produced by moving the ultrasound transducer over the skin surface.

Contact sensitivity. A type of delayed hypersensitivity reaction in which sensitivity to simple chemical compounds is manifested by skin reactivity.

Containment. May be defined as the physical features of facilities for preventing the accidental escape of the fission products formed during reactor operation, or authorized channels limiting the access to nuclear materials.

Containment system. Means the components of the packaging intended to retain the radioactive contents during transportation.

Contamination. Accidental spread of unwanted radioactivity to an area where it does not belong.

Contamination monitor. An instrument used to detect radioactive contamination of laboratory working surfaces. A probe unit containing a counter is connected by a flexible cable to the main control unit. For beta and gamma radioactivities a thin-walled Geiger counter is commonly used (with a shutter to enable the two activities to be distinguished), while a scintillation counter employing a zinc sulfide-coated screen as a phosphor is used for alpha particles.

Continence. Ability to refrain; incontinence: inability to refrain from desire or urging, inability to control the release of urine.

Contingency table. A classification of qualitative data into r rows and c columns (to which a chi-square test of association can be applied).

Continuous acquisition. A mode of acquisition in single photon emission computerized tomography (SPECT), where the motion of the rotating gantry is continuous. The data are acquired continuously during the entire rotation without interruption. The data acquisition is very similar to that of a dynamic study where the data are also acquired continuously. In a SPECT acquisition all the data acquired during predefined angular intervals (defined by angular step parameter) are stored in consecutive frames. For example, if the angular step is set to 6°, all the counts collected between 0 and 6° will be stored in the first frame. Between 6 and 12°, the counts will be stored in the second frame, and so on.

Continuous data. Data representing an infinite number of possible points along a continuum.

Continuous discharge. That portion of the charge collected vs. voltage region in which, once initial ionization occurs, the ions are accelerated to such an extent that they impinge on the wall of the chamber, producing further ions, which continue the process indefinitely.

Continuous wave. A wave in which cycles repeat indefinitely, not pulsed. A technique of NMR spectroscopy that utilizes continuous radiofrequency irradiation as opposed to pulsed radiofrequency irradiation.

Continuous-wave Doppler. In this mode, two crystals function continuously: one to transmit and the other to receive signals. With this technique, high velocity flow can be measured accurately. A wave of a most constant amplitude which persists for a large number of cycles and is used for sampling Doppler shifts regardless of distance form the transducer. There is no sampling limitation or inherent limitation on peak detected velocity, as there is for range gated Doppler.

Continuous waveform. A waveform in which the amplitude modulation factor is less than or equal to 5%.

Contractility. The ability to respond to stimulus with mechanical action. Myocardial fibers respond mechanically to electrical stimulation by contracting. Several indices help quantity contractility; ejection fraction, the velocity with which the ventricular wall contracts, and the velocity with which blood is ejected into the aorta.

Contrast. Contrast can be defined as the relative difference of the signal intensities in two adjacent regions. In a general sense, we can consider image contrast, where the strength of the image intensity in adjacent regions of the image is compared, or object contrast, where the relative values of a parameter affecting the image (such as spin density or relaxation time) in corresponding adjacent regions of the object are compared. If the two intensities are J_1 and J_2, a useful quantitative definition of contrast is $(J_1 - J_2)/(J_1 + J_2)$. Relating image contrast to object contrast is more difficult in NMR imaging than in conventional radiography, as there are more object parameters affecting the image and their relative contributions are very dependent on the particular imaging technique used. As in other kinds of imaging, image contrast in NMR will also depend on region size, as reflected through the modulation transfer function (MTF) characteristics.

Contrast echocardiography. This is an extension of the routine examination. Gaseous microbubbles are intense reflectors of ultrasound and act as an acoustic contrast agent. When , during echocardiographic examination, a bolus of a biologically compatible fluid (usually 5% dextrose) is injected into a peripheral vein, the microbubbles within the bolus are seen to opacify the right heart; they are filtered out in the pulmonary circuit and, in the absence of a right-to-left shunt, do not enter the left heart. Opacification of the left heart is thus diagnostic of a right-to-left shunt and the site of opacification indicates the level of the shunt.

Contrast enhancement. Accentuates differences between high and low count areas of an image by compressing the intensity display (gray scale) to a narrow range of information.

Contrast media. Compound used to produce density differences in tissues, organs, or vessels to permit their imaging. X-ray contrast media are largely iodinated organic molecules that are either selectively excreted by a particular organ after intravenous injection or are injected intravascularly; their high iodine content strongly absorbs X-rays and attenuates the beam.

Contrast resolution. Contrast resolution is that contrast which is detectable with a certain confidence in an image with a certain signal-to-noise ratio. Spatial resolution relates to the "size" detectability of an object, contrast resolution relates to the "amplitude" detectability of an object.

Contrast sensitivity. The ability to detect small contrast differences.

Control. The purposeful variation of the reactivity of a reactor. Absorber control is obtained by variation of the amount of neutron absorbers within the reactor. Configuration control is obtained by changing the geometry of the reactor.

Control bus. In computing, a group of connecting paths which conveys signals that control the operation of the computer.

Control character. A character entered by holding down the CTRL key and pressing a typing key. Many application programs allow to enter control characters for such functions as moving the cursor and manipulating data. Control characters generally are not used as data in text files, and they do not represent displayable characters in the ASCII character set. When they must be represented in writing, they are prefixed with a caret (^) or with the word CTRL.

Control group. A group of organisms, animals, or persons which are maintained under "normal" conditions to serve as a basis for comparison with the experimental group.

Controlled area. A specified area in which exposure of personnel to radiation or radioactive material is controlled and which is under the supervision of a person who has knowledge of the appropriate radiation protection practices, including pertinent regulations, and who has responsibility for applying them.

Controlled thermonuclear reaction. The attempt to use fusion reactions, especially of heavy hydrogen isotopes, in a controlled manner for generating power. The basic physics associated with this work is called plasma physics and temperatures of at least 20 million degrees K are necessary to enforce quickly the fusion reactions in sufficient number.

Control rod. A rod in a nuclear reactor which is used for controlling the effective neutron multi-plication constant. In a thermal reactor the rod is composed of neutron-absorbing materials, such as cadmium, boron, or hafnium. It is situated in the core or reflector of a reactor and when it is withdrawn from either of these the neutron which would have been absorbed in the rod is then preferentially captured in the fuel, and thus there is an increase in reactivity. In a fast reactor where the neutrons are not readily absorbed in most materials, fuel rods in the core or movable reflectors are used as control rods.

Control samples. Samples of known composition run to check accuracy or correct for reaction vectors.

Control system. A coordinated group of components designed to exert a directing influence on other components. (Reactor engineering) A system of apparatus for controlling the rate of reaction in a nuclear reactor. The term may refer to all apparatuses provided for this purpose or to one of several essentially independent arrangements, such as a regulating system and safety system. A reaction may be controlled automatically by a servo system that adjusts the control elements as necessary to hold the flux level close to a desired value. A reactor may have a tendency toward stability because of self-regulation, but the quality of stability ordinarily is not considered part of the control system.

Control unit. A part of the computer in the central processing unit which performs the control functions. It is responsible for decoding microprogrammed instructions and then generating the internal control signals that perform the operations required.

Convection. This usually refers to the convection of heat, which is the transfer of heat from one part of a fluid to another by flow of the fluid from the hotter to the colder parts.

Converging hole collimator. The converging hole collimator allows relatively small objects to have increased image size. This is particularly useful with large field of view (large diameter detector) gamma cameras where organs such as the heart, thyroid, testes, and brain can be visualized more easily with improved sensitivity. The field of view over the zone near the collimator decreases with increasing object distance and results in a reduction in spatial resolution.

Conversation. The interaction between user and computer processor to list a set of instructions to be carried out by the computer system.

Conversion coefficient. The probability of the

de-excitation of a given nuclear state by internal conversion, relative to that for decay by gamma emission.

Conversion electron. Orbital electron that has been excited (ionized) by internal conversion of an excited atom.

Conversion factor. A factor required for conversion of one system of units to another.

Conversion time. The time it takes for analog-to-digital converter to convert the analog signals to digital numbers.

Converter. A device placed in a flux of slow neutrons to produce fast neutrons. In isotope separation, the assembly containing the separative elements of one stage of a gaseous diffusion cascade.

Converter reactor. A nuclear reactor that converts fertile atoms into fuel by neutron capture. Two different ways of using the words converter and breeder are in use at present: a converter is a reactor that uses one kind of fuel and produces another (e.g., consumes ^{235}U and produces Pu from ^{238}U; a breeder is a converter that produces more fissionable atoms than it consumes.

Convolution. A mathematical operation used in image processing that describes a filtering process in real space.

Coolant. A substance, ordinarily fluid, used for cooling any part of a reactor in which heat is generated. Such parts include not only the core, but also the reflector, shield, and other elements that may be heated by absorption of radiation.

Cooling. In reactor and health physics this term is used to imply the reduction of radioactivity by decay of the active species. It is a very powerful method of avoiding handling and shielding problems by the simple expedient of introducing a waiting period, since on the whole the highest energy radiations, which are most difficult to shield against, are emitted by the shortest-lived isotopes.

Coombs' test. (Antiglobulin test) The direct Comb's test is an agglutination test for detecting serum components absorbed to cells; principally incomplete antibodies bound specifically to red blood cell membrane antigens.

Coordinate covalent bond. Covalent bond formed by two atoms in which one atom donates both electrons for the bond.

Coordination number. The number of atoms bound to the central atom of a coordination compound by, usually, nonionic bonds. The number of nearest neighbors to any particular atom in a crystal lattice.

Copper. Element symbol Cu (cuprum), atomic number 29, atomic weight 63. 546.

Coprecipitation. The precipitation of a trace substance along with weighable quantity of another precipitating substance.

Copy protection. The practice of making a diskette uncopyable by storing data on it in a nonstandard way. Software vendors often copy protect their distribution diskettes to prevent a purchaser from copying the diskettes and reselling the copies.

Cord. Any long, rounded, flexible, anatomical structure; umbilical cord of the fetus; spermatic cord.

Core. In a nuclear reactor, the region containing the fissionable material. The body of fuel or moderator and fuel in a nuclear reactor. It does not include the fuel outside the active section in a circulating reactor. Identical with active lattices in a reactor. In a heterogeneous reactor, the region containing fuel-bearing cells. In a computer, a special type of early digital memory consisting of arrays of ferrite rings (cores) which are magnetized to represent either a binary digit (bit) of value 0 or 1.

Core memory. Main memory storage used by the central processing unit, in which binary data are represented by the switching polarity of magnetic cores.

Core temperature. The temperature inside the body itself, usually estimated accurately by obtaining the rectal temperature. Oral or mouth temperatures are often falsely low as a measure of core temperature.

Coriolis force. The deflects, relative to the earth, a body moving with constant space velocity above the earth.

Cornea. The transparent part of the sclerotic that forms the front surface of the eye.

Coronary. Applying to structures that encircle a part or organ, in a crownlike manner, as, for example, the coronary arteries encircling the base of the heart.

Coronary angiography. Selective examination of the right and left coronary arteries supplying the heart is the most common current indication for coronary angiography.

Coronary arteries. The right and left coronary arteries, which branch off the aorta to supply the heart muscle with oxygen and nutrients.

Coronary heart disease. (CHD) An abnormal condition of the coronary arteries that impedes the adequate supply of blood to the heart tissues.

Coronary perfusion. Blood flows through the coronary arteries mainly during the diastole.

During systole the pressure developed by the ventricle produces a resistance that is too high to be overcome. Owing to the pressure existing in the heart chamber during diastole there is a pressure gradient between the subendocardial and the subepicardial parenchyma. The resultant reduced perfusion of the subendocardial tissue is physiologically compensated by an active increase of resistance in the precapillaries of the subepicardium. If there is a blood flow deficit due to coronary artery disease, however, the epicardium is prefused to the maximum degree possible, which creates a perfusion deficit in the subendocardium. In addition, the end-diastolic pressure is increased by coronary heart disease, with the result that the inequality is magnified.

Coronary spasm. This term denotes the active contraction of a coronary vessel segment which leads to inadequate perfusion and consequent pain. Spasm develops preferentially at the level of an atheromatous narrowing of the coronary lumen, but about 10% of the cases it can cause an attack also in the presence of normal coronaries.

Coronary stenosis. A narrowing of the lumen by more than 50% leads during increased cardiac work to a pressure drop distal to the stenosis, hence to a subendocardial perfusion deficit. The extent of this blood flow disturbance increases with increasing stenosis and with the length of the stenotic region. Several successive stenoses reduce the volume of blood flow also at rest. The ischemia results in a dilatation of the physiologically developed anastomoses, which are then able to offset the perfusion deficit in part.

Corpus. A discrete mass of material, corpus collosum.

Corpuscle. Small mass or body; formed elements of the blood; after cell type.

Correlation coefficient. In statistics, a measure of the tendency of two random variable having a linear relationship to vary together. Its value must lie between +1 and −1, ±1 denoting complete dependence of one characteristic of the other, and 0 denoting no association between them.

Correlation time. (τ_c) It is the characteristic "average" time between two molecular orientations for a molecule undergoing some kind of motion through interaction of a particular type, e.g., dipolar interaction correlation time, such as diffusional correlational time, rotational correlational time, etc.

Correlative. (Legal) Having a mutual or reciprocal relation, in such sense that the existence of one necessarily implies the existence of the other. (Left and right, up and down, duty and right.)

Corruption. Corruption occurs when computer information is accidentally lost, changed, or disorganized by equipment failure or an error in a program, user error, or other problem.

Cortex. The outer or superficial part of an organ or body structure; especially the outer layer of gray matter of the brain and cerebellum.

Cortical. Of, relating to, or consisting of the cortex.

Corticosterone. Compound isolated from the adrenal cortex.

Corticotropin. One of the hormones secreted by the adenophypophysis.

Cortisol. A hormone of the adrenal cortex.

Cosmic abundance. The relative abundance of the chemical elements throughout the universe. Theory seeks to account for the relative abundance of the elements in terms of nuclear properties, on the assumption that all the elements were built up from hydrogen by a succession of nuclear reactions.

Cosmic rays. High-energy particles and electromagnetic radiations which bombard the earth from outer space. The particles hitting the outer atmosphere are mostly protons, but, as a result of collisions with atmospheric nuclei, other forms of radiation are produced with a wide range of energies and penetrating power.

Cosmotron. A proton-synchrotron. The magnets of the Brookhaven machine weigh 2200 tons.

Coulomb. Unit of electrical charge in the practical system of units. A quantity of electricity equal to 3×10^9 electrostatic units of charge.

Coulomb barrier. That region surrounding the nucleus near the maximum of the potential energy for a positively charged particle. The combined effects of the long-range repulsive coulomb force and the short-range attractive nuclear force result in that maximum in the potential energy.

Coulomb excitation. The excitation of a nucleus by the electric field of a passing charged particle. The bombardment of nuclei with charged particles, of insufficient energy to penetrate the coulomb barrier, can result in the excitation of low-lying energy levels of the nuclei. Since barrier penetration is impossible, the excitation must be caused by coulomb, rather than specifically nuclear, forces.

Coulomb force. The electrostatic force of attraction or repulsion exhibited between charged particles.

Coulomb's law. Basic law of electrostatics, which states that

$$F = \frac{q_1 q_2}{4\pi\epsilon r^2} \quad \text{or} \quad F = \frac{qq'}{r^2}$$

Coulter counter. This is a trade name for a particle counter which calculates a number of characteristics of blood samples. The essential element in the device is a cell counter (hemocytometer) which causes blood cells to pass through a small aperture through which an electric current is being passed between electrodes each side of the aperture. As a cell passes through there will be a transient change in the electrical resistance, since the resistance of a blood cell will be higher than the electrolyte in which it is suspended.

Count. (Radiation measurements) The external indication of a device designed to enumerate ionizing events. It may refer to a single detected event or to the total registered in a given period of time. The term often is erroneously used to designate a disintegration ionizing event, or voltage pulse.

Counter. A detector of radiation which gives an instantaneous, discrete, electrical signal upon passage of a single-charged particle through it. Counters may be of various types, the most important being the pulse ionization chamber, proportional counter, Geiger counter, and scintillation counter.

Counterpulsation. A form of circulatory assistance by which the main pressure wave occurs in diastole rather than systole and hence is opposite to the normal arterial pulsations. An example of a device using counter pulsation is the intraaortic balloon, which consists of a sausage-shaped balloon at the end of a catheter. The device is passed through the femoral artery and lies just distal to the left subclavian artery in the descending thoracic aorta. The balloon is alternately inflated and deflated, with timing determined by the electrocardiogram. Rapid inflation occurs during diastole and produces a pressure pulse wave in the aorta that helps to propel blood distally while increasing the perfusion pressure of the coronary arteries. Rapid deflation of the balloon during systole reduces the pressure (afterload) against which the heart must pump. Reducing afterload, in turn, increases the forward stroke volume of the ventricle. Counterpulsation is an effective means of maintaining coronary blood flow, or of increasing coronary blood flow, in patients who are very hypotensive.

Counting efficiency. Counts per minute per disintegrations per minute $\times$ 100 = efficiency.

Counting error. The statistical uncertainty associated with counting a radioactive sample based upon the radiation detected in a time interval much shorter than the physical half-life of the radionulcide. The standard deviation for an N count determination equals the square root of N. (For a standard deviation of 1%, 10,000 counts must be recorded.)

Counting loss. Because of the random occurrence of nuclear events, as, for example, in radioactive decay, some events will not be recorded by a detecting system, such as a Geiger counter, due to its inherent resolving time. Any two or more events occurring within that time will only be recorded as one. The counting loss will obviously increase with counting rate.

Counting rate meter. A device which gives a continuous indication of the average rate of ionizing events.

Counting statistics. In counting radioactivity, this refers to statistical variability of counts or count rate.

Count rate. The rate at which decay events are seen by a detector. Also, the absolute rate (counts per second) of decay events for a standard source.

Coupling. The condensing or "coupling" of two molecules of diiodotyrosine (DIT) or DIT and monoiodotyrosine (MIT) to form the iodothyronines, thyroxine (T-4) and triiodothyronine (T-3).

Coupling medium. Oil or gel used to provide a good, sound path between the transducer and the skin.

Covalent bond. A type of chemical bond which involves transfer of electrons between the atoms forming the molecule.

Covalent compound. Compound held together by covalent bonds.

Covariance. For each x,y pair of data, the x deviation from the mean of all x's (i.e., $x - X$) is multiplied by the y deviation from the mean of all y's (i.e., $y - y$). These products are then summed for all pairs. Thus,

$$\frac{\Sigma(x - x)(y - y)}{n - 1}$$

$$\frac{\Sigma(x - x)^2}{n - 1} \quad \text{or} \quad \frac{\Sigma(y - y)^2}{n - 1}$$

Cow. (Popular term) A generator for short-lived isotopes based upon successively eluting or otherwise separating a short-lived radioactive daughter from a longer-lived parent. Examples: ^{99m}Tc from ^{99m}Mo or ^{113m}In from ^{113m}Sn.

Cranium. The part of the skull which encloses the brain.

Crash. A hardware crash is the failure of a particular computer device to operate; the operation of an entire computer system may be affected. A software crash is the result of an operating system malfunction; the system's protection mechanisms may have failed, or the software may not have executed correctly.

C-reactive protein. (CRP) A β-globulin found in the serum of patients with diverse inflammatory diseases.

Creatine. A compound present in muscle tissue. Creatine phosphate acts as an energy storage substance; a nitrogenous waste product.

Creatine phosphokinase. (CK) An enzyme important in phases of cellular metabolism found in many body tissues, but in highest concentrations in heart and skeletal muscle. Rapid elevation in serum levels occurs in a number of conditions, including muscle injury and infarction.

Creatinine. A substance present in urine, blood and muscle, formed from creatine. It is the end product of muscle metabolism.

Crenation. Formation of notching on edge of a cell.

Crescendo angina. This term refers to angina pectoris in which the painful attacks increase in severity within weeks to months. This may be true of the intensity and duration of the symptoms as well as of the lower level of exertion that can provoke attacks. In such a situation coronary perfusion must be assumed to become increasingly critical and the development of a myocardial infarction must be anticipated.

Crest. A projection or ridge surmounting a bone or organ; also crista.

Crevice. A longitudinal fissure.

Crime. (Legal) An offense prosecuted by the state for conduct prohibited by law or failure to comply with requirement of law. The essential feature is the existence of legislation or regulation requiring or prohibiting a specific act or conduct.

Critical. Critical or criticality are the terms used to describe the condition in which a chain reaction is being maintained at a constant rate, i.e., it is just self-sustaining.

Critical angle reflection. When a sound beam strikes a smooth acoustical interface at angles other than the perpendicular, more of the energy is reflected and less is transmitted. An angle will eventually be reached, depending upon the velocity charge across the interface, where the refracted sound travels along the interface. Beyond this critical angle, the sound is completely important when evaluating acoustic shadowing.

Critical experiment. A test or series of tests performed with an assembly of reactor materials which can be gradually brought to the critical state for the purpose of determining the nuclear characteristics of a reactor. The experiment is usually performed at very low power.

Criticality accident. The release of energy as a result of accidentally producing a self-sustaining or divergent neutron chain reaction.

Critical mass. The mass of fissionable material required to sustain a nuclear reaction.

Critical moisture content. The water content of a solid when it contains only its water crystallization. The word *critical* has here no nuclear connotation.

Critical organ. The organ or tissue that receives the largest dose of radiation in a procedure; this depends on radionuclide concentration by the organ, geometric factors, and the effective retention in that organ. Organ of interest most affected by a technique.

Critical pressure ratio. When a gas is flowing under steady-state conditions from a reservoir at high pressure through a nozzle into a region of lower pressure, there is a finite pressure difference at which the flow velocity in the throat of the nozzle becomes equal to the velocity of sound under the conditions ruling in the throat.

The ratio of the high to the low pressure is called the critical pressure ratio. If the pressure outside the reservoir is decreased further, no increase occurs in flow velocity at the minimum cross-sectional area of flow, and with well-rounded nozzles there is no increase in fluid discharge.

Critical ratio. A statistic test, formed from the sampling outcome, which indicates the significance of the sampling result.

Critical size. Any one of a set of physical dimensions of the core and reflector of a nuclear reactor maintaining a critical chain reaction, the material and structure of the core and the reflector having been specified.

Critical tissues. Human tissues which are most sensitive to radiation and which therefore must be most closely guarded against the deleterious effects of radiation.

Critical volume. The volume corresponding to the critical size.

Crohn's disease. Chronic inflammation of the lower part of the ileum.

Cross-assembler. Program to translate the same instructions for different computers.

Cross bombardment. A method for assigning the mass to a radioactive nuclide by producing it in different nuclear reactions.

Crossed-coil. Coil pair arranged with their magnetic fields at right angles to each other in such a way as to minimize their mutual electromagnetic interaction. (NMR.)

Crossing-over. An exchange process during meiosis in which homologous chromosomes undergo synapsis and exchange segments, resulting in the production of new combinations of linked genes.

Cross-reacting antibodies. Antibodies which react with various antigens of similar structure in contrast with specific antibodies which only react with their specific antigen.

Cross-reacting antigen. Antigen capable of combining with antibody produced in response to a different antigen. A type of tumor antigen present on all tumors induced by the same or a similar carcinogen.

Cross-reaction. The reaction of an antibody with an antigen other than the one that induced its formation.

Cross-reactivity. The reaction of a molecule with an immunoglobulin directed toward another substance.

Cross section. A measure of the probability of a specified interaction between an incident radi-

ation and a target particle or system of particles. It is the reaction rate per target particle for a specified process divided by the particle flux density of the incident radiation (cross section, microscopic). In reactor physics the term is sometimes applied to a specified group of target particles, e.g., those per unit volume (cross section, macroscopic), or per unit mass, or those in a specified body. The unit of cross section, is the barn; $1\ b = 10^{-24}\ cm^2$.

Cryobiology. Science dealing with the effect of low temperatures on biological systems.

Cryogenics. The use of extreme cold, often near absolute zero, in order to make use of the phenomena of superconductivity, particularly advantages for very fast microelectronic circuits.

Cryogenic stabilization. A superconductor-stabilizer configuration where the superconductor will be below the critical temperature even when all current is diverted to the stabilizer.

Cryoglobulin. A protein that has the property of forming a precipitate of gel in the cold.

Cryomagnet. Superconducting magnet that can operate without external electrical power once the field is established. At very low temperatures (less than 23°K) some substances become superconducting, i.e., zero resistance. A cryomagnet needs to be kept at these very low temperatures by using liquid helium.

Cryopumping. The process of removing gas from a system by condensing it on a surface maintained at very low temperatures.

Cryoshims. The superconducting correction coils (shim coils) used in the superconducting magnet for adjustment of the homogeneity of the field.

Cryostat. An apparatus for maintaining a constant low temperature (as by means of liquid helium). Requires vacuum chambers to help with thermal isolation.

Cryotron. A device based upon the principle that superconductivity established at temperatures near absolute zero is destroyed by the application of a magnetic field.

Crystal counter. If an electric field is applied to a crystal such as diamond or cadmium sulfide, then the passage of an ionizing particle through the crystal makes it counducting and produces a voltage pulse at the electrodes.

Crystallography. This is the science of the crystalline state. Modern crystallography includes morphology, or the study of crystal shape, structural crystallography, which deals with the geometrical arrangement of the atoms in crystals, crystal chemistry, and crystal physics.

CT scan (abdomen / pelvis). Evaluation of the liver, spleen, pancreas, adrenals, and kidneys is the usual indication for abdominal CT scanning. The extent of lymph node disease in the abdomen or pelvis is perhaps best evaluated by CT and it is quite useful in the follow-up of patients undergoing chemotherapy or radiotherapy for known malignant intraabdominal disease. It is frequently necessary to administer i.v. contrast and in addition to this it is necessary to opacify all of the loops of bowel in the abdomen with orally administered contrast to prevent misidentification of fluid-filled loops of bowel as potential masses. Because of the precise degree of localization on CT, small suspected malignant masses (particularly retroperitoneal) can accurately be localized and, furthermore, can accurately undergo needle biopsy once they have been localized.

CT scan (chest). CT of the chest can basically be divided into examination of the lungs and mediastinum (heart, esophagus, lymph nodes, and central vascular structures of the chest). CT scanning of the lungs is usually limited to examination for the presence of small nodules associated with widespread or early spread of metastatic malignant disease. Examination of the mediastinum has been greatly simplified by CT since mediastinal structures are poorly depicted on conventional radiographs or tomographs. To a large extent the cross-sectional (axial) anatomy depicted on CT has simplified the evaluation of these structures. Usually axial sections are taken at 1-cm intervals from the clavicle through to the diaphragm.

CT scan (head). The three primary indications for CT examination of the brain are intracranial hemorrhage, head trauma, and suspected brain tumor. There are numerous secondary indications including hydrocephalus, congenital abnormalities, as well as numerous rare and obscure neurologic diseases including degenerative disease of the brain and spinal cord. A plain (or nonenhanced) scan is performed without administration of iodinecontaining contrast material. Frequently, if a vascular abnormality or vascular neoplasm is suspected (e.g., meningioma), iodine-containing material will be given i.v. and the lesion in question will be observed as quite dense on the subsequent scan.

Culture. Propagation of microorganism or cells in defined media.

Cumulative distribution. A statistical distribution of ordered data cumulated successively. The cumulative number (or percent) indicates that portion of the population which has a certain X value or less.

Cumulative dose. The total dose resulting from repeated exposures to the same region of the whole body.

Cumulative ionization. The ions formed in a device such as a gas discharge tube are accelerated towards the electrodes by the electric field. If the gas pressure is not too low the ions will collide with gas atoms and may cause them to be ionized. These secondary ions may in turn produce other ions. Under certain conditions of gas pressure and applied voltage the effect is cumulative, giving rise to a sustained discharge.

Curie. A non-SI unit of radioactivity defined as 3.70×10^{10} disintegrations per second. One gram of radium has an activity of 1 Ci. (Abbreviated Ci, several fractions of the curie are in common usage). The curie has now been superseded by the SI unit, the becquerel (one disintegration per second).

Curie point. All ferromagnetic substances have a definite temperature of transition at which the phenomena of ferromagnetism disappear and the substances become merely paramagnetic. This temperature is called the "Curie point" and is usually lower than the melting point.

Curie's law. The intensity of magnetization

$$I = AH/T$$

where H is the magnetic field strength, T the absolute temperature, and A Curie's constant. Used for paramagnetic substances.

Curium. Element symbol Cm, atomic number 96, atomic weight ~247.

Current directory. The directory that a disk operation system (DOS) refers to when a file specification or a drive name is entered with no directory name. At any time, the disk on each disk drive has its own current directory. When DOS is started or a new disk is mounted, the disk's root directory is made the current directory.

Current (electric). The rate of transfer of electricity. The transfer at the rate of 1 ESU of electricity in 1 s is the electrostatic unit of current. The electromagnetic unit of current is a current of such strength that 1 cm of the wire in which it flows is pushed sideways with a force of 1 dyn when the wire is at right angles to a magnetic field of unit intensity. The practical unit of current is the ampere, a transfer of 1 C/s, which is one tenth of the electromagnetic unit. The international ampere is the unvarying electric current which, when passed through a solution of silver nitrate in accordance with certain specifications, deposits silver at the rate of 0.001118 g/s. The international ampere is equivalent to 0.999835 absolute ampere.

Current ionization chamber. When a charged particle passes through a gas it loses energy in ionizing some of the atoms of the gas; its electric field transfers energy to atomic electrons which are ejected from the atoms, leaving positively charged ions. The current ionization chamber is a detector of radiation which employs the effect.

Cursor. A symbol on a computer's display that marks the place where the next thing to type will appear.

Curve. An x-, y-based grid plot of one subject based upon its relation to another. Usually generated from a selected region of interest applied to a series of images (e.g., time-activity curve).

Curve fitting. In competitive radioassay, the plotting in various ways of the fraction of tracer bound as a function of test substance concentration in the assay standards. Commonly, mathematical transformations are used to linearize these curves, which tend to be exponential, the most popular methods being Scatchard plots, logit, and hyperbolic transforms.

Curve generation of radionuclide imaging. There are several techniques in which nuclear medicine image data are displayed in the form of curves. The first method is the generation of a profile across an image, with the subsequent formation of a curve that reflects the change in counts with spatial position. The second technique is to use a region of interest (ROI) to monitor the change of counts with time within a restricted area of a "dynamic" set of images. The third and final type of curve may be the result of an analytical technique, such as deconvolution or phase and amplitude analysis which can present the data from a "dynamic" study in a modified form and may reflect a physiological parameter.

Since curves may be formed from data contained within a ROI, they may be subject to normalization processes and their accuracy governed by the statistical quality of the image data from which they were generated. The display of the curve is usually achieved by finding the maximum ordinate value, and normalizing all other curve data relative to this value on the monitor. For a curve generated from "dynamic" data, each point on the curve represents the average pixel value or total counts within the ROI for each frame or image in the study. In studies with more than one time zone, data are usually normalized for different acquisition times, thus avoiding sharp discontinuities between time segments.

Curve math. Math manipulations of one or more curves; for example: smooth, add, subtract, normalize, multiply, divide, take the log or exponential of curves.

Cushing's disease. A condition caused by the oversecretion of hormones of the adrenal cortex which may be due to a tumor in the adrenal or pituitary glands.

Customer support. All the services that are obtained from a dealer before and after purchasing hardware or software. Customer support includes advice on what to buy, expert help in installing a product, and adapting it to particular needs, training, and repair.

Cut. The fraction of the feed into a stage or an isotope separation plant which is either withdrawn as product or passed on to the next stage towards the product end of the system.

Cutie pie. (Colloquial) Portable ionization chamber for determining relatively stable dose rates.

Cutoff frequency. Some manufacturers define the cutoff frequency of single photon emission tomography reconstruction at the point where a filter value drops to zero, others define the cutoff frequency as the point where the filter magnitude drops below a given value. The meaning of the term cutoff frequency may also differ for different kinds of filters (even the same manufacturer). It is also important to define the units being used when speaking of frequencies. Frequencies may be defined as cycles/pixel, cycles/centimeter, or in any number of other units. Unless it is clear which units are being used and how the cutoff frequency is defined, inappropriate values may be used to define filters, resulting in improper filtering.

Cyanosis. Bluish-purple discoloration of the skin and/or mucous membranes due to deficient oxygenation of the blood and consequently high concentration of reduced (oxygen-lacking) hemoglobin.

Cycle. Complete variation of an acoustic variable.

Cycle average intensity. (I_a) The intensity of the wave average over one cycle. In such a wave the instantaneous peak intensity (I_p) is twice the value of I_a, i.e., $I_p = 2I_a$.

Cycle length window. The range of cardiac cycle times (R-R interval times) that will be accepted in a gated radionuclide ventriculogram.

Cycle-specific drugs. Cytotoxic or immuno-suppressive drugs that kill both mitotic and resting cells.

Cycle time. The time to run through one operation; from the call for, to the delivery of information.

Cyclic adenosine monophosphate. (cAMP) Associated with the response of cells to hormones.

Cyclotron. Since its invention by E. O. Lawrence in 1931, the cyclotron has been the nuclear particle accelerator of choice for the production of radioisotopes by charged-particle-induced nuclear reactions. Nuclear reactors, which produce neutron-rich radioisotopes by neutron bombardment, supplanted cyclotrons in the 1950s and 1960s as the major producers of radioisotopes, but the latter are still the dominant producers of neutron-deficient radioisotopes. As a result of significant improvements in cyclotron technology, the number of cyclotrons in dedicated use in biomedical applications has increased rapidly. This trend to increased utilization of cyclotrons has been reinforced by the recent development of positron emission tomography, a procedure which enables complex physiological and biochemical processes to be studied *in vivo*. The neutron-deficient (and hence positron-emitting) radioisotopes ^{11}C, ^{13}N, ^{15}O, and ^{18}F have been especially useful in these studies of function and metabolism. As the longest lived of these isotopes, ^{18}F has a half-life of only 110 min; hospitals and research institutions that undertake positron emission tomography programs need a cyclotron nearby.

Cyclotron (or gyro) frequency. Frequency of gyration of a charged particle in a magnetic field

$$\Omega = Zeb \text{ // } m \text{ (radian/s)}$$

where Ze = particle charge (C), B = magnetic field strength (T), and m = particle mass (kg).

Cyclotron principle. If q and m are, respectively, the charge and mass of a particle moving with velocity v in an arc of radius r, in a plane normal to a uniform magnetic field B, the equation of motion of the particle, by Newton's second law, is $qvB = mv^2/r$. An ex-

pression for the rotational frequency f of the particle follows directly from $f = qB/2\pi m$ and the kinetic energy E of the particle is $E = B^2r^2q^2/2m$.

It is clear from that, that the frequency of rotation of the particle is independent of its speeds. This fact underlies the principle of the cyclotron: the same electrodes can be used over and over again to give a series of impulses that are regularly spaced in time and which thus accelerate particles to energies many times that represented by the maximum potential at the electrodes.

Cyclotron radiation. Electromagnetic radiation emitted by charged particles due to their natural gyration in a magnetic field (also called "synchrotron radiation").

Cyclotron resonance heating. Radio-frequency heating of a plasma in a magnetic field near the ion or electron cyclotron frequency or low multiples thereof.

Cyclotrons level I. ($E_{p,d} \leq 10$ MeV) These are single-particle machines, deuterons being included because of the historical importance of several 8-MeV deuteron machines that have been used in biomedical research. The burgeoning interest over the past decade in positron tomography has stimulated intensive interest in the techniques for producing the radioisotopes ^{11}C, ^{13}N, ^{15}O, and ^{18}F (CNOF). It is now clear that these nuclides can all be produced by proton-only cyclotrons with isotopically enriched targets.

Cyclotrons level II. ($E_p \leq 20$ MeV These are generally multiple-particle machines, that is, they produce beams of protons and deuterons; some provide ^{3}He and ^{4}He, also. A multiplicity of cyclotrons of this class is commercially available. In general, the proton and deuteron output currents are specified in 50 μA. Although the primary application of level ll cyclotrons is CNOF production, all of these machines produce proton beams in the upper part of the energy range (16 or 17 MeV).

Cyclotrons level III. ($E_p \leq 45$MeV) Cyclotrons in the level III class are multiple ion machines providing all four particles (protons, deuterons, ^{3}He, ^{4}He). The potential applications cover the full range of biomedical research and production possibilities. Copious quantities of CNOF can be produced as well as other important radionuclides such as ^{67}Ga, ^{111}In, ^{201}T1, and ^{123}I. This class of machine is also being used in cancer therapy.

Cyclotrons level IV. ($E_p \leq 200$ MeV) Machines

have produced in the proton energy range 50 to 60 MeV. The application considerations are similar to those machines at the upper end of level III.

Cylinder. The part of a computer disk that can be read from and written to with the disk drive's read/write head(s) in one position. The number of tracks per cylinder depends on the number of recording surfaces a disk has. A diskette has one or two tracks per cylinder; a hard disk may have more, since it may consist of a stack of platters on a single spindle, each platter having its own pair of read/write heads.

Cyst. Closed cavity or sac filled with liquid or semisolid materials; may be due to infection or presence of foreign material.

Cystography. A catheter is placed through the urethra into the bladder and contrast material is allowed to enter and fill the bladder to capacity (cystogram).This outlines the interior of the bladder and helpful in evaluation of bladder size and in looking for the presence of reflux of urine to either ureter. This latter abnormality is associated with recurrent episodes of kidney infection.

Cystometrogram. In this examination an evaluation is made of the amount of contrast material necessary to distend the bladder (through a catheter) and subsequently the amount of pressure the bladder can generate when voiding is initiated. It is of value in the determination of the presence or absence of a neurological deficit in the bladder and, in general, is a rough guide to degree of bladder tonicity.

Cystoscope. An endoscope designed for the examination of the urinary bladder.

Cytochrome. One of a number of iron-containing proteins found in cells which take part in electron transport systems; yellow pigment that transfers electrons in cellular respiration.

Cytogenetics. Science of cellular constituents concerned with heredity and chromosomes.

Cytokinesis. Changes in the cytoplasm of a cell during cell division.

Cytology. Study of cells, their origin, structure, and chemical properties.

Cytoplasm. A protein complex outside the nucleus of a cell, and surrounded by the cell membrane.

Cytoskeleton. Filamentous network of proteins in the cytoplasm.

Cytosol. Liquid portion of the cytoplasm.

Cytotoxic drugs. Drugs that are toxic to cells. They may be used to treat certain types of cancer, cells often being more vulnerable to such drugs than normal cells.

Cytropic antibodies. Antibodies of the IgG and IgE classes that sensitize cells for subsequent anaphylaxis.

D

Dacryocystogram. Dacryocystography is the evaluation of the nasolacrimal (tear) duct that connects the eye with the nose and which is responsible for drainage of tears from the eye.

Daisy wheel. An interchangeable typing element used in certain printers. Characters on the element are raised outlines at the ends of spokes sticking out of a central rod, like petals on a daisy. The rod rotates at high speed; when the desired character is in position, a hammer hits it. The outline is typed on the page.

Damping. Material placed behind the far face of a transducer element to reduce pulse duration; also, the process of pulse duration reduction.

Danger. (Legal) The possibility of injury. This is inherent to a given situation and there is no liability for danger as such. Dangerous procedures are made feasible by the careful conduct of a physician.

Dark adaptation goggles. Red-tinted goggles used to aid adaptation for fluoroscopy.

Dark current. The current (due to thermal or other effects) that flows through a photomultiplier or other photoelectric detector, when all light is excluded.

Dark-field illumination. Illumination of an object in a microscope in such a way that only light diffracted by the object reaches the eye. The objects appear as bright images against a dark background.

Data. Data are any kind of information put into, processed by, or taken out of a computer. Data processing is what the computer does when it sorts, manipulates, and stores information. "Data" is plural; "datum" is the singular form.

Data access arrangement. (DAA) A mechanism sometimes required by the telephone company that goes between a device and the telephone line on which the device will transmit or receive. Its claimed purpose is to prevent electrical damage to the telephone system.

Data acquisition system. In computing, a system which captures data from various sources and converts it into binary codes for subsequent use by the computer.

Data base. An organized collection of interrelated data items that allows one or more applications to process the items while disregarding physical storage locations.

Data base management system. (DBMS) An application program that processes information organized as a set of records, each record consisting of fields of data. A DBMS can display and print reports derived from a data base and can perform various kinds of processing, such as sorting records, totaling fields from groups of records, and selecting records on the basis of the values of fields.

Data bus. A group of connections which conveys data to and from the central processing unit, memory storage, and peripheral devices of a computer.

Data definition language. (DDL) A special group of commands used in data base management systems that allows the definition of the structure and contents of the data base.

Data link. Communication lines that transport data between different locations. For example: telephone line, satellite, or radio station.

Data management language. (DML) A group of commands that gives a programmer a standard method of storing and retrieving data when using a data base system.

Data processing consultant. An expert in the use of computers in specific applications environments, e.g., business data processing consultant, medical data processing consultant.

Data structure. How information is stored in memory: by arrays, files, lists, stacks, and other methods or organization.

Dating. Carbon-14 is continuously generated in the atmosphere by the action of the cosmic radiation. It is gradually distributed over the carbon reservoir, consisting principally of the bicarbonate in the sea, the carbonaceous materials of the biosphere, and the atmospheric carbon dioxide; a dynamic equilibrium is established between these parts of the reservoir. Living matter, trees, for example, maintain isotopic equilibrium with the atmospheric carbon dioxide, but once the subject dies equilibration ceases so that the radiocarbon content of dead material gradually falls according to the decay of its ^{14}C content, which is no longer replenished after death. A comparison of the specific activity of the dead material, e.g., wood, charcoal, paper, with that of living material thus permits a calculation of the time elapsing since death, i.e., since isotopic equilibration caused, using the half-life of ^{14}C. In view of the half-life of ^{14}C, which is 5730 years, the procedure is most useful for determining the time elapsing since the death of organic materials between 1,000 and 30,000 years ago.

Daughter product. A nuclide formed by the decay of a radionuclide. A daughter product may be either radioactive or stable. Synonym for decay product.

Day. The duration of one rotation of the earth, or another celestial body, on its axis. A day is measured by successive transits of a reference point on the celestial sphere over the meridian, and each type takes its name from the reference used. Thus, for a solar day the reference is the sun; a mean solar day if the mean sun; and an apparent solar day if the apparent sun. For a lunar day the reference is the moon, for a sidereal day the vernal equinox; for a constituent day as astre fictif or fictitious star. The expression lunar day refers also to the duration of one rotation of the moon with respect to the sun. A Julian day is the consecutive number of each day, beginning with January 1, 4713 BC. A period of 24 h beginning at a specific time, as the civil day beginning at midnight, or the astronomical day beginning at noon.

dB/dt. The rate of change of the amagnetic field (induction) with time. Because changing magnetic fields can induce electrical fields, this is one area of potential concern for safety limits. (NMR.)

D-D. Symbol for reaction between nuclei of two deuterium atoms.

Dead space. The space in the air-conducting system of the respiratory tract where no gas exchange occurs. It consists of the nose, pharynx, trachea, bronchi, and conducting bronchioles.

Dead time. Time during which receiver is unable to receive the signal in a pulsed NMR spectrometer. The time interval following a radioactive even in which the detecting apparatus remains unresponsive to further events. Same as pulse resolving time.

Dead zone. Distance closest to an ultrasound transducer in which imaging cannot be performed.

Death. Cessation of life; legally "the irreversible cessation of total cerebral function, spontaneous function of the respiratory system, and spontaneous function of the circulatory system."

Deblocking factor. An antibody that, when mixed with blocking factors, neutralizes their activity.

Debride. To remove foreign material or contaminated tissue from wound with a scalpel.

De Broglie wavelength. The wavelength associated with a moving particle of mass m, momentum p, and velocity v, derived by equating the expressions $E = mc^2$ and $E = hv$.

Debug. A jargon word to indicate the deletion and correction of errors in a computer program.

Debusser. Device used to erase material from a computer or recording tape.

Debye length. A theoretical length which describes the maximum separation at which a given electron will be influenced by the electric field of a given positive ion. Sometimes referred to as the Debye shielding distance or plasma length. It is well known that charged particles interact through their own electric fields. In addition, Debye has shown that the attractive force between an electron and ion which would otherwise exist for very large separations is indeed cut off for a critical separation due to the presence of other positive and negative charges in-between. This critical separation or Debye length decreases for increased plasma density.

Decade. A group of ten storage locations — ten places in memory, each of which can hold a single computer "word". A decade is the minimum amount of data that can be called up from a computer's memory.

Decade scaler. A recording instrument having a scaling factor of ten.

Decarboxylation. Removal of CO_2 from the carboxyl group (–COOH) of an organic acid.

Decay. When a radioactive atom disintegrates it is said to decay. What remains is a different element. Thus, an atom of polonium decays to form lead, ejecting an alpha particle in the process. In a mass of a particular radioisotope a number of atoms will disintegrate or decay every second — and this number is characteristic of the isotope concerned. The spontaneous transformation of a radionuclide, resulting in a decrease with time of the number of radioactive events in a sample.

Decay branching. Radioactive decay which can proceed in two or more different ways.

Decay constant. The fraction of the number of atoms of a radioactive nuclide which decay in a unit time. Symbol: $\lambda = 0.693 +_{1/2}$ is the half-life of a radionuclide. It may also be noted that λ is the reciprocal of the mean of average life of the radioactive nuclide.

Decay curve. The decay curve of a radioactive substance is the activity plotted against the time. Since the activity is given by the equation

$$A = A_o \exp(-\lambda t)$$

where A_o is the activity at time $t = o$ and λ is the decay constant, it follows that a plot of the logarithm of A vs. t will give a straight line when we are dealing with a single radioactive substance. When two radioactive materials are involved the composite decay curve comprises two linear portions corresponding to the two radioactive nuclides present.

Decay law. Of a radioactive nuclide is the law which states that the number of atoms decaying in unit time is proportional to the number present.

Decay product. A nuclide resulting from the radioactive disintegration of a radionuclide, being formed either directly as the result of successive transformations in a radioactive series. A decay product may be either radioactive or stable.

Decay scheme. Diagram showing the decay mode or modes of a radionuclide.

Decay series. Synonym for decay chain. A series of radioactive decompositions in which radioactive daughters are produced; these radioactive daughters then become parents by producing radioactive daughters of their own.

Decibel. One tenth of a bel: the number of decibels denoting the nature of the two amounts of power being ten times the logarithm to the base 10 of this ratio; db is the commonly used abbreviation for decibel.

Deciles. Values that divide a distribution of ordered data into ten equal parts.

Decimal numbers. The base-10 number system. This is the standard number system.

Decimal representation. Using characters in the range 0 to 9 to represent symbols.

Decision tree. A graphical representation of a complex decision process, showing the alternative choices and the expected outcome and consequences thereof.

Deck. A pack of punched computer cards that can contain a program or a file of information.

Decommissioning. Those actions to be taken by a nuclear facility licensee to (1) decontaminate the structures and equipment, (2) remove sources of radioactivity or render them inaccessible, and (3) return the site to such a condition that it may be either safely returned to unrestricted use or maintained under the security and surveillance required for the protection of public health and safety.

Decomposition. Is the chemical separation of a substance into two or more substances, which may differ from each other and from the original substances.

Decontamination. This term is commonly used to denote the removal of radioactive contaminating material from surfaces of one kind or another. It is rarely used in connection with the cleaning up of gases or liquids. Everyday examples of decontamination requirements include the surfaces of laboratory benches, floors, and walls, laboratory apparatuses, including glove boxes and hot cells, and the skin, usually the hands of personnel.

Decontamination factor. The ratio of the amount of undesired radioactive material initially present to the amount remaining after a suitable processing step has been completed. Decontamination factors may refer to the reduction of some particular type of radiation, or of the gross measurable radioactivity.

Deconvolution. A mathematical technique which is the inverse of convolution. One application is to eliminate the "blurring" effect of tracer circulation or organ time — activity histograms and compensate for poor bolus injection.

Decrement. An instruction to decrease a storage location, usually by one step.

Dedicated. A computer system or other machine assigned to one particular user or application.

Dee. A D-shaped hollow metal electrode used in the cyclotron and synchrocyclotron particle accelerators to obtain the necessary electric field for acceleration.

Dee lines. Tubes used to support the dees in a cyclotron or synchro-cyclotron. They are usually made part of a 1/4-wavelength transmission line into which is fed the radio-frequency power used for particle acceleration.

Default. A default value, default image, or default operation is the value, image, or operation that is used if a particular value, image, or operation is not specified.

Default drive. The disk drive that a disk operating system (DOS) or a command uses to read from or write to a file when the drive name has been omitted from a file specification. The name of the current default drive is displayed in the standard DOS command line prompt.

Deferent. Conveying away from a center.

Defibrillation. The process of abolishing atrial or ventricular fibrillation to allow the resumption of normal heart rhythm. It is achieved by passing an electric current through the heart.

Defibrillator. An apparatus used to counteract fibrillation (very rapid, irregular contractions of the muscle fibers of the heart) by application of electric impulses to the heart.

Definite proportions. In every sample of each compound substance the proportions by weight of the constituent elements are always the same.

Degranulation. A process whereby cytoplasmic granules of phagocytic cells fuse with phagosomes and discharge their contents into the phagolysosome thus formed.

Degree. Angle subtended at the center by a circular arc which is 1/360 of the circumference.

Degree of association. $(1 - \alpha)$ The degree of association of an electrolytic solution is the percentage of ions associated into nonconducting species, such as ion pairs.

Degree of dissociation. (α) The degree of dissociation (or ionization) of an electrolytic solution is the percentage of solution (or electrolyte) in the dissociated (or ionized) state in solution. Classically, this degree is obtained from conductance measurements from the ratio, A/A, where A is the equivalent conductance an electrolytic solution would have at some finite concentration if it were completely dissociated into ions at that concentration. This symbol is also used to denote the fraction of free ions in a solution when simple ions, ion paris, and clusters higher than ion pairs are present.

Degrees of freedom. (df) Number of independent contributions to a theoretical statistical sampling distribution (such as χ^2, t, and F distribution).

Dehydration. Removal of water from a substance, condition when water content of the body falls below normal.

Deiodinate. Removal of iodine from a compound.

Delayed coincidence. Two signals are said to be in delayed coincidence if the second occurs at a definite time after the first.

Delayed heat. Biphasic burst of heat liberated from isometrically contracting muscle during the recovery period, after the muscle has relaxed; first phase is oxygen independent, the second phase requires oxygen, is longer lasting, and liberates the most heat.

Delayed neutrons. Neutrons emitted by nuclei in excited states which have been formed in the process of beta decay. (The neutron emission itself is prompt, so that the observed delay is that of the preceding beta emission or emissions.)

Delay tanks. Used to hold radioactive gas or liquid for a period either to allow short-lived activity to decay or to allow sampling. Shielding of the tank will probably be necessary since the device is generally used to reduce very high levels of very short-lived radionuclides. For sampling, the liquid is allowed to flow into one of a series of two or more delay tanks and when one is full the flow is diverted to another. Samples are then taken and assayed so as to know what treatment is required.

Delimiter. An instruction to indicate the beginning or end of a section of a computer program.

Delta host functions. (DHF) Refers primarily to the commands passed to and used by the host computer.

Delta-ray. When an ionizing particle passes through matter some electons are emitted, from the molecule hit, with sufficient energy to cause further ionization. In cloud chambers, for example, short tracks of these electrons or Δ-rays can be seen coming from the track of the ionizing particle. Also called Δ-electrons.

Dementia. Mental deterioration of intellectual function from disease of the brain.

Demodulation. Converting voltage pulses from one form to another.

Demodulator. Another term for detector, by analogy to broadcast radio receivers.

Demonstration reactor. A reactor designed to demonstrate the technical feasibility and explore the economical potential of a given reactor type. It may, in some cases, also serve as the prototype.

Demyelination. The removal or destruction of the myelin surrounding nerve axons.

Denaturation. Destruction of the usual nature of a substance; a change in the tertiary or secondary structure of protein which causes it to lose its unique properties.

Dendrite. Any of the usual branching protoplasmic processes that conduct impulses toward the body of a nerve cell. They have synapses with, and receive impulses from, axons of other nerve cells.

Densitometer. An instrument utilizing the photoelectric principle to determine the degree of darkening of developed photographic film.

Density. Density is used to denote the degree of darkening of photographic film. Is the concentration of mass. It is the mass divided by the volume taken up by the mass (mass per unit volume).

$$\text{density (kg/m}^3\text{)} = \text{mass (kg)/volume (m}^3\text{)}$$

2-Deoxy-D-glucose. (2-DG) Commonly referred to as DG.

2-Deoxy-2-fluro-D-glucose. (2-FDG) Commonly referred to as FDG.

Deoxyribonucleic acid. (DNA) The nucleic acid in which the genetic information of the cell is stored. It also mediates the functional activity of the cell. The DNA molecule is composed of a deoxyribose phosphate backbone arranged in a right-handed helix structure held together by hydrogen bonds between pairs of purine and pyrimidine bases.

Depleted uranium. Uranium having less than the natural content, namely, 0.7% of the easily fissionable uranium ^{235}U, e.g., the residue from a diffusion plant or a reactor.

Depletion. Reduction of the concentration of one or more specified isotopes in a material or one of its constituents.

Depolarization. The removal of any alignment in space (polarization) of the elementary electric or magnetic dipoles in a substance, or in a beam of particules. Reduction in the resting membrane potential, especially in an axon or muscle fiber during the development of an action potential (impulse).

Depolymerization. The breaking down of an organic compound into two or more molecules of less complex structure.

Depth compensation. The compensation of attenuation due to losses and geometrical divergence of acoustic signals along the propagating pathway. When accomplished electronically, this is called time gain compensation (TGC), depth compensation, or swept gain.

Depth dose. The radiation dose delivered at a particular depth beneath the surface of the body. It is usually expressed as a percentage of surface dose or as a percentage of air dose. Depth of penetration.

Depth of field. A photographic concept that finds application with focused collimators. It is the longitudinal distance, in the field of view, over which resolution is acceptable.

Depth of focus. The distance along the beam axis, for a focusing transducer assembly, from the point where the beam cross-sectional area first becomes equal to four times the focal area to the point beyond the focal surface where the beam cross-sectional area again becomes equal to four times the focal area.

Derivative. Rate of change of one variable with respect to another.

Derivative analysis. A method of analysis depending upon the production of a radioactive derivative of the substance to be assayed.

Derived limits. Upper levels of radioactive contamination or of concentrations of airborne radionuclides, laid down by the competent authority and not to be exceeded. Derived working limits from the basic recommendations of the International Commission on Radiological Protection for maximum permissible doses and dose limits.

Dermatitis. Lesions affecting the epithelium of the skin; includes dryness, scaliness, hyper-pigmentation, and peeling of the skin.

Dermis. Lower layer of the skin, containing specialized nerve endings for touch, temperature, and pain and rich plexuses of blood vessels. The hair follicles and skin glands also originate in the dermis.

Descriptive statistics. Methods used to describe or summarize a set of data which do not involve generalization to a larger set of data.

Desensitization. The act of depressing or abolishing a hypersensitivity state by administering a specific antigen or hapten.

Desiccation. With reference to blood coagulation, a surgical technique based on straightforward ohmic heating of tissue by placing an active electrode in contact with the tissue.

Design. Description of a special form material, a package, or packaging that enables those items to be fully identified. The description may include specifications, engineering drawings, reports showing compliance with regulatory requirements, and other relevant documentation.

Desorption. The reverse process of adsorption whereby adsorbed matter is removed from the adsorbent.

Desquamation. A shedding of the superficial epithelium, renal tubules, mucous membranes, and skin.

Destructive read. To read information is to retrieve it from memory. In a destructive read, the act of reading the data erases it from memory. This is what happens when reading data from a computer core memory.

Detective quantum efficiency. A measure of the accuracy of quality of data transfer in imaging systems, expressed in terms of noise, the detective quantum efficiency being equal to the ratio $(\text{noise in})^2/(\text{noise out})^2$.

Detector. Portion of the receiver that demodulates the radio frequency (rf) NMR signal and converts it to a lower frequency signal. Most detectors now are phase sensitive (e.g., quadrature demodulator/detector), and will also give phase information about the rf signal. A measuring chamber which detects incoming X-rays and indicates them quantitatively. Materials used for the detectors in computerized tomography are highly compressed gasses (e.g., xenon) or solid matter (e.g., iodide or germante crystals). An instrument for detecting the presence of radioactivity by converting the energy absorbed into some form such as sound or light.

Detector geometry. The detector to sample distance, and the sample and detector sizes define a solid angle that is a percentage of the total events radiated by the source. This geometry helps to define the efficiency of the detector.

Detector noise. Continuous background of very small, random pulses or noise produced by a nuclear detector in the absence of any incident particles. This occurs, for example, in the use of scintillation detectors in which the light produced by the scintillator releases photoelectrons from the sensitive cathode or an electron multiplier which multiplies the signal so that an output pulse of several volts may be produced. Inevitably thermal agitation also releases electrons from the various sensitive surfaces, and these are also multiplied to produce a continuous background of small pulses, or noise, at the output stage. This detector noise can be reduced by cooling the photomultiplier tube. The level of the noise sets a lower limit to the energy of the radiation which can be studied with a scintillation spectrometer.

Detector of radiation. Nuclear particles in motion, and also γ- and X-rays, may be detected by their interaction with matter through which they pass. A detector of radiation is a device in which this interaction is readily translated into some measurable physical quantity. The process which provides the bases of all detectors is the excitation of an atom of the detection medium by the electric field of a charged nuclear particle which passes nearby.

Determinant groups. Individual chemical structures present on macromolecular antigens that determine antigenic specificity.

Deterministic. As pertaining to a cause-and-effect relationship, not a statistical description.

Detoxify. Process, usually consisting of a series of reactions, by which a substance foreign to the body is changed to a compound or compounds more readily excreted.

Deuterium. The isotope of hydrogen of mass number 2, heavy hydrogen, or deuterium that consists of a proton and a neutron bound together by nuclear forces. Symbol D or $_1H^2$.

Device. A computer accessory that is used for input or output, such as a disk drive, a printer, or a keyboard. Also called an "I/O" device.

Device handler. A software routine that services and controls the hardware activities of an input/output (I/O) device.

Device name. A name used by a disk operating system (DOS) to identify a peripheral device like a serial interface or a console. It always ends with a colon. For example, in the command copy con: b: example.txt {ENTER}, "con:" is a device name that refers to the console.

Dextran-coated charcoal. Solution of cross-linked dextrans and activated charcoal used to separate bound from free in radiobinding assay (RBA) absorbing free ligand.

Dextrans. Polysaccharides composed of a single sugar.

Diabatic process. A process in a thermodynamic system in which there is a transfer of heat across the boundaries of the system. Diabatic process is preferred to nonadiabatic process.

Diabetes insipidus. A condition characterized by thirst and the passage of a large amount of urine.

Diabetes mellitus. Pathologic condition with an absolute or relative insulin deficiency accompanied by elevated levels of glucose in the blood and urine.

Diagnosis. Referring to determination of the disease; analysis of symptoms; pertaining to the detection and isolation of a malfunction (hardware) or mistake (software).

Diagnostic program. A set of programming steps the computer uses to diagnose its own function. Computers use diagnostics to test themselves, find faults, and signal the operator that there is trouble. Some diagnostic programs even allow the computer to correct the problem itself.

Diagnostic-type protective tube housing. Housing so constructed that at every specified rating of the X-ray tube, the leakage radiation at a focal distance of 1 m does not exceed 100 mr in 1 h.

Dialysis. Process of separating materials by their relative permeability through a membrane.

Diamagnetic materials. Those within which an externally applied magnetic field is slightly reduced because of an alteration of the atomic electron orbits produced by the field. Diamagnetism is an atomic-scale consequence of the Lenz law of induction. The permeability of diagmagnetic materials is slightly less than that of empty space, e.g., aluminum is diamagnetic.

Diamagnetism. Many substances, when they are subjected to a magnetization force, become magnetized in such a direction as to oppose that force, i.e., exhibiting negative suscepti-

bility. This property is referred to as diamagnetism.

Diapedesis. The outward passage of cells through intact vessel walls.

Diaphragm. Muscular membrane separating the thorax and abdomen; involved in breathing. In general, membrane or shutter.

Diaphragmatic breathing. Breathing caused by contraction and relaxation of the diaphragm. As the diaphragm contracts during inhalation, it moves toward the abdomen, enlarging the lung cavity and drawing air into the lungs. The abdominal contents are simultaneously pushed outward and down. As the diaphragm relaxes, it moves upward, reducing the volume of the lungs and expelled air from them (exhalation).

Diaphysis. Portion of long bone between the articulate ends; shaft.

Diarrhea. Abnormal frequency and fluidity of fecal material.

Diastasis. In surgery, injury to a bone involving separation of an epiphysis. (A center for ossification of each extremity of long bones.)

Diastole. The stage of the cardiac cycle during which the ventricles fill with blood. The relaxation, or period of relaxation, of the heart, especially of the ventricles.

Diastolic blood pressure. The pressure of blood in the arteries during diastole. The average diastolic pressure in the brachial artery of a young adult is 70 to 90 mmHg.

Diathermy. Heating of tissue by high-frequency electromagnetic radiation.

Dicrotic. Having a double beat; being or relating to the second expansion of the artery that occurs during the diastole of the heart (hence dicrotic notch in the blood pressure wave).

Dielectric. A material having a relatively low electrical conductivity; an insulator; a substance that contains few or no free electrons and that can support electrostatic stresses. The principal properties of a dielectric are its dielectric constant (the factor by which the electric field strength in a vacuum exceeds that in the dielectric for the same distribution of charge), its dielectric loss (the amount of energy it dissipates at heat when placed in a varying electric field), and its dielectric strength (the maximum potential gradient it can stand without breaking down).

In an electromagnetic field, the centers of the nonpolar molecules of a dielectric are displaced, and the polar molecules become oriented close to the field. The net effect is the appearance of charges at the boundaries of the dielectric. The frictional work done in orientation absorbs energy from the field, which appears as heat. When the field is removed the orientation is lost by thermal agitation and so the energy is not regained. If free-charge carriers are present they too can absorb energy.

A good dielectric is one in which the absorption is a minimum. A vacuum is the only perfect dielectric. The quality of an imperfect dielectric is its dielectric strength; and the accumulation of charges within an imperfect dielectric is termed dielectric absorption.

Dielectric aborption. Strong microwave electrified absorption by polar liquids, e.g., water.

Diethylenetriaminepentaacetic acid. (Pentetic acid, DTPA) Chelating agent that can be labeled with ^{99m}Tc and used for scintigraphy (renography).

Differential absorption ratio. The ratio of the concentration of an isotope in a given organ or tissue to the concentration that would be obtained if the same administered quantity of this isotope were uniformly distributed throughout the body.

Differential cross section. The cross section for an interaction process involving one or more outgoing particles with specified direction or energy per unit interval of solid angle or energy.

Differential particle flux density. That part of the particle flux density resulting from particles or photons having a specified direction, energy, or both per unit interval of solid angle, energy, or both.

Differentiation. Process of acquiring individual fixed characteristics for a cell or tissue; cancers are sometimes characterized by an apparent reversal of this process in specific cells. Count rate changes over a computer image or across images. Used to highlight changes occurring at edges of organ structures, i.e., edge detectors.

Diffraction. That phenomena produced by the spreading of waves around and past obstacles which are comparable in size to their wavelength.

Diffraction of alpha- and gamma-rays. Since the wavelengths of α-rays and soft γ-rays are of the same order of magnitude as the spacing of lattice planes in a crystal, diffraction effects are observed when these radiations are passed through a crystal.

Diffuse reflection. Scattering at all angles from the point of reflection.

Diffuse scattering. When a "rough" surface intercepts a sound beam, the sound is scattered in many directions in a random fashion. The designation, rough, refers to a surface texture of many wavelengths so that a few millimeters of roughness are needed at diagnostic frequencies. Although the signal amplitude is generally greatest when the interface is normal to the beam, it is much smaller than with the smooth reflector because energy is scattered away from the transducer. Unlike the smooth reflector, this interface returns energy to the transducer over a much wider range of inclinations.

Diffusing capacity. The rate at which a gas passes from the alveoli into the blood at a partial-pressure difference of 1 mmHg.

Diffusion. The process by which molecules or other particles intermingle and migrate due to their random thermal motion. NMR provides a sensitive technique for measuring diffusion of some substances. Net movement of a solute or gas from a region of higher to a region of lower concentration. A method of isotope separation. In nuclear physics, the passage of particles through matter in such a way that the probability of scattering is large compared with that of capture.

Diffusion barrier. In isotope separation, a porous structure or membrane, which because of its small pore size restricts ordinary gas flow, but permits diffuse flow, thereby explaining mass differences for isotope separation.

Diffusion exchange. The process by which a radioactive molecule is substituted for a stable molecule, allowing an influx of the tagged material into a target area. Brain imaging with lypophilic cerebral agents is accomplished in this manner.

Diffusion of gases and particulates. When considering the consequences of any release of radioactivity to the atmosphere, whether intentioanl or accidental, it is necessary to be able to calculate the concentration which is likely to exist at some distance from the point of release.

Digit. A character used to represent one of the nonnegative integers smaller than the radix (for example, in decimal notation, one of the characters 0 to 9; in octal notation, one of the characters 0 to 7; in binary notation, one of the character 0 or 1). A finger or toe.

Digital. Pertaining to digits or to the representation of data or physical quantities by digits. In direct contrast to analog signals, digital information can assume only a finite number of discrete values.

Digital autofluoroscope. A camera device for detecting gamma emissions for diagnosis. It consists of a matrix of individually collimated crystals and related electronic circuits producing a display on an oscilloscope screen.

Digital camera. A camera in which the spatial position of the output of each event is adjusted according to a predetermined lattice. This lattice is a map of the response to a narrow beam source for each lattic location over the detector's field of view.

Digital cassette drives. Cheap storage devices similar to cassette tape recorders. The magnetic tape stores information in the digital mode to be read sequentially and in computer terms, slowly.

Digital computer. A device that performs calculations and manipulates data composed of discrete elements such as numbers. Most modern digital computers work in the binary number system.

Digitalis. The dried leaf of the foxglove plant. A cardiac stimulant that acts indirectly as a diuretic. Its main active ingredient is digitoxin.

Digital mode. Compared with the constantly varying electric signals carrying messages down the wires of the present-day telephone, the "digital mode" uses pulses of current to convert speech to binary numbers for transmission. Equally, the pulses of current could be pulse of light transmitted down fiber optic cables.

Digital radiography. Acquisition or display of radiographic images using digital techniques includes digital video-fluoroscopy and scan-projection radiography (SPR). Also includes digital subtraction and angiography (DSA), digital intravenous angiography (DIVA), and computed tomography (CT).

Digital recording system. A system in which counts collected for a predetermined period of time (e.g., time constant) are recorded as actual numbers. There is no conversion into count rate as in analog rate-meter systems. These true primary digits may be printed as numbers graphed on a chart, or stored on magnetic tape for later recovery and portrayal.

Digital scan converter. A type of scan converter where the image is stored in binary code in a solid-state computer memory.

Digital stabilization. The monitoring of two windows or regions of a spectrum, one for gain and one for zero, to correct for drift in the detector system electronics. Stabilization is usually done in the digital domain, to avoid changing amplifier gain and zero which would induce extra noise.

Digital subtraction angiography. Radiologic technique that uses computer-enhanced video images to display vascular opacification after intravenous or intraarterial administration of contrast media.

Digital-to-analog conversion. (DAC) The transformation of digital word or numbers to analog representation, usually using voltage conversion proportional to the value of the words or numbers received.

Diiodotyrosine. (DIT) An iodotyrosine that is formed by the incorporation of activated iodine into the 3- and 5-positions of the amino acid tyrosine.

Diluent. Chemically inert solvent added to complexing solvent to facilitate solvent extraction. Usually reduces extraction coefficient but may also reduce viscosity etc., and permit more convenient extraction.

Dilution. The difference in concentration of test substance between steps in a standard curve. The addition of diluent to test sample to match the concentration of standard(s) more closely or minimize the effect of interfering substances.

Dilution analysis. A method of analysis based upon the fact that, after dilution, the tracer concentration is reduced by the dilution factor; applied to the determination of volumes (e.g., blood volume) and body composition (e.g., total exchangeable sodium).

Dimer. A compound formed by the union of two radicals or two molecules of a simpler compound. More specifically, a polymer formed from two molecules of a monomer.

Dimercaptosuccinic acid. (DMSA) A chelating agent that can be labeled with ^{99m}Tc for imaging the renal cortex.

Diode. An electronic device which allows current to flow in only one direction in a circuit. A diode can convert AC current to DC current.

Diode detector. A type of detection used in radios and NMR spectrometers using simple iodes. They are nonlinear under some conditions. They are amplitude detectors and carry no phase information.

Diopter. A unit, the reciprocal of the meter, used to express the power of a lens, i.e., the reciprocal of the focal length of the lens.

Diphosphonate. Organic phosphate compound that can be labeled with ^{99m}Tc and used for bone scintigraphy.

Diploid. Having a double set of chromosomes. This is the normal condition of the nuclei of the somatic (nonreproductive) cells of animals an higher plants, as distinct from the haploid condition of the gametes (reproductive cells), which have only a single set of chromosomes.

Diplopic vision. Double vision, i.e., the appearance of single objects as double.

Dipolar correlation time. It is the characteristic "average" time taken by a spin system to change between two molecular orientations by "through-space" interactions with neighboring spins.

Dipolar interactions. Magnetic interaction between two spins possessing magnetic moments. This interaction is due to the magnetic field produced by one spin acting on the other.

Dipole. A combination of two electrically or magnetically charged particles of opposite sign which are separated by a very small distance. Any system of charges, such as a circulating current, which has the following properties: (1) no forces act on it in a uniform field; (2) a torque proportional to sin θ, where θ is the angle between the dipole axis and a uniform field, does act on it; (3) it produces a potential which is proportional to the inverse square of the distance from it.

Dipole moment. The dipole moment of a charge distribution, in which there are equal amounts of positive and negative charges, is the sum of the moments of all the charges about any point.

Dipole radiation. This is the simplest and most important form of electromagnetic radiation from a system of oscillating charges and currents. It is useful to distinguish between the radiation from an oscillating electric dipole (e.g., a pair of equal and opposite charges oscillating along the line joining them about their fixed center of mass) and an oscillating magnetic dipole (e.g., an alternating current flowing in a loop).

Direct address. A direct address represents a location in memory in terms of the machine code that the computer can understand. Such an address does not require any manipulation or translation by the computer.

Direct agglutination. The agglutination of red cells, microorganisms, or other substances directly by serum antibody.

Direct-connect modem. A type of modem that connects to the telephone system by plugging directly into a modular wall jack.

Direct current. (DC) An electric current in a circuit that does not change its direction or polarity with time.

Direct-cycle reactor. A reactor in which the primary coolant is used directly to produce useful power.

Direct immunofluorescence. The detection of antigens by fluorescently labeled antibody.

Directly ionizing particles. Charged particles having sufficient kinetic energy to produce ionization by collision.

Directly ionizing radiation. Radiation consisting of directly ionizing particles.

Direct memory access. (DMA) A device's ability to move data into and out of main computer memory without central processor interaction.

Directory. An area on a disk that records the names and locations of the files on the computer disk. Display (list of contents) of the occupied storage places (files) for recalling an individual computed tomogram.

Direct radiation. Radiation proceeding directly from a source.

Discrete data. Discontinuous data.

Discrete fourier transform. Sampled data representation of the Fourier transform which converts a waveform from the time to the frequency domain.

Discriminant function. A mathematical expression by which one variable may be classified based on the values of other variables.

Discriminator. A circuit which supplies a standard output pulse only when the input pulse is greater than a certain amplitude, called the discriminator bias, which is usually variable. Such a circuit is used to discriminate against pulses of less than a specified height. The instrument is useful in eliminating noise and low pulse-height background.

Disintegration. A spontaneous process in which the nucleus of an atom changes its form or its energy state, by emitting either particulate or electromagnetic radiation, or by electron capture.

Disintegration constant. The fraction of the number of atoms of a radioactive nuclide which decay in unit time; λ in the equation $N = N_o e^{-\lambda t}$, where N is the initial number of atoms present, and N_o is the number of atoms present after some time, t.

Disintegration energy. The energy which is released in the radioactive decay of a nucleus. For example, in α decay, it is the sum of the kinetic energy of the α particle and the recoil energy of the daughter nucleus, when the daughter nucleus is formed in the ground state. In nuclear reactions, the disintegration energy is more commonly termed the Q value of the reaction. The Q value may be positive or negative.

Disintegration family. A number of radioactive nuclides each, except the first, being the daughter product of the previous one.

Disintegration rate. The number of disintegrations per unit time (disintegrations per second). The standard unit is the bacquerel, which equals one disintegration per second.

Disk. A memory based on a rotating disk, similar to a music record, which is covered with a magnetic ferric coating. Binary numbers of computer data are recorded as patterns of magnetization on the disk surface. Floppy disks are small, flexible, plastic disks that can be slotted into a disk read/write unit for transfer of data. Winchester disks are rigid disks of large capacity. The size of a disk is usually expressed in terms of megabytes of storage capacity.

Disk drives. A generic name for "hardware" having moving mechanical parts and designed to store data on magnetic media.

Floppy disk drives: The storage medium is somewhat like a small gramophone record sealed inside a card sleeve with a window to allow the tracks of the disk to be read or written on by a read/write head moving radially across the tracks. Data can be stored on both sides of some disks, thus storage capacity can vary from 100 kilobytes to 1 megabyte.

Hard disk drive: The storage medium is a sealed hard disk storing considerably more data than the floppy disk and having a longer life. Today's microcomputer systems can use hard disk storing 10 or more megabytes of information. They can be read or written onto at much greater speeds than in the case of the floppy disk. A commonly mentioned hard disk is the Winchester disk.

Diskette. Sometimes called floppy disks or flexible disks. A diskette is an oxide-coated, flexible-lastic, magnetic recording medium. Access time is slow — often exceeding 100 ms, and capacity is small — usually less than 1 Mb. However, diskettes are relatively inexpensive.

Disk operating system. (DOS) An executive software system or set of programs which utilize a disk for temporary storage resulting in faster and more efficient operations. This program controls the operation of the computer. The acronym DOS generically refers to many different operating systems on different computers.

Disordering. Any process by which atoms are displaced form their positions in a crystal lattice to positions which are not part of the lattice, e.g., by ionizing radiation. When this displacement is caused by radiation it is often referred to as the Wigner effect.

Dispenser or dispenser/diluter. A mechanical device to dispense reagents and/or dilute samples or standards as an aid in laboratory benchwork.

Dispersion. Colloidal system of one phase dispersed in another, e.g., smoke from solid particles in gas phase or emulsion formed from two immiscible liquid phases. The difference between the index of refraction of any substance for any two wavelengths is a measure of the dispersion for those wavelengths, called the coefficient of dispersion.

Displacement. Distance that an object has moved.

Displacement analysis. One of several general terms for competitive binding assay, most often used to refer to a variant technique wherein the addition of tracer is delayed to enhance assay sensitivity.

Displacement factor. The correction factor used to calculate the true absorbed dose (or dose equivalent) at a point in a phantom when a dose meter that was calibrated in air with respect to exposure is used to measure radiation intensity at that point in the phantom.

Displacement law. Originally established empirically, this connects the type of radioactive decay (alpha or beta) with the displacement, caused by the change in nuclear charge, of the daughter relative to the parent in the periodic table of elements. Thus, β decay leads to the isotope of an element one place to the right of the parent element in the periodic table, but of the same number: β^+ decay to the isotope of an element one place to the left and α decay to an isotope of mass number four less than the parent of an element two places to the left in the periodic table.

Displacement transducer. Distance moved, or position, may be measured by a potentiometer (e.g., as used to determine the position and orientation of some ultrasonic B-scan transducers) or the ratio of inductive coupling between two coils may be varied by the movement of a third coil or ferrite core. Displacement transducers may also be used as velocity or acceleration transducers with suitable electronics.

Disposal of radioactive waste. The disposal of unwanted radioactive waste by-products presents a problem which is common to many industries. To deal with it safely is often both difficult and costly. The emphasis on safe disposal methods is reinforced by the extensive legislation devised to limit, for example, the pollution of the environment.

Radioactive waste disposal in the nuclear power industry is of such importance that it has not only affected the choice of atomic energy sites, but has required for its solution as much scientific manpower as any other major aspect of the work.

Dissection. To cut apart into sections.

Dissociation-field effect. The increased dissociation (or ionization) of the molecules of weak electrolytes under the influence of high electrical fields (potential gradients).

Distal. Farthest from the center from a medial line or from the trunk. Away from the point of origin. Remote; opposite of proximal.

Distributed processing. Refers to the utilization of a mix of local and remote computer power, available for the solution of a user's problem.

Distribution. A function which describes the probability that a random sample of a variable will assume any given value.

Distribution law. A substance distributes itself between two immiscible solvents so that the ratio of its concentrations in the two solvents is approximately a constant (and equal to the ratio of the solubilities of the substance in each solvent). The above statement requires modification if more than one molecular species is formed.

Disturbed flow. A pattern of flow with a disorganized velocity distribution. It is characterized by marked differences in direction and speed of blood cells within a vessel. The term turbulence can be mathematically defined but has been generally used interchangeably with disturbed flow.

Diuretic. An agent that promotes the excretion, or increases the amount of urine.

Divergence. A chain reaction is said to diverge when the number of neutrons produced increases in each succeeding generation.

Diverging hole collimator. The diverging hole collimator has been principally used with small field of view (small diameter detector) gamma cameras to enable large organs to be visualized on a single image. Larger objects can be encompassed within the increasing field of view, but the spatial resolution is not constant with increasing object distance.

Documentation. User documentation: an instruction manual or its equivalent that provides users with sufficient information to use and instrument a system. System documentation: description of hardware and software, contained in a variety of manuals. Program documentation: a concise, complete exposé of what a program does and how it does it, on both an overall basis and a detailed basis. Documentation is most important when someone other than the original programmer must correct or extend a program.

Doerner-Hoskins distribution law. A law explaining the logarithmic distribution of activity occurring in certain cases of coprecipitation.

Domestic safeguards. Measures employed by a nation to prevent or detect the diversion of nuclear material and to protect against the sabotage of facilities.

Donor. In transistors, the N-type semiconductor, the electrode containing impurities which increase the number of available electrons.

Doppler blood pressure monitor. Arterial blood pressure has a peak (systolic) pressure occurring when the heart pumps and a trough (diastolic) just before the next pumping stroke. These two pressures are commonly detected using a stethoscope placed below the sphigmomanoter's inflatable cuff. The stethoscope can be replaced by a thin ultrasonic transducer placed under the inflatable cuff which detects the movement of the artery wall. The Doppler signals are detected and fed to a pattern recognition circuit which identifies the characteristic signals occurring as the cuff pressure falls past the systolic and diastolic pressures.

Doppler broadening. The broadening of either an emission line or an absorption line due to random motions of molecules of the gas that is emitting or absorbing the radiant energy. In the case of an emitting gas, for example, those molecules which are approaching the observer as they emit quanta of radiant energy will, because of the Doppler effect, appear to send out a train of waves of slightly shorter wavelength than that characteristic of a stationary molecule, while receding molecules will appear to emit slightly longer wavelengths. The net effect, averaged over many molecules, is to superimpose, on the natural line width, a bell-shaped broadening that is proportional to the square root of the absolute temperature of the gas.

Doppler echocardiography. Analysis of intracardiac or intravascular flow by ultrasonic techniques involving the Doppler effect with or without a spatial reference by A-mode, M-mode, two-dimensional imaging, or auditory signals for the localization of the site being sampled.

Doppler effect. The Doppler effect, first described by Christian Johann Doppler in 1843, refers to the change in frequency of a waveform when the source and receiver are moving with respect to each other. This effect is observed with any waveform, including sound waves. Thus, if an observer moves toward a sound source, he will hear a sound with a higher pitch (frequency) than when he is at rest. If he moves away from the source he will hear a sound with a lower frequency. This change in the frequency is also known as the "Doppler shift". A commonly observed example of this phenomenon is the change in the pitch of a siren from an ambulance as it approaches and passes by. In Doppler echocardiography, a hand-held transducer, which emits ultrasound, is placed on the chest. This sound will be reflected from all accoustic interfaces. When the interface is moving (red blood cells), the sound will be reflected with a slightly higher or lower frequency than the transmitted frequency. Conversely, if flow is away from the transducer, the reflected frequency will be lower. Thus, the direction of blood flow can be accurately determined.

Doppler examination modes. Three modes of Doppler examination are currently used: continuous wave, pulsed wave, and color flow imaging. These three modes are complementary. In the pulsed and continuous-wave modes, the Doppler shift is rapidly analyzed and presented to the examiner in two ways: as an audible sound and as a graphic display which can be recorded on paper or videotape. In the graphic display flow toward the transducer is recorded above the zero reference line, while flow away from the transducer is shown below the reference line. The velocity of blood flow is displayed in meters per second (m/s) or centimeters per second (cm/s). The electrocardiogram can be used to time the Doppler signal.

Doppler frequency shift. The difference in frequencies of transmitted and received sound energy. This difference is directly proportional to the velocity of relative motion between the transducer and reflectors and the interrogation frequency. It is inversely proportional to the velocity of sound in the intervening medium.

$$\Delta F = \frac{V \times 2F_0 \times \cos\theta}{\text{velocity of sound}}$$

$$V = \frac{\Delta F \times \text{velocity of sound}}{2F_0 \times \cos\theta}$$

where V = velocity ΔF = frequency shift, F_0 = frequency of interrogation (mHz), and θ = angle of incidence between the direction of motion of the scatters and the direction of interrogation.

Doppler image (D) — mode flow map. A display method in which only areas containing moving targets are displayed. It is a Doppler imaging technique in which the flow information can be shown as an overlay on the image to denote areas with flow. A spatial plot of Doppler flow may be superimposed upon the two-dimensional image with the direction and spectral content of flow shown either by color coding or gray scale overlay and the area of flow denoted by specific overlay on the image itself.

Doppler interrogation frequency. The frequency of the transmitted acoustic energy relative to which a Doppler frequency shift is measured. This frequency is usually, but not necessarily, the nominal transducer frequency.

D-orbital. Electron orbital or wave function which has an orbital angular momentum of 1/2. Electrons in the d-orbital give rise to paramagnetism of transitional metal ions, e.g., 3d electrons in iron group transformation metals.

Dorsal. Pertaining to the back.

Dose. The radiation delivered to the whole human body or to a specified area or volume of the body. A general term denoting the quantity of radiation or energy absorbed in a specified mass. For special purposes, its meaning should be appropriately stated, e.g., absorbed dose. The SI unit of absorbed dose is the gray (Gy). The term is also used loosely for the amount of radioactivity administered. In competitive binding assay, the amount of test substance added to any given reference standard.

Dose commitment. (D_c) The total dose equivalent to a part of the body that will result from retention of radioactive material in the body.

Dose distribution factor. A factor used in computing dose equivalent to account for the nonuniform distribution of internally deposited radionuclides.

Dose equivalent. (H) The absorbed dose multiplied by factors to allow for the different biological effect produced, for equal energy absorption, by different types of radiation as well as other modifying effects. Thus, the dose equivalent H is defined as H $\equiv$ DQN, where D is the absorbed dose, Q is the quality factor, and N is the product of all other modifying factors (currently assigned the value 1). If D is given in J/kg then so is H, since Q is dimensionless. The J/kg has the special name gray (Gy) when applied to absorbed dose, but has the special name sievert (Sv) when applied to dose equivalent. However, the situation is one in which two different quantities (D and H) are stated in terms of the same units.

Dose equivalent index. The absorbed dose index at a point in a field of ionizing radiation is defined as the maximum dose equivalent occurring within a 30-cm-diameter sphere (simulating the body) centered at the point, and consisting of material equivalent to soft tissue with a density of 1 g/cm^3. The preferred unit is the sievert (Sv).

Dose equivalent limit. (DEL) The numerical values recommended by the International Commission of Radiological Protection to be the controlling limits of radiation dose which should not be exceeded by radiation workers or by any maximally exposed group of the general public. The DEL supersedes the MPD (maximum permissible dose).

Dose fractionation. The delivery of the total dose in a number of fractions separated by time intervals. For example, in radiotherapy a course of treatment usually consists of a number of daily treatments extending over a period of up to 6 weeks. In general, the biological effect achieved by a given total dose delivered singly in a short period is greater than that achieved when the same dose is fractionated or protracted.

Dose limits. The recommended dose limits for controlling the exposure of members of the public to ionizing radiations. Generally, the figures recommended for individuals in the population are one tenth of the corresponding maximum permissible doses for workers.

Dose rate. The dose of radiation received per unit of time.

Dose rate meter. An instrument for measuring radiation dose rate. Such instruments commonly comprise an ionization chamber followed by an electrometer valve circuit feeding an output microammeter graduated to read the dose rate in gray per second. Instruments of this type are used for providing detailed information about the radiation intensities in different parts of a laboratory where radioactive materials are handled, or where machines producing ionizing radiations are in use. They may be used in a fixed position (they are then called installed dose rate meters), or they may be portable and used for the measurement of radiation dose rate at a variety of different locations. Instruments of this latter type are often called survey meters.

Dose response curve. Curve indicating percent response to a specified (log) dose or less. The curve may represent an increasing percentage of animals responding to a drug or an increasing magnitude of response within an individual animal or tissue. The graphic relationship between counts bound and amount of standard added in a radioimmunoassay; a standard curve.

Dose threshold. The minimum absorbed dose that will produce a specified effect.

Dose transit. A measure of the primary radiation transmitted through a patient and measured along the central ray at some point beyond the patient.

Dose volume. The product of absorbed dose and the volume of the absorbing mass.

Dosimeter. Instrument used to detect and measure an accumulated dosage of radiation; in common usage it is a pencil-size ionization chamber with a built-in self-reading electrometer; used for personnel monitoring.

Dosimeter charging unit. Condenser pocket ionization or chambers and quartz-fiber electroscopes are used for the measurement of total dose received during a period of time (usually a working day). In order to use these devices the ionization chambers must be charged by connecting the electrodes of the chamber momentarily to a battery, or other source of voltage.

Dosimetry. The measurement of the quantity of radiation absorbed by a substance or a living organism. Instruments used for such measurements are known as dosimeters. In many cases it is not possible to make a direct measurement of the dose and resort must be had to calculation which may range from a simple approximation to the precise computation of isodose curves which is used in radiotherapy.

Dot matrix. An array of dots (often in 7×5 format) forming a number or character symbol. Generated by a dot printer, which can be a computer peripheral.

Dot-matrix printer. A kind of printer whose print head contains a vertical row of pins that points at the paper through an inked ribbon. The printer forms printed characters by striking the paper with the wires through the ribbon as the print head moves across the paper.

Dot scan. A display, on paper, of equidense dots in a manner that reproduces the spatial distribution of radioactivity in the area desired to be visualized.

Double-antibody technique. A technique of recovering bound tracer for measurement of competitive binding assay system wherein the separation agent is antibody, heterologous to the primary binding agent antibody.

Double beta decay. A mode of decay involving the almost simultaneous emission of two beta particles. For certain nuclei containing an even number of protons this is the only form of beta decay energetically possible. The event has not yet been detected experimentally with complete certainty owing to the very long lifetime ($>10^{15}$ years).

Double-blind testing. A clinical trial in which medicaments (one of which may be a placebo) are administered to each of a group of patients and the physician does not know what particular patients have received.

Double compton effect. The production of two scattered quanta as a result of the interaction between a photon and a free electron.

Double label. The use of two tracer species (usually different radioisotopes in an assay system).

Doubling time. The time taken, under given conditions, for the neutron flux, and hence power, of a nuclear reactor to increase by a factor of 2.

Doughnut. A term used in connection with particle accelerators to describe the evacuated ring-shaped chamber in which the particles are made to orbit.

Download. To move code from one computer to another computer's memory for execution of some task via a communication line.

Downtime. Period of time during which an instrument, equipment, or a computer system is not functioning. Scheduled downtime is the time during which the system is not available, not because it has failed, but because it is performing functions such as backup, or because preventive hardware maintenance is being done. Unscheduled downtime: unexpected system failure because of a bug, crash, power failure, or other problem.

Drift. The output of an electric circuit tends to change slowly over a period of time. This is known as drift. Causes of drift include fluctuations in system voltage and changes in environmental conditions.

Drive name. Formally known as a "drive specifier", a drive name is the name of a computer disk drive, used alone or as a prefix to a file specification. For example, in the command copy b: example.txt a: {ENTER}, "b:" and "a:" are drive names.

Driving pressure. The pressure difference between the two ends of any section of a blood vessel.

Dual-head gamma camera. Dual-head gamma cameras have been designed to assist in single-photon emission computed tomography and whole body area scanning. Gamma cameras with dual heads can be used either to decrease imaging times, or conversely to improve quality of images for similar imaging times. The setting-up procedures, however, are more complex.

Dual-in-line package. (DIP) An integrated circuit housed in a protective casing that includes pin connections for plugging chips into a circuit board.

Dual temperature-exchange separation process. A process for the separation of isotopes based on the change in the separation factor of two isotopes in a mixture of two compounds as the temperature is changed.

Dual-use reactor. A reactor from which useful power is produced by utilization of heat from the primary and secondary coolant circuits.

Duct. A passage with well-defined walls or a tube for excretions or secretions.

Dulong and Petit law. The specific heats of the several elements are inversely proportional to their atomic weights. The atomic heats of solid elements are constant and approximately equal to 6.3. Certain elements of low atomic weight and high melting point have, however, much lower atomic heats at ordinary temperatures.

Dumb terminal. A computer terminal that does not possess any intrinsic data processing capability and that acts as a pure input and/or output device.

Dump. An operation in which the contents of a computer's memory are transferred to another memory or to an output device such as a line printer. Dumping clears the memory and stores its data elsewhere.

Dump tank effluent. Dump tanks or delay tanks are used to store radioactive fluids until their activity no longer constitutes a radiation hazard, or until they can be disposed of safely. The effluent from such a tank is usually called the dump tank effluent.

Duplex. A data communications line or device that allows transmission of information in both directions at the same time.

Duplex scanner. An ultrasound scanning system, usually real time, which contains a Doppler transducer in or alongside the scanning head, so that Doppler information may be obtained from a known point in the image.

Dural. Pertaining to the dura mater, the outermost membrane covering the spinal cord.

Duty. (Legal) The obligation to meet the expectations of another as to his person, his possessions, and his actions, such as are recognized by custom, by law, or by agreement. There is no duty unless there is a identifiable person with a right to receive the obligation.

Duty cycle. Ratio of the pulse duration to the pulse repetition time in ultrasound.

Duty factor. Fraction of time that pulsed ultrasound is actually on.

Dwell time. The time between the beginning of sampling one data point and the beginning of sampling of the next successive point in the free induction decay. (FID.) (NMR.)

Dynamic-condenser electrometer. A vibrating-reed electrometer used as a direct-current votage amplifier by converting DC to AC, amplifying the AC voltage and rectifying the amplified voltage back to DC.

Dynamic display. The ratio between the largest and the smallest acceptable signals measured at the input to the display and expressed in decibels. In B-mode, the dynamic range is determined by the smallest signal levels which produce the maximum brightness and a barely detectable spot, respectively.

Dynamic radionuclide image acquisition. A dynamic acquisition is a series of images that are recorded to reflect changes within the radioactive distribution with time. The acquisition may monitor changes in concentration of the radiopharmaceutical, transfer of radioactivity, changes in shape or volume of organs, transient perfusion effects, or the excretion of a radionuclide. For the purpose of clarity it should be noted that, although in emission computer tomography (ECT) and whole body imaging the gamma camera is in motion, the images acquired usually reflect a static distribution. Dynamic studies may follow changes in radioactive distribution in time ranging from seconds to many hours, and introduce an extra dimension into imaging. It is often the case that a dynamic study will be performed in only one projection, and therefore it is important from the outset to identify the view which will yield the best information. The view that gives the least attenuation and hence the maximum detected photon rate should be chosen. A dynamic acquisition can be recorded either as a series of analog or digital images. With analog images and the use of electronic format devices a sequence of images can be generated on a single film, the number and size of images being interrelated.

Dynamic range. Refers to the range of values over which image information is stored or displayed. In conventional radiographic imaging, it refers to the maximum minus minimum detectable radiation exposure. For a digital system, the range of radiation exposures that may be recorded is limited by the number of bits used to store the information. Expressed in decibels, the dynamic range of an ultrasound amplifier is specified as the ratio of the maximum input signal which can be processed without reaching saturation to the smallest input signal which can be identified above the noise levels.

Dynamic response. A measure of output/input ratio as a function of signal frequency for a system.

Dynamic stabilization. A superconductor-stabilizer configuration where normal transitions of the superconductor briefly divert a portion of the current to the stabilizer, followed by complete recovery of superconductivity.

Dyne. The unit of force that, when acting upon a mass of 1 g, will produce an acceleration of 1 cm/s.

Dynode. An electrode in a photomultiplier tube that undergoes secondary emission upon bombardment by electrons.

Dysarthria. Speech impairment, e.g., stammering or stuttering, caused by disease of the central nervous system.

Dyskinesis. Impairment of motor function or activity.

Dysphagia. Inability to swallow or difficulty in swallowing.

Dysplasia. An abnormal development of tissue in the body.

Dyspnea. Labored breathing; breathing is difficult and conscious effort is involved.

Dyspraxia. An impairment of the ability to perform coordinated movements.

Dysprosium. Element symbol Dy, atomic number 66, atomic weight 162.50.

Dysrhythmia. Disordered rhythm, especially of heart beats.

Dystrophia. Dystrophy, defective or faulty function; muscular dystrophy, degeneration of muscle structure, sometimes hereditary.

Dysuria. Pain upon irination.

E

Ecchymosis. A form of macula appearing in large, irregularly formed hemorrhagic areas of the skin.

Echo. Acoustic energy received from scattering elements or a specular reflector.

Echocardiography. Examination of the heart by diagnostic ultrasound, principally using M-mode and real-time cross-sectional displays. An ultrasonic record of the dimension and movement of the heart and its valves.

Echogenic. Pertains to properties of a structure or medium (e.g., tissue) that produce echoes, in contrast to a structure or medium that is free of echo-producing properties. Commonly used to infer the production of excessively high amplitude echoes.

Echography. The use of ultrasound to obtain diagnostic images. Strictly speaking, should be restricted to B-scan images.

Echolucent. Transonic and echo free.

Echo planar imaging. A technique of planar imaging in which a complete planar image is obtained from one selective excitation pulse. The free induction decay (FID) is observed while periodically switching the y-gradient field in the presence of a static x-gradient field. The Fourier transform of the resulting spin echo train can be used to produce an image of the excited plane. (NMR.)

Echo poor. A term used to describe a tissue that produces unusually low amplitude echoes.

Echo time. Period between the 90° pulse and the peak of the echo in either a spin echo sequence of inversion recovery sequence employing the 180° rephasing pulse. The period between the 90° and 180° pulses is half TE. (NMR.)

Ectoderm. The outermost of three primary germ layers of the embryo; origin of epidermis, nails, hair, glands, nervous system, ear, and membranes of mouth and anus.

Ectopic. Located away from the normal position.

Ectopic beat. A contraction of the heart originating at some point in the heart other than the sinoatrial node. Also known as extrasystole.

Eddy currents. Electric currents induced in a conductor by a changing magnetic field or by motion of the conductor through a magnetic field. One of the sources of concern about potential hazard to subjects in very high magnetic fields or rapidly varying gradient or main magnetic fields. Can be a practical problem in the cryostat of superconducting magnets.

Edema. An excessive accumulation of fluid in the intracellular tissue spaces of the body due to a disturbance in the fluid-exchanging mechanism.

Edetic acid. (erhylenediaminetetraacetic acid, EDTA) Chelating agent.

Edge effect. Loss of resolution and sensitivity near the boundaries of the field of view of a scintillation imaging system.

Edit. To arrange and/or modify the format of alphanumeric data; for example, to insert or delete characters.

Editor. A program that allows the user to enter text into the computer and edit it. Editors are language independent and will edit anything in character representation.

Effective atomic number. For a material containing two or more elements, it is the number that replaces the atomic number in the calculation of the interaction of that material with a given radiation.

Effective cutoff energy. For a specific absorbing cover surrounding a given detector in a given experimental configuration, that energy value which satisfies the condition that if the cover were replaced by a hypothetical cover back to neutrons with energy below this value and transparent to neutrons with energy above this value, the observed detector response would be unchanged. (The specific value depends on the geometry and thickness of the cover, the geometry and thickness of the absorbing sample, the nature of the energy variation of the cross section of the sample, and the neutron velocity distribution.)

Effective half-life. (T_e) Time required for an administered dose to be reduced to one half due to both physical decay and biologic elimination of a radionuclide. It is given by $T_e = (T_p \times T_b)/(T_p + T_b)$, where T_e is the effective half-life, and T_p and T_b are the physical and biologic half-lives, respectively.

Effective neutron cycle time. The lifetime of an average neutron within a reactor from the time it is produced to the time it is fission captured. This average takes into account delayed as well as prompt neutrons.

Effective reflecting area. The area of a reflector from which sound is received by a transducer.

Effective relaxation length. The distance within a material in which the radiation intensity is reduced to l/e of its initial value. This term includes geometric effects.

Effective resolution. The lateral resolution of the sound beam at a given power threshold level. Greater input powers and lower thresholds give poorer resolution.

Effective wavelength. Wavelength of monochromatic X-rays which would undergo the same percentage attenuation in a specified filter as the heterogeneous beam under consideration.

Effector cells. A term that usually denotes T cells capable of mediating cytotoxicity suppression or helper function.

Effector nerves. Nerves which effect the functioning of muscles and glands.

Efferent. Conducting impulses from the central nervous system to the periphery; motor output. Conveying away from a center.

Efficiency. The percentage of decay events from a standard sample that are seen and stored by the multichannel analyzer (MCA) system. Used to calibrate the MCA system for quantitative analyses. Also used to specify germanium detectors, here being the relative efficiency of the germanium detector when compared to a standard NaI(T1) detector. (Counters): A measure of the probability that a count will be recorded when radiation is incident on a detector. Usage varies considerably so that it is well to make sure which factors (window transmission, sensitive volume, energy dependence, etc.) are included in a given case.

Effluent monitor. An equipment for measuring radioactivity of fluids, either liquid or gaseous. They may be either recirculating or flowing out from a plant for disposal.

Effusion. Escape of fluid into a part, as the pleural cavity, such as pyothorax (pus), hydrothorax (serum), hemathorax (blood), chylothorax (lymph), pneumothorax (air), hydropneumothorax (serum and air), and pyopneumothorax (pus and air).

Einsteinium. Element symbol Es, atomic number 99, atomic weight ~252.

Einstein's mass-energy equation. $E = mc^2$, which quantitatively relates the equivalence of mass and energy and can be used to calculate how much energy (E) is released in a nuclear reaction (e.g., fission) from the loss of mass (m) which occurs (c = velocity of light).

Einthoven's triangle. A hypothetical triangle in the frontal plane of the body, used in electrocardiography to describe the cardiac vector. The three apices of the triangle represent the right arm, the left leg, and the left arm.

Ejection fraction. A measure of the ability of the left ventricle to expel blood. The ejection fraction equals the stroke volume divided by the end-diastolic volume. A normal left ventricular ejection (LVEF) fraction is approximately 0.67, a value that indicates that the left ventricle can expel two thirds of its volume into the aorta with each contraction. The ejection fraction falls with the onset of heart fail-

ure, and it may reach as low as 0.10 in the more severe cases.

EKG (ECG) trigger. A method to initiate the start of data acquisition using the patient's electrocardiogram as the synchronizer.

Elastance. Reciprocal of the compliance.

Elastic collision. A collision between two particles is described as an elastic collision if neither of the particles absorb energy internally. Although either of the particles may gain or lose energy during the collision, the sum of the kinetic energies of the participating particles remains unchanged as a result of the collision.

Elastic cross section. A cross section which is a measure of the probability for the occurrence of a particular elastic scattering process. The differential cross section expresses the probability that a particle will be elastically scattered into unit solid angle about a particular direction.

Elasticity. The property by virtue of which a body resists and recovers from deformation produced by force.

Elastic scattering. Scattering effected through the agency of elastic collisions and therefore with conservation of kinetic energy of the system.

Elastic tissue. A type of connective tissue, containing elastic fibers.

Electrical activity. The initiation and transmission of impulses by the heart's intrinsic electrical system that prepares the heart to contract.

Electrical charge. Quantity of electricity.

Electrical pulse. A brief excursion of electrical voltage from its normal value.

Electric dipole. A pair of equal and opposite charges an infinitesimal distance apart.

Electrocardiogram. (ECG or EKG) A graph, recorded over time, of variations in voltage produced by the heart during different phases of the cardiac cycle; the record of the heart's electrical activity.

Electrocardiograph. An instrument used for the measurement of the electrical activity of the heart.

Electrocautery. The application of a wire loop, heated by an electric current, to living tissue, in order to destroy the tissue or seal bleeding vessels.

Electrochemical process. Chemical process involving oxidation and reduction of the reaction constituents.

Electrode. The positive (+, anode) or negative (–, cathode) terminal of an electrical system. To record the ECG, EEG, EMG, etc. electrodes must be used as transducers to convert an ionic flow of current in the body to an electronic flow along a wire. These are usually made of metal. Two important characteristics of electrodes are electrode potential and contact impedance. Good electrodes will have low stable figures for both of the above characteristics. Electrode potential arises because a metal electrode in contact with an electrolyte (body fluids) forms a half-cell with a potential dependent upon the metal in use and the ions in the electrolyte. The most widely used electrodes for biomedical applications are silver electrodes which have been coated with silver chloride by electrolyzing them for a short time in a sodium chloride solution. When chlorided the surface is black and has a very large surface area. A pair of such electrodes might have a combined electrode potential below 5 mV. Many types of recording electrodes exist including metal disks, needles, suction electrodes, glass microelectrodes, fetal scalp clips or screws. etc. Electrodes are also used to inject electricity into the body as in faradism, surgical diathermy, and physiotherapy diathermy.

Electroencephalogram. (EEG) A record of the electrical activity of the brain. Used for recognition of certain patterns, frequency analysis, evoked potentials, and so on. Measured with surface electrodes on the scalp and with needle electrodes just beneath the surface or driven into specific locations within the brain.

Electroencephalograph. An instrument for measuring and recording electrical activity from the brain (brain waves).

Electrogastrogram. A record of muscle potentials associated with motility of the gastrointestinal tract.

Electroimmunodiffusion. (Counterimmunoelectrophoresis) An immunodiffusion technique in which antigen and antibody are driven toward each other in an electrical field and then precipitate.

Electrolysis. If a current, i, flows for a time, t, and deposits a metal whose electrochemical equivalent is e, the mass, m, of metal deposited is m = eit. The value of e is usually given for mass in grams, i in amperes, and t in seconds.

Electrolyte. A substance that dissociates into ions in solution, and thus becomes capable of conducting electricity. For example, sodium chloride (NaCl) dissociates into Na^+ and Cl^- in solution.

Electrolytic capacitor. A basic component that stores electricity, usually for the purpose of timing, filtering, or coupling electrical signals.

Electrolytic dissociation or ionization theory.

When an acid, base, or salt is dissolved in water or any other dissociating solvent, a part or all of the molecules of the dissolved substance are broken up into parts called ions, some of which are charged with positive electricity and are called cations, and an equivalent number of which are charged with negative electricity and are called anions.

Electrolytic reactions. Oxidation-reduction reactions.

Electromagnet. A type of magnet which is energized by electrical power.

Electromagnetic radiation. Electrical and magnetic energy in the form of waves of energy called photons traveling through space at the speed of light; the spectrum of electromagnetic radiation ranges from long-wavelength, low-energy radio waves to very high-energy, short-wavelength X-rays and γ-rays.

Electromagnetic separation process. A process for separating isotopes that utilizes their behavior in an electromagnetic field.

Electromagnetic spectrum. The ordered array of known electromagnetic radiations, extending from the shortest cosmic rays, through γ-rays, X-rays, ultraviolet radiation, visible radiation, infrared radiation, and including microwave and all other wavelengths of radio energy. The division of this continuum of wavelengths (or frequencies) into a number of named subportions is rather arbitrary and, with one or two exceptions, the boundaries of the several subportions are only vaguely defined. Nevertheless, to each of the commonly identified subportions there correspond characteristic types of physical systems capable of emitting radiation of those wavelengths. Thus, γ-rays are emitted from the nuclei of atoms as they undergo any of several types of nuclear rearrangements; visible light is emitted, for the most part, by atoms whose planetary electrons are undergoing transitions to lower energy states; infrared radiations are associated with characteristic molecular vibrations and rotations; and radio waves, broadly speaking, are emitted by virtue of the accelerations of free electrons as, for example, the moving electrons in a radio antenna wire.

Electrometer. Electrostatic instrument for measuring the difference in potential between two points. Used to measure change of electric potential of charged electrodes resulting from ionization produced by radiation.

Electromotive force. (EMF) Potential difference across electrodes tending to produce an electric current.

Electromyogram. (EMG) A record of muscle potentials, usually from skeletal muscle. Electrical potentials: 50 µV to 1 mV peak amplitude. Required frequency response: 10 to 300 Hz. Used as indicator of muscle action, for measuring fatigue, and so on. Measured with surface electrodes or needle electrodes penetrating the muscle fibers.

Electromyography. The technique of recording the action potentials generated by muscle as a result of either voluntary muscular contraction or spontaneous muscle-fiber activity, or in response to stimulation of the nerve supplying the muscle.

Electron. A fundamental particle with negative charge constituent of all atoms. Electrons take up most of the volume of the atom but little of the mass. The mass of the electron is 9.11×10^{-28} g.

The term electron is also used collectively to include both the negative particle, also called negatron or negaton, and the positive particle of equal mass and charge, the positron or position. Both types may be emitted in β decay but the lifetime of the positron is very short. The electrons in an atom occur in bound states around the central nucleus known as shells, denoted by the letters K, L, M, N, etc., corresponding to the quantum numbers n = 1, 2, 3, 4, etc., the total number of electrons permitted in each shell by the Pauli exclusion principle being $2n^2$ (i.e., 2 in the K shell, 8 in the L shell, etc). The number of electrons is determined by the nuclear charge which it must neutralize and the electrons normally fill the shells from the lowest quantum number upwards. The electrons in the outer shell determine the chemical behavior of the atom. Beta particles, positrons, Auger, and internal conversion electrons have a range in tissue from a few micrometers to a few millimeters. However, the electron, in losing energy, follows a tortuous path and the mean range is typically a fifth of the maximum range. Energy losses are principally by excitation and ionization, but the interaction is less strong than for α particles because of the much smaller mass and single electronic charge. For example, a 1-MeV β-particle creates about 20 ion pairs per millimeter at the start of its track and has linear energy transfer of 0.25 keV mm^{-1}.

Electron accelerators. Machine used to accelerate electrons using potential differences.

Electron-beam therapy. The treatment of deep-seated malignant tumors by beams of electrons.

Electron capture. Radioactive transformation in which an inner orbital electron is captured by an atom's nucleus. The capture of an electron by the nucleus leaves a vacancy in one of the inner electron shells. As a result the product atom, and not the nucleus, has an energy above the ground state. This excess energy is lost either by the emission of the characteristic X radiation of the daughter, or by the transfer of the excess energy to an outer electron, thereby ejecting it as an Auger electron. The X-rays and Auger electron have much lower energies than the particle emissions since the former result from extranuclear processes and the latter from intranuclear processes. Electron capture is more likely to occur than positron decay for nuclides with high Z in which the K shell is closer to the nucleus. Positron decay will be predominant at low Z provided there is an energy difference of at least 1.02 MeV between the parent and daughter nuclides.

Electron configuration. Refers to the space relationships of electrons in an atom.

Electron density. The number of electrons per unit volume, at some point in space (for example, near the nucleus of an atom).

Electronegativity. Tendency of a neutral atom to acquire electrons, measured relative to that of fluorine.

Electron gun. A device, consisting of a heated cathode focusing electrodes and an anode, which produces a beam of electrons suitable for injection into a high-energy accelerator. A similar device is used to produce a focused beam in the conventional cathode ray tube.

Electronic structure. Structure of the orbital electrons in an atom that satisfies the quantum mechanical Schrödinger equation.

Electron microprobe analysis. A technique used to determine the concentration of chemical elements within microscopic regions of a specimen. A finely focused beam of electrons is directed onto the sample and the X-rays generated within the region are analyzed spectroscopically. Also known as X-ray microanalysis.

Electron microscope. A microscope in which visible light is replaced by a beam of electrons, electric or magnetic lenses being substituted for the optical ones. The electron lenses contain shaped electric or magnetic fields which deflect the electronic rays in such a manner as to focus the electrons and produce an enlarged image of a specimen which is placed at an appropriate point in the beam. The image is rendered visible by the use of a fluorescent screen which emits visible light under electronic bombardment, and so converts the electronic image into a visible one.

Electron-multiplier tube. A device by which small light flashes (photons) are amplified electronically by a cascade process employing secondary emission of electrons. This device detects and amplifies the scintillations produced by the interactions of γ-rays and the crystal in a scanner. Also called a photomultiplier tube.

Electron positron pair. The formation of an electron and a positron (or generally of a particle and its antiparticle, which is then designated pair production) through the interaction of a photon or a fast particle with the field of an atomic nucleus or other particles, or through de-excitation of an excited nucleus.

Electron shell. A set of atomic energy levels with approximately equal energies, denoted by the letters K, L, M, N, etc.

Electron spin-echo spectroscopy. Technique exactly similar to nuclear spin-echo spectroscopy except that one observes electron spin echoes. In this technique, pairs of microwave pulses of high strength are applied to the electron spins in a paramagnetic sample in the same way as in a nuclear spin-echo experiment and an electon spin echo is observed. (NMR.)

Electron spin-lattice relaxation time (T_1). The characteristic time constant taken by the electron spins to reach thermal equilibrium through interaction with the fluctuating local electrical fields surrounding these spins (lattice). (NMR.)

Electron spin resonance. (ESR) Spectroscopic technique that determines structural features of a molecule based on electron resonance in a magnetic field.

Electron spin-spin relaxation time (T_2). The characteristic time constant taken by the electron spins to lose phase coherence, i.e., return to the equilibrium value through interaction with neighboring spins in an electron spin resonance (ESR) experiment. It is inversely related to the line widths of the resonance and its origin is similar to the "uncertainty broadening" observed in other forms of spectroscopy. (NMR.)

Electron transfer. The transfer of electrons from a lower oxidation state of an element to a higher oxidation state. The exchange of one or more electrons between an ion and a neutral molecule or atom.

Electronvolt. (eV) A unit of energy equivalent to the amount of energy gained by an electron in passing through a potential difference of 1 V. Larger multiple units of the electronvolt are frequently used, viz, keV for thousand or kilo-

electronvolts; MeV for million or megaelectronvolts. 1 eV = 1.602×10^{-19} J. The joule (J) is the SI unit of energy.

Electrooculogram. A record of corneal-retinal potentials associated with eye movements.

Electroosmosis. The movement of liquid through a semipermeable membrane due to a difference in the electric potentials of liquids on opposite sides of the membrane. The converse of streaming potential.

Electrophoresis. A process by which different kinds of organic molecules in a solution are separated from each other when an electric potential is applied across the solution. Electrophoresis utilizes the property of ions to move under the influence of an electric charge. Components of a sample will move at different rates along a strip of paper or gel medium according to their charge and ionic mobility. As such, this technique finds use in a number of applications such as the determination of radioactive iodide in iodopharmaceuticals. The electrophoretograms are measured in the same manner as thin-layer and paper chromatograms.

Electrophoretic effect. The slowing down owing to interionic attraction and repulsion, of the movement of an ion with its solvent molecules in the forward direction by ions of opposite charge with their solvent molecules moving in the reverse direction under an applied electrical field (potential gradient).

Electrophysiology. The science of physiology in its relations to electricity; the study of the electric reactions of the body in health.

Electroretinogram. A record of potentials from the retina.

Electroscope. Instrument for detecting the presence of electric charges by the deflection of charged bodies. If an insulated conductor with an attached light-flexible member (e.g., a gold leaf) is charged, then this member will move away from the conductor under the mutual coulomb repulsion of the shared charge and will reach equilibrium under electrostatic and gravitational forces. The charge is reduced if the air near the leaf is ionized and the leaf then moves toward the conductor. The rate at which the leaf moves is proportional to the rate of production of ions.

Electrostatic field. The region surrounding an electric charge in which another electric charge experiences a force.

Electrostatic unit. In the cgs system, the measure of electrostatic charge, defined as a charge which, if concentrated at one point in a vacuum, would repel, with a force of 1 dyn, and equal a like charge placed 1 cm away. A system of electrical units based on the electrostatic unit.

Electrosurgery. A surgical technique that uses high-frequency, high-density currents to cut tissue and/or coagulate blood. The technique is also known as surgical diathermy.

Element. Pure substance, consisting of atoms of the same atomic number, that cannot be decomposed by ordinary chemical methods, e.g., hydrogen.

Elemental composition. The composition of a mixture or compound expressed in terms of the constituent elements.

Elementary particles. Particles which are believed to be the basic "building bricks" of all matter. Over 200 are known; the majority have only very short lives before they decay or are annihilated.

Elution. A method of extraction of an adsorbed substance from a solid adsorbing matter (such as ion-exchange resin) with a liquid. Elutriation.

Embolism. Blocking of a blood vessel by a clot or air bubbles that have been transported through the blood.

Embolus. A relatively large blood clot released from a blood vessel and lodged in a smaller vessel so as to obstruct blood circulation. An embolus can also be an abnormal particle of air or fat disrupting blood flow.

Embryo. A human or animal offspring prior to emergence from the womb or egg; hence, a beginning or undeveloped stage of anything.

Emergency dose. The absorbed dose, when the maximum permissible dose equivalent is exceeded, knowingly incurred in the performance of an unusual task to protect individuals or valuable property.

Emergency shutdown. The act of shutting down a reactor suddenly to prevent or minimize a dangerous condition.

Emesis. Vomiting.

Emission. The process in which photons from any particular radionuclide leave the place in which the radionuclide is deposited.

Emission computed tomography. (ECT) Tomographic projections are nothing more than a series of planar images taken at different angles around the patient. These images are then backprojected into transaxial images. The transaxial images can then be reoriented to produce sagittal, coronal, or oblique angle images. As with planar images, tomographic projection data include a certain amount of noise. This noise, however, is amplified in the backprojection

technique and causes the resultant transaxial information to appear different from the radioactive distribution being studied. More specifically, the goal of tomographic reconstruction is to provide a blur-corrected transaxial tomogram from processed planar projections. The solution to this problem in frequency space involves the application of filters to the frequency components of each projection. Once filtered, each projection is transformed back into the conventional spatial domain and then backprojected to form the blur-corrected transaxial tomograms. Positron emission tomography (PET) is a specialized area of research which uses banks of detectors or two opposing detectors to record the annihilation photons from the positron-electron interaction. Annihilation photon counting systems make use of the two 511-keV γ-rays traveling in exactly opposite directions which result from positron-electron annihilation interactions. If these two γ-rays are detected simultaneously, in coincidence, by two detectors, then the point of origin of the γ-rays must be on a line joining the two detectors. The activity along a series of lines through a slice can therefore be determined using a set of coincidence detectors. At present development of PET has been limited to centers with on-site cyclotrons, and has been of great importance in the research of physiological processes, particularly metabolic activity in the heart and brain. Single photon emission computed tomography (SPECT) has developed in many centers with the use of rotating gamma cameras and other methods exist to reconstruct images using either slant hole or multipinhole collimators. Scanners can be used to traverse focused detectors across a patient. The detectors are then rotated through a small angle and traversed again. This process is repeated until all directions and positions have been covered. The effect can also be achieved by causing a γ camera to rotate around a patient. This has the advantage that emission data are gathered simultaneously from a set of slices.

Emission rate. Of a given radiation source, the number of particles of given type and energy leaving the source per unit time.

Emission spectrum. The array of wavelengths are relative intensities of electromagnetic radiation emitted by a given radiator. Each radiating substance has a unique, characteristic emission spectrum, just as every medium of transmission has its individual absorption spectrum.

Emphysema. A chronic condition characterized by loss of lung elasticity, collapse of the terminal bronchioles, and production of a thick, viscous mucus. Distension of the lungs due to the presence of air in the intraalveolar tissue.

Empirical. Based on experience, not theory.

Empirical formula. Chemical formula that reflects only the simplest molar ratio of the elements in the compound, not the actual molar ratio.

Emulator. A hardware device or software program that permits a program written for a specific computer system to be run on a different type of computer system.

Emulsion.   Mixture of two liquids, one suspended within another; colloid system; suspended mixture where one of the components is gelatin-like.

(Photographic) A suspension of a sensitive silver salt of mixture of silver halides in a viscous medium (as a gelatin solution) forming a coating on photographic plates, film, or paper. (Nuclear) A photographic emulsion specially designed to permit observation of the individual tracks of ionizing particles.

Enabled. A condition that allows the computer central processing unit (CPU) to be started.

Encapsulation. A quasi-immunologic phenomenon in which foreign material is walled off within the tissues of invertebrates.

Encephalopathy. Disease of the brain, the cause of which may be vascular or degenerative or due to local disease of the cerebrum.

Echoencephalography. Examination of the brain by diagnositc ultrasound, principally by using A-mode.

Encoding. Sometimes it is easier to process data if they are prepared for machine handling by converting the English names of diseases to codes. This process is called encoding.

End-diastolic volume. A value representing the amount of blood in the left ventricle just prior to contraction. With the onset of heart failure, end-diastolic volume increases as the ventricle dilates. End-diastolic volume is an index of preload.

Endocarditis. Inflammation of the endothelial lining of the heart, caused by either microbial infection or by a generalized inflammatory disorder.

Endocardium. A thin, smooth membrane forming the inner surface of the heart.

Endocrine.   Internal secretion; pertaining to ductless glands that secrete substances (hormones) directly into the bloodstream.

Endocrinology.   Study of hormonal secretion and of the endocrine glands.

Endocytosis. The process whereby material external to a cell is internalized within a particular cell. It consists of pinocytosis and phagocytosis.

Endodermal cells. Cells forming the inner germ layer of the embryo (the endoderm). They give rise to the epithelial cells of the digestive tract and its outgrowths — the lungs, liver, and pancreas.

Endoergic. A term usually employed in connection with endoergic processes, which are nuclear processes in which energy is consumed.

Endogenous. Produced within or as a result of internal causes; applied to the formation of cells or of spores within the parent cell.

Endometrium. Mucous membrane lining the uterus.

Endoplasmic reticulum. A system of membranes present in many types of cells extending outward through large regions of cytoplasm from the cell's nuclear envelope to the cell membrane. One of its main functions is to transport proteins, complex lipids, and polysaccharides to their sites of utilization or storage.

Endoscope. Instrument, tubular in nature, carrying an illumination source (fiber optics), inserted into a body cavity to permit visual inspection.

Endoscopy. Visual examination of the interior of a hollow organ of the body by the insertion of an illuminating instrument, usually through a natural channel.

Endosteum. Membrane lining of a hollow bone.

Endothelium. A form of squamous epithelium consisting of flat cells that line the blood and lymphatic vessels, the heart, and various body cavities. It is derived from mesoderm.

Endothermic reaction. Reaction which absorbs energy specifically in the form of heat.

Endotoxin. Lipopolysaccharides that are derived from the cell walls of Gram-negative microorganisms and have toxic and pyrogenic effects when injected *in vivo*.

End product. The end product of a radioactive series is the stable nuclide which is its final member.

Energy. The capacity to do work. Potential energy is the energy inherent in mass because of its position with reference to other masses. Kinetic energy is the energy possessed by mass because of its motion. Nuclear energy results from the equivalence of mass and energy according to the relationship stated by Einstein, $E = mc^2$.

Energy dependence. The characteristic response

of a radiation detector to a given range of radiation energies or wavelengths as compared with the response of a standard free air chamber.

Energy deposition. A term commonly used in radiation chemistry and physics. When a solid, liquid, or gas is irradiated it may absorb energy by interaction with the incident radiation; this process is described as energy deposition, which is conveniently expressed in milliwatts per gram of material.

Energy dissipation. Energy existing in an organized form, such as mechanical motion or the kinetic energy of a beam of particles, is said to be dissipated when it is converted to heat (degraded) and removed from the system.

Energy fluence. The quotient dE_f/dA where dE_f is the sum of the energies, exclusive of rest energies, of all the particles which enter a sphere of cross-sectional area dA.

Energy flux density. The quotient dF/dt where dF is the energy fluence in time dt.

Energy imparted to matter. The difference between the sum of the energies of all the ionizing particles or photons which have entered a volume and the sum of the energy equivalent of any increase in rest mass that took place in nuclear or elementary particle reactions within the volume. It is identical with the integral absorbed dose in the volume.

Energy level. The stable energy states that an atom or molecule can take up or the nuclear or electron spins take up in the presence of the applied magnetic field. The lowest energy states are occupied while the higher energy states are partially occupied. Only discrete sets of energy levels exist according to quantum mechanical principles.

Energy-range relation. The relation between the range of a particle in a specified material and its kinetic energy.

Energy resolution. The ability of the detector to discriminate between photons of adjacent energies.

Energy transferred. The kinetic energy received by charged particles in a specified finite volume, regardless of where or how they in turn spend that energy.

Enhancement. Improved survival of tumor cells in animals that have been previously immunized to the antigens of a given tumor. Increase in ultrasound relection amplitude from reflectors that lie behind a weakly attenuating structure.

Enrich. To increase the abundance of a particular isotope in a mixture of the isotopes of an element.

Enriched material. Material containing an element in which the abundance of one of the isotopes has been increased above that found in the naturally occurring material. It is commonly used to describe uranium or uranium compounds containing more than the natural ratio of ^{235}U. Also called enriched fuel.

Enrichment factor. The ratio proportion or the fraction of atoms of a particular isotope (expressed as a percentage) in a mixture enriched in that isotope, to the fraction of atoms of that isotope in a mixture of natural composition.

Enter key. Key on the computer's keyboard. It is also called the "return key", since its function resembles that of a typewriter's carriage return key.

Entrainment. The suspension of liquid droplets, gas bubbles of fine solid particles being carried by stream of fluid.

Entropy. A measure of the extent to which the energy of a system is unavailable. A mathematically defined thermodynamic function of state, the increase in which gives a measure of the energy of a system which has ceased to be available for work during a certain process.

$$ds = (du + pdv)/T \geq dq/T$$

where s is specific entropy, us is specific internal energy, p is pressure, v is specific volume, T is Kelvin temperature, and q is heat per unit mass. For reversible processes,

$$ds = dq/T$$

in terms of potential temperature 0,

$$ds = c_p(d\theta/\theta)$$

where cp is the specific heat at constant pressure.

In an adiabatic process, the entropy increases if the process is irreversible and remains unchanged if the process is reversible. Thus, since all natural processes are irreversible, it is said that in an isolated system the entropy is always increasing as the system tends toward equilibrium, a statement which may be considered a form of the second law of thermodynamics. In communication theory, average information content.

Envelope. A waveform which connects the relative maxima on the absolute value of the instantaneous acoustic pressure waveform.

Environment string. A string of text in the environment that contains a piece of information for a particular computer program.

Enzyme. An organic compound, frequently a protein, that accelerates (catalyzes) specific transformations of material as in the digestion of foods.

Eosinophil chemotactic factor. (ECF) A lymphokine which is chemotactic for eosinophils.

Eosinophils. Circulating granulocytes characterized by large eosinophilic cytoplasmic granules; they migrate to sites of anaphylactic reactions where they release histaminase and prostaglandins that modulate mast cell degranulation. Eosinophils kill certain animal parasites by a C-unrelated antibody-dependent contact mechanism.

Epidemiology. The science dealing with the factors which determine the frequency and distribution of a disease in a human community.

Epidermis. The outermost layer of cells of the skin.

Epigastrium. Space in the abdomen just below the ribs, over the stomach.

Epilation. The removal of hair by the roots. If the hair follicles are destroyed in the process, regrowth cannot take place.

Epilepsy. A disorder of the brain, resulting from excessive or disordered discharge of cerebral neurons. It is characterized by transient, uncontrollable episodes of abnormal mental or neurological function, or both, usually with clouding of consciousness.

Epinephrine. One of the important hormones, made chiefly in the adrenal gland, required for function of the symphathetic nervous system. Adrenaline.

Epiphysis. Wide end of long bones just before the joint; usual region of growth.

Epithelium. Tissue covering the internal and external surfaces of the body, including the lining of vessels, hollow organs, ducts, and respiratory passages.

Epithermal. Having energy just above the energy of thermal agitation and comparable with chemical bond energies. Epithermal neutrons have speeds and energies intermediate between those of fast and thermal ones.

Equilibration. The process of establishing isotopic homogeneity throughout a system in which allobars have been mixed. Equilibration is also used to denote the process of establishing equilibria between phases, for example, between vapor and liquid in a fractional distillation column, and especially of a solute between two liquid phases.

Equilibrium. The stage in a reaction where the concentration of the reactive species is no longer changing.

(Chemical) A condition in which a chemical reaction and its reverse reaction are taking place at equal velocities, so that the concentrations of reacting substances remain constant.

Equilibrium absorbed dose constant. The energy emitted per disintegration in the form of i-type radiation; it is denoted by Δ_i.

Equilibrium constant. True constant that relates the concentration of products and reactants in a reversible chemical system when no further net change is occurring in those concentrations.

Equilibrium dialysis. A technique for measuring the strength or affinity with which antibody binds to antigen.

Equilibrium time. The time required for the mole fraction at each separation stage of a cascade to reach 99.9% of its asymptotic value.

Equivalence. A ratio of antigen-antibody concentration where maximal precipitation occurs.

Equivalent. Weight of a chemical species that contains either 1 mol of electrons and 1 mol of replaceable hydrogen, or combines with exactly 8 g of oxygen.

Equivalent activity. Of a radiation source, the activity of a point source of the same radionuclide which will give the same exposure rate at the same distance from the center of the source.

Equivalent residual dose. (ERD) The accumulated dose corrected or such physiological recovery as has occurred at a specific time. It is based on the ability of the body to recover to some degree from radiation injury following exposure. It is used only to predict immediate effects.

Equivalent square beam. Or equivalent field. A radiation beam that has a square beam profile and gives the same values of percentage depth dose, tissue/air ratio, tissue/maximum ratio, or tissue/phantom ratio as a given rectangular, circular, or irregular beam profile of the same radiation spectrum.

Erasable programmable read-only memory. (EPROM) A memory chip that can be reprogrammed after exposure to ultraviolet light; often used for circuit design, rather than routine computer application.

Erbium. Element symbol Er, atomic number 68, atomic weight 167.26.

Erg. A unit of energy corresponding to the work that is done when a force of 1 dyn produces a displacement of 1 cm in the direction of the force.

Ergometer. Instrument used for measuring energy expended.

Ergonomics. The study of how the properties of the human body and mind affect the design of tools and equipment used in work.

Erythema. An abnormal redness of the skin due to congestion of the capillaries with blood. It can be caused by many different agents; e.g., heat, certain drugs, ultraviolet rays, ionizing radiation.

Erythroblast. Immature red blood cell in the red bone marrow giving origin to erythrocytes.

Erythrocyte. The blood cell whose oxygen-carrying pigment, hemoglobin, is responsible for the red color of fresh blood; thus also called red blood cell.

Erythrocytosis. Increase in red blood cells from a known stimulant.

Erythropoiesis. The production of red blood cells by red bone marrow.

Erythropoietin. A hormone produced by the kidney that stimulates erythropoiesis.

ESC key. A key on the computer's keyboard labeled "ESC". It is pronounced "escape". Many application programs let you use ESC to escape from an error condition or to change the program from one mode of operation to another.

Esophagus. The canal which runs from the pharnyx to the stomach, along which food passes.

Esters. Organic compound formed by the action of an acid with an alcohol; contains the functional group

$$\begin{matrix} & \text{O} \\ & \| \\ -\text{C} & -\text{O} - \text{C} - \end{matrix}$$

Estimated maximum heart rate. The calculated rate determined by subtracting one's age from 220.

Estimated radiation dose. The amount of absorbed radiation energy frequently cannot be determined precisely in any one patient study but can be predicted or "estimated" rather accurately.

Estrogen. A female sex hormone secreted by the ovaries.

Etiology. The study of the cause or origin of disease or disorder.

Euglobulin. A class of globulin proteins that are insoluble in water but soluble in salt solutions.

Eupnea. Normal, quiet breathing.

Euratom. The European Atomic Energy community set up by the Rome Treaty of 1957.

Europium. Element symbol Eu, atomic number 63, atomic weight 151.96.

Eustachian tube. The passage connecting the ear to the throat, serving to equalize the pressure on either side of the tympanic membrane.

Euthyroidism. A condition in which the thyroid gland is functioning normally.

Evaporative centrifuge. One of the three methods of using a centrifuge for separating mixtures of isotopes. In the evaporation centrifuge the mixture to be separated is in the liquid phase at the periphery of the centrifuge. The vapors are removed from a point near the axis of the centrifuge, having been separated by diffusion through the centrifuge field.

Even-even nuclei. Nuclei containing an even number of protons and an even number of neutrons. The mass number is therefore even.

Even-odd nuclei. Nuclei containing an even number of protons and an odd number of neutrons. The atomic weight is therefore also odd. Even-odd nuclei tend to be more unstable than even-even nuclei.

Event. An occurrence or happening. An occurrence of significance to a task; typically, the completion of an asynchronous operation, such as an input/output operation.

Evidence. (Legal) The content of legal presentation in court — records, documents, objects or verbal accounts — for the purpose of inducing judge and jury to believe the contentions of the parties to the trial of an issue.

Exanthem. Any skin eruption or rash; visible skin lesions often accompanied by fever.

Exchange distillation. A process for the separation of isotopes by distillation of a compound that gives a dissociated vapor.

Exchange force. A force between two particles due to a potential that interchanges some of their coordinates, of space, of spin, or of charge.

Exchange reaction. The transfer of atoms, radioactive or stable, of the same element, between molecules, or from one site to another on the same molecule.

Excitability. The ability to respond to an impulse or stimulus. Atrial and ventricular myocardial fibers respond to the impulse generated by the pacemaker cells of the cardiac conduction system by depolarization and repolarization.

Excitation. Transference of energy into the spin system: process by which nuclei are put into a higher energy state. If a net transverse magnetization is produced, the response of an excited system can be observed (NMR); A stimulation which is followed by increased activity.

Excitation energy. Atoms, molecules, and nuclei possess internal energy associated with the kinetic energy of motion of the particles of which they are composed. Normally, the internal energy adjusts itself to a minimum value and in this condition the system (atom, molecule, or nucleus) is said to be in its ground or normal state. The internal energy can be increased above this level by collision with other particles, or by absorbing electromagnetic radiation (light γ-rays), and the system is then said to be in an excited state. This excess internal energy which the system has acquired above its normal state is called the excitation energy.

Excited state. If the internal energy of an atom, molecule, or nucleus exceeds the minimum possible value, it is said to be in an excited state.

Exclusion area. The area around a nuclear or radiation facility to which access is controlled.

Exclusive or. A logic circuit that selects "either, but not both" of two input signals.

Excretion. The elimination of waste products.

Excretion monitoring. One method of detecting the presence of radioactive material in the body and of estimating what the quantity is by assaying the excreta.

Execute. To perform an instruction or run a program on the computer.

Exenteration. Surgical removal of the organs, commonly used to indicate radical excision of the contents of the pelvis.

Exercise or stress EKG test. Measurement of the electrocardiogram and other cardiovascular functions during exercise. It is usually performed on a treadmill or bicycle with gradual increase in the level of exercise performed.

Exergonic process. A biochemical reaction in which the end products possess less free energy than the starting products.

Exit dose. Dose of radiation at surface of body opposite to that on which the beam is incident.

Exocrine. Pertaining to glands that deliver their secretion or excretion to an epithelial surface, either directly or by means of ducts.

Exoergic. That which liberates energy.

Exogenous. Originating outside an organ or part.

Exophthalmos. Protusion of the eyeballs from the orbit.

Exophytic. Growing outward; a cauliflower-like growth proliferating on the exterior or surface of an organ or structure in which the growth originated.

Exostosis. A bony growth that arises from the surface of a bone, often involving the ossification of muscular attachments.

Exothermic reactions. Chemical or nuclear reactions in which energy is liberated. To be contrasted with endothermic reactions in which energy is required to initiate them.

Expansion. A method of making a displayed image one, two, four, or eight times its original size by increasing the size of the pixels; zooming.

Expansion cloud chamber. A very early type of nuclear detector, in which a mixture of gas and a saturated condensible vapor is contained in a cylinder by a piston. By moving the piston out rapidly the volume is increased adiabatically and the temperature drop of the mixture is sufficient to make the vapor supersaturated. In this condition the vapor will condense on ions formed by the passage of an ionizing particle and grow to droplet size. With suitable illumination and photography the track of the ionizing particle through the gas-vapor is recorded.

Expected number. Number expected in a particular category in a sample under the assumption of the null hypothesis (no true difference exists).

Experimental reactor. A reactor operated primarily to obtain reactor physics or engineering data for the design or development of a reactor type. Reactors in this class include: zero-power reactor (may also be a research reactor); prototype reactor.

Expert witness. (Legal) An individual competent to give expert testimony because of special knowledge, skill, or experience not likely to be possessed by the ordinary layman. Where an ordinary witness may give testimony only to what he has experienced by his five senses, the expert is entitled to give an opinion or an inference. The jury determines his credibility.

Expiratory reserve volume. (ERV) The maximum volume of air that can be additionally expired after a normal expiration.

Exponential decay. A decay process in which the decay decreases exponentically with time. The most common example of this process is the decay of activity of a radioactive substance with time, in accordance with the equation

$$A = A_o e^{-\lambda t}$$

where A and A_o are the activities present at times t and zero, respectively, and λ is the characteristic decay constant.

Exponential experiment. A subcritical lattice

of fuel and moderator with an external source of neutrons. By measuring the neutron population, one can calculate the critical size of the lattice.

Exponential function. A mathematical function arising in the solution of linear differential equations with constant coefficients; of particular importance, therefore, in radioactive decay and multicompartment tracer analysis.

Exponential law of attenuation. The law of attenuation which applies to all processes where a constant fraction of the quantity being measured is lost per unit of distance traveled.

Exposure. A measure of the ionization produced in air by X- or γ-radiation. It is the sum of the electrical charges on all the ions of one sign produced in air when all electrons liberated by photons in a volume element of air are completely stopped in the air, divided by the mass of the air in the volume element. The SI unit of exposure is the coulomb per kilogram (C/kg). A person is said to be subject to radiation exposure if he/she is in a situation where his/her body or part of it has radiation incident on it. If the radiation can reach all or most of the body it is said to be whole-body exposure and if only certain parts are exposed, such as an organ or the extremities, it is partial exposure. Exposure can be from radiation arising outside the body or from material thatthat has been taken into the body by ingestion or inhalation or through a wound. Depending on its duration it may be acute exposure or chronic exposure.

Exposure angle. The angle through which the X-ray beam (or central ray) moves during exposure: the equivalent movement of object and film with a fixed tube system.

Exposure rate. The exposure in a small time interval, divided by that time interval. The SI unit of exposure rate is the coulomb per kilogram per second (C kg^{-1} s^{-1}); the non-SI unit is the roentgen per second (R s^{-1}).

$$1 \text{ C kg}^{-1} \text{ s}^{-1} = 3, 876 \text{ R s}^{-1}$$

$$1 \text{ R s}^{-1} = 2.58 ¥ 10^{-4} \text{ C kg}^{-1} \text{ s}^{-1}$$

$$= 0.258 \text{ m kg}^{-1} \text{ s}^{-1}$$

Exposure rate constant. The exposure rate due to the mission of X- and γ-rays from a specific radionuclide of activity 1 Bq at a distance of 1 m. The "exposure rate constant" replaced the former "specific γ-ray constant", and has, in turn, beeen replaced by the "air kerma-rate con-

stant". The term exposure rate constant has been retained, however, because adequate data in respect of the new quantity are not yet available.

The SI unit of exposure rate constant is the coulomb square meter per kilogram per becquerel per second (C m^2 kg^{-1} Bq^{-1} s^{-1}); the non-SI unit is the roentgen square meter per curie per hour (R m^2 Ci^{-1} h^{-1}).

$$1 \text{ C m}^2 \text{ kg}^{-1} \text{ Bq}^{-1} \text{ s}^{-1}$$
$$= 5.16 \times 10^{17} \text{ R m}^2 \text{ Ci}^{-1} \text{ h}^{-1}$$

$$1 \text{ R m}^2 \text{ Ci}^{-1} \text{ h}^{-1}$$
$$= 1.94 \times 10^{18} \text{ C m}^2 \text{ kg}^{-1} \text{ Bq}^{-1} \text{ s}^{-1}$$

Exposure time. The total amount of time the transducer assembly is delivering ultrasonic energy to the subject.

External contamination. Radioactive material on the body surface. Usually refers to unsealed radionuclides.

External exposure. Exposure from any radiation source outside the body or object of interest. An object subjected to external exposure has been "irradiated".

External lock. In a high-resolution NMR technique, and NMR signal from another substance other than the actual substance under investigation is used to control the field-frequency ratio of the spectrometer. If the material giving rise to the locking signal is located outside the sample tube, it is referred to as an external lock.

External radiation. Radiation that arises from some source outside the body in contradistinction to internal radiation which arises from radioactive material which is inside the body.

External reference. In high-resolution NMR spectroscopy, the chemical shifts are measured with reference to the position of a selected standard material in the NMR spectrum. If this reference compound is not dissolved in the same phase as the sample under investigation, it is referred to as an external reference.

External respiration. Movement of gases in and out of lungs.

External storage. A storage medium other than main computer memory, for example, a disk or tape.

Extirpation. Complete removal.

Extracellular. Situated or occurring outside a cell or the cells of the body.

Extracorporeal. Situated or occurring outside the body.

Extracorporeal circulation. The circulation of blood outside the body by means of an external agent, e.g., a heart-lung machine.

Extractor. Device that removes something; liquid that removes another substance with it.

Extranuclear. Referring to the space in an atom outside of the nucleus.

Extrapolation ionization chamber. An ionization chamber with electrodes whose spacing can be adjusted and accurately determined to permit extrapolation of its reading to zero chamber volume.

Extrasystole. Heartbeats that come earlier than expected (premature beats), causing an irregularity of the heartbeat or pulse, which may be felt as palpitations. Premature beats may be single or repetitve, occasional or very frequent. They may arise from many parts of the heart and often may be accurately diagnosed by electrocardiography.

Extraterrestrial radiation. In general, solar radiation received just outside the earth's atmosphere.

Extremity arteriography. Evaluation of the arterial structures in the arms or legs is done by percutaneous puncture of the appropriate vessel to an extremity, insertion of a small catheter, and subsequent injection of an appropriate radionuclide or contrast material. The two most common indications are arterial narrowing (arteriosclerosis) and trauma.

Extremity venography. Usually performed through the feet but occasionally in the arm, this procedure involves percutaneous injection of an appropriate radionuclide or water-soluble contrast material through a superficial vein specifically to look for evidence of deep venous thrombosis (DVT) or thrombophlebitis in regional veins.

Extrinsic spatial resolution. Overall system resolution of gamma camera with an appropriate collimator and scatter.

Exudate. Escaping fluid or semifluid material that oozes out of a blood vessel (usually as a result of inflammation), which may contain serum, pus, and cellular debris.

F

Fab. An antigen-binding fragment produced by enzymatic digestion of an IgG molecule with papain.

F(ab')$_2$. A fragment obtained by pepsin digestion of immunoglobulin molecules containing the 2H and 2L chains linked by disulfide bonds.

It contains antigen-binding activity. An $(F(ab')^2$ fragment and an Fc fragment comprise an entire monomeric immunoglobulin molecule.

Facilitated diffusion. Diffusion in which a carrier molecule transports a substance across a membrane.

Facsimile. The process of scanning a picture or page of text and converting it to signals that can be sent over a telephone line or other communications channel. A machine at the receiving end picks up the signals and converts them back to their original form to produce a copy of the original image.

Fail safe. Refers to a principle of design by which, in the event of any failure in a system, the system takes up a safe condition.

Fail soft. A fail-soft computer system is designed to shut itself down in case of a serious error or malfunction. Fail-soft systems remain shut down until the defect is corrected, and they accomplish this with no loss of data and no additional damage to the system.

Fallopian tube. Pair of slender tubes through which ova from the ovaries pass to the uterus; oviduct.

Fallout. The term refers to radioactive material deposited following the explosion of nuclear weapons. The amount of fission product activity resulting from the explosion of a nuclear weapon is roughly proportional to the magnitude of the explosion, and the physical form and distribution of the debris depend to a large extent on the mode of firing the weapons and the power of the explosion. It is considered that, in general, H-bomb debris is distributed as smaller particles, proceeds higher into the atmosphere, remains there longer, and falls more uniformly over the earth's surface than the A-bomb debris.

Families. Sets of elements that have the same valence-shell electronic configurations.

Farad. (Unit of electric capacitance) The capacitance of a capacitor between the plates of which there appears a difference of potential of 1 when it is charged by a quantity of electricity equal to 1 C.

Faraday cage. In environments with high levels of electrostatic noise it is sometimes desirable to make a whole room which is impervious to electrostatic fields. This can be achieved by including a metal mesh in the doors, walls, ceiling, floor, and (if they must be present) the windows. All of the mesh must be connected together and grounded to earth.

Faraday constant. (Symbol F) The product of

the Avogadro constant N_A and the elementary charge e, $F = N_A e = 96.489 \pm 2$ C/mol.

Faraday effect. The rotation of the plane of polarization produced when plane-polarized light is passed through a substance in a magnetic field, the light traveling in a direction parallel to the lines of force. For a given substance, the rotation is proportional to the thickness traversed by the light and to the magnetic field strength.

Faraday shield. Electrical conductor interposed between transmitter and/or receiver coil and patient to block out electric fields. (NMR.)

Faraday's law. States that time-dependent flux induces a voltage in a conductor crossing the flux lines.

Far zone. The region of a sound beam in which the beam diameter increases as the distance from the transducer increases.

Fast fission. Fission induced by "fast" neutrons.

Fast Fourier transform. (FFT) Fast Fourier transform is a computational algorithm which reduces the computational time required from Fourier analysis by digital computer. For a function which does not have a closed-form Fourier transform and which has N separate digital data points, the computational time required to determine the N sinusoidal amplitudes, the digital computer requires N^2. However, in the Cooley and Tukey FFT algorithm this time becomes proportional to $N \log_2 N^2$ computations, thus reducing the total time.

Fast neutrons. Neutrons having energies in excess of about 100 keV are often referred to as fast neutrons. As neutrons do not exist as free particles in nature, they must be released from nuclei in some kind of nuclear reaction. The probability that a neutron having an energy less than a few kiloelectronvolts will escape from a nucleus in such a reaction is very small. Therefore, for all practical purposes, neutrons are produced initially as fast neutrons. If slow neutrons are required, the fast neutrons must be slowed down in a moderator.

Fast reactor. A nuclear reactor in which there is little moderation and fission is induced primarily by fast neutrons, that have lost relatively little of the energy with which they were released. The slowing down of neutrons that does occur is due largely to inelastic scattering instead of elastic scattering. About 100 keV is regarded as the minimum value of mean energy of neutrons inducing fission for a reactor to be considered fast, with 0.5 to 0.3 Mev more common. Sometimes the fission threshold of

^{238}U is taken as the lower limit of the fast range.

Fat. Chemical compounds that share a common property, the inability to dissolve in water or various body fluids. They are an important source of food and energy as well as structural materials of all body cells and tissues. Cholesterol and triglycerides are the most important fats.

Fatigue fracture. A brittle fracture due to fatigue caused by cyclic stressing of a metal. Usually possesses two distinct zones, one with a bright, smooth surface and the other fibrous and dull. The former indicates the area of the initial fatigue fracture and the latter is the area of instantaneous final fracture. To a certain extent, the same principle could be applied to bone stress fractures.

Fatty acids. Compounds composed of long chains of carbon atoms that serve as an important source of energy for the body. Fatty acids are part of the triglyceride molecule and are stored in fat tissue in this form. Fatty acids are "saturated" when all the bonds between the carbon atoms are filled and "unsaturated" when the bonds are incomplete.

Fault. (Legal) Any deviation from prudence, duty, or rectitude; any shortcoming or neglect of care, of performance resulting from inattention, incapacity, or perversity.

Fc fragment. A crystallizable fragment obtained by papain digestion of IgG molecules that consists of the C-terminal half of 2H chains linked by disulfide bonds. It contains no antigen-binding capability but determines important biologic characteristics of the intact molecule.

Fc receptor. A receptor present on various subclasses of lymphocytes for the Fc fragment of immunoglobulins.

F distribution. The distribution followed by the ratio of two independent sample estimates of a population variance, i.e.,

$$F = s_1^2/s_2^2$$

The shape of the distribution depends on two degrees of freedom values associated, respectively, with

$$s_1^2 \quad \text{and} \quad s_2^2$$

Feather analysis. A technique first described by N. Feather in 1938 for measuring the range of beta particles by comparison with beta particles of known energy distribution, usually

^{210}Bi (range—501 mg/cm^2).

Feather rule. A rule or equation for the maximum range R of beta particles. The equation is

$$R(g/cm^2) = 0.536\ E_{max} - 0.165$$

This equation may be rewritten as

$$E_{max} = 1.84R + 0.294$$

The range expressed in these units does not vary widely with the atomic number of the absorber. Thus, the range of a 1-MeV beta particle in aluminum (Z = 13) and gold (Z = 79) is 400 and 500 mg/cm^2, respectively.

Feedback. Feedback helps computers to change their course of action based on the progress of their current operations. Feedback is the use of information produced at one step in a program to determine how the next step will proceed.

Feedback signal. An attenuated signal fed back from the output of an amplifier to the input, in antiphase with the input. With such a feedback amplifier the resultant gain depends on the feedback ratio (the ratio by which a feedback signal was attenuated). If the gain is made to be very much less than the gain without feedback the feedback amplifier has high gain stability.

Fermi age theory. A theory of the slowing down of neurons by elastic collisions, in which it is assumed that the slowing down takes place by a very large number of very small energy changes.

Fermium. Element symbol Fm, atomic number 100, atomic weight ~257.

Ferrimagnetic materials. Those in which the magnetic moments of atoms or ions tend to assume an ordered but nonparallel arrangement in zero applied field, below a characteristic temperature called the Neel point. In the usual case, within a magnetic domain, a substantial net magnetization results from the antiparallel alignment of neighboring nonequivalent sublattices. The macroscopic behavior is similar to that in ferromagnetism. Above the Neel point, these materials become paramagnetic.

Ferrokinetics. Study of iron metabolism within the body.

Ferromagnetism. The phenomenon whereby certain materials exhibit a high degree of magnetism in weak fields and possess a very high permeability.

Ferromagnetic materials. Those in which the magnetic moments of atoms or ions in a magnetic domain tend to be aligned parallel to one another in zero applied field, below a char-

acteristic temperature called the Curie point. Complete ordering is achieved only at the absolute zero of temperature. Within a magnetic domain, at absolute zero, the magnetization is equal to the sum of the magnetic moments of the atoms or ions per unit volume. Bulk matter, consisting of many small magnetic domains, has a net magnetization which depends upon the magnetic history of the specimen (hysteresis effect). The permeability depends on the magnetic field, and can reach values of the order of 10^6 times that of free space. Above the Curie point, these materials become paramagnetic.

Fertile. Of a nuclide, capable of being transformed, directly or indirectly, into a fissile nuclide by neutron capture. Of a material, containing one or more fertile nuclides.

Fetal antigen. A type of tumor-associated antigen that is normally present on embryonic but not adult tissues and which is reexpressed during the neoplastic process.

Fetch. A command to take the next instruction from a computer memory.

Fetus. Unborn offspring after major structures have been defined from the embryo.

F factor. If the exposure level (coulomb per kilogram) at a certain location is multiplied by the f factor, the absorbed dose (gray) delivered to a person at that location can be estimated. The f factor is different for soft tissue and bone and varies as a function of the energy.

Fiber optics. The use of glass fibers for the transmission of optical images.

Fibrillation. Random, ineffective, disordered contractions of the heart muscle. Atrial fibrillation: fibrillation present in the upper heart chambers, the atria. Ventricular fibrillation: fibrillation present in the lower or pumping chambers, the ventricles. Unless immediately reversed, ventricular fibrillation is fatal.

Fibrin. An insoluble protein formed from fibrinogen (coagulation factor I) during normal clotting of blood. Fibrin is the essential portion of the blood clot.

Fibrinogen. A protein found in blood plasma which is converted by thrombin into fibrin.

Fibrinolysis. Dissolution of splitting of fibrin.

Fibroblast. Connective tissue cell; immature form of collagen-producing cells that synthesize collagen and elastin and form the fibrous tissues of the body.

Fibrosis. An abnormal increase in the amount of fibrous connective tissue in an organ or in the skin; the narrowing or closing of minute arteries and capillaries by inflammatory internal fibrosis.

Fick principle. The Fick principle states that blood flow through organs can be estimated if a measurable substance is either removed or added as blood flows through them. Thus, cardiac output f can be measured using the equation

$$Q/t = f(C_A - C_V)$$

where Q is the subject's oxygen consumption measured by the spirometric collection of expired air, C_A is the oxygen concentration of a systemic arterial blood sample, and C_V is the oxygen concentration of a mixed venous blood sample from the pulmonary artery. The oxygen content of arterial blood is greater than the oxygen content of venous (pulmonary arterial) blood due to oxygen inhaled and transferred to the blood via the lungs. The concentration of oxygen in arterial blood is also relatively uniform, but this is not true of venous blood: each tissue may utilize varying quantities of oxygen, and the blood oxygen content in the superior vena cava thus differs from that in the inferior vena cava. Also, mixing is incomplete in the right atrium and only in the pulmonary artery can a truly mixed sample be obtained. This method therefore requires right-heart catheterization, arterial blood sampling, and meticulous expired air collection. It is likely that data will have an error of at least 10%. For example, if an oxygen consumption of 300 ml min−1 results in a systemic arterial blood oxygen concentration of 19 ml oxygen per 100 ml blood, and the venous oxygen concentration is found to be 14 ml/100 ml, then $(C_A - C_V) = 5$ ml oxygen per 100 ml blood. Thus,

$$f = \frac{Q}{t(C_A - C_V)} = \frac{300}{5} \times \frac{100}{1} \text{ ml min}^{-1}$$

$$= 61 \text{ min}^{-1}$$

The Fick principle was the first to allow repeated and reasonably accurate measurement of cardiac output. However, it has now been superseded by other techniques.

Field. Basic element of a computer file that can be stored or retrieved with one read or write operation.

Field effect transistor. (FET) A transistor with operating characteristics similar to that of a vacuum tube.

Field emission. Emission of electrons by a cold conductor due to the presence of a very high local electric field, for example, at a sharp point.

Field gradient. Defines the rate of change of the magnetic field. It is also used as an inexact definition of an auxiliary field which brings about a spatial change in the field strength of a previously homogeneous magnetic field. (NMR.)

Field lock. A feedback control used to maintain the static magnetic field at a constant strength, usually by monitoring the resonance frequency of a reference sample or line in the spectrum. (NMR.)

Field nonuniformity. Uniformity requirements for single photon emission computerized tomography (SPECT) are more stringent and require further correction than for planar projections. The greatest sources of image field nonuniformities in SPECT are "imperfect" collimators. A local nonuniformity from a collimator is propagated in the reconstructed transaxial slice in the form of a circular or "ring" artifact, since the same nonuniformity is backprojected at each of the angles of acquisition. The higher the number of acquired counts for that slice the more prominent the artifact since it rides above the random noise error. Also, the closer the local nonuniformity is to the axis of rotation the higher the amplitude of the artifact, since the backprojected lines are closer together there is more overlapping of the count values. Uniformity correction for SPECT usually requires imaging a ^{57}Co flood source for 30 million counts in order to reduce the error due to nonuniformity to less than 1%. For this reason it is important that the flood source used have a variation of radionuclide concentration less that 1%. Normalization factors are determined from this image and applied to each of the projection views. Importantly, the 30 million-count rule assumes a 64×64 matrix used to reconstruct a 1 million-count slice. A 128×128 matrix will require four times the 30 million-count flood in order to maintain the same variation.

Field of view. The area which can be "seen" by an optical system. It may be expressed as an angle or as a diameter; it defines the volume from which emitted activity may be detected.

Field sweep. One mode of observing the nuclear magnetic resonance (NMR) spectrum by systematically varying (sweeping) the applied static field and keeping the frequency of the radio-frequency (rf) radiation constant. By varying the magnetic field strength, NMR transitions of different energies can be brought into resonance successively. In this kind of experiment, the NMR spectrum consists of signal intensity vs. the magnetic field strength.

Field uniformity correction. The compensation for changes in the sensitivity of a detector to achieve a uniform response.

Figure of merit. A measure of performance of a detection system that combines sensitivity and ability to record rapid or discontinuous spatial changes in source intensity.

File. A logical collection of data that is treated as a unit, occupies one or more blocks on a mass storage volume, and has an associated file name and type. Computers store information under files. Since a file may be too big to store in a computer's memory as a single unit, it may be divided into records, blocks, or other smaller segments.

File maintenance. The activity of keeping a mass storage volume and its directory up to date by adding, changing, or deleting files.

File name. The alphanumeric character string assigned by a user to identify a file. A file name has a fixed maximum length that is system dependent.

File name extension. The second part of a file name, which describes the type of data in the file.

Filling factor. A measure of the geometrical relationship of the radio-frequency (rf) coil and the body. If affects the efficiency of irradiating the body and detecting NMR signals, thereby affecting the signal-to-noise ratio and, ultimately, image quality. Achieving a high filling factor requires fitting the coil closely to the body, thus potentially decreasing patient comfort.

Film badge. A simple type of personnel radiation monitor that can be issued to individuals likely to be exposed to significant radiation doses. It consists of a metal or plastic case with a clip or pin for fastening to the outside of protective clothing, and holding a piece of photographic film (similar to that used for dental X-ray) wrapped in a light-tight envelope. Part of the film is covered by a thin metal screen. The unscreened portion is affected by β-, γ-, and X-rays, while the screened part containing a set of absorber filters is affected by the more energetic γ- and X-rays. When the film is developed, the blackening of the two parts due to radiation exposure enables an estimate to be made of the beta dose and the gamma plus X-ray dose to which the wearer has been exposed. Films are usually issued for a fixed period such as a week or a month, after which they are col-

lected, processed, and radiation doses calculated with the aid of a densitometer by measuring the degree of blackening of the film.

Film ring. A film badge in the form of a finger ring.

Filter. Metallic plate (usually aluminum or copper) at the aperture of the X-ray tube through which the rays must pass before striking the object to be examined or treated. A hardware device or software algorithm that modifies data for easier processing or reading. For instance, filtering enhances image quality without significantly altering diagnostic capability by reducing high-frequency noise and/or low-frequency background. A filter for removing particulate matter from gases. The filter has a collection efficiency of at least 99.97% (by weight) for particles in the size range from 0.3 to 1.0 μm. Electronic device that lets through only certain frequencies and is characterized by a bandwidth (Δv) or window.

Filtered back projection. Mathematical technique used in reconstruction from projections to create images from a set of multiple projection profiles. It essentially involves an algorithm to reconstruct the projection profiles by convolving them with a suitable mathematical filter and then backprojecting the filtered projections into image space. Widely used in computerized tomography (transmission and emission) and nuclear magnetic resonance.

Filtered backprojection reconstruction. This method can be defined in various ways. The most straightforward conceptually is the two-dimensional frequency space approach. This means reconstructing an image by simple backprojection, then generating Fourier transform of that image. Since the amplitude of the image at each frequency has been suppressed in proportion to the frequency value, correction must be made for this effect by multiplying each of the amplitudes by its frequency (ω), boosting the high-frequency components and suppressing the low ones. Here the term ω is the two-dimensional form of the well-known Ramp filter. The resulting filtered image in frequency space is converted to a real space image via the inverse Fourier transform. A more popular approach that is computationally more efficient involves filtering of the individual projections before backprojection. Doing a Fourier transform on each projection, multiplying the resulting frequency space function by the one-dimensional Ramp (ω), then inverse Fourier transforms the result to obtain the filtered projection in real space. The filtered projections are then backprojected to obtain the reconstructed image. In theory, filtered backprojection will produce perfect reconstructions given an infinite number of continuous noise-free projections. In reality, there is a rather limited number of projections available, each consisting of discretely sampled values rather than being continuous, and each of these values being subject to random noise.

Filter house. The container in which a filter is mounted. When radioactive materials are to be processed, such a house may be heavily shielded and incorporate facilities for remotely replacing the filters.

Filtering. A process used extensively on nuclear medicine images to reduce statistical noise, enhance edges for edge detection, and in the reconstruction of tomographic images. Filtering can be performed in either the spatial domain or in frequency space. Frequency domain methods of image enhancement deal with the spatial frequencies (cycles/centimeter or cycles/pixel) which make up the image. An image can be decomposed into a summation of different spatial frequencies. Spatial frequencies relate to the rapidity of change in intensity (counts) with distance. The high-frequency components define edges, areas where there is a rapid change in intensity from bright to dark. Regions in an image where the changes are more gradual are primarily due to the lower-frequency components. In order to convert an image into its frequency components it is necessary to use an image transform, such as a Fourier transform, to transfer the image to frequency space. The Fourier transform yields the frequencies that are present in the image and the amplitude of each frequency. An inverse Fourier transform transfers the image back into the spatial domain, which is the conventional format for representing images. Filtering in frequency space is accomplished by removing, or altering, the magnitude of selected frequency components. Each specific frequency is multiplied by a factor assigned by the filter. If a particular frequency needs to be totally suppressed, the factor assigned to that frequency is set to zero. Filters that place emphasis on the low-frequency components while reducing the high-frequency components are called low-pass filters. If the opposite effect is desired, a high-pass filter is applied which reduces the low frequencies. A bandpass filter reduces both low and high frequencies allowing only a band of frequencies in-between to remain.

Firmware. Instructions, routines, and programs that today are typically implemented in read-only memory (ROM) and are available for execution but not for alteration. Synonymous with microcode.

First derivative. The instantaneous rate of change of a function with respect to the variable. Two special interpretations: (1) as the slope of a curve; (2) as the speed of a moving particle.

First in/first out. (FIFO) A data manipulation method in which the first item stored is the first item processed by the computer.

First transit study. Examination of the first passage of a bolus of radioactivity through an organ. Usually refers to examination of the cardiovascular system.

Fisher t test. Determination of whether two sets of data come from similar populations where any differences in means are the result of random error.

Fishtail collimator. The "fishtail" collimator has been designed to achieve a whole body scan with a moving camera. The fishtail has diverging channels, to encompass the width of the patient while the channels are parallel in the direction of motion of the gamma camera. The solution across orthogonal axes of the collimator is different but has similar changes in overall spatial resolution as the parallel hole collimator synonym of area scan collimator.

Fissile. The term is loosely applied to any nucleus that can be made to undergo fission. However, it is normally taken to mean fissionable by thermal neutrons.

Fissile material. Means any material consisting of or containing one or more fissile radionuclides. Fissile radionuclides are ^{238}Pu, ^{239}Pu, ^{241}Pu, ^{233}U, and ^{235}U. Neither natural nor depleted uranium is fissile material.

Fission. The splitting of a heavy nucleus into two (or, very rarely, more) approximately equal fragments — the fission products. Fission is accompanied by the emission of neutrons and the release of energy. It can be spontaneous, or it can be caused by the impact of a neutron, a fast charged particle, or a photon. This process provides the energy for the atomic bomb and nuclear reactors.

Fission chamber. A counter containing fissile material that is used to detect the occurrence of a fission in that material. When this occurs the of a fission in that material. When this occurs the fission fragments are emitted with considerable energy and can initiate an electrical pulse usually by ionizing a gas.

Fission fragment. In a fission event the nucleus breaks up into two lighter nuclei each about half the original atomic weight. These two halves, called fragments, take away nearly the whole of the energy from fission in the form of kinetic energy.

Fission neutrons. Neutrons originating in the fission process that have retained their original energy.

Fission poison. Fission products that absorb neutrons unproductively; especially used for those having high absorption cross sections, e.g., xenon.

Fission products. The nuclides produced either by fission or by the subsequent radioactive decay of the nuclides thus formed.

Fission spectrum. The wide range of elements and isotopes formed in fission is called the fission spectrum. Up to 35 elements may be formed — but some such as ^{137}Cs and ^{90}Sr are much more abundant than others. The energy spectrum of the neutrons or of the prompt γ radiation produced in fission.

Fission yield. The fraction of fissions giving rise to one particular group of fission products all having the same mass number.

Fissure. Term for cleft or groove in organ.

Fistula. An abnormal opening or passageway generally caused by disease or radiation necrosis between one hollow organ and another or to the skin.

Fix. To definitely determine ones position.

Fixation. The incorporation of radioactive elements, usually fission products, into solid materials in such a way as to insure no significant release over long periods of exposure to the natural environment.

Fixed link. A fixed communications path, which is always available whether or not it is in use. Also referred to as a leased line.

Flag. A variable used to record the status of a computer program or device.

Flame emission spectroscopy. An analytical technique in which an atomized sample is introduced into an oxyhydrogen or oxyacetylene flame to produce a line emission spectrum.

Flat-field collimator. A collimator constructed so as to permit a broad area to be visualized by a radiation detector. It is usually made of lead with a single aperture that is either cylindrical or slightly conical in shape.

Flexor reflex. Contraction of the flexor muscles in response to a harmful or unpleasant stimulus, resulting in a rapid withdrawal of the stimulated limb or flexions of the torso.

Flip angle. Amount of rotation of the macroscopic magnetization vector produced by a radio-frequency (rf) pulse, with respect to the direction of the static magnetic field. (NMR.)

Flip-flop. A two-state electronic circuit that can be electrically flipped from one to the other and then flopped back. The flip-flop is a convenient way to represent 1 bit.

Floating point. A number system in which the position of the radix point is indicated by the exponent part of a number, and another part represents the significant digits or fractional portion of a number. For example, 5.39×10^8 — decimal; 137.3×8^4 — octal; 101.10×2^{13} — binary.

Flood field. A uniform source of activity used to test the uniformity of response of a radiation detector.

Floor monitor. A floor monitor is a special type of contamination monitor. In laboratories and workshops where radioactive materials are handled it is necessary to provide monitoring equipment so that any contamination can be detected and located should spills occur. If the contamination falls on the ground it may be dispersed over a large area, and a very sensitive instrument is necessary that can scan the suspected area as quickly as possible.

Floppy disk. A type of magnetic disk which is flexible in structure. Floppy disks are usually slower in data transfer rates and smaller in storage capacity than rigid disks. An informal name for a flexible disk or diskette.

Floppy disk drive. A machine that plugs into a computer for information storage on floppy disks. Inside the drive, the disk spins at high speed while a record/play head takes information off the disk's surface and feeds it to the computer. The disk drive can also receive information from the computer and store it on the disk.

Flow chart. A graphical representation for the definition, analysis, or solution of a problem in logical steps where symbols are used to represent operations, data, flow, and equipment.

Flow counter. A counter in which an appropriate atmosphere is maintained in a counter tube by allowing a suitable gas to flow through it. Such counters are operated in either the Geiger-Müller region or the proportional region. The source to be assayed is usually placed in the counter volume. The method is therefore particularly applicable to low-energy β-emitters and α-emitters. Flow counters operating in the proportional region are often used when a very high precision of measurement is required.

Fluence. A measure of particle flux integrated with respect to time, and usually expressed in particles per square centimeter.

Fluid thioglycollate. Medium that provides conditions for growth of aerobic and anaerobic bacteria; used in microbiologic sterility testing of radiopharmaceuticals.

Fluor. In liquid scintillation counting, an organic compound that reacts indirectly to the energy of beta (or equivalent) radiation from sample material and in turn emanates light photons. In gamma counters the luminescent material is usually inorganic and referred to as scintillator or crystal.

Fluorescence. The property of a substance to emit radiation in the visible portion of the electromagnetic spectrum after exposure to electromagnetic radiations such as X-rays. The frequency of the light emitted may be the same or lower than that of the absorbed light. In radioassay, a term often used to denote intrinsic luminescence noted in liquid scintillation counting independent of sample radioactivity. Phosphorescence is also used similarly.

Fluorescence yield. The probability that an excited atom will decay by X-ray emission rather than by ejecting an Auger electron. The fluorescence yield lies between 0 and 1.

Fluorescent screen. A sheet of material coated with a substance such as calcium tungstate or zinc sulfide which will emit visible light when irradiated with ionizing radiation.

Fluorescent X-rays. When a beam of X-rays passes through an absorber, part of the absorption is due to the ejection of electrons from the K-shell of the absorber atoms. The vacancies thus created are then filled by other electrons and the atoms radiate. This radiation, which for a heavy absorber is in the X-ray band, is referred to as fluorescent X-radiation and is characteristic of the particular absorber used.

Fluorimeters. Several elements of importance, including uranium and beryllium, can be determined by measurement of the fluorescence of a solution or solid containing the element. The instrument used for this purpose is called a fluorimeter. The fluorescence is excited by an energetic light beam, usually in the ultraviolet frequency region. The sample is viewed, either subjectively or more satisfactorily objectively,

with a photosensitive device and some form of wavelength selection from a direction normal to the incident excitation beam. It is a very sensitive method and has been employed particularly for the examination of urine samples from persons working with uranium and its salts (and ores).

Fluorine. Element symbol F, atomic number 9, atomic weight 18.998.

Fluorography. Photography of an image produced on a fluorescent screen by X- or γ-radiation. Also known as photofluorography.

Fluoroscope. A fluoroscope is a screen device for use with an X-ray generator to make visible an X-ray shadowgraphy similar to that obtained by the photographic process. It consists essentially of a card of suitable size coated on the viewer's side with a material, such as zinc sulfide, which fluoresces under the action of the radiation. In order to protect the viewer from the radiation the fluorescent screen is covered with a sheet of transparent lead-bearing glass.

Fluoroscopy. Fluoroscopy is the use of a fluoroscope either in medical diagnosis or for industrial inspection purposes. When handling of the patient or object is necessary, lead-bearing rubber gloves should be worn or, in industrial work where the X-rays energy is usually greater, it may be necessary to provide some form of remote-handling equipment or viewing on a TV screen after intensification.

Flux. The product of the number of radiant energy, particles, or photons per unit time through a unit volume normal to the direction of motion of the particles.

Focal length. In ultrasound, it is the distance from focused transducer to center of focal region or to the location of the spatial peak intensity.

Focal plane. The plane perpendicular to the axis of symmetry of a collimator that contains the focal point.

Focal point. The theoretical spot in front of a focused collimator at which all channels converge. This is the point of maximum sensitivity and resolution.

Focal spot. (X-rays) The part of the target of the X-ray tube which is struck by the main electron stream.

Focal zone. The narrowest portion of the ultrasound beam produced by a focused transducer. Also called as focal surface.

Focus. To concentrate a sound, light, photon beam into a smaller beam area that could exist without focusing.

Focused collimator. A collimator constructed to as to permit only a restricted area to be visualized at one time. It is usually made of lead with holes arranged in a honeycomb fashion and converging at some point distant to the face of the collimator.

Focusing transducer. An ultrasound transducer assembly in which the ratio of the smallest of all beam cross-sections, to the radiating cross-sectional area, is less than one fourth.

Foil detector. Leaves or thin plates of metal which can be used as neutron detectors. The foils are irradiated in a neutron flux and their resulting β-ray and/or γ-ray activity counted with a suitable detector, e.g., Geiger counter or scintillation counter. A large number of different metals are used, the most common being gold, indium, silver, copper, manganese, and uranium.

Foldover. A term used in pulsed Fourier NMR spectroscopy when single phase detection is used. Because of this type of detection, a single spectral line can be detected at two different frequencies symmetrically located at about the carrier frequency (v_o). The process of reflecting the line at, for example, $v_o + \Delta v$ to $v_o - \Delta v$ is called foldover.

Folic acid. Vitamin essential for the normal growth and maturation of erythrocyte and a growth-promoting agent. Also called pteroglutamic acid.

Follicle. A small secretory or excretory sac or gland.

Follicle-stimulating hormone. (FSH) Anterior pituitary hormone that stimulates follicle growth in the ovaries and spermatogenesis in the testes.

Fonar. One type of imaging technique called field focusing NMR, developed by Damadian in which the field is focused at a point on the object called a saddle point. In this technique, the volume of interest can be localized with the aid of an inhomogeneous magnetic field which produces a saddle-shaped profile.

Fontanelle. The soft space in the skull of an infant. The spot ossifies completely within the first 1 or 2 years of life.

Food irradiation. Irradiation process of any food commodity up to an overall dose of 10 kGy (100 rads) with electron beams, γ-, or X-rays as a method of food preservation. This technology has the potential of extending the food harvest and alleviating world hunger without any apparent toxicologic hazard nor specific microbiologic problems. On the contrary, this process has shown to minimize changes in color, flavor, and texture while retaining the nutritional value of food, thus proving to be superior to canning or freezing. The commercial name for food irradiation is known as RADURA, for radiation durability.

Foramen. A natural opening or passage through a bone or tissue.

Foramen magnum. Large opening in the occipital bone between the cranial cavity and the vertebral canal.

Forbidden clone theory. The theory proposed to explain autoimmunity that postulates that lymphocytes capable of self-sensitization and effector function are present in tolerant animals, since they were not eliminated during embryogenesis.

Force. Forces change the state of rest or motion of matter. If there were no forces, everything would be in a state of rest or steady motion.

Forced expiratory flow. ($FEF_{200-1200}$) the average rate of flow for a specified portion of the forced expiratory volume, usually between 200 and 1200 ml (formerly called maximum expiratory flow rate).

Forced expiratory volume. (FEV_t) The volume of air expired per unit time during forced expiration following full inspiration.

Forced midexpiratory flow. ($FEF_{25-75\%}$) The average rate of flow during the middle half of the forced expiratory volume.

Forced vital capacity. (FVC) The maximum volume of gas that can be expelled as forcefully and rapidly as possible after maximum inspiration.

Foreground. Pertaining to the computer, a program that runs at the highest priority. Pertaining to the user, a program which requires operator interaction.

Forensic medicine. The application of medical evidence or opinion to legal problems.

Formation cross section. Cross section for the formation of a certain nuclide or compound nucleus; it is used, e.g., when different nuclides are formed from the same nuclide through different nuclear reactions.

Formatting. The process of writing a special pattern of data over the recording surface of a disk. You must format a disk before you can use it to store data.

Form feed. A printer operation that advances the printer's paper to the top of a new sheet (if the paper is correctly positioned). The control character a computer sends to a printer to make it do a form feed is also called a "form feed" or a "form feed character".

FORTRAN. (*FOR*mula *TRAN*slator) High-level

user computer programming language. A language similar to English that is particularly useful for mathematical expressions and calculations. FORTRAN is now by far the most widely used procedure-oriented language and is being effectively employed in certain businesses as well as scientific applications. The essential element of the FORTRAN language is the assignment statement; e.g., $Z = X + Y$ causes the current values of the variable X and Y to be added together and their sum to replace the previous value of the variable Z.

Fossa. A small depression in the surface of a part of the body, especially in bone.

Fourier series. An infinite series of sine and cosine functions of integer multiples of a variable (e.g., time). The series can be used to represent a periodic function.

Fourier transform analysis. Mathematical treatment of spatially or temporally varying data that considers frequency variations as the sum of a number of sine/cosine functions. Used in tomographic image reconstruction (CT, ECT, NMR) and for analyzing temporally varying data, such as cardiac chamber volume changes.

Four-pi counter. A counter which measures the radiation emitted in any direction (4π) from a radioactive material.

Fovea. With reference to the eye, the small central area of the retina where the photoreceptor cells (cones only) are most densely packed and, hence, the area where visual acuity is greatest. Also known as the yellow spot; term for small pit on the surface of an organ.

Fractional rate of elimination. The ratio of the rate of removal of a substance from a living system by biological processes to the quantity of the substance therein.

Fractional turnover rate. The percentage of plasma pool catabolized and cleared into the urine per day.

Fractionating column. A vertical column attached to a still filled with rings or intersected with bubble plates. An internal reflux takes place, resulting in a gradual separation between the high and low boiling-point fractions inside the column, with the result that the fractions with lowest boiling point distill over.

Fractionation. Of a radiation dose. The prolongation of delivery of a given total radiation dose by substituting a set of shorter exposures of the same intensity which are separated in time.

Fragmentation. Fragmentation occurs when information is placed in the computer's memory in such a way that there are a number of unused portions of memory that, individually, are too small to be useful.

Frame. A section of image memory which can be addressed separately. Synonymous with image.

Frame freeze. A technique that allows the production of still frames from a real time sequence.

Frame of reference. That system of coordinates which is chosen for the description or analysis of a physical process, especially scattering.

Frame rate. Number of frames displayed per unit time.

Francium. Element symbol Fr, atomic number 87, atomic weight ~223.

Free. In competitive binding assay, the fraction of tracer test substance not bound at reaction completion.

Free air ionization chamber. An ionization chamber in which a delimited beam of radiation passes between the electrodes without striking them or other internal parts of the equipment. The electric field is maintained perpendicular to the electrodes in the collection region; as a result, the ionized volume can be accurately determined from the dimensions of the collection electrode and the limiting diaphragm. This is the basic standard instrument of X-ray dosimetry.

Free induction decay. (FID) Transient nuclear signal induced in the NMR coil after a radio-frequency pulse has excited the nuclear spin system in pulsed NMR techniques. This is referred to as free induction decay signal because the signal is induced by the free precession of the nuclear spins around the static field after the radio-frequency pulse has been turned off.

Free radical. Any atom or molecule which possesses one unpaired electron. Such a radical usually exhibits considerable additive properties and high reactivity. It is considered that radicals of the type OH (hydroxyl), HO_2 (perhydroxyl), CH_2 (methylene), CH_3 (methyl), etc. are capable of existence in the free state for very brief periods of time under suitable chemical conditions, and that they initiate or otherwise take part in many kinds of chemical reactions. Organic free radicals would appear to play an important part in polymerization reaction and in biochemistry. Free radicals are often formed when an excited molecule decomposes by rupture of chemical bonds; they are generally involved in the propagation of chain reactions and polymerizations.

Free thyroxine. (Free T-4) The minute fraction of thyroxine (0.05%) which is unbound to protein. Free thyroxine is believed to be the active form of thyroxine.

Freeze-drying. (Lyophilization) The process of rapidly freezing a solution and removing the solvent by sublimation under vacuum.

Freeze-fracture replication. A technique used to prepare cells and cell organelles for electron microscopy. A hydrated specimen is rapidly frozen and cleaved in vacuo to expose a fracture face which is then shadowed with a heavy metal and coated with a layer or carbon. The carbon layer is then examined in the microscope.

Fremitus. Vibration tremors, especially those felt through the chest wall by palpation.

Frequency. Characteristic quantity of a magnetic or electrical field which is changing its direction alternatively at a regular interval. It is equal to the reciprocal of the period of this periodic motion. It is measured in hertz (Hz) which is 1 cps. Number of individuals with value X (or in the xth class interval). A weighting factor in calculations.

Frequency distribution. Arrangement of data indicating the frequency of specified X values.

Frequency of emission. When a particular radionuclide is selected for imaging it is important to note the number of useful gamma emissions per disintegration. For example, the frequency of emission of the 159- and 429-keV photons in the decay of ^{123}I is 84%. Hence it would be very inefficient to perform imaging of this radionuclide with the discriminators set about the higher energy level. Some radionuclides such as ^{67}Ga have complex decay schemes with many gamma emissions. In such cases, it is often necessary in terms of imaging efficiency to have equipment with multiple energy window discrimination. Thus, discriminators can be set to record events from the 93-, 185-, and 300-keV photons which have frequency of emission per disintegration of 38, 24, and 16%, respectively.

Frequency polygon. A many-sided figure. Formed by straight lines which connect the points representing the frequencies of the X values. In grouped data, the frequencies are plotted at the midpoints of the class intervals.

Frequency response curve. The data output curve from an imaging system in response to input of varying spatial or temporal frequency.

Frequency sweep. One mode of observing the NMR spectrum by systematically varying the frequency of the radio-frequency (rf) radiation and keeping the static field strength constant.

This can also be done by varying the frequency of the modulation side band of the applied rf field. By varying the frequency of the applied rf radiation, NMR transitions of different energies can be brought into resonance successively. In this kind of experiment, the NMR spectrum consists of signal intensity vs. frequency of the applied rf.

Fresnel. A measure of frequency, defined as equal to 10^{12} cycles/second.

Friction factor. If the friction head loss for a fluid in any pipe is written in the form

$$hr = f\frac{1}{d}h\nu$$

then f is a function of the velocity v, the diameter d, and the kinematic viscosity of the fluid provided only that the pipes are all in the same internal condition of roughness. The term f is called the friction factor.

Fritted glass. Smitered (ground glass melted into a porous mat) glass used in filtration.

Front end. The front end is the part of the computer that the user works — keyboard, terminals, small processors, and so forth. A front-end processor usually does simple, routine work such as sorting information or translating programs into machine language, while the main processor handles more difficult tasks — storage, program execution, and mathematical calculations.

F test. A test of the equality of two variances. For the test we use the F ratio

$$(F \text{ ratio} = s_1^2/s_2^2)$$

which is compared with the F distribution (i.e., the distribution of the ratio of two independent sample estimates of a population variance).

ft value. In the theory of nuclear beta decay, a constant equal to the product of the half-life t with a quantity f, which is known function of the maximum energy of the beta particles and of the nuclear charge (for heavy nuclei), proportional to the amount of phase space available.

Fuel. Fissionable material of reasonably long life, used or usable in producing energy in a nuclear reactor. The term frequently is applied to a mixture, such as natural uranium, in which only part of the atoms are fissionable, if it can maintain a self-sustaining chain reaction under the proper conditions.

Fuel-cooling installation. A large container or cell, usually filled with water, in which spent fuel is set aside until its radioactivity has decreased to a desired level.

Fuel cycle. The sequence of steps, such as utilization, reprocessing, and refabrication, through which nuclear fuel passes.

Fuel element. A unit of nuclear fuel for use in a reactor — generally uranium, as metal or oxide, enclosed in a can that may have an extended surface area, e.g., fins, to assist heat transfer. If rod shaped, it is called fuel rod. Short fuel rods are called slugs.

Fuel rating. The rate of heat production per unit weight of fuel. Generally expressed in megawatts per tonne (MW/t).

Fulgaration. A technique for coagulating blood. An electrode supplied with high-frequency current is placed close to the tissue. Electric sparks generated between the electrode and the tissue char and destroy the tissue locally.

Full backup. A backup of all the files on a computer disk.

Full duplex. In communication, pertaining to a simultaneous, two-way, independent transmission.

Full width at half maximum or full width at tenth maximum. (FWHM or FWTM) Of the line spread function (LSF) or point spread function (PSF) ($\Delta v_{1/2}$). Is usually used to specify spatial resolution of scintillation and positron cameras.

Fulminate. Occurring suddenly and with severity. (A fulminating anoxia is a sudden reduction in the oxygen content of the blood causing collapse.

Fume cupboard. A box-like enclosure having a sliding sash in front and in which chemical and radioactive handling work may be done. There is an extract of air from the top or back of the fume cupboard so as to prevent fumes or dust from from coming out into the laboratory.

Function. A small program or section of a computer program that will reach a specific solution with information given (or passed) to it and return that solution to the main program or calling routine.

Functional group. Portion of a molecule responsible for its specific chemical properties.

Functional image. An image in which intensity reflects a physiologic parameter rather than activity; a derived image formed according to some mathematical rule. For example, intensity may be proportional to blood flow or to ejection fraction. Parametric image.

Functional residual capacity. (FRC) The volume of air in the lungs at the resting expiratory level.

Fundamental particle. Any particle of matter not composed of simpler units. Several such particles are known. Three — the electron, the proton, and the neutrino — are stable; the remainder decay spontaneously into fundamental particles of lower mass.

Fundus. The posterior portion of the interior of a body cavity; the bottom or base of an organ, or farthest from the entrance.

Fusion. If an isotope of a heavy element (uranium or plutonium) is encouraged to break up into two medium mass elements, the combined mass of which is less than the original mass, then the process is known as fission. The energy is released in the form of energetic neutrons and ultimately appears as heat which can be abstracted from reactor by more or less conventional means. Since the medium mass nuclei are the most tightly bound (i.e., have the smallest ratio of actual to nominal atomic weight), then it is possible to release energy also by fusing together lighter elements. The results of this fusion process when it is carried out rapidly and with the release of energy are represented by the hydrogen bomb. The major problem in the practical peaceful applications of this process is to release the energy slowly and in a controlled way. Naturally, this is the way that immense energy is generated in the sun.

G

Gadolinium. Element symbol Gd, atomic number 64, atomic weight 157.25.

Gain. Ratio of output to input electrical power. Control of amplification of echoes.

Gallium. Element symbol Ga, atomic number 31, atomic weight 69.72.

Galvanic current. Uninterrupted current derived from a chemical battery.

Galvanic skin response. (GSR) Measurements of the electrical resistance of the skin and tissue path between two electrodes. A variation of resistance from 1000 to over 500,000 Ω. Variations are associated with activity of the autonomic nervous system. Used to measure autonomic responses. Principle behind "lie detection" equipment. Variations occur with bandwidth from 0.1 to 5 Hz. Measured with surface electrodes.

Gamete. One of the reproductive cells (spermatozoids and eggs) which fuse at fertilization. Each contains only a single set of chromosomes in its nucleus.

Gamma. A term used pertaining to gamma (i.e., γ) radiation (e.g., γ-quantum, γ-absorption, γ-scattering, γ-spectrum, γ-source).

Gamma camera. An imaging apparatus used to visualize the distribution of radionuclides within the body. The majority of gamma cameras in clinical use operate on the principle devised originally by H. O. Anger at the Donner Laboratory in Berkeley in 1956. Radiation emanating from the patient is detected by a single, large, circular NaI(Tl) scintillation crystal. An array of (37, 61, or 91) photomultiplier tubes detects the light quanta emitted by the crystal and converts their energies into electrical pulses. Associated electronic circuitry determines the x, y coordinates of each scintillation event, the outputs of all the tubes being summed to provide a z pulse, the amplitude of which corresponds to the total energy of the scintillation event. The distribution of radioactivity is usually displayed on an oscilloscope. For quantitative analysis, the gamma camera is connected to a dedicated microcomputer, radioactive distributions being displayed either on a monochrome TV monitor as a gray scale range of tones or on a color TV monitor as a color scale.

Gamma counter. Solid scintillation counter (solid NaI crystal) used for counting radiation from gamma emitters.

Gamma emission. Nuclear process in which an excited nuclide deexcites by emission of a nuclear photon. (Electromagnetic wave.)

Gamma flux. The intensity of gamma radiation at a point, usually measured in coulomb per kilogram second.

Gamma globulin. (Ig) Serum protein with gamma mobility in electrophoresis that comprises the majority of immunoglobulins and antibodies. (IgA, IgE, IgG, IgM, and IgD.)

Gamma quantum. A gamma photon, i.e., a unit amount of gamma energy of magnitude hv where h is Planck's constant and v is the frequency of the gamma radiation.

Gamma radiation. (γ radiation or γ-rays) Electromagnetic radiation of a short wavelength that is emitted by the nucleus of a radionuclide during radioactive decay. The wave length of a γ-ray may be from 10^{-9} to 10^{-12} cm. Radioactive materials emit three types of radiation. The three types are called α-rays, β-rays, and γ-rays, respectively. Of the three radiations γ-rays are the most penetrating and require several inches of heavy material to reduce their intensity appreciably. It is now definitely established that γ-rays bear a similar relationship to the atomic nucleus as do α-rays to the atom itself. α-Rays originate when transitions between the electronic levels of the atom take place; γ-rays originate from transitions between the nuclear levels.

Gamma-ray detector. To be detected γ-rays must first interact with matter to produce energetic particles and the three interactions of importance are the photoelectric effect, the Compton effect, and pair production.

At low energies (<100 keV) the photoelectric effect in heavy elements is the most effective method of absorbing γ-rays. Between 100 keV and 1 MeV, either the photoelectric effect in heavy elements or the Compton effect in light elements is most useful. Above 1 MeV the Compton effect is the major process, but pair production increases rapidly in heavy elements and becomes dominant at 10 MeV. Detectors of γ-rays may be divided into three categories. (1) Counters. These permit the detection of individual quanta, and in the case of proportional detectors, e.g., proportional counter and scintillation counter, may also be used as γ-ray spectrometers. (2) Mean level detectors or monitors. These indicate the rate of arrival of γ-rays at the detector and may be employed as health monitors and as components in reactor instrumentation. (3) Dosimeters. These record the total amount of γ radiation incident upon the detector over a period of time. They may be used, for example, by personnel to measure the amount of radiation received.

Gamma-ray spectrometer. This is the name given to an instrument which measures the energy spectrum of γ-rays. The instruments in use at the present time, of which there are many, fall into two main groups: (1) those based upon the diffraction of γ-rays by crystals; (2) those based upon the measurement of the energies of the secondary electrons emitted in the three interactions of γ-rays with matter, the photoelectric effect, Compton scattering, and pair production.

Gamma source. A material from which γ-rays are emitted constitutes a γ-ray source. Generally, a γ-ray source refers to some radioactive material which emits γ-rays, in which case the γ-rays consist of discrete energy groups. The term is also applied, however, to a source of bremsstrahlung, which is emitted in the passage of high-speed particles through matter. This source has a continuous energy distribution.

Ganglion. Any collection or mass of nerve cells outside the central nervous system that serves as a center of nervous influence.

Gantry. The cylindrical opening located at or near the center of an imaging scanner into which the subject is placed.

Gas. A state of matter in which the molecules are practically unrestricted by cohesive forces. A gas has neither definite shape nor volume.

Gas amplification. The release of additional ions from neutral atoms; the release is caused by collisions of electrons that are freed by ionizing radiation. As applied to gas ionization radiation detecting instruments, the ratio of the charge collected to the charge produced by the initial ionizing event. This is a phenomenon seen in proportional counters.

Gas centrifuge process. A method of isotopic separation in which heavy gaseous atoms or molecules are separated from lighter ones by centrifugal force.

Gas chromatography. Various chemicals, whether in the gas or liquid phase, absorb energy from specific regions of the electromagnetic radiation spectrum. Thus, infrared radiation passed through two parallel chambers to a detection device may be used to record the difference in infrared absorption. The difference is sometimes detected in a Golay cell which consists of two infrared absorption chambers separated by a diaphragm whose movement is detected by a capacitance change with respect to an adjacent electrode. The infrared radiation is passed through a chopping disk so that each cell in turn receives the radiation, causing alternating displacement of the diaphragm in the Golay cell. The diaphragm will be displaced to one side or other depending on the relative quantities of infrared light reaching the absorption chambers. An electronic circuit to amplify, demodulate, and linearize the output is connected to the capacitance transducer. One of the cells is filled with a reference gas while the other is filled with a background gas plus a small flowthrough of the gas being sampled. The modification in absorption is used to detect the molar fraction of the sample gases.

Gas entrainment. The transportation of fine particles of solid or liquid by a gas stream; a serious problem in radioactive plants.

Gaseous diffusion. The kinetic process whereby gaseous molecules intermingle and become uniformly scattered throughout a volume. This comes about because all molecules in a gas are in constant motion. They thus collide with one another, and, according to kinetic theory, the rates of diffusion of different gases at the same temperature are in inverse proportion to the square root of the molecular weights. Light molecules thus diffuse more rapidly through a mixture of gases than heavy molecules. A method of separating isotopes, by causing a gaseous compound to diffuse through a porous membrane; the lighter molecules diffuse faster than the heavy ones and consequently their concentration increases on passing through the membrane, for the initial portions of gas.

Gas-filled detector. Type of ionization detector that converts absorbed radiation into electrical current. Includes ionization chamber (i.e., dose calibrators), proportional counters, and Geiger-Müller counters (survey meters).

Gas flow counter. A radiation counter in which an appropriate atmosphere is maintained in the counter tube by allowing a suitable gas to flow slowly through the volume. The source is usually placed inside the counting volume. A very high stability is obtainable if a gas proportional counter is operated in this way.

Gas multiplication. Multiplication of the ionization produced in the gas of a nuclear counter by an ionizing particle. Each electron produced by the initial ionizing particle produces several secondary electrons before reaching the anode, and each secondary electron in turn produces several more, and so on. This process produces a multiplication of the original quantity of ionization and a corresponding increase in the size of the negative pulse appearing at the anode.

Gastrin. A hormone secreted by the pyloric mucosa of the stomach.

Gastrointestinal tract. The digestive system comprises the mouth, esophagus, stomach, and small and large intestines, and associated structures. This is a convoluted tube in which food materials are chemically converted into simpler substance for absorption as nourishment by the process of digestion. Some 8 m long, this tube is called the gastrointestinal tract, or digestive tract. The lining of the canal is a mucosa which varies in character in different regions, many of its cells being highly specialized for secreting enzymes or ferments; also the lubricant mucus.

Gastrulation. The complex movement of those

cells in the embryo whose descendants will form the future internal organs.

Gate. A circuit that produces an output only when certain input conditions are met. Gates provide the basic logic circuits (e.g., and, or, not) of a computer.

Gated image. An image made from data acquired only over a brief, selected, physiologic interval, usually a selected portion of the cardiac cycle, such as end-systole or end-diastole; the image data acquisition is triggered or gated by the R wave for short 10- to 40-ms periods at a selected interval or intervals from the R wave to coincide with end-systole (downslope of T wave) and end-diastole (r wave itself); sufficient cycles are repetitively gated to build up data for a diagnostic image. This provides for removal or organ motion artifacts by imaging only during specific portions of the organ cycle.

Gating. (Pulsed Doppler) Passing only short pulses of voltage to the transducer from the voltage generator.

Gating receiver. Passing only sound reflections that arrive at a certain time after the transducer produces a pulse.

Gauss. A unit of magnetic flux density in the older (CGS) system. The earth's magnetic field is approximately 1/2 to 1 G, depending on location. The currently preferred (SI) unit is the tesla (T) (1 T = 10,000 G).

Gaussian distribution. (Normal distribution) A mathematical function describing the distribution of events in terms of the mean and standard deviation of the population or events under observation; produces a bell-shaped curve when plotted graphically.

Geiger-Müller counter. (G-M tube) A highly sensitive gas-filled tube with collecting electrode (anode) maintained at high voltage to collect, multiply, and measure the ions produced by entering ionizing radiation. It is based upon the avalanche effect which is observed when ions are accelerated by an electric field under appropriate conditions.

Geiger-Müller region. In an ionization radiation detector, the operating voltage interval in which the charge collected per ionizing event is essentially independent of the number of primary ions produced in the initial ionizing event.

Geiger-Müller threshold. The lowest voltage applied to a Geiger-Müller counter at which the output pulse is for the most part independent of the initial ionization. It corresponds to the start of the plateau.

Gel. A colloid in a solid or semisolid form.

Gel immunodiffusion tests. Precipitin techniques for identifying and measuring antigens (Ags) and antibodies (Abs) by allowing them to diffuse in various patterns through gels to form precipitates.

Gel permeation. Gel permeation is used to separate large molecules from small molecules by a sieving effect. Large molecules have difficulty penetrating the pores of gels and are eluted in a column separation procedure more rapidly than small molecules. Quantification can be obtained by passing the eluate through a radioactive counter, but is usually effected by fraction collecting and counting.

Geminate. Growing in pairs or couples.

Gene. The basic hereditary unit which, singly or in combination, determines inherited characteristics. The genes are located at certain specific points along the chromosomes.

General label. General or randomly labeled compounds are nonuniformly labeled compounds where the position of the radioactive atom in the molecule varies from one molecule to the other.

Generator. A device in which a short-lived daughter is separated chemically and periodically from a long-lived parent absorbed on adsorbent material (usually an inorganic resin). For example, ^{99m}Tc is eluted from the ^{99}Mo generator by means of saline solution. Commonly described as a "cow" and the elution as "milking".

Generic. Public or common name for a chemical.

Genetically significant dose. That radiation dose which, if received by every member of a defined population, would be expected to produce the same total genetic injury to the population as do the actual doses received by its various individuals.

Genetic code. The genetic information in the nucleotide sequences in DNA that determines the amount and type of proteins produced in a cell. There are 64 nucleotide triplet sequences or codons, each codon specifying one amino acid, and a chain of codons (averaging 100 codons) specifying a protein.

Genetic effects of radiation. Inheritable changes (mutations) produced by the absorption of ionizing radiation. Mutations are abrupt changes in genes, the most characteristic feature of which is that the gene is permanently altered and handed down in the changed form, so that the character difference caused by the mutation is inherited. All ionizing radiations, and also ultraviolet light, have been found to cause mutation. Quantitative studies have established the important fact that the frequency of mutation shows a linear relationship with the dose of ionizing radiation and is independent of its intensity. There is no threshold dose, with the result that numerous small doses of such radiations are just as effective in causing mutation as are only a few large doses, provided the total dose is the same. The linear relationship is taken to imply that mutation is caused by a single hit by an ionization path, though whether the effect is a direct physical action, or indirect through the formation of some mutagenic chemical, is uncertain.

Genetics. The branch of biology dealing with the phenomena of heredity.

Genetic switch hypothesis. A hypothesis that postulates that there is a switch in the gene controlling heavy chain synthesis in plasma cells during the development of an immune response.

Genitalia. The reproductive organs.

Genome. The complex set of self-reproducing particles upon which cell inheritance depends.

Genotype. The fundamental hereditary (genetic) constitution of an organism.

Geological age. Soon after the discovery of radioactivity it was pointed out that since the rate of decay of radioactive minerals set in the earth's crust was unaltered by drastic physical and chemical changes, these naturally occurring radioactive substances provide us with chronometers of exquisite accuracy. Measuring the amount of daughter product formed and the amount of the parent substance present when the decay rate is known can determine the age of a material.

Theoretically, every radioactive element should be able to act as a geochronometer. Uranium, thorium, rubidium, and potassium have been most widely used because they are relatively abundant and their decay constants are known.

Geometric mean. Antilog of the mean of logarithmic data.

Geometry. Refers to the geometric relationship between the detector and activity to be measured which determines the fraction of total emitted radiation that can be detected.

Geometry factor. That fraction of the total radiation emitted from a point source that impinges on the detector.

Germ. A pathogenic or harmful microorganism.

Germanium. Element symbol Ge, atomic number 32, atomic weight 72.61.

Germ cells. The cells of an organism whose function it is to reproduce its kind. (Genetic cells.)

Germinal centers. A collection of metabolically active lymphoblasts, macrophages, and plasma cells that appears within the primary follicle of lymphoid tissues following antigenic stimulation.

Gestation. Period of development before birth.

G force. Centrifugal force.

Gland. Group of cells specialized to secrete or excrete biochemical materials.

Glass. (For shielding) To provide viewing points for heavily shielded apparatuses, thick blocks, made from a glass with a high lead content, are used. Their value as shielding is intermediate between that of iron and concrete.

Glass dosimeters. Comprise a piece of glass of a special kind which fluoresces under ultraviolet light following γ irradiation. Glass dosimeters are not direct-reading, but must be read with a separate instrument comprising an ultraviolet lamp with suitable light filters and a photocell detector to measure the fluorescence.

Glia. The web of supporting tissue of the central nervous system surrounding cell bodies, dendrites, and axons of the neutrons. It consists mainly of cells with long fibrous processes, and mesodermal cells. Also known as neuroglia.

Glitch. Slang for an electrical disturbance that interferes with a circuit.

Global radiation. The total of direct solar radiation and diffuse sky radiation received by a unit horizontal surface.

Globin. Protein component of hemoglobin.

Globule. A small spherical mass; small spherical bodies in cells or secretions.

Globulin. One of a class of proteins present in blood plasma that is insoluble in water but soluble in saline; important in the immune response.

Glomerular filtration rate. The volume of plasma filtered through the glomerular capillaries of the kidneys per minute.

Glomerulus. A tuft of fine blood capillaries in the nephron, which acts as a filter.

Glove box. A form of protection enclosure used when working with certain radioactive materials. Gloves fixed to parts in the walls of a box allow manipulation of work within the box. The box is usually kept under slight negative pressure and ventilation is through high-efficiency filters.

Glucocorticoid. Hormone secreted by the adrenal cortex stimulating the conversion of proteins to carbohydrates.

Glucoheptonate. Chelating molecule that can bind ^{99m}Tc and be used as an imaging agent.

Gluconeogenesis. The synthesis of glycogen from noncarbohydrate sources, such as amino or fatty acids.

Glucose. Six-carbon monosaccharide found in fruit and other foods and in the blood of all animals; chief source of energy for most living organism.

Glucosuria. The presence of glucose in the urine.

Glycogen. The storage form of sugar, primarily in the muscles and the liver. It is broken down to glucose to meet the body's energy needs.

Glycogenesis. Synthesis of glycogen from glucose.

Glycogenolysis. The conversion of glycogen to glucose.

Glycolysis. The breakdown of glucose by enzymes to give lactic and pyruvic acids with the liberation of energy.

Glycoprotein. Protein and a carbohydrate that does not contain phosphoric acid, purine, or pyrimidine.

Goiter. Any enlargement of the thyroid gland beyond normal size. The goiter may be diffuse (generally homogeneous enlargement) or nodular. Goiter may be associated with normal (euthyroid goiter), decreased, or increased thyroid function.

Golay coil. Term commonly used for a particular kind of gradient coil, commonly used to create gradient magnetic fields, perpendicular to the main magnetic field. (NMR.)

Gold. Element symbol Au (aurum), atomic number 79, atomic weight 196.966.

Gonad. Reproductive organ (testis or ovary) in which the gametes (spermatozoids or eggs) are formed. The sex gland.

Gonadal dose. The absorbed dose (or dose equivalent) to the gonads, i.e., the testes or ovaries, averaged over the total gonadal volume.

Goodness of fit test. A chi-square test of qualitative data in which a sample distribution is compared with a theoretical or population distribution. Has $(r - 1)$ df. An additional df is subtracted for each parameter of the theoretical distribution estimated from the sample itself.

Gradient. Change of the individual components of a vector quantity along a given spatial coordinate. The amount and direction of rate of change in space of some quantity, such as magnetic field strength.

Gradient coils. Current carrying coils designed to produce a desired gradient magnetic field (so that the magnetic field will be stronger in some locations than others). Proper design of the size and configuration of the coils is necessary to produce a controlled and uniform gradient.

Gradient magnetic field. A magnetic field which changes in strength in a certain given direction. Such fields are used in NMR imaging with selective excitation to select a region for imaging and also to encode the location of NMR signals received from the object being imaged. Measured (e.g.) in teslas per meter and expressed by the symbols G_x, G_y, and G_z.

Graft. Tissue or organ for transplantation to another site or another individual.

Graft-vs.-host. (GVH reaction) The clinical and pathologic sequelae of the reactions of immunocompetent cells in a graft against the cells of the histoincompatible and immunodeficient recipient.

Graft-vs.-host disease. (GVHD) (Secondary disease, runt disease, allogeneic disease) A disease, either acute or chronic, that results from an immunologic graft-vs.-host attack by donor lymphocytes.

Gram atomic weight. A mass in grams numerically equal to the atomic weight of an element.

Gram equivalent. (Of a substance) Is the weight of a substance displacing or otherwise reacting with 1.008 g of hydrogen or combining with one half of a gram atomic weight (8.00 g) of oxygen.

Gram molecular weight. (Gram-mole) Mass is grams numerically equal to the molecular weight of a chemical compound.

Granule. Small particle of grain; nonsoluble particles in cells; breadlike masses of tissue.

Granulocyte. Granule-containing cells, especially the leukocytes with basophil, eosinophil, or neutrophil granules in their cytoplasm.

Granuloma. A tumor-like mass of granular appearance; granulomas are of many diverse types and causes.

Granulopoietin. (Colony-stimulating factor) A glycoprotein with a molecular weight of 45,000 derived from monocytes that controls the production of granulocytes by the bone marrow.

Graphics. Any form of computer-based drawings; i.e., graphs, histograms, maps, diagrams. These may be displayed on an oscilloscope device in black and white or in color, or may be drawn out by a graph plotter.

Graphite. A form of carbon in which the atoms are hexagonally arranged in planes. The form of carbon commonly used for moderators because it can be made in compact, fairly strong blocks and can be machine easily to close tolerances and because the prolonged baking at high temperature used in its manufacture contributes to elimination of impurities that might absorb neutrons.

Graveyard. A place for burying unwanted radioactive objects to prevent the escape of their radiations. In this case the earth acts as a shield. It is usual to place such objects in water-tight noncorrosive containers so that the radioactive contamination cannot escape by leaching or other means and contaminate underground water supplies.

Gravitation. Force of attraction existing between all material bodies in the universe. The magnitude of the force between any two bodies is proportional to the product of the masses of the two bodies and inversely proportional to the square of the distance between them.

Gray. The SI unit of absorbed dose of ionizing radiation; 1 gray (Gy) = 1 J/kg.

Gray matter. Tissue of the central nervous system containing nerve cell bodies, dendrites, and the cell synapses.

Gray scale. A series of tones ranging in steps from black to white, used to represent values of a variable on a display screen.

Gray scale display. A type of display or paper recorder utilizing varying intensity to indicate a third parameter. This is best known in medical equipment in gray scale display of ultrasonic images in which the brightness is used to indicate the intensity of the echo. Gray scale displays on cathode ray tube (CRTs) can be achieved using a conventional CRT for real-time scanning or using scan converters with TV-type displays. Fiber-optic recorders can also achieve gray scale printing of such images on photographic paper.

Grenz rays. X-rays produced in the region of 5 to 20 kV.

Grid. A system of fine conducting wires which is used to produce an electric field, thus controlling the flow of electrons in a thermionic valve or other electronic device.

Ground. The state of a nucleus, an atom, or a molecule when it has its lowest energy. All other states are termed excited.

Ground disposal of effluent. A method for the disposal of radioactive liquid wastes by passage into suitable strata in the ground.

Growth. A normal process of increase in mass; or an abnormal tissue mass, normal or malignant cells.

Growth curve. When a radioactive nuclide has

a radioactive daughter whose half-life is short compared with the parent, the quantity of daughter product present will gradually grow until it is equal, when measured in becquerel (or curie) units, to that of the parent.

G value. An expression denoting the yield of products of radiolysis. The number of radicals or molecules formed or destroyed per 100 eV of radiation energy absorbed. A characteristic number which denotes the size of the magnetic moment of a paramagnetic species. The electron spin resonance (ESR) spectrum of a paramagnetic species occurs at a position in the frequency domain determined by the g value of the species. The g value of the free electron is 2.0023. (NMR.)

Gyromagnetic ratio. Constant of proportionality relating the angular frequency of precession of a nucleus to the magnetic field strength: has a value which is both constant and specific to a particular isotope. Also called magnetogyric ratio, defined by the Larmor equation.

Gyrus. Infolding of the surface of the brain.

H

Hafnium. Element symbol Hf, atomic number 72, atomic weight 178.49.

Hahn emanation technique. A radioactive technique, named after its originator, which has been widely used for studying the solid state. Very small quantities of a radium isotope, for example, ^{226}Ra or ^{224}Ra are uniformly incorporated into the material being examined. The radium decays to give the inert gas emanations radon or thoron and the rate of evolution of these gases is used as a qualitative measure of the reactions, rearrangements, or other crystalline changes occurring in the solid materials under various treatments.

Half duplex. A computer communications linkage that can send and receive — but not simultaneously. Sometimes the term simplex is used for a linkage that can only send or receive.

Half-life. (Tp or $T_{1/2}$) A unique characteristic of a radionuclide, defined by the time during which an initial activity of a radionuclide is reduced to one half. It is related to the decay constant λ by $t_{1/2} = 0.693\ \lambda$. Half-lives may vary from less than a millionth of a second to millions of years, according to the isotope and element concerned. Biologic refers to the time for the body or an organ to eliminate one half the original material; physical refers to physical radioactive decay of nuclei to one half their original numbers; effective refers to the combined effects of biological elimination and physical decay, which result in an observed half life shorter than either of these two values individually.

Half-reaction. Term used in an electrochemical reaction to describe either the oxidation process or the reduction process as a separate entity.

Half-time of exchange. In a chemical reaction involving the exchange of atoms, the time required for one half of the atoms to be measurably exchanged.

Half-value layer. (HVL) The thickness of any absorbing material required to reduce the intensity or exposure of a radiation beam to one half of the initial value when placed in the path of the beam. Synonym for half-thickness. This thickness T may be related to the linear absorption coefficient μ by the equation $T = 0.693/\mu$.

Half-value layer of sound. A term used to express the role of attenuation of sound in tissue is the half-value layer, which is defined as the thickness of tissue, in centimeters, required to reduce the intensity of the beam by half. Not all tissues are isotropic in their attenuation. For example, attenuation in muscle may be different by a factor of 2.5. This depends upon whether the sound beam passes along or across its fibers. In general, the echoes arriving back at the emitting transducer are substantially smaller than the initially transmitted pulse because of the low reflection coefficients and high attenuation.

Hall probe. A device used for measuring magnetic fields. A Hall probe is used with wideline NMR and electron spin resonance (ESR) instruments for stabilizing the magnetic field produced by the electromagnets.

Halo. A luminous or colored circle seen in the light around an object.

Halogenation. A combination of a halogen molecule with a microbial cell wall that results in microbial damage.

Halogen counter. A Geiger counter in which the self-quenching action is provided by the admixture of a halogen gas such as chlorine or bromine. These are corrosive and careful construction is needed. After dissociation in the quenching process, however, the diatomic halogen molecules reform, and thus a halogen counter has a long life.

Halogens. Family of chemical elements of similar electron structure (that is, the valence shell is completely filled except for one electron) — fluorine, chlorine, bromine, iodine, and asta-

tine.

Hamiltonian. (H) The hamiltonian is a mathematical operator used in quantum mechanical treatment of some phenomena (e.g., magnetic resonance). It represents the sum of the kinetic and potential energies of a particle or a system. It can be represented as a function of momentum and position coordinates of the particle. It can be expressed as $H = p^2/2m + V(r)$, where p is the momentum operator, $V(r)$ is the potential energy as a function of position operator r, and m is the mass of the particle.

Hands and clothing monitor. In most laboratories where radioactive materials are handled it is necessary to take the most stringent precautions to prevent the spread of contamination and to ensure that operators do not allow radioactivity picked up accidentally on their person or clothing to remain there. One of the most useful instruments to include in the laboratory monitoring room is the hands and clothing monitor. It is provided with probes, sensitive to β-, γ-, and α-radiation, for general-purpose monitoring.

Handshaking. Back and forth exchange of control signals, usually between a computer and peripheral devices.

Hann filter. A common filter used in nuclear medicine image processing. This low-pass filter is usually called a Hanning filter. The filter has a magnitude of one at the lowest frequencies and decreases to zero at a frequency known as the cutoff frequency. A Hann filter with a cutoff frequency of 0.5 cycles/pixel removes this and higher-frequency components from the image. When this filter multiplies the same input image spectrum it can be seen that the 0.5-cycles/pixel frequency of the input image has been removed in both the filtered spectrum and image. The amplitude of the frequencies lower than 0.5 is reduced by the product of the filter value at those frequencies and objects related to these frequencies do not have as much contrast in the output image as in the input image.

Haploid. Having one set of chromosomes.

Haplotype. That portion of the phenotype determined by closely linked genes of a single chromosome inherited from one parent.

Hapten. A substance which is antigenic when combined with a protein but cannot on its own induce the production of antibodies. It is the part of an antigenic complex that determines immunological specificity. A substance that is not immunogenic but can react with an antibody of appropriate specificity.

Hard component. Cosmic radiation can be roughly separated into two components, a hard or penetrating component and a soft component. At sea level the hard component is defined as that which penetrates through 10 cm of lead and consists mainly of mu-mesons.

Hard copy. Computer output printed on paper or film. Hard copy provides a permanent record that the user can read and store for visual inspection or analysis.

Hard disk. In computing, a disk of a rigid alloy plate coated with Mylar, a magnetizable compound; used for data storage. Its storage capacity (megabytes) is much greater than that of a floppy disk.

Hard disk drive. A type of disk drive that uses a rigid (hard) disk. The hard disk is usually permanently sealed into the drive to protect it from contamination by dust. Hard disk drives tend to have greater capacity, speed, and reliability than diskette drives, and also tend to be more expensive.

Hardness. (X-rays) A term referring to the penetrating power of X-rays. Soft X-rays, of lower frequency and hence lower energy, are less penetrating. Hard X-rays, having a higher frequency and greater energy, are more penetrating.

Hard radiation. Ionizing radiation of high energy which has high penetrating ability.

Hardware. Physical computer equipment, such as mechanical, electrical, or electronic devices.

Hard-wired. Physically (and usually permanently) connected to a computer, usually by an electronic conductor. Hard-wired programs: on old computers, programs actualized in the form of interconnections of wires on patchboards. A method still used on analog computers to process continuous signals instead of digital (numeric) information.

Harmonic. A sinusoidal quantity whose frequency is an integral multiple of some fundamental frequency, that is, given a quantity, $x(t)$, where

$$x(t) = A \cos (\omega t + \o)$$

Its harmonics, $h_n(x)$, are of the form

$$h_n(x) = A_B \cos(n\ \omega t + \o_n)$$

where n is an integer larger than 1.

Hash code. A number determined by an algorithm from name, etc., and used for locating a file.

Haversian system. System of canals in the bones where the blood vessels branch out.

Head. An electromagnet used to record, receive, or erase information stored on magnetic tapes, disks, cassettes, or drums.

Health monitor. Monitoring has been defined as the periodic or continuous determination of the amount of ionizing radiation or radioactive contamination present in a specified region (designated area monitoring), in or upon a person or his clothing (designated personnel monitoring), or in the air (designated air monitoring), or in water (designated water monitoring). Monitoring may be carried out as a safety measure for purposes of health protection, or to assess and sometimes control the operation of a given machine or process. The term health monitor is used to cover the instrument employed for these various purposes.

Health physics. A division of occupational health dealing particularly with protection of personnel from the harmful effects of ionizing radiation.

Heart. The pumping organ that maintains the circulation of the blood in the vascular system.

Heart block. A state in which the atrium and ventricle beat unnaturally and independently owing to inefficient conduction of electrical stimuli along the specialized conduction tissue of the heart.

Heart-lung machine. A device which takes over the pumping and gas-exchange functions of the heart and lungs during cardiac surgery.

Heart murmurs. Sounds heard through the stethoscope when listening to the heart. In most cases produced by increasing turbulence of the blood as it passes through the heart chambers. Some murmurs are benign or functional. (There is no underlying structural abnormality of the heart to account for them.) Other murmurs are organic and are caused by structural abnormalities within the heart.

Heat. It is the type of energy due to thermal molecular motion.

Heat capacity. That quantity of heat required to increase the temperature of a system of substance 1° of temperature. It is usually expressed in cal/°C or J/°C. Molar heat capacity is the quantity of heat necessary to raise the temperature of one molecular weight of the substance 1°.

Heat fatigue. Transient deterioration in performance from exposure to heat and humidity, and resulting in relative state of dehydration and salt depletion.

Heat-sensitive printer. Type of printer that imprints characters on special sensitized paper by use of heat, without the use of an ink ribbon.

Heat transfer. (Or transmission) The study of heat transfer is concerned with the means by which heat can be exchanged. The natural flow of heat is caused by temperature difference, the direction of flow being from high to low temperature.

Heavy chain. (H chain) One pair of identical polypeptide chains making up an immunoglobulin molecule. The heavy chain contains approximately twice the number of amino acids and is twice the molecular weight of the light chain.

Heavy elements. A term often used with reference to the actinide elements, especially thorium and uranium. Atomic weights range from 232 (thorium) upwards.

Heavy hydrogen. (Deuterium, D_2, H_2) The isotope of hydrogen of mass number 2; hydrogen of mass number 1 being known as light hydrogen and that of mass number 3 as tritium. Deuterium is prominent for its efficiency, in the form of heavy water — $(H_2)D_2O$ — as a moderator in fusion reactions.

Heavy ions. A term used with reference to such ions as are formed by ^{12}C, ^{13}C, ^{14}N, ^{15}N, ^{16}O, etc.

Heavy particles. Neutrons and charged particles with a mass of 1 or greater.

Heavy water. Water consisting of molecules in which the hydrogen is replaced by deuterium, or heavy hydrogen. It is present in ordinary water as about 1 part in 5000. It is used as moderator because it has a low neutron absorption cross section. Its density is greater than that of H_2O. Density = 1.076 g/ml at 20°C.

Heisenberg's theory of atomic structure. The currently accepted view of the structure of atom, formulated by Heisenberg in 1934, according to which the atomic nuclei are built of nucleons, which may be protons or neutrons, while the extranuclear shells consist of electrons only. The nucleons are held together by nuclear forces of attraction, with exchange forces operating between them. The number of protons is equal to the atomic number (Z) of the element; the number of neutrons is equal to the difference between the mass number and the atomic number (A − Z). The number of excess neutrons, i.e., the excess of neutrons over protons, is of paramount importance for the radioactive properties or stability of the element.

Helium. Element symbol He, atomic number 2, atomic weight 4.0026.

Helmoltz coils. Two circular, parallel coils of the same radius separated by a distance equal to their radius. $\Delta v_{1/2} = 1/\pi T_2$ is the characteristic time constant for the decay of the free induction decay signal. They produce a region of constant magnetic field on either side of the midpoint between the two coils. (NMR.)

Help. A computer system for medical decision making.

Helper T cells. A subtype of T lymphocytes that cooperates with B cells in antibody formation.

Hemagglutination inhibition. A technique for detecting small amounts of antigen in which homologous antigen inhibits the agglutination of red cells or other particles coated with antigen by specific antibody.

Hemagglutinin. An antibody which reacts with antigen-determinant sites on red blood cells to cause agglutination of the red cells.

Hemarthrosis. Bloody effusion into the cavity of a joint.

Hematemesis. Vomiting of blood.

Hematocrit. (Hct) An expression of the volume of the red blood cells per unit volume of circulating blood, 46% in males and 43% in females, or the centrifuge used to separate the cells from the plasma to determine this fractional volume.

Hematology. Study of the diseases of blood and blood-forming organs.

Hematoma. A swelling or mass of blood (usually clotted) confined to an organ, tissue, or space and caused by a break in a blood vessel.

Hematopoiesis. Formation of blood cells.

Hematopoietic system. All tissues responsible for production of the cellular elements of peripheral blood. This term usually excludes strictly lymphocytopoietic tissue such as lymph nodes.

Hematuria. The presence of blood or red blood cells in the urine.

Heme. Nonprotein iron protoporphyrin ring compound of hemoglobin and other respiratory pigments.

Hemilateral. Affecting only one side.

Hemiparesis. Partial paralysis of one side of the body.

Hemiplegia. Paralysis of one side of the body.

Hemocytometer. Instrument used to count blood cells.

Hemodialysis. The removal (separation) of waste materials from blood by dialysis. Most commonly, the circulating blood is passed extracorporeally through an artificial kidney — essentially a hollow device made of semipermeable membranous material immersed in dialysate.

Hemodynamics. A branch of fluid dynamics dealing with the motion of the blood and the forces involved in its circulation.

Hemoglobin. Proteinaceous pigment of red blood cells. Combines loosely with oxygen to form oxyhemoglobin, whereby oxygen is transported to the tissues.

Hemolysin. An antibody or other substance capable of lysing red blood cells.

Hemolysis. Red blood cell destruction; escape of hemoglobin within the bloodstream.

Hemophilia. A condition characterized by a bleeding tendency.

Hemopoietic tissue. Blood cells do not live indefinitely, and as the different varieties die or wear out new cells have continually to be provided by the hemopoietic, or blood-forming, tissues. The bone marrow and lymph glands are the main tissues. The bone marrow and lymph glands are the main tissues concerned. Deaths due to acute irradiation can usually be attributed to a damaged hemopoietic system. For the most part, the cells which make the blood cells are damaged rather than the blood cells themselves, the chief exception to this rule being the lymphocyte which dies in the circulating blood.

The lymphocytes of the blood are reduced in numbers a few hours after irradiation. The granulocytes decrease in numbers during the first few days and reach a minimum during the second week after doses which result in a mortality of 50%. A sufficiently marked reduction in the numbers of granulocytes makes the irradiated individual liable to severe infections.

The platelets are the next cells to be reduced in numbers and as they are important in the control of bleeding, hemorrhages tend to develop, usually between 2 and 6 weeks after exposure. Small areas of bleeding, if sufficiently numerous, will reduce the numbers of red cells in the circulation and the anemia which follows acute radiation is primarily due to the shortage of platelets. The bone marrow cells which produce red cells are very radiosensitive and the damage which they suffer also contributes to the postirradiation anemia.

Hemoptysis. Act of coughing up blood; caused by lesion of the lungs, trachea, or larynx.

Hemorheology. The study of blood flow, especially non-Newtonian flow.

Hemorrhage. The escape of blood from the blood vessels; bleeding.

Hemostasis. The stopping or slowing down of blood flow or blood loss.

Hemostat. A small surgical tool for clamping off blood vessels.

Hemothorax. Blood fluid in the pleural cavity caused by the rupture of small blood vessels, owing to inflammation of the lungs in pneumonia and pulmonary tuberculosis, to a malignant growth, or trauma.

Henry. (Unit of electric inductance) The inductance of a closed circuit in which an electromotive force of 1 V is produced when the electric current in the circuit varies uniformly at a rate of 1 A/s.

Heparin. A naturally occurring substance found most abundantly in the liver. Produced chemically, it serves as an anticoagulant by inhibiting the conversion of prothrombin in the blood into thrombin.

Hepatoportal. Pertaining to the portal or venous side of the liver circulation.

Heptasulfide. Technetium heptasulfide: $^{99m}Tc_2S_7$ coprecipitates with colloidal sulfur particles stabilized with gelatin in ^{99m}Tc-sulfur colloid preparation.

Heredity. Transmission of characters and traits from parent to offspring.

Hernia. Protrusion of a loop of an organ through an abnormal opening; weakness of the abdominal wall allowing protrusion of a segment of intestine.

Herpes. A skin disease in which small blisters appear, often in clusters. (Herpes simplex may be referred to as cold sores or fever blisters and is caused by a virus infection involving mostly the lip borders and the nose. Herpes zoster, shingles, is also a virus infection but involving nerve trunk areas.)

Hertz. (Hz) The standard (SI) unit of frequency. One cycle or pulse per second; unit of pulse repetition frequency.

Heterocytotropic antibodies. An antibody that can passively sensitize tissues of species other than those in which the antibody is present.

Heterogeneous. A term used to describe a structure or medium which has an uneven texture.

Heterogeneous population. Population can be subdivided on the basis of a characteristic other than the one under consideration into subgroups that differ significantly among themselves with respect to the item being measured.

Heterogeneous reactor. The fissionable material and moderator are arranged as discrete bodies (usually according to a regular pattern) of such dimensions that a nonhomogeneous medium is presented to the neutrons.

Heterologous antigen. An antigen that participates in a cross-reaction.

Heteronuclear decoupling. A technique used in high-resolution NMR spectroscopy for elimination of spin-spin interactions between nuclei of different types, irradiating with high radio-frequency (rf) power at the resonance frequency of the heteronucleus; e.g., coupling between ^{31}P and ^{1}H spins is eliminated by irradiating, at the ^{1}H NMR frequency of the protons, couples to ^{31}P nucleus under observation.

Heterozygous. Refers to the situation where the two members of a pair of genes are different.

Heuristic. Approaching a problem by using general principles (in contrast to the precise rules of an algorithm).

Hexadecimal. Pertaining to the number system with a radix of 16. Note: Hexadecimal numerals are frequently used as a "shorthand" representation for binary numbers, with each hexadecimal digit representing a group of four bits (binary digits); e.g., the binary numeral 1001 0111 0100 can be represented as hexadecimal 974. The hexadecimal numbering system includes: 0, 1, 2, 3, 4, 5, 6, 7, 8, 9, A, B, C, D, E, F.

Hexane. Alkane with the molecular formula C_6H_{14}.

H_o. Conventional symbol historically used for the constant magnetic field in an NMR system; it is physically more correct to use B_o. A magnet provides a field strength, H; however, at a point in an object, the spins experience the magnetic induction, B.

H_1. Conventional symbol historically used for the radio-frequency magnetic field in an NMR system; it is physically more correct to use B_1. It is useful to consider it as composed of two oppositely rotating vectors. At the Larmor frequency, the vector rotating in the same direction as the precessing spins will interact strongly with the spins.

Hiatus. Term for gap, cleft, or opening; opening in diaphragm through which aorta and thoracic duct pass.

High attenuation. On the diasonography, a way of producing low sensitivity; the attenuation can be applied to the transducer or to the ultrasound echo signals.

High-current accelerator. The demands for very intense beams of high-energy particles in thermonuclear work and other subjects have led to the development of accelerators capable of currents of the order of 1 A at tens of kilovolts of energy.

High-dose (high-zone) tolerance. Classic immunologic unresponsiveness produced by repeated injections of large amounts of antigen.

High-endothelial venules. Specialized venules in lymphoid structures that allow the selective passage of lymphocytes across the endothelial barrier.

High flux reactor. A nuclear reactor in which the thermal neutron flux is $>10^{14}$ neutrons/cm^2/s. The term is most frequently used when considering research reactors.

High gain. In ultrasound. Increasing amplification of the echoes to increase sensitivities by better displaying the small echoes. This is one way of achieving "high sensitivity".

High-level language. These are sophisticated computer languages that closely resemble plain English. FORTRAN, COBOL, and BASIC are three popular high-level languages. Although the computer must translate these high-level languages into machine language, they are easier to use than the more primitive assembly languages.

Highlighting. In highlighting, selectable ranges of density are made to appear light, as a result of which they stand out clearly from the gray shades of the computed tomogram, regardless of the window setting.

High-order byte. The most significant byte in a word. The high-order byte occupies bit positions 8 through 15 of a 16-bit word (starting at zero).

High-pressure recombination. In a device (e.g., a gas discharge tube or an ionization chamber) in which ions formed in a gas are attracted toward electrodes by an electric field, some of the ions will collide with gas atoms and will be slowed down. If the gas pressure is high (or the accelerating field low) many of the collisions will occur before the ions have been accelerated sufficiently to cause further ionization. These ions will eventually recombine. Thus, a gas is a better insulator at a high pressure than at a low one. This property is made use of in a Van de Graaff accelerator.

High-pulse repetition frequency Doppler. A method of achieving high sampling rates: multiple pulses and their return signals from within the heart are present at any point in time, and Doppler shifts along the beam are summed along sample volume depths which are multiples of the initial sample volume depth to give a signal output.

High resolution collimator. A collimator designed to maximize spatial resolution by using small, long holes; as a result, sensitivity is reduced.

High-resolution computerized tomography. (HR/CT) The picture elements in areas of the image (usually central) can be diminished in size by reducing the scan field or narrowing the distance between the detectors, i.e., the spatial resolution can be improved. At present, picture element diameters of 0.2 mm can already be achieved. Diminishing the size of the picture or volume element leads to an increase in image noise, so that particularly high-contrast structures, e.g., bones, can be clearly demonstrated by HR/CT. For the same reason, longer scanning times must be chosen for soft-tissue structures. Since small measuring fields are usually employed, this is also referred to as a sector scan.

High-resolution gamma spectroscopy. High-resolution gamma spectroscopy utilizing a high-purity germanium crystal is a basic tool in the estimation of radionuclidic impurities. It allows many gamma emitting impurities to be resolved, identified, and quantified at very low levels.

High-resolution NMR spectroscopy. An NMR spectrometer that is capable of producing very narrow NMR lines for the nucleus of a given isotope, i.e., lines with widths that are less than the majority of chemical shifts and coupling constants for that isotope.

High sensitivity. Demonstration of a high range of echoes from those of low amplitude, possibly including those in the noise level, to those of high amplitude. A collimator designed to achieve high count rates by using large, short holes.

High-temperature reactor. Roughly, the temperature may be considered high in this connection if it is high enough to permit the generation of mechanical power at good efficiency.

Hilar. Pertaining to a hilus; hilar nodes are those nodes surrounding a hilus, such as those in the mediastinum.

Hilum. Or hilus, a depression or pit at that part of an organ where the vessels and nerves enter.

Histamine. Amine produced by damaged cells, and by eosinophils and mast cells; potent vasodilator, increases gastric secretion, smooth muscle contraction, and capillary permeability. Antihistamine drugs reduce or prevent those reactions.

Histamine-releasing factor. A lymphokine released from sensitized lymphocytes or antigenic stimulation that causes basophil histamine release.

Histochemical. Referring to the deposit of chemical components in cells.

Histocompatibility antigens. (Transplantation Ags) Cell-surface Ags of major importance in allograft rejection; controlled largely by a single gene complex called the MHC.

Histocompatible. Sharing transplantation antigens.

Histogram. A plot of frequency of samples falling into each of a series of bins representing a range of values. A bar graph for grouped data. Assuming equal class intervals, the frequency of a class is represented by the height and the class interval by the width of the bar.

Histogram mode matrix. Acquisition of a dynamic study such as a radionuclide angiocardiogram into a predefined number of frames and framing rate.

Histology. Study of the form and structure of tissues or of a part of the body.

Hold-back agent. A term used in precipitation separation processes to describe substances added to a mixture to prevent or hold back precipitation of an undesired element present at tracer concentration, while enabling precipitation of the required element to occur. An example is the separation of traces of radium B (a lead isotope) from radium by co-deposition of the radium B on copper sulfide, making use of barium as a hold-back agent for the radium. Synonym: hold-back carrier.

Holder of the authority. A person, organization, or institution having control over one or more radioactive sources and to whom an authority has been issued by the competent authority.

Holmium. Element symbol Ho, atomic number 67, atomic weight 164.930.

Hologram. A recording or picture of a three-dimensional wavefront.

Holography. A recording and viewing process which allows reconstruction of three-dimensional images of diffuse objects.

Holter monitor/analyzer. A device for ambulatory monitoring of patients over a 24-h period during which a diary of activities is kept. The monitor records the electrocardiogram during this time on a recording device that is subsequently scanned and analyzed for rate, rhythm, and conduction disturbances of the heart. Modern digital monitors record the EKG tracings, while the analyzer selects aberrant complexes automatically in accordance with clinical significance.

Homeostasis. State of biological equilibrium of the internal environment of the body that is maintained by dynamic processes of feedback and regulation.

Homocytotropic antibody. An antibody that attaches to cells of animals of the same species.

Homogeneity. Uniformity. In NMR, the homogeneity of the static magnetic field is an important criterion of the quality of the magnet. Homogeneity requirements for NMR imaging are generally lower than the homogeneity requirements for NMR spectroscopy, but for most imaging techniques must be maintained over a larger region.

Homogeneity spoil pulse. One of the techniques used in pulsed Fourier transform NMR spectroscopy. In this technique, a temporary deterioration of the homogeneity of the static magnetic field (B) is deliberately introduced in a pulsed mode.

Homogeneous. A term used to describe a structure or medium that has an even texture or distribution.

Homogeneous population. No further subdivision of population is necessary for appropriate statistical analysis.

Homogeneous reactor. A nuclear reactor in which the fissionable material and moderator (if used) are combined in a mixture such that an effectively homogeneous medium is presented to the neutrons. Such a mixture is represented either by a solution of fuel in moderator or by discrete particles having dimensions small in comparison with the neutron mean free path.

Homologous antigen. An antigen that induces an antibody and reacts specifically with it.

Homonuclear decoupling. A technique used in high-resolution NMR spectroscopy for the elimination of spin-spin interactions between the nuclei of the same type by irradiation with high radio-frequency (rf) power at the resonance frequency of one of them. Very useful in the assignment of lines in NMR spectra, e.g., by the decoupling of one proton from another adjacent to it in a molecule.

Homonuclear lock. A lock signal in high-resolution NMR spectrometer which is obtained from the same nuclide that is being observed.

Homopolymer. A molecule consisting of repeating units of a single amino acid.

Homozygous. Refers to the situation where the two members of a pair of genes are the same.

Hormesis. The beneficial stimulation of biological system using small doses of substance or radiation which in large doses are normally harmful.

Hormonal cross-reactions. In hormonal cross-reactions the antibody reacts with an entirely different biologically active hormone of the same species.

Hormone. Substance secreted by the endocrine, or ductless, glands that influences the activity of the various organs of the body and thus regulates the metabolic processes. Chemically, this represents a diverse group of compounds and can be divided into three classes:

1. Polypeptide or protein hormones — those secreted by pituitary, parathyroid, and pancreas (for example, thyrotropin, TSH, growth hormone, HGH, follicle-stimulating hormone, FSH, parathormone, calcitonin, and insulin).
2. Steroid hormone — those produced by the adrenal cortex and gonads (for example, aldosterone, corticosterone, testosterone, progesterone, and estrogens).
3. Simple hormones — those produced by adrenal medulla and thyroid. These are neither protein nor steroid, but simple amino acid derivatives (for example, epinephrine, triiodothyronine [T_3], and thyroxine [T_4]).

Host. An animal or plant that harbors or nourishes another organism or parasite.

Host (master) computer. The main processor running the operating system the user interacts with.

Host-vs.-graft reaction. (HVG) An immunologic reaction mounted by a graft recipient against a graft; HVG reactions of any appreciable intensity are largely limited to allogeneic and xenogeneic systems.

Hot. A colloquial expression commonly used to mean "highly radioactive".

Hot antigen suicide. A technique in which an antigen is labeled with a high-specific-activity radioisotope (^{131}I). It is used either *in vivo* or *in vitro* to inhibit specific lymphocyte function by attachment to an antigen-binding lymphocyte, subsequently killing it by radiolysis.

Hot atom. An atom which has an excited energy state or kinetic energy above the thermal level of its surroundings, usually as a result of a nuclear process such as beta decay or neutron capture.

Hot atom chemistry. The chemical reactions and processes of hot atoms, ions, and radicals.

Hot cell. Heavily shielded enclosure or laboratories to protect personnel working with large amounts of substances emitting gamma radiation. Such a cell may be of concrete construction, or lead may be used as the shielding medium. Facilities incorporated in a hot cell include lead glass or zinc bromide window, service plugs, material transfer ports and doors, together with equipment for remote handling of the radioactive materials. This includes powered manipulators and master-slave manipulators. It will be provided with special facilities including ventilation, fume cupboards, glove boxes (these are sometimes known as hot boxes), and, for large quantities of gamma emitters, shielded boxes called hot cells. Special drainage will be provided and wall, floors, and fittings will be given a smooth, impervious finish to facilitate decontamination.

Hot spot. Focal area of increased activity in scintigraphy.

Hot trap. A device for removing impurities from fluid systems by raising the temperature to the point at which the impurities react with a solid substance.

Hue. The property of a color that enables an observer to classify it as corresponding to a particular wavelength of visible light, e.g., red, green, yellow, etc.

Human albumin microspheres. (HAM) Used for lung perfusion scanning.

Human leukocyte antigen. (HLA) The major histocompatibility genetic region in man.

Human serum albumin. (HSA) When labeled by a radioactive substance can be used for radionuclide compartmental scintigraphy and *in vitro* studies.

Humoral. Pertaining to molecules in solution in a body fluid, particularly antibody and complement.

Hybrid. Animal or plant produced from parents different in kind; cell made by fusion of two cell types.

Hybridoma. Transformed cell line or clone of hybrid cells grown *in vivo* or *in vitro* which is a somatic hybrid of two parent cell lines and contains genetic material from both.

Hydrocarbon. Compound containing carbon and hydrogen exclusively.

Hydrogen. Element symbol H, atomic number 1, atomic weight 1.00794. The lightest and simplest element, the nucleus of which is simply a proton. It has unit mass.

Hydrogen ion concentration. The concentration of hydrogen ions in solution when the concentration is expressed as gram-ionic weights per liter. A convenient form of expressing hydrogen ion concentration is in terms of the negative logarithm of this concentration. The negative logarithm of the hydrogen ion concentration is called pH. Water at 25°C has a concentration of H ion of 10^{-7} and of OH ion of 10^{-7} mol/l. Thus, the pH of water is 7 at 24°C. A greater accuracy is obtained if one substitutes the thermodynamic activity of the ion for its concentration.

Hydrolysis. A process in which a compound splits into two components by reacting with water when water is used as the solvent.

Hydronephrosis. Distention of the renal urinary collecting system caused by an obstruction to urinary drainage in the outflow tract.

Hydrophone. A small transducer element mounted on the end of a narrow tube.

Hydrostatic pressure. Pressure exerted by fluids (water, blood).

Hydroxide. The ion OH^-.

Hydroxyapatite. A natural mineral structure similar to the crystal lattice of bones and teeth $Ca_{10}(PO_4)_6(OH)_2$.

8-Hydroxyquinoline (Oxine). Compound that can form a complex with indium and gallium and be used to label blood cells.

Hyperacute rejection. An accelerated form of graft rejection that is associated with circulating antibody in the serum of the recipient and which can react with donor cells.

Hypercapnia. Increased amount of carbon dioxide in the blood.

Hyperemia. Excess blood in any part of the body; congestion.

Hyperfine splitting. Splittings in the lines of an electron spin resonance spectrum arising due to the interaction of the nuclei in the vicinity of an unpaired electron with the unpaired electron under observation. This parameter can be used for determining the structure of a free radical or in identifying the ligands of a paramagnetic ion.

Hyperglycemia. An abnormally high blood glucose level.

Hyperkalemia. Abnormally high level of potassium in the blood.

Hyperlipidemia. Any abnormally high level of one or more lipids, such as triglycerides or cholesterol, in the blood.

Hypermetropia. Long-sightedness — a condition of the eye by which the image of an object is formed behind the retina.

Hyperon. Any article with mass intermediate between that of the neutron and the deuteron.

Hyperplasia. The abnormal multiplication or increase in the number of normal cells in the normal arrangement of the tissue.

Hyperpnea. Increased rate and depth of breathing.

Hypersensitive. Abnormally high sensitivity. A state of increased capacity to respond specifically to an antigen or hapten.

Hypertension. Persistently high arterial blood pressure. A condition in which the individual has a higher blood pressure than that judged to be normal.

Hyperthyroidism. The result of a hyperplastic, overactive thyroid gland that secretes an excess of hormone into the circulation.

Hypertonic. Above-normal tension or strength.

Hypertrophy. Enlargement or overgrowth of an organ due to increase in size of its constituent cells.

Hyperventilation. Abnormally prolonged deep and rapid breathing, often leading to hypocapnia. It can be induced by overbreathing oxygen at high pressures.

Hypocapnia. A deficiency of carbon dioxide in the blood.

Hypochondrium. Upper lateral area of abdomen below the rib cage.

Hypogammaglobulinemia. (Agammaglobulinemia) A deficiency of all major classes of serum immunoglobulins.

Hypoglycemia. Deficiency of sugar in the blood. A condition in which the glucose in the blood is abnormally low.

Hypokalemia. Abnormally low level of potassium in the blood.

Hypokinesia. Decreased motor reaction or function to stimulus.

Hypokinetic disease. The debilitating effects of insufficient physical activity. The whole spectrum of inactivity-induced somatic and mental derangements.

Hypophysis. Pituitary gland.

Hypopituitarism. Insufficient secretion of the pituitary.

Hypoplasia. Incomplete development of an organ because of too few cells.

Hypotension. Low arterial blood pressure.

Hypothalamus. A part of the brain, forming the floor and part of the lateral wall of the third ventricle. It exerts control over visceral activities, water balance, temperature, sleep, etc.

Hypothyroidism. A clinical state resulting from deficiency in thyroid activity and lack of thyroid hormone. A symptom complex including weight gain, sluggishness, weakness, intolerance to cold, general slowing of all intellectual functions, puffiness of the face, enlargement of the tongue, constipation, pallor, dryness, thickening and flakiness of the skin, brittleness of fingernails, dryness, brittleness, and excessive falling out of hair, alteration of the established menstrual pattern, huskiness of the voice, psychological or behavioral changes

from mild hyperirritability to depression (actual psychosis — "myxedema madness"), and a variety of other clinical findings due to deficient thyroid hormone.

Hypotonic. Pertaining to defective muscular tone or tension. A solution of lower osmotic pressure than another.

Hypoventilation. Decrease of air in the lungs below the normal amount.

Hypoxia. Oxygen deficiency; any state wherein a physiologically inadequate amount of oxygen is available to or utilized by tissue without respect to cause or degree.

Hysteresis. The magnetization of a sample of iron or steel due to a magnetic field which is made to vary through a cycle of values; lags behind the field. This phenomenon is called hysteresis.

Hysterosalpingography. The fallopian tubes (salpinges) are connected to the uterus at its sides and allow for the passage of ova from the ovaries to the uterine cavity. One of the known causes of infertility is an obstruction to the fallopian tubes. To evaluate the tubary patency an iodinated contrast can be injected into the system and flow studied by X-rays. A radionuclide (usually ^{99m}Tc-macro aggregate albumin) can be used to evaluate the patency of the fallopian tubes in a more functional and less invasive way by following the pattern of flow (of the radiopharmaceutical) from images obtained with a gamma camera.

I

Idiopathic. Relating to any disorder that is of unknown origin or apparently of spontaneous origin; self-originating.

Ileum. The distal portion of the small intestine, ending at the cecum of the large intestine.

Image. A picture or conception with more or less likeness to objective reality. Also, a general name for the visual presentation of anatomic or physiologic data.

Image acquisition time. Time required to carry out an imaging procedure comprising only the data acquisition time. The additional image reconstruction time will also be important to determine how quickly the image can be viewed. In comparing sequential plane imaging and volume techniques, the equivalent image acquisition time per slice must be considered, as well as the actual image acquisition time.

Image artifacts. The accuracy and level of confidence in interpreting an image is reduced when artifacts are introduced into an image. Image artifacts can originate from several distinct sources. It should be part of an overall quality assurance program that operators of equipment reduce to a minimum the possibility of image artifacts occurring, while the diagnostician should recognize and allow for the possibility of artifacts being present in an image. These are some of the circumstances that may generate image artifacts: malfunction of equipment, incorrect operation of equipment, lack of quality control, patient-generated artifacts, technique-generated image artifacts.

Image evaluation. Objective data can be gained from an acquired image by simple mathematical operations. The evaluation of an image is facilitated by an interactive display.

Image filing. The image data contained in the temporary disk store can be recalled to the monitor and recorded photographically. This permanently fixes the window level and width (image reproduction) of the computed graphic display. The magnetic tape and the floppy disk are long-term electronic (digital) storage media on which the entire information pertinent to a study is stored. This means that, on later recall of an image, the window level and width can be set and other processes of image evaluation performed.

Image filtration. Each individual point of an image can be subjected to a computing operation which takes account of the extent and importance of the surrounding points. Image noise, definition, and contours can be optically altered by different image filters. Image filtration, which takes the already processed image as its basis and can be repeated at will (secondary image filtration), should not be confused with the primary filtration of image reconstruction.

Image formatter. A device for displaying images in specific locations on a screen or film to permit multiple images on a single film.

Image intensifier. This is an integral part of any diagnostic X-ray set which can produce a fluoroscopic image on a video monitor or on cine film. X-rays can cause a fluorescent screen to glow in the form of the X-ray image, and early fluoroscopes employed this principle to provide moving pictures which had to be viewed in total darkness. The image intensifier enhances the brightness of the image many times (e.g., ×1000 to ×5000) so that it can be televised or filmed for daylight viewing. The image intensifier itself is an electronic device contained in a large evacuated glass envelope. It comprises a fluorescent screen onto which the X-ray falls, and this is in contact with a second layer (photocathode), which emits electrons in response to light from the fluorescent screen. The rest of the image intensifier is an electron accelerator and focusing system which produces a smaller, brighter image on a second phosphorescent screen similar to a cathode ray tube (CRT) screen.

Image interpolation. A generated condition under which one matrix may be increased to a larger matrix by the calculation of a progression relating the change from one point to the next and the interposing of sufficient data based upon that progression to fill voids created by the expansion.

Image matrix. Depending on the type of scanner, the image matrix may be composed of 64 × 64, 128 × 128, 256 × 256, or 512 × 512 picture elements, or pixels, arranged in rows and columns, and is usually quadratic. The individual pixels are unequivocally defined by the coordinate system. By general agreement, pixels on the axes (x, y) are counted from the top left-hand corner of the matrix.

Image memory. A large block of memory made up of random-access memory (RAM) in which images are temporarily held for viewing and/or processing.

Image noise. Statistical inaccuracy of the density value of an individual pixel caused by the statistical variation in the photon flow.

Image nonlinearity. When straight-line objects (i.e., a test pattern) appear as curved-line images. Causes include poor sensitivity of photomultiplier tubes, resistance network, and optical light guide nonuniformity.

Image reconstruction. Image reconstruction is a process of computation which produces the computed tomogram from the data acquired. The algebraic methods have now been replaced by faster convolution algorithms. These involve subjecting the absorption profiles to a filtering function (convolution core) and then superimposing them in the direction from which they were measured (backprojection). The filtering function (core) is necessary to suppress the blurring which occurs at the boundaries of the object on backprojection. It can be applied in various ways and be adapted to certain problems. The impression of the image alters as a result.

Image redundancy. Multiple storage of the same image.

Image reproduction. In the case of computed tomography or other imaging systems, image reproduction consists of a grid of numerical values covering a scale of, for instance, 2000 units. Since under normal evaluation conditions only 15 to 20 shades of gray can be distinguished with the naked eye, each shade would represent about 50 units if the gray scale is to be extended over the entire density scale. The image window was introduced so that fine differences in density could be recognized while allowing evaluation of high-contrast structures. Using the window, the gray scale can be extended over selectable density ranges (window width). The window level (center) within the density scale determines which density value will be represented by the middle shade of gray. The choice of window setting depends on the diagnostic query. Narrow window settings involve the risk of structures outside the frame not being seen and thus of being excluded from the diagnosis. Wide window settings homogenize and mask slight differences in density.

Image technology. Techniques for the design and construction of pictorial information such as television pictures of "graphical displays". Examples of the use of image processing occur in computer-aided tomography and radionuclide scintigraphy.

Iminodiacetic acid. (IDA) Chelating group capable of binding technetium so that it can be attached to biologically active molecules, such as "hepatic" N,N'-(2,6-dimethylphenyl) carbamolmethyl iminodiacetic acid (HIDA), *para*-isopropyl iminodiacetic acid (PIPIDA), diethyl iminodiacetic acid (DIDA), diisopropyl iminodiacetic acid (DISIDA), or parabutyl iminodiacetic acid (BIDA), which are all used as hepatobiliary radionuclide imaging agents.

Immediate hypersensitivity. An unusual immunologic sensitivity to antigens that manifests itself by tissue reactions occurring within minutes after the antigen combines with its appropriate antibody.

Immersion dose. When a person is surrounded by a mixture of air and a radioactive gas or aerosol his body will receive radiation both from the gas in his lungs and from that surrounding him. In case of a large cloud containing gamma-emitting gas the external radiation is the important contribution and the dose received in this way is called the immersion dose.

Immersion scanning. A method of coupling an ultrasonic transducer to a subject or tissue by placing the subject or tissue to be examined, as well as the transducer, into a bath of coupling medium.

Immune complexes. (ICs) Complexes (soluble or insoluble) containing antigen (Ag), antibody (Ab).

Immune elimination. The enhanced clearance of an injected antigen from the circulation as a result of immunity to that antigen brought about the enhanced phagocytosis of the reticuloendothelial system.

Immune response. Initially used to designate a response, either specific or nonspecific, that leads to immunity. However, unless specified otherwise, the term is currently used to designate the total specific response involving the production of both antibodies (Abs) and immune cells, irrespective of whether protective immunity against a harmful agent(s) results.

Immune response genes. (Ir genes) Genes that control immune responses to specific antigens.

Immune surveillance. A theory that holds that the immune system destroys tumor cells, which are constantly arising during the life of the individual.

Immunity. Response to antigenic or foreign material in the body; protection against disease. The state of being protected against injury by virtue of being able to resist and/or overcome harmful agents. (Immune.)

Immunize. The act of inducing either active or passive protective immunity.

Immunoactive. Immunity produced by stimulation of antibody-producing mechanisms.

Immunoadsorption. The procedure of fixing antigens or antibodies on a column for absorbing antigens or antibodies, respectively, from fluids passed through the column.

Immunochemistry. With special reference to competitive binding assay, biochemical techniques and concepts applied to the production, purification, and characterization of antigens and antibodies and to the manipulation of antigen/antibody reactions for analytic purposes.

Immunocompetent cells. Mature antibody-producing cells.

Immunocyte. A cell capable of proliferation and antibody production.

Immunodominant. That part of an antigenic determinant which is dominant in binding with antibody.

Immunoelectrophoresis. A technique combining an initial electrophoretic separation of proteins followed by immunodiffusion with resultant precipitation arcs.

Immunofluorescence. A histo- or cytochemical technique for the detection and localization of antigens in which specific antibody is conjugated with fluorescent compounds, resulting in a sensitive tracer that can be detected by fluorometric measurements.

Immunogen. A substance that elicits a general immune response, one that triggers the response mechanism without necessarily resulting in the production of specific antibody. Often synonymous with antigen but sometimes referring only to functional immunity against a pathogen.

Immunogenicity. The property of a substance making it capable of inducing a detectable immune response.

Immunoglobulin. A glycoprotein, isolated from the globulin fraction of serum having a characteristic shape and the ability to bind to molecules that are not endogenous to the species producing the immunoglobulin. All antibodies are immunoglobulins, but it is not certain that all immunoglobulins have antibody function.

Immunoglobulin class. A subdivision of immunoglobulin molecules based on unique antigenic determinants in the Fc region of the H chains. In man there are five classes of immunoglobulins designated:

1. IgA. The predominant immunoglobulin class present in secretions
2. IgD. The predominant immunoglobulin class present on human B lymphocytes
3. IgE. A reaginic antibody involved in immediate hypersensitivity reactions
4. IgG. The predominant immunoglobulin class present in human serum
5. IgM. A pentameric immunoglobulin comprising approximately 10% normal human serum immunoglobulins, with a molecular weight of 900,000 a sedimentation coefficient of 195

Immunoglobulin subclass. A subdivision of the classes of immunoglobulins based on structural and antigenic differences in the H chains. For human IgG there are four subclasses: IgG1, IgG2, IgG3, and IgG4.

Immunologic enhancement. Enhanced survival of allografts and tumors protected from the forces of rejection by specific antibodies (enhancing antibodies).

Immunology. The biology and chemistry of the immune response, including the phenomena of antibody production, of the development of immunity, and of the mechanisms of immunologic tolerance.

Immunopotency. The capacity of a region of an antigen molecule to serve as an antigenic determinant and thereby induce the formation of specific antibody.

Immunoradiometric assay. A technique similar to radioimmunoassay in which radioactive antibodies, rather than radioactive antigens, are used.

Immunoreaction. Reaction taking place between an antigen and its antibody.

Immunoscintigraphy. The ability to image abnormal tissue using radiolabeled monoclonal and polyclonal antibodies directed against specific antigens. Examples of this technique are the visualization of some types of tumors, inflammatory lesions, or myocardial infarction, by directing radiolabeled antibodies against tumor antigens, human granulocytes, or myocardial myosin, respectively.

Immunosorbent. An artificial solid phase form of immunochemical reagent made by coupling antigen or antibody to a polymer or other insoluble matrix; used for either preparative or analytic purposes.

Immunosuppressant. Any external agent that can nonspecifically suppress the immune system, e.g., X-ray or drugs.

Immunotherapy. Treatment of diseases by stimulating the formation of antibodies that attack the organisms which cause the diseased conditions.

Impatency. Being closed or obstructed.

Impedance. A measure of afterload that equals instantaneous pressure divided by instantaneous flow in the aorta. Impedance is closely related to systematic vascular resistance, but is not so widely used in clinical practice. Density multiplied by sound propagation speed.

Impedance plethysmography. A noninvasive technique which can be used to monitor changes in cardiac output. It is an indirect measurement allowing changes in blood flow to be followed qualitatively. The values, however, may differ markedly from the absolute values obtained by invasive methods.

Impermeable. Not allowing passage.

Implant. A radiotherapeutic technique in which discrete radioactive sources such as radium needles or seeds are inserted into a malignant tumor. Radioactive tantalum wire and radioactive gold seeds are commonly used. The distribution of the sources is carefully planned so as to achieve a suitable degree of homogeneity of dose throughout the tissue. Material inserted or grafted to the body.

Impulse. An action potential that is propagated along a membrane, e.g., that of an axon.

Impulse generator. A system for generating high voltages by charging a series of condensers in parallel and then effectively connecting them in series by simultaneously discharging a number of spark gaps.

In-air dose. The dose measured in free air by means of a device which does not significantly disturb the radiation field. It will differ from and is to be distinguished from the dose measured at the surface of a body placed at the same position in the same field.

Incidence angle. Angle between incident sound direction and line perpendicular to media boundary.

Incision. A cut produced by a sharp instrument.

Inclusion. A particle in the cell cytoplasm.

Incoherent scattering. Scattering of photons of particles in which the scattering elements act independently of one another so that there are no definite phase relationships among the different parts of the scattered beam. The intensity of the scattered radiation at any point is obtained by adding the intensities of the scattered radiation reaching this point from the independent scattering elements.

Incontinent. Unable to control excretory functions.

Incremental addition. A technique for preparing standards for a standard curve so that the last in a row of tubes contains the highest concentration of known test substances.

Incubate. To provide proper conditions for growth or a reaction to occur.

Independent events. Events either of whose occurrence in no way influences the probability of occurrence of the other.

Independent samples. Samples whose values are independent of each other because they represent measurements on entirely different individuals or are otherwise unrelated.

Indeterminacy principle. (Uncertainty principle) The postulate that it is impossible to determine simultaneously both the exact position and the exact momentum of an electron. So this aspect of electronics can only be expressed as a probability.

Index register. Contains address information that can be modified without affecting the instruction in the computer memory.

Indicator dilution methods. The volume of fluid in any container can be calculated if a known quantity of indicator (e.g., dye, cold saline, or radioisotope) is added and the concentration of indicator measured after it has been uniformly dispersed throughout the fluid. This technique was developed and refined by Steward and Hamilton. A suitable indicator is one which can be detected and measured, and which remains within the circulation during at least its first circuit. Subsequent removal from the circulation is an advantage.

Indicators. Substances which change from one color to another when the hydrogen ion concentration reaches a certain value, different for each indicator.

Indirect immunofluorescence. A technique whereby unlabeled antibody is incubated with substrate and then overlaid with fluorescently conjugated antiimmunoglobulin to form a sandwich. Also known as double antibody immunofluorescence.

Indirectly ionizing particles. Uncharged particles or photons which can liberate directly ionizing particles or can initiate a nuclear transformation.

Indirectly ionizing radiation. Radiation consisting of indirectly ionizing particles.

Indirect or passive agglutination. The agglutination of particles or red blood cells to which antigens have been coupled chemically.

Indium. Element symbol In, atomic number 49, atomic weight 114.82.

Induced nuclear disintegration. A process occurring when a nucleus comes into contact with a photon, an elementary particle, or another nucleus. In many cases the reaction can be represented by

$$X + a \rightarrow y + b$$

in which X is the target nucleus, a is the incident particle or photon, b is the emitted particle or photon, and y is the product nucleus. an example is the reaction

$$_7N^{14} + {}_2He^4 \rightarrow {}_8O^{17} + {}_1H^1.$$

Induced radioactivity. That radioactivity produced in a substance after bombardment with neutrons or other particles.

Inductance. Measure of the magnetic coupling between two current-carrying loops (mutual) (reflecting their spatial relationship) or of a loop (such as a coil) with itself (self). One of the principal determinants of the resonance frequency of a radio-frequency (rf) circuit.

Induction. Any change in the intensity or direction of a magnetic field causes an electromotive force in any conductor in the field. The induced electromotive force generates an induced current if the conductor forms a closed circuit.

Indurated. Firm, hard.

Industrial applications of isotopes. The industrial applications of radioactive isotopes fall roughly into two main groups: those in which the isotope is simply a source of radiation such as thickness gauging and radiography of castings, and those in which the isotope traces the movement and behavior of a material by being incorporated with it.

Inelastic collision. A collision in which there are changes both in the internal energy of one or more of the colliding systems and in the sums of the kinetic energies of translation before and after collision.

Inelastic scattering. Scattering effected by inelastic collisions, such as are involved in the Compton effect.

Inert. Lacking activity.

Inertia. The resistance offered by a body to a change of its state of rest or motion; a fundamental property of matter.

Infarct. An area of tissue in an organ or part that undergoes necrosis following cessation of blood supply. May result from occlusion or stenosis of the supplying artery.

Infection. Invasion and multiplication of microorganisms in the body.

Inference. Statistical estimation of population values (parameters) from sample data.

Inferential statistics. Methods used to summarize a relatively small set of data (e.g., a sample) in order to make generalizations concerning a much larger set of possible data (e.g., a population).

Inferior. Used medically in reference to the undersurface of an organ or indicating a structure below another structure.

Inferior vena cava. The venous trunk for the lower extremities and the pelvic and abdominal organs, which empties into the right atrium of the heart.

Inflammation. Local protective response to injury, characterized by redness, swelling, heat, pain.

Information content. Containing or transmitting data involving new knowledge. When applied to waves or wavefronts, it includes both amplitude and phase of all parts of a wavefront at a given instant of time.

Information density. A measure of the number of recorded events per unit area, such as the number of counts per square centimeter, that are recorded in the field of interest within a particular image. The effect of statistical fluctuations decreases with increasing information density. Usually measured per square centimeter of gamma camera crystal face.

Information theory of antibody synthesis. A theory that predicts that antigen dictates the specific structure of the antibody molecule.

Infrared radiation. Invisible radiation of a thermal nature whose wave is longer than the red segment of the visible spectrum.

Infusion. The steeping of a substance or drug in water to extract its medicinal benefit; to introduce fluid or blood into a vein.

Ingest. To take foods into the body; to take in.

Inguinal. Relating to the groin region.

Inherent filtration. The "filtering" effect of the walls of the X-ray tube on the less penetrating component of the X-ray beam before it exits to the air. This is to be distinguished from the added filters, usually made of aluminum or copper.

Inhibitor. Substance preventing or interfering with a chemical reaction.

Inhomogeneity. Degree of lack of homogeneity, for example, the fractional deviation of the local magnetic field from the average value of the field.

Initial attenuation. The electronic attenuation relative to full gain put on the received signal and indicates the (initial) level of sound attenuation before further modification occurs by slope control.

Initial binding. ($\%B_O$) The percent of radioimmunoassay (RIA) binding with zero or no standard and should be between 30 and 70% of the total activity. A change of greater than 5% throughout the life of the kit indicates a problem with antibody affinity, incubation time, or separation method. Maximum binding.

Initialize. To set computer counters, switches, or addresses to starting values at prescribed points in the execution of a program, particularly in preparation for reexecution of a sequence code. To format a volume in a particular file-structured format in preparation for use by an operating system.

Injury. (Legal) Any wrong or damage done to another, either in his person, rights, reputation, or property.

Innate. Inborn, hereditary, congenital; present at birth.

Innate or constitutive immunity. Immunity which is native or constitutive for the species as distinct from acquired immunity. It does not result from previous experiences with external agents.

Inner bremsstrahlung. The radiation produced by the interaction of a charged particle (usually an electron) with the coulomb field of the nucleus or atom in which it originated. Inner bremsstrahlung radiation is also produced in the transition of an electron to the nucleus in electron capture.

Inoculation. The introduction of an antigen or antiserum into an animal in order to confer immunity by stimulation of antibody production.

Inorganic chemistry. Branch of chemistry having to do with compounds and processes that do not involve carbon.

Inotropic. Affecting the force or energy of muscular contractions. An intervention that increases contractility has positive inotropic effects, while one that decreases contractility has negative inotropic effects.

Input. Transfer of data from auxiliary or external storage into the internal storage of a computer: the result of the processing is the output.

Input device. A machine capable of accepting data and making it available for processing in a form acceptable to a computer.

Input/output device. (I/O) A device attached to a computer that makes it possible to bring information into the computer or get information out. A typical input would be the alphanumeric keyboard consisting of a full set of letters, numerals, particular signs for drawing and charting, and punctuation marks. The object of all input devices is data entry. Typical outputs are visual display units (VDUs) and printers, both designed to bring computer-processed data to the user. Input and output devices may also be called terminals or peripherals.

Input/output (I/O) error. Any error associated with an I/O operation. One example of an I/O error is a disk error, which occurs when the computer is typing to read or write data on a disk.

In situ. In the natural or normal place; confined to the site of origin without invasion of neighboring tissues.

Insolubilized antibody. Antibody converted to insoluble form, such as a polymer before the radioimmunoassay (RIA) reaction (incubation) as a convenience in separating bound and free tracer.

Inspiratory capacity. The maximal volume of gas that can be inspired from the resting expiratory level.

Inspiratory reserve volume. The maximum volume of air that can be additionally inspired after a normal inspiration.

Instruction. A single order that tells the computer to carry out some specific task. An instruction in a program might tell the computer to operate a line printer, add two numbers together, store information in memory, or to perform any one of a number of other functions.

Each instruction must be retrieved from memory, decoded, and executed by the computer's central processing unit. A program is simply a series of instructions designed to solve a problem or accomplish a task.

Instruction length. The number of words needed to store an instruction.

Instruction register. The register that contains the instruction being executed by the central processor.

Insufflation. The act of blowing powder, vapor, gas, or air into a body cavity.

Insulators. Materials which have a high resistivity to the flow of electrical current.

Insulin. A hormone, produced by the the beta cells of the islets of Langerhans in the pancreas, that controls the metabolism of glucose in the body. Insulin lowers the blood glucose by accelerating the passage of glucose into cells for storage as glycogen or exidation to yield energy; deficiency causes diabetes mellitus.

Integral. A quantitative measure of the relative intensities of the NMR signals. The integral is given by the area of the spectral line and is usually presented as a step function in which the heights of the steps are proportional to the intensities of the resonance line, if integration is done in the analog mode. If the integration is done digitally, it is obtained by summing the amplitudes of the digital data points that define the envelope of each NMR line. The results of those summations are usually displayed either as a normalized total number of digital counts for each line or as a step function superimposed on the spectrum.

Integral absorbed dose. The integral of the absorbed dose over the mass of irradiated matter in the volume under consideration. It is identical with the energy imparted to matter in that volume.

Integral dose. The total energy absorbed during an exposure to radiation.

Integral experiment. An experiment giving information about the total (integral) effect of several parameters or processes in a system rather than about their separate (differential) effects.

Integrated circuit. (IC) A miniature electronic circuit imprinted or etched on the surface of a silicon chip. Components on the chip are linked by an imprinted pathway of conductive material rather than wires and soldered electrical connections.

Integrated dose meter. An instrument for measuring the total or integrated radiation dose over a period of time. Such an instrument is often called a dosimeter, and the most popular form of instrument is the quartz-fiber dosimeter which comprises an ionization chamber and a quartz-fiber electroscope.

Integrating circuit. An electronic circuit that records, at any time, an average value for the number of ionization events occurring per unit time, or an electrical circuit that records the total number of ions collected in a given time.

Integrating dosimeter. Ionization chamber and measuring system designed for determining total radiation administered during an exposure. In medical radiology the chamber is usually designed to be placed on the patients skin. A device may be included to terminate the exposure when it has reached a desired value.

Integrity. Preservation of information content of data.

Intelligent terminal. A terminal containing a microprocessor to perform limited data manipulations and save the time of a main computer.

Intensitometer. A device for determining the relative X-ray intensities during radiography.

Intensity. The intensity of any form of radiation (heat, light, sound, nuclear particles) is defined as the amount of radiant energy falling on or crossing unit area per second. One sometimes speaks of a source of radiation having a certain intensity. In this case the intensity means the total energy radiated per second by the source.

Intensity of magnetization. Given by the quotient of the magnetic moment of a magnet by its volume. Unit intensity of magnetization is the intensity of a magnet which has unit magnetic moment per cubic centimeter.

Intensity of sound. Depends upon the energy of the wave motion. The intensity is measured by the energy in ergs transmitted per second through 1 cm^3 of surface.

Intensity reflection coefficient. Reflected intensity divided by incident intensity.

Intensity transmission coefficient. Transmitted intensity divided by incident intensity.

Interaction broadening. Electron spin resonance (ESR) lines in an ESR spectrum can be broadened by magnetic interactions between paramagnetic molecules. This interaction is dependent on the concentration of the paramagnetic species. (NMR.)

Interaction process. Any process in which two particles approach each other closely enough to affect each other in any way. An interaction may involve an exchange of energy, spin, par-

ity, a disintegration into other particles, or merely a change in the direction of motion of the particles.

Interactive display. Individual pixels of the image matrix can be marked on the monitor screen by means of light pencils (joy stick, roller ball). The site of the pixels is recorded visually, which obviates the need to note the coordinate intercepts (x_1, y_1) (image matrix). The marked pixels may represent the midpoints of circular areas and rectangles, the surface areas of which can be varied (regular region of interest). Freely selectable areas are recorded by drawing around the corresponding areas of the image with the light pencil (irregular region of interest).

Interactive mode. A method of computer use in which the computer responds promptly to the user's commands so that a "dialogue" can be set up between computer and user.

Interactive terminal. Typically, a visual display unit with a keyboard, which is not only a display conveying information from the computer to the user, but one that permits the user to input data in response to the information displayed. There are a wide variety of other ways of responding to the display such as light pens and touch-sensitive panels.

Interassay precision. Determined by assaying the same sample n times in multiple assays.

Interatrial septum. The thin muscular wall that separates the two atria of the heart.

Interface. That part which is intended to provide the connection between one item of equipment to another which ensures compatible flow. The specification of an interface should include the characteristics of signals (amplitude, duration, timing) and of the signal path (e.g., impedance, timing) and the nature of any control sequences. In computing, a common boundary between adjacent systems enabling them to interact.

Interference pattern. The pattern of light and dark fringes produced when two or more coherent waves interfere or intersect.

Interferon. A heterogeneous group of low-molecular-weight proteins elaborated by infected host cells that protect noninfected cells from viral infection.

Interlaced video. Standard 525 line video frames are formed from two independent video fields which are displaced vertically with respect to one another (interlaced). Positive interlace implies accurate positioning of the two fields and random interlace implies no precise positioning.

Interlock. A device, usually electrical and (or) mechanical in nature, to prevent activation of a control unit unless a preliminary condition has been met, or to prevent hazardous operations. Its purpose usually is safety of personnel or equipment.

Intermediate neutrons. Neutrons having kinetic energies greater than those of thermal neutrons but less than those of fast ones, i.e., energies of approximately 100 to 100,000 eV.

Intermediate reactor. Fission is induced predominantly by neutrons whose energies are greater than thermal, but much less than the energy with which neutrons are released in fission. From 0.5 to 100,000 eV may be taken roughly as the energy range of neutrons inducing fission in intermediate reactors. The neutron absorption resonances of the fuel may be important in this range.

Internal absorption. The absorption of radiation within the source from which it originates.

Internal command. A command that is part of a disk operating system (DOS) and is therefore kept in the random access memory (RAM) whenever DOS is running.

Internal conversion. In some decay schemes the energy of the excited daughter is not emitted as gamma radiation, but is transferred to an inner orbital electron which is ejected. This process is called internal conversion and the emitted electron is called the internal conversion electron. The filling of the resultant vacancy gives rise to characteristic X-rays of the daughter or to Auger electrons. The probability of internal conversion taking place increases with increasing atomic number, the closeness of the energy of the transition to the electron's binding energy, and the lifetime of the excited state.

Internal conversion coefficient. The ratio of the number of transitions in which internal conversion takes place to the remaining number of transitions between two given nuclear states.

Internal memory. The storage facilities in a computer system where programs and data are placed immediately before execution. It is usually the highest-speed memory in a computer system, although sometimes small higher-speed cache memories are made part of the internal memory.

Internal radiation. Exposure to ionizing radiation when the radiation source is within the body as a result of deposition of radioelements in body tissue.

Internal reference. A reference substance that is dissolved in the same phase as the sample. The primary internal reference for proton spectra and $_{13}C$ spectra of nonaqueous solutions is tetramethylsilane (TMS). A concentration of 1% is recommended. For proton spectra of aqueous solutions, the recommended internal reference is sodium salt of 2,2,3,3,-tetradeutro-4,4-dimethyl-4-silapentanoic acid (TSP-d4). For $_{13}C$ spectra of aqueous solutions, secondary standards such as dioxane have been found satisfactory. (NMR.)

Internal refresh. Self-contained system for maintaining data in a dynamic storage medium, i.e., a storage medium which would otherwise lose its pattern without replenishment.

International Atomic Energy Agency. (IAEA) An independent United Nations organization, which promotes the peaceful uses of atomic energy and establishes international standards of safety.

International Atomic Energy (IAEA) Special Form. A test specification for sealed sources given in the International Atomic Energy Agency (IAEA) transport regulations (IAEA Safety Series No. 6) It is used in determining the maximum acceptable activities for various types of transport containers.

International Commission on Radiological Protection. (ICRP) First set up in 1928, its members are chosen on the basis of their recognized activity in the fields of radiology, radiation, protection, physics, biology, genetics, biochemistry, and biophysics. The Commission functions under the auspices of the International Congress of Radiology, and its purpose is to make recommendations on radiation safety standards.

International Commission Radiological Units and Measurements. (ICRUM) First organized in 1925 under the auspices of the International Congress of Radiology: its members are chosen on the basis of their recognized activity in the field of radiological units, standards, and measurements, but the Commission must include at least three medical radiologists and three physicists. It is responsible for developing the specification of radiation treatment and the basic principles needed in radiation dosimetry. It also collects and evaluates the latest data and information pertinent to the problems of radiation measurement and dosimetry, and recommends the most acceptable values for current use. In addition, the Commission considers and makes recommendations on radiation units and measurements necessary in the field of radiation protection.

International Organization for Standardization Classification. (ISO) Has produced a system of classification of sealed radioactive sources based on safety requirements for typical uses. This system provides a manufacturer of sealed radioactive sources with a set of tests to evaluate the safety of his products under working conditions. It also assists a user of such sealed sources to select types which suit the application he has in mind, especially where protection against the release of radioactive material is concerned.

International reference materials. International biological standard — a reference material of an international source serving as the prime reference or standard against which other reference preparations may be standardized. International reference preparation — a reference preparation standardized against the international biologic standard may be used directly in an assay system.

International safeguards. Measures used to detect and deter the diversion of nuclear material from uses permitted by law or treaty, to give timely indication of possible diversion or credible assurance that no diversion has occurred, and to verify the declared operation of the facility.

Interphase. The period between two divisions of a cell, during which genetic material is duplicated.

Interpolation. The process of obtaining intermediate terms, usually by the method of linear proportioning.

Interpreter. Translates a higher-level language instruction-by-instruction as the program runs. Unlike a compiler which translates the whole program before the program is run, an interpreter translates each instruction as it is needed. If the same instruction is executed repeatedly in the program it must be translated each time it is encountered.

Interpulse time. Time between successive radio-frequency (rf) pulses used in pulse sequences. Particularly important are the inversion time (T1) in inversion recovery, and the time between a 90° pulse and the subsequent 180° pulse to produce a spin echo, which will be approximately one half the spin echo time (TE). The time between repetitions of pulse sequences is the repetition time (TR). (NMR.)

Interrupt. Suspension of a computer operation to have it perform another function. At the completion of the function, the computer returns to the main program and resumes from the interrupt point.

Interspace. Space between one objective plane and another; space between one film and another.

Interstices. Small gaps between tissues or structures.

Interstitial. Pertaining to or situated in the interspaces of a tissue.

Interventricular septum. The muscular wall that separates the two ventricles of the heart.

Intima. Innermost part of a structure.

Intraassay precision. Determined by assaying the same sample n times in a single assay.

Intrapulmonary blood volume. The volume of blood contained between the origin of the pulmonary artery and the junction of the pulmonary veins with the left atrium.

Intrathecal. Within a sheath, particularly within the meninges into the subarachnoid space. Applied to the cerebrospinal fluid cavity.

Intravascular pressure. The ratio of the blood pressure in any part of the blood vessel to the atmospheric pressure.

Intravenous. Within a vein or veins.

Intravenous pyelography. (IVP) This commonly used procedure involves the i.v. administration of a water-soluble iodine-containing contrast material which is primarily concentrated and excreted by the kidneys. It also allows visualization of the ureters and the bladder.

Intrinsic angular momentum. That part of the total angular momentum which cannot be described as orbital, e.g., due to the spin of an electron, proton, or neutron. The term is sometimes applied to any part of the angular momentum which it is not convenient to analyze further, e.g., that of a nucleus in a nuclear reaction.

Intrinsic count rate performance. Count rate performance characterizes a scintillation camera's ability to accurately function at count rates which are near the maximum rate of camera operation.

Intrinsic efficiency. Fraction of radiation striking a detector that also interacts with it. Depends on type and energy of radiation, attenuation coefficient, and thickness of detector.

Intrinsic energy resolution. Intrinsic energy resolution is a parameter of a scintillation camera which characterizes its ability to accurately identify the photopeak events. This parameter in a scintillation camera determines its ability to distinguish between primary gamma events and scattered events. This test is intrinsic and one without a collimator.

Intrinsic factor. A substance normally present in the gastric juice of humans. Its presence makes absorption of vitamin B_{12} possible. Absence of this factor leads to vitamin B_{12} deficiency and pernicious anemia.

Intrinsic flood field uniformity. Intrinsic flood field uniformity is a parameter of a scintillation camera which characterizes the variability to observe count density with a homogeneous flux.

Intrinsic spatial linearity. Spatial linearity is a parameter of a scintillation camera which characterizes the amount of positional distortion caused by the camera with respect to incident gamma events entering the detector.

Intrinsic spatial resolution. Intrinsic means the basic scintillation camera without variables such as collimators, which may change its inherent characteristics.

Intrinsic tracer. An isotope, present naturally in a given sample, that may be used to trace a given element through chemical and physical processes.

Inulin. Polysaccharide that on hydrolysis yields levulose, which can be used to test kidney function.

Inverse bremsstrahlung. Absorption of photons by electrons in the presence of the Coulomb field of a nucleus.

Inverse-square law. Rule by which the radiation intensity of any source decreases inversely as the square of the distance between the source and the detector.

Inversion. An excited or nonequilibrium state in which the net magnetization vector is in a direction opposite to that of the main field. (NMR.) Turning inside out of an organ. Reversal of normal relationship.

Inversion recovery. A radio-frequency pulse sequence which inverts the magnetization and then measures the rate of recovery as the nuclei of interest return to equilibrium magnetization. The rate of recovery depends upon T_1. (NMR.)

Inversion recovery sequence. A type of pulse sequence in which the magnetization is inverted by means of a 180° radio-frequency (rf) pulse, and recovery from this is monitored by means of a 90° rf pulse applied after a time τ. This sequence is commonly used for measurement of T_1 (*in vivo* and *in vitro*) in biological systems. (NMR.)

Inversion time. (T1) Time between inversion and subsequent 90° pulse to elicit NMR signal in inversion recovery.

In vitro. Observable in a test tube; removed from the natural environment; excised.

In vivo. Within the living body.

Iodide trap or pump. The iodide concentration mechanism of the thyroid gland.

Iodination. Addition of iodine to a compound.

Iodine. Element symbol I, atomic number 53, atomic weight 126.904.

Iodine escape peak. Photoelectric interaction of photons in the NaI crystal usually results in a 28-keV K X-ray, which may escape the crystal, resulting in a peak 28 keV below the primary photopeak.

Iodohippurate. (Hippuran) Orthoiodohippurate salt excreted by the kidneys via tubular secretion with ~80% efficiency and used to measure effective renal plasma flow. The remaining ~20% is excreted by glomerular filtration.

Iodothyronines. Iodinated thyronines formed through the oxidative coupling of the precursor iodothyrosines, monoiodotyrosines (MIT) and diiodotyrosines (DIT), in varying combinations. The principal iodothyronines are thyroxine (T-4) and triiodothyronine (T-3).

Iodotyrosines. Compounds formed by the incorporation of activated iodine into a tyrosine moiety. Monoiodotyrosine (MIT) is formed by incorporating activated iodine into the 3-position of a tyrosine moiety. Another iodine is then added to the 5-position to form diiodotyrosine. (DIT).

Ion. An atom or group of atoms bearing a positive (cation) or negative (anion) electric charge as a result of having lost or gained one or more electrons.

Ion exchange. A chemical process involving the reversible interchange of ions between a solution and a particular solid material, such as an ion exchange resin consisting of a matrix of insoluble material interspersed with fixed ions of opposite charge. The process is used for purifying water (removing hardness), or in a radioisotope generator, i.e., ^{99}Mo-^{99m}Tc.

Ionic compound. Compound held together by purely electrostatic forces.

Ionic inhibitors. (Thiocyanate, perchlorate) Substances which interfere with the concentration of the iodide ion by the thyroid gland.

Ionic radius. Ions in crystals packed together like rigid spheres of definite radii. Since cations touch neighboring anions ionic radii can be found from interionic distances once one ionic radius is known absolutely. The effective radius of an ion does vary slightly according to the number, charge, and size of its neighbors.

Ionic strength. One half the sum of the terms obtained by multiplying the molarity of each ion by the square of its valence.

Ionic yield. The number of ion pairs produced per incident particle or quantum.

Ion implantation. A technique used especially in the manufacture of semiconductors for introducing impurities to produce a desired characteristic. The ions may be accelerated electromagnetically and injected into the semiconductors.

Ionization. The process in which an atom or molecule separates into two parts (ions) which have opposite electrical charge. Two general types of ionization can be distinguished. First, there is that which occurs when a salt is dissolved in water and which results in the formation of two atomic or molecule ions in solution. Second, there is that which occurs when one or more electrons become detached from an atom or molecule.

Ionization of an atom or molecule requires that one or more electrons in the atom or molecule is raised from a bound to an unbound state. For an electron to become detached then, a certain minimum amount of energy, equal to the electron's binding energy, has to be transferred to the atom or molecule. This energy varies from element to element, ranging from about 5 eV for the alkali metals to about 20 eV for the rare gases.

The energy needed to produce ionization can be supplied when another particle collides with the atom or molecule. The colliding particle must in some way disturb the electrical field in the atom or molecule. For this reason suitable projectiles are other atoms, ions, γ-rays, and all the charged elementary particles. Other particles, like neutrons and neutrinos, produce negligible ionization because any electromagnetic interaction associated with them is very weak.

Ionization chamber. Ionizing radiation can be detected by the small electric current which can be made to flow between two electrodes when particles of the gas between them become ionized. The electrodes and gas are often in a sealed glass envelope to allow the gas pressure to be reduced, which makes the device more sensitive. The Geiger-Müller (GM) tube is a special type of ionization chamber which contains low-pressure neon or argon, and a very high voltage is applied between specially shaped electrodes. Ionization chambers are used to measure X-ray and γ-ray radiation levels.

Ionization current. The passage of a charged particle through a gas causes ionization; if an electric field is applied across the gas a current (due to the motion of the ions produced) flows between the electrodes. Certain detectors of radiation use this phenomenon.

Ionization density. The density of the ionization, produced in the path of a charged particle passing through matter, depends upon the amount of charge, the velocity of the particle, and the nature of the matter.

Ionization loss. The loss of energy incurred by a charged particle due to the ionization it produces in matter.

Ionization potential. The energy (in electron volts) which is required to remove a particular electron from an atom is measured by its ionization potential (in volts). For the outermost electrons in almost all atoms the ionization potentials lie between 5 and 20 V, while those of the most tightly bound inner electrons in the heaviest atoms approach 100 kV.

Ionization track. In certain detectors of radiation the track of a charged particle may be shown by the ionization which is produced in its path. The detectors which are used in this way are the cloud chamber, bubble chamber, and nuclear plates. Also called ionization path.

Ionizing energy. The energy which must be given to an electron in an atom to cause ionization, i.e., to remove the electrons from the atom. It is generally measured as an ionization potential.

Ionizing event. The interaction of very high energy radiation (e.g., a cosmic ray) with matter in a detector such as a cloud chamber or nuclear plates, which results in the production of one or more energetic charged particles.

Ionizing particle. Any charged particle possessing sufficient energy to produce ion pairs.

Ionizing radiation. Electromagnetic and particulate radiations may have sufficient energy to remove electrons from atoms (ionization). The energy of electromagnetic radiation is related to the frequency (or wavelength). Ionization of some atoms begins with rays of about 10 eV which corresponds to waves in the ultraviolet region. Thus, visible light (1 eV), microwaves (0.0001 eV), and lower frequencies may be considered to be nonionizing. Ionization in human tissues is caused deliberately in radiotherapy using X-rays (0.1 to 10 MeV) and γ-

rays (up to 100 MeV). Particulate radiation of beta particles (electrons), alpha particles, neutrons, and heavy nuclei may be used.

Ionography. An electrostatic imaging technique, used in mammography, in which a layer of high atomic number gas contained in a thin disk-shaped chamber is ionized by X-rays emerging from the breast.

Ion pair. Two particles of opposite charge, usually referring to the electron and positive atomic or molecular residue resulting after the interaction of ionizing radiation with the orbital electrons of atoms.

Ion source. A device which produces ionized atoms suitable for use in high-energy accelerators or mass spectrometers.

Ipsilateral. Referring to structures on the same side of the body.

I region. That portion of the major histocompatiblity complex which contains genes that control immune responses.

Iridium. Element symbol Ir, atomic number 77, atomic weight 192.2.

Iron. Element symbol Fe (ferrum), atomic number 26, atom weight 55.847.

Irradiance. A measure of the rate of energy falling on a given area.

Irradiation. A term meaning exposure to radiation. Irradiation may be accomplished by exposure of the sample to the radiation from a radioactive substance, the radiation from a particle accelerator, or in the case of neutron irradiation by placing the sample in a nuclear reactor. Application of a radioactive source for therapy or diagnosis.

Irradiation reactor. A reactor used primarily as a source of ionizing radiation for irradiation of materials or for medical purposes. Reactor types in this case include: chemonuclear reactor, materials processing reactor, biomedical irradiation reactor, materials testing reactor.

Irrigation. Washing with a stream of water or saline.

Ischemia. The state of a tissue that is receiving insufficient blood to meet its metabolic needs. Ischemia may be reversible or irreversible depending upon the cause of the insufficiency.

Ischemic damage. Damage from constriction of a blood vessel, leading to necrosis of tissue.

Is genes. Genes that control development of specific suppressor T lymphocytes.

Isoagglutinin. An agglutinating antibody capable of agglutinating cells of other individuals of the same species in which it is found.

Isoallotypic determinants. Genetic markers that act as allotypic determinants within a specific immunoglobulin subclass and also appear on all members of at least one other subclass of IgG.

Isoantibody. An antibody that is capable of reacting with an antigen derived from a member of the same species as that in which it is raised.

Isobar. One of a group of nuclides having the same atomic mass number (A) so that the total number of particles (neutrons and protons) in the nucleus is the same, but with these particles so proportioned as to result in different values of Z; for example, ^3H and ^3He, therefore, there are different elements.

Isocenter. The intersection of the beam axis of a radiation therapy machine and the axis of rotation of that machine.

Isocount curves. Curves showing the distribution of radiation in a medium by means of lines or surfaces drawn through points receiving equal doses.

Isodiaphere. In a nucleus there are N neutron and Z protons. The term isodiaphere relates to nuclei which have the same number (N – Z).

Isodose. Descriptive of a locus at every point of which the absorbed dose is the same.

Isodose chart. Chart showing the distribution of radiation in a medium by means of lines or surfaces drawn through points receiving equal doses. Isodose charts have been determined for beams of X-rays transversing the body, for radium applicators used for intracavitary or interstitial therapy, and for working areas where X-rays or radioactive isotopes are employed.

Isodose curve. A curve depicting loci of identical radiation dosage in a structure.

Isodose surface. A surface all points of which receive the same dose. For example, the isodose surfaces due to a point source of radiation embedded in a uniform medium are concentric spheres centered on the source.

Isoelectric. Uniformly electric throughout; having the same electric potential, and hence giving off no current.

Isoelectric point. The pH at which, in the course of the titration of a protein from the completely acidic to the completely basic form, the mean charge on the protein is zero. In electrophoresis, that pH at which the protein does not migrate.

Isoenzyme. One of several forms in which an enzyme may exist in a species. For example, lactic dehydrogenase (LDH) may exist in five different forms, with differing concentrations in different tissues.

Isohemagglutinins. Antibodies to major red cell antigens present in members of a given species and directed against antigenic determinants on red cells from other members of the species.

Isomer. One of two or more nuclides having the same mass number A and atomic number Z, but existing for measurable times in different states of energy. The state of lowest energy is the ground state. Those of higher energy are metastable states. It is usual to indicate the metastable isomer by adding the letter m to the mass number in the symbol for nuclide (^{99m}Tc).

Isomeric state. An excited nuclear state having a measurable lifetime.

Isomeric transition. (IT) The process by which a nuclide decays to an isomeric nuclide of lower energy state. Isomeric transitions proceed by γ-ray and/or internal conversion electron emission.

Isomer separation. The chemical separation of isomers made possible when the radiation emitted in their formation has different effects on chemical bonds.

Isometric. Having the same length: a muscle acts isometrically when it applies a force without changing its length.

Isometric contraction. Contraction of a muscle in which shortening or lengthening is prevented. Tension is developed but no mechanical work is performed, all energy being liberated as heat.

Isonitriles. Hexakis (alkylisonitrile) ^{99m}Tc complexes such as ^{99m}Tc-carbomethoxyisopropyl isonitrile (CPI) or ^{99m}Tc-methoxyisobutyl isonitrile (MIBI) are used to study myocardial blood flow for the scintigraphic assessment of coronary artery disease and myocardial infarction.

Isopleth. Graph showing frequency of an event as a function of two variables.

Isopters. Lines on a field-of-vision chart which pass through points of equal visual acuity.

Isoresponse curve. Representation in cross section of surfaces of constant efficiency of detection for a focused-collimator imaging system. A diagram comparing the system's (i.e., the collimator's) efficiency for detection of off-focus radioactive decay with its efficiency for detection of focal events.

Isosbestic points. The points of intersection in a spectrum observed when one species is converted to a spectrally distinct species.

Isosmotic. Solutions with the same osmolarity and osmotic pressure.

Isotachophoresis. This technique is based on the ability to separate mixtures of compounds according to their electrophoretic mobility in various media.

Isotone. Any one of several nuclides having the same number of neutrons in the nucleus but differing in the number of protons and therefore a different mass number.

Isotonic. Descriptive of solutions having identical concentrations of solvent and solute molecules and hence the same osmotic pressure as the solution with which it is compared. Having the same tone: a muscle acts isotonically when it changes length without appreciably changing the force it exerts.

Isotonic exercise. Contraction of a muscle during which the force of resistance to the movement remains constant throughout the range of motion.

Isotope. One of several nuclides having the same number of protons in their nuclei, and hence having the same atomic number, but differing in the number of neutrons, and therefore in the mass number. Almost identical chemical properties exist between isotopes of a particular element, for example, $^{11/6}$C, $^{12/6}$C, $^{13/6}$C, $^{14/6}$C are isotopes of carbon. The use of this term as a synonym for nuclide is not recommended. Nuclides are distinct nuclear species, while isotopes are nuclides of the same element.

Isotope dilution analysis. A method of analysis whereby the amount of a particular element in a specimen is found by observing how the isotopic composition of that element is changed by the addition of a known amount of one of the isotopes of the element. The method can be used both mass spectroscopically with stable isotopes or radiometrically with radioactive isotopes.

Isotope effect. Differences that may be detectable in the chemical or physical behavior of two isotopes or their compounds.

Isotope separation. Process in which a mixture of isotopes of an element is separated into its component isotopes or in which the abundance of isotopes in such a mixture is changed.

Isotope separation value. A measure of the difficulty of preparing a given quantity of one isotopic composition from a given quantity of another isotopic composition.

Isotope shift. The spectra produced from, and the electronic structure of, different isotopes are not quite identical. Differences arise because the different isotopic masses give different reduced masses for the electrons and because the slightly different nuclear sizes produce differences between the electric fields felt by the electrons when they pass within the nucleus.

Isotope tracer. A radioactive or sometimes stable isotope used to follow the behavior of a particular element in a system. The isotope must be in the same chemical form as the inactive compound. For example, many organic compounds are labeled with ^{14}C and are widely used in medical and biological work.

Isotopic. Containing different isotopes of the same element or elements.

Isotopic abundance. The number of atoms of a particular isotope in a mixture of the isotopes of an element, expressed as a fraction of all the atoms of the element.

Isotopic analysis. Determination of the concentration of different isotopes in a sample of a chemical element. It is usually accomplished by mass spectrography.

Isotopic labeling. It refers to a compound in which an atom has been replaced by an isotope of the same element, in the same position, and without any other change in the molecule; it also refers to compounds in which more than one atom has been replaced under the same conditions.

Isotopic level detector. Determining the level in a tank containing a liquid that is either under pressure or is hermetically sealed to prevent contact with the atmosphere is often difficult. A technique has been evolved in which a ^{60}Co source is placed on a small float, so it can rise and fall with the level of the liquid. A counting tube is mounted in the roof of the tank and a meter is calibrated so that measurement of the count rate gives a reading in terms of the liquid level in the tank.

Isotopic mass. The atomic weight of an isotope.

Isotopic number. The excess of neutrons over protons in a nuclide. If the nuclide has atomic number Z and mass number A, the isotopic number is equal to $A - 2Z$.

Isotopic power generator. A device for generating useful power from the heat produced by the radioactive decay of a radionuclide. The heat is usually converted to electricity by thermoelectric or thermionic devices.

Isotropic. If a property is the same in every direction, for example, while the proton NMR spectrum of liver tissue is isotropic, that of muscle may depend on the direction of the fibers with respect to the applied magnetic field. Contrast with anisotropy where the property is not the same in all directions, e.g., anisotropy of T_2 in muscle tissue.

Isotropic motion. Motion that is equally probable in all directions, e.g., random rotational motion of a molecule about the three axes of a molecule.

Isotropic spectrum. Electron spin resonance (ESR) or NMR spectrum in which the molecular motion is so fast that any anisotropy in the spectrum is averaged out, e.g., ESR spectrum of a spin label in a liquid or NMR spectrum of bulk water.

J

Jaundice. Yellowness of skin, secretions, and mucous membranes because of bile pigments in the blood.

J chain. A glycopeptide chain that is normally found in polymeric immunoglobulins, particularly IgA and Igm.

Jeener-Broekaert phase shifted-pulse pair sequence. A type of pulse sequence used in pulsed NMR experiments to measure T_{1D}, the spin-lattice relaxation time in the dipolar field. In this method, pulse sequence used is $90° - \tau_1 - (45°)_0 - \tau_2 - (45°)_{90}$ - echo. The subscripts 0 and 90 refer to 0° and 90° phase shifts introduced into the radio-frequency (rf) pulse, τ_1 and τ_2 are time delays between pulses.

Jejunum. The portion of the small intestine lying between the duodenum and the ileum.

Jet. A very high (unphysiologic) velocity area downstream from an obstruction where laminar flow proceeds at high velocity.

Job. A group of data and control statements that does a unit of work. A program and all of its related subroutines, data, and control statements is an example.

Joint (compound) probability. Probability that two or more events, a, b, c, ..., n, will occur simultaneously.

Joule. A unit of energy, work, equivalent to newton meter or in SI base units, m^2 kg s^{-2}.

Joy stick. An input device with a lever mounted on a universal joint that moves in all directions. The joy stick lets the user move a cursor, or electronic blip, on a computer screen.

J-spectra. In high-resolution Fourier transform NMR spectroscopy, Fourier transformation of the Carr-Purcell spin-echo sequence gives spectra called J-spectra, consisting of lines which have their natural line width and are separated only by coupling constants. Chemical shifts do not appear in the spectra. J-spectra are useful for measurement of very small coupling constants.

Jump. Instruction that tells the computer to depart from the normal sequence of instructions, then to return to continue the program.

Juxtaglomerular apparatus. Specialized cells in the afferent arterioles of the kidney glomeruli and the distal kidney tubules; this apparatus produces renin.

K

K absorption edge. The abrupt increase in the photoelectric effect and, therefore, the coefficient of absorption at photon energies corresponding to the K shell binding energy.

Karyogram. A chart of the numbers and shapes of the chromosomes in the cell of an individual.

K cell. A killer cell responsible for antibody-dependent cell-mediated cytotoxicity.

K-edge subtraction. The same technique as employed in dual-energy subtraction with the added requirement that energies are selected to be just below and just above the K-edge of iodine (33 keV).

K-electron. One of the two electrons in the K-shell, the innermost electron shell in an atom.

K-electron capture. The radioactive decay process in which an orbital electron from the K-shell of the atom is captured by the nucleus, resulting in the production of X-rays characteristic of the daughter atom.

Keloid. A new growth or tumor of the skin, consisting of whitish ridges, nodules, and plates of dense tissue; these growths tend to recur after removal and are sometimes tender and painful; they generally arise in the area of a mending surgical incision, burns, or irradiation.

Kelvin. (K) The unit of thermodynamic temperature, is the fraction 1/273.16 or the thermodynamic temperature of the triple point of water.

Keratin. Fibrillar protein composed of closely bonded polypeptide chains. It is the chief structural material of the outermost layer of the skin, hair, and nails.

Kerma. Kinetic energy released in material. Nonstochastic quantity relevant only in the fields of indirectly ionizing radiations (photons or neutrons) or for any ionizing radiation source distributed within the absorbing medium. Thus, the kerma is the expectation value of the energy transferred to charged particles per unit mass at a point of interest, including radiative-loss energy but excluding energy passed from one charged particle to another.

Kerma can be expressed in units erg/g, rad, or J/kg. The latter unit is also the gray (Gy). The rad is still commonly employed for kerma and absorbed dose, but J/kg is to be preferred as it is an SI unit: $1 \text{ Gy} = 1 \text{ J/kg} = 10^2 \text{ rad} = 10^4 \text{ erg/g}$.

Kerma components. The kerma of X- or γ-rays consists of the energy transferred to electrons and positrons per unit mass of medium. The kinetic energy of a fast electron may be spent in two ways:

1. Coulomb-force interactions with atomic electrons of the absorbing material, resulting in the local dissipation of the energy as ionization and excitation in or near the electron track. These are called collision interactions.
2. Radiative interactions with the coulomb force field of atomic nuclei, in which X-ray photons (bremsstrahlung) are emitted as the electron decelerates. These X-ray photons are relatively penetrating compared to electrons and they carry their quantum energy far away from the charged-particle track.

In addition, a positron can lose an appreciable fraction of its kinetic energy through in-flight annihilation, in which the kinetic energy possessed by the particle at the instant of annihilation appears as extra quantum energy in the resulting photons. Hence, this is also a type of radiative loss of kinetic energy, in which the resulting photons can carry kinetic energy away from the charged-particle track.

Kerma rate. The kerma rate at a given point and time is expressed as J/kg·s (Gy/s) or in the non-SI units erg/g·s or rad/s, with other time units often substituted.

Kernel. The particular filter function used in the convolution operation. For example, a smoothing kernel might have values of 1/4, 1/2, 1/4. (These are frequently known as weighting values.) In the case of reconstruction tomography, the kernel is a sharpening kernel such as −1/4, 1, −1/4. Note: The convolution operation with this kernel on a projection array will result in each projection pixel value being modified by subtracting from it 1/4th the count value of the pixel on either side to compensate for the blurring generated during the backprojection operation. For two dimensions the kernel is two-dimensional; for example, 3 × 3 picture smoothing can be accomplished by a kernel with weightings of 1/4 in the center and 1/16 in the surrounding eight elements.

Ketone. Organic molecule with a carbon-oxygen double bond separating two alkyl portions

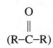

Ketone bodies. Products of fatty acid metabolism including acetoacetic acid, β-hydroxybutyric acid, and acetone.

Ketosis. An excess of ketone bodies in blood, characteristic of diabetes mellitus and starvation.

Key. A digit or digits used as a label that lets the computer locate or identify a collection of information (a record) stored in memory. The key is not necessarily attached to the record.

Keyboard. A typewriter-like device used for entering information and instructions into the computer. The keyboard includes keys representing numbers, letters, and symbols, plus special-function keys that instruct the computer to do specialized tasks such as interrupting a program or erasing the memory.

Keypunch. A keyboard device for producing cards with punched holes.

Keystroke. The amount of data that you can enter through a keyboard by pressing one typing key.

Kicksorter. Popular term for a pulse height analyzer which is an electronic device useful for identifying radioactive isotopes by the type and energy of the radiation they emit. It distinguishes isotopes by the different characteristic energy "kicks" which their radiation give and thus sorts them one from another.

Kilo. A prefix meaning 1000. Thus, a kilo-electronvolt (keV) is 1000 eV.

Kilogram. (kg) The unit of mass; it is equal to the mass of the international prototype of the kilogram.

Kiloton. A measure of nuclear weapon energy. A 1-k ton weapon releases the same amount of energy as would 1000 tons of TNT.

Kilovolts peak. (KVP) The crest value of the potential wave in kilovolts. When only one half of the wave is used, the crest value is to be measured on this half of the wave.

Kinetic energy. The energy of translational motion of a particle or system of particles.

Kinetics. Those features of a physical process determined solely by the fundamental conservation laws of energy, linear momentum, and angular momentum; e.g., the relation between the energy and angle of a scattered particle. Pertaining to or consisting of motion.

Kinin. A peptide that increases vascular permeability and is formed by the action of esterases on kallikreins, which then act as vasodilators.

Kit. A complete system of calibrated reagents and aids prepackaged for convenient performance of an assay.

Klein-Nishina formula. A formula which expresses the cross section of an unbound electron for scattering of a photon in the Compton effect as a function of the energy of the photon. The term usually refers to the integral Klein-Nishina formula, which gives the total cross section of the process.

K-L ratio. The ratio of the number of internal conversion electrons from the K-shell to the number of internal conversion electrons from the L-shell, emitted in the deexcitation of a nucleus.

Klystron. A velocity-modulated electron beam tube used to generate very-high-frequency oscillations at high power. It consists of an electron gun, drift tunnel (with usually not less than two resonant cavities), and a beam collector.

K-meson. A charged or neutral elementary particle having a mass about 966 electron masses. It is unstable and decays in a variety of ways. Until recently each mode of decay was identified with a different particle.

Knocked-on atom. An atom which recoils owing to collision with an energetic particle.

Knock-on. The process whereby a particle, on being struck by a fast-moving particle or photon, is set in motion; also used as an adjective to describe the particle so set in motion.

Korotkoff sounds. Sounds produced by sudden pulsation of blood being forced through a partially occluded artery and heard during auscultatory blood pressure determination.

Krypton. Element symbol Kr, atomic number 36, atomic weight 83.80.

Krypton-81m. Short, 13-s-half-life radionuclide of the inert gas krypton, which can be obtained from a $^{81}Rb/^{81m}Kr$ generator and used in studying and imaging the ventilation of the lungs. In solution in dextrose it can be injected intravenously or intraarterially to define the extent of perfusion of the tissues drained or supplied by the infused blood vessel.

K-shell. Inner orbital electron path adjacent to the nucleus.

Kupffer cells. Fixed mononuclear phagocytes of the reticuloendothelial system that are present within the sinusoids of the liver.

L

Label. The process by which a substance or compound is charged by the addition of a stable nuclide (for example, ^{13}C in place of ^{12}C) or a radioactive nuclide (^{14}C in place of ^{12}C); in the latter situation the changed substance or compound has been radiolabeled. The incorporation of a tracer isotope, radioactive or stable, into a molecular species or macroscopic sample for purposes of detection. By observations of radioactivity or isotopic composition this compound or its fragments may be followed or traced through physical, chemical, or biological processes. One or more characters used to identify a source language statement or line in a computer program.

Labile. A term used in chemistry, meaning unstable or liable to change. Frequently applied to compounds readily participating in isotopic exchange reactions.

Labyrinth. The interconnecting system of cavities of the inner ear; system of interconnecting cavities or canals.

Lactase. An enzyme splitting lactose into glucose and galactose.

Lacteals. The lymphatic vessels of the small intestine which contain milk-white fluid during the process of digestion and convey it into the blood through the thoracic duct.

Lactic acid. A colorless, syrupy liquid formed in milk, sauerkraut, and in certain types of pickles by the fermentation of the sugars by microorganisms. It is also formed in muscles during activity by an aerobic breakdown of glycogen.

Lactic dehydrogenase. (LDH) An enzyme found in varying concentrations in all tissues of the body, with increase occurring following tissue injury.

Lactoferrin. An iron-containing compound that exerts a slight antimicrobial action by binding iron necessary for microbial growth.

Lactose. (Milk sugar) A double sugar (disaccharide).

Lacuna. A small space, depression, or defect in the body.

Lag. A term usually employed to mean time lag. Thus, in the case of a counter, the time lag is the time between the occurrence of the primary ionizing event and the occurrence of the count.

Lamella. Thin leaf or plate, as of bone.

Lamina. Thin, flat plate or layer; composite structure.

Laminar flow. The flow of a fluid in a channel is said to be laminar or streamline when all the fluid particles move regularly in paths parallel with the walls of the channel.

Landau damping. The damping of a space charge wave by electrons which move at the phase velocity of the wave and gain energy transferred from the wave.

Language. A means of communication between the machine and the user. It consists of a set of various conventions and rules to convey meaning. Thus it is a code.

Machine code — A fundamental technical set of instructions peculiar to each design of computer. A computer operates on one machine code instruction at a time.

High level language — A language, such as BASIC, FORTRAN, ALGOL, etc. consisting of a set of statements which correspond to fixed sets of machine code instructions. These statements have been designed with particular users in mind and are compiled to aid certain types of functions. The importance of a high level language is that one "statement" in it is translated into (typically) terms of machine instructions.

Lanthanides. The term refers to the rare earth section of elements in the periodic table, and derives from the first member of the rare earth series, namely lanthanum. Atomic numbers range from 57 to 71. The actinide series of elements shows a resemblance in some respects to the lanthanides.

Lanthanum. Element symbol La, atomic number 57, atomic weight 138.9055.

Laparoscopy. The endoscopic examination of the abdominal cavity.

Laparotomy. Surgical incision through the flank; less correctly, but more generally, abdominal section at any point.

Large-scale integration. The technology of producing circuits (usually more than 1000) on a single chip.

Larmor equation. The equation defining the resonance condition in magnetic resonance phenomena. The Larmor equation is $\omega_0 = \gamma B_0$, where ω_0 is the Larmor frequency in radiations per second, γ is the gyromagnetic ratio, and B_0 is the magnetic field (induction) strength.

Larmor frequency. (ω_0) Resonant frequency defined by the Larmor equation. Expressed in hertz (f_0) or radians per second (ω_0); $\omega_0 = 2\pi f_0$. The frequency at which magnetic resonance can be excited; given by the Larmor equation. By varying the magnetic field across the body with a gradient magnetic field, the corresponding variation of the Larmor frequency can be used to encode position. For protons (hydrogen nuclei), the Larmor frequency is 42.58 MHz/T.

Larmor precession. The precessional motion of an orbiting charged particle when the particle is exposed to a magnetic field. The particle precesses about the direction of the field. For an electron orbiting about an atomic nucleus the precessional angular velocity is given by eH/2mc, where e is the charge on the electron, m its mass, c the speed of light, and H the magnetic field strength.

Larmor radius. The radius of gyration of a charged particle in a magnetic field: $r_L = v/\Omega$, where v is the velocity of the particle perpendicular to the magnetic field and Ω is the cyclotron frequency.

Laser fusion amplifier. A device that increases the light intensity of a laser beam level suitable for compressing and heating an inertial confinement target.

Last in/first out. (LIFO) A data manipulation method in which the last item stored is the first item processed; a pushdown stack.

Latch. Circuit that holds and stores information within the computer for future use.

Late effects. Effects of radiation which do not become evident until a period of many months or even years following completion of irradiation.

Latency. Time delay between stimulus and response. The period or state of seeming inactivity between the time of exposure of tissue to an injurious agent and the beginning of the response.

Lateral. Toward the outer margins of the body.

Lateral resolution of ultrasound. The smallest separation of two objects that can be distinguished in a plane normal to axis of the ultrasound beam; approximately equal to the diameter of the beam.

Lattice. Magnetic and thermal environment with which nuclei exchange energy during longitudinal relaxation.

Lattice energy. The energy required to separate the ions of a crystal to an infinite distance from each other.

Lavage. The wash from inside an organ; or to wash out toxic material.

Law of constant composition. If two (or more) elements combine chemically to form a compound, the relative number of moles of each constituent elements will always be in a constant proportion to each other. (Law of definite proportions.)

Law of mass action. The velocity of the chemical reaction is proportional to the masses of the reactants.

Law of multiple proportions. If two elements form more than one compound, the number of moles of one element in the first compound is proportional to the number of moles of the same element in the second compound.

Law of reciprocal proportions. Two chemical elements unite with a third element in proportions that are multiples of the union of the first two elements.

Lawrencium. Element symbol Lr, atomic number 103, atomic weight ~260.

Lead. Element symbol Pb (plumbum), atomic number 82, atomic weight 207.19.

Lead age. A determination of the age of a mineral by measuring the amount of radiogenic lead which it contains.

Lead castle. The production of a wide range of standard sized and shaped lead bricks has made possible the erection of small compounds, with or without viewing or handling facilities, to enclose small radioactive sources used in experimental work. Such a structure is known loosely as a lead castle.

Lead equivalent. The thickness of lead, which, under specified conditions or irradiation, affords the same protection as the material under consideration. The lead equivalent of a substance, such as lead-glass or lead-rubber, which attenuates the radiation essentially by its lead content, is largely independent of the quality of the radiation. The lead equivalent of all other protective materials and also building materials for protective walls (concrete, brick, etc.) and barium protective glass show a dependence on the quality of the radiation.

Leading edge. The upward deflection of each echo on an A-mode display.

Leakage radiation. All radiation, except the useful beam, coming from the tube or source housing.

Leak detectors. Instruments used, generally in conjunction with a tracer substance, for finding small holes or cracks in the walls of a vessel. The type of leak detector used for a given test depends on the degree of tightness needed on the vessel.

Least detectable value. The value at 2 SDs from the zero standard value that can be significantly differentiated from zero. Most results should never be reported as zero, but as less than the least detectable value.

Least squares method. A method of fitting a regression line to a set of data so as to minimize the sum of squared vertical deviation of the y values around that line.

Le Châelier's principle. If a system is initially at equilibrium and is forced away from equilibrium when a parameter is changed, the system will spontaneously return to a new equilibrium.

Left ventricular filling pressure. The equivalent of left atrial pressure, i.e., the pressure of blood in the left atrium before it passes to the left ventricle. As left atrial pressure rises, pulmonary congestion occurs, producing the characteristic symptom of shortness of breath. Left ventricular filling pressure expresses the concept of "backward heart failure" numerically. It is also an index of the preload of the left ventricle.

Leg. The logical sequence of events in a routine or subroutine that is part of a larger program. Legs are the different paths a computer program can travel along, depending on which routines and subroutines it selects and follows.

L-electron. One of the eight electrons in the L-shell of an atom.

Lens. Clear biconvex part of the eye through which light passes.

Lepton. Term derived from word for smallest Greek coin which refers to the group of small particles, the electron, positron, and neutrino.

Lesion. Any change in the structure of a bodily part due to injury or disease.

Lethal dose-50%. (LD_{50}) Synonym for median lethal dose.

Lethal dose-50/30. ($LD_{50/30}$) A dose of a substance that, when administered to a group of any living species, kills 50% of the group in 30 days.

Lethal mutation. A mutation which leads to the death of the individual who carries it, usually at an early stage of development. If recessive, the lethal mutation must be present in both the appropriate homologous chromosomes for its effects to be manifest.

Letter-quality printer. A printer that forms characters by striking a raised type element against the paper through a ribbon. Letter-quality printers produce high-quality output but operate at moderate speeds.

Leukemia. A disease in which there is great overproduction of white blood cells, or a relative overproduction of immature white cells, and great enlargement of the spleen. The disease is variable, at times running a more chronic course in adults than in children. It is almost always fatal. It can be produced in some animals by long-continued exposure to low intensities of ionizing radiation.

Leukocyte. White blood cell or corpuscle; numerous functional types; leukocytes.

Leukocyte inhibitory factor. (LIF) A lymphokine that inhibits the migration of polymorphonuclear leukocytes.

Leukocyte mitogenic factor. (LMF) A lymphokine that will induce normal lymphocytes to undergo blast transformation and DNA synthesis.

Leukocytosis. Abnormal increase in the number of leukocytes (white blood cells), usually reflecting the presence of an acute inflammation or infection.

Leukopenia. Less than the normal number of white blood cells.

Leukotaxine. Crystalline nitrogen substance appearing when tissue is injured.

Level. A nucleus can possess only certain discrete amounts of internal energy. These values are those of the nuclear energy levels. The level with the least energy is termed the ground state; the energies of the other levels are usually given relative to it.

Level density. The number of energy levels of a nucleus per unit energy interval, at a particular energy.

Level spacing. The average separation between nuclear energy levels at a particular excitation energy; it is the reciprocal of the level density.

Levitron. A toroidal plasma confinement system formed by a combination of magnetic fields, one field being produced by current flowing through a metal ring suspended inside the plasma chamber. The ring is kept away from the walls of the chamber by magnetic forces.

Lewis concept. An acid is an electron-pair acceptor and a base is an electron-pair donor.

Liable. (Legal) To be bound or obligated to make satisfaction, compensation, or restitution for an injury to another as determined by rules of law or equity.

Library. Organized collection of computer programs, books.

Lifetime. The mean time between the appearance and disappearance (birth and death) of a particle. An excited state of an atom or nucleus also has a lifetime, which determines the rate at which it decays to another state. The term is also used for the lifetime of a carrier in a semiconductor.

Ligament. A band or sheet of fibrous tissues which connects two or more bones, usually within a joint.

Ligand. An atom or small molecule binding to an atom or molecule of interest. The binding can be either covalent binding (e.g., nitrogens or oxygen to a metal ion) or noncovalent binding of a small molecule to a big molecule (e.g., binding of a substrate to an enzyme). In radioimmunoassay, ligand usually means an antigen or small molecule that binds to a native carrier protein.

Ligation. Tying off, especially arteries, veins, or ducts.

Light chain. A polypeptide chain present in all

immunoglobulin molecules. Two types exist in most species and are termed kappa (κ) and lambda (λ).

Light-emitting diode. (LED) A semiconductor component; and on/off indicating device that emits light when a current is passed through it. A source of light commonly used to form digits in an alphanumeric display.

Light pen. Instructions may be given to a computer by the use of a light pen. This is a hand-held probe which has a light detector at its tip which is connected to the computer. If the pen is held to the face of the visual display unit the position on the screen is known to the computer by the time at which the light pen receives the pulse of light from the scanning spot as it passes underneath it. Depending on the type of computer program it is thus possible to enter graphical information into the computer or answer questions by touching particular spots on the display. Light pens are now sometimes used with ultrasonic B-scanners and with some nuclear imaging apparatus to draw around a particular organ or region of interest seen on the display. Such images of the body are normally held in a computer memory and so are readily accessible for data processing.

Light pipe. Plastic interface between camera crystal and photomultiplier tubes to maximize light transfer. Also reduces nonuniformity (and spatial resolution). Optical contact between the surfaces of the scintillator, light-piper, and photomultiplier is then made with a mineral oil of suitable refractive index. Good light transmission is aided by internal reflection from the polished sides of the rod.

Limbic system. Part of cerebral cortex involved in emotion and behavior.

Limited proportionality region. The region of operation of a gas counter below the Geiger threshold and above the proportional region. The gas amplification depends upon the initial ionization, and strict proportionality as in the proportional region no longer exists.

Limulus test. A lysate of the circulating amebocytes of the horseshoe crab. (Limulus polyphemus.) It reacts with Gram-negative bacterial endotoxins in low concentrations to form an opaque gel. *In vitro* test for pyrogens, particularly suitable for testing short-lived radiopharmaceuticals.

Line amplitude. The height of the spectral line in an NMR spectrum as measured from the baseline.

Linear absorption coefficient. Of a thin parallel beam of indirectly ionizing radiation passing through a uniform absorber, the fractional decrease of the beam's intensity per unit length of absorber traversed.

Linear accelerator. Electrons can be accelerated to high velocities (up to 99% of the speed of light) in a straight wave guide driven by a microwave (e.g., 10 GHz) generator. Electrons are fed from a thermionic source into the evacuated wave guide which contains a series of metal diaphragms with a hole in the middle so that with each wave the electrons move from one diaphragm to the next. The spacing of the diaphragms is increased down the length of the tube as the velocity of the electrons increases. At the far end they strike an X-ray target from which high-energy X-rays (6 to 20 MeV) are produced, or pass through a window to allow direct electron treatment. The resultant X-ray beam is attenuated by a beam-flattening filter, a circular piece of metal, thicker in the center than at the edge, which is introduced into the beam to produce a uniform X-ray intensity. The beam size is controlled by metal shutters, usually adjustable over the range 4 to 30 cm. Beam intensity may be modified by a variety of metal filters, the most common being wedge shaped, which attenuate uniformly from one side of the beam to the other. Such devices are used in the treatment of deep cancers since these high-energy rays have good penetration properties.

Linear amplifier. An electronic device of special design for amplifying pulses so that the size of the output pulse will be proportioned to the size of the input pulse.

Linear array. Array made up of rectangular elements in a line consisting of a row of up to 400 small transducers side by side which are triggered sequentially to produce parallel lines of information.

Linear array scanning. The most common type of moving picture ultrasonic scanning uses a linear array transducer. This is a large transducer which has a contact area with the skin of approximately 1×10 cm. Inside the transducer the piezoelectric element is divided into many parallel elements along the 10-cm length and these are connected by electronic switching so that only a small area (e.g., 1×1 cm) of the transducer is active at any time. With the active area at one end of the transducer an ultrasonic pulse is transmitted, and echoes are detected from the tissue immediately beneath this area. On the B-scan display this produces a line of bright dots. Then the active area commutates along the transducer repeating the process so that many parallel lines of scan are produced on the screen. The process is repeated so that the complete scan is refreshed onto the screen at greater than the flicker frequency of the eye, thus producing a moving picture. Moving picture scans have a number of advantages particularly where there is rapid movement of the structures in the scanning plane (e.g., heart). The scan is a "simple" scan in that each point in the tissue is interrogated from one direction only, so that theoretically some information may be lost. However, the diagnostic information is usually greater than with the static B-scanners except where a large field of view is required or where the skin surface cannot be flattened to accommodate the large contact area. Most modern scanners include a frame freeze module in which the level of brightness (echo amplitude) at every point on the picture is stored in a computer memory so that the motion of the picture can be arrested for examination or recording.

Linear attenuation coefficient. The fractional number of photons removed from a beam of radiation per unit thickness of a material through which it is passing due to all absorption and scattering processes.

Linear energy transfer. (LET) Energy deposited by radiation per unit length of matter through which the radiation passes. Its usual unit is keV/μm.

Linear phased array. Linear array operated by applying voltage pulses to all elements, sequentially with small time differences.

Line intensity. Area under the spectral line in an NMR spectrum. Under certain conditions, the intensity is an index of the number of nuclei giving rise to this resonance line.

Line number. A number that identifies a line in a text file.

Line of force. A term employed in the description of an electric or magnetic field. A line such that its direction at every point is the same as the direction of the force which would act on a small positive charge (or pole) placed at that point. A line of force is defined as starting from a positive charge (or pole) and ending on a negative charge (or pole). The line (or force) is also used as a unit of magnetic flux, equivalent to the Maxwell.

Line pairs. Used to specify the spatial resolution of imaging systems. The largest number of observable alternating black and white lines in a given distance is a measure of the system resolution.

Line printer. A high-speed output computer de-

vice in which the text is printed a line at a time rather than character by character.

Line scanning. One type of NMR imaging technique in which the spin density distribution is sampled one line at a time. A line is scanned sequentially through the sample to obtain the complete image. This method is also referred to as the "sensitive line" or "multiple sensitive point" imaging.

Line scanning radiography. An imaging system which uses a linear array of detectors and an X-ray fan-beam which is scanned over the patient to produce an image. Detector arrays may be scintillator/photodiodes or high-pressure xenon detector arrays.

Line shape. Shape of a spectral line, i.e., the variation of the height of the line as a function of frequency.

Line space. The distance between lines of dots on a dot or photo scan; usually expressed in centimeters.

Line spread function. (LSF) The full spatial response of an imaging system to a line source of activity. The contribution of the imaging device to the resolution of an image is specified by the shape and width of the LSF.

Line width. Width of line in spectrum; related to the reciprocal of the transverse relaxation time (T2* in practical systems). Measured in units of frequency, generally at the half-maximum points. (NMR.)

Lingula. Small tonguelike structure.

Link. A pointer from one item in a file to another.

Linkage. The location of two genes close together on a chromosome so that they are passed on as one characteristic (rather than two) from parent to offspring.

Linkage disequilibrium. An unexpected association of linked genes in a population.

Linker. A program which takes object files and combines these with library routines to resolve references between them, thus creating a linked file.

Lipase. An enzyme which catalyzes the hydrolysis of fats, breaking the ester bonds of fatty acids.

Lipid. Fats or fat-like substances found in living tissue. They contain one or more fatty acids.

Lipopolysaccharide. (also called endotoxin) A compound derived from a variety of Gram-negative enteric bacteria that have various biologic functions including mitogenic activity for B lymphocytes.

Lipoproteins. Combination of a lipid and a protein.

Liquid. A state of matter in which the molecules are relatively free to change their positions with respect to each other, but restricted by cohesive forces so as to maintain a relatively fixed volume.

Liquid crystal display. (LCD) A method for creating an alphanumeric display, commonly used in digital watches, which consumes little power. It forms the desired digit by reflecting outside light.

Liquid drop model. A model of the nucleus which has had considerable success in accounting theoretically for many of the details of nuclear fission and which forms the basis of the semiempirical mass formula. In this model, the nucleus is regarded as having properties similar to that drop of incompressible liquid.

Liquid emulsion technique. Nuclear photographic emulsion manufactured in gel form so that after heating it can be poured to the desired shape at the desired time.

Liquid scintillation counter. γ-Rays of less than 20 keV and β-rays of less than 500 keV cannot be counted by the usual sodium iodide type of scintillation counter. This problem is overcome in the liquid scintillation counter (also known as a beta counter) by mixing the scintillator with the sample and using photomultiplier (PM) tubes to count the scintillations. The scintillators used are fluorescent complex organic molecules, and secondary scintillators may be used to convert the wavelength to match the PM tube. The sample and the PM tubes must be housed in a light-tight box. The PM tube itself produces emission of electrons which may affect the results and so the sample is often cooled (e.g., to 5°C) and only scintillations detected simultaneously by two tubes are counted. Normally several hundred samples are counted in turn by use of an automatic sample changer, and calibration and background samples are included, to enable computer correction factors to be included in the results. These devices are intended for counting low-energy isotopes such as ^{125}I, tritium, and ^{14}C. They are used for radioimmunoassay (RIA) or competitive binding analysis.

List. A sequence of instructions, or command to print every relevant item or data.

Listing. The printed copy generated by a printer or terminal.

List mode acquisition. List mode acquisition is a method of recording data on an image processor at very high data rates and without necessarily presuming a predefined image format (as required for dynamic acquisitions or gated studies). However, in the latter instance, most studies are acquired using a list mode-like structure which is subsequently and automatically formatted into image matrices.

When data are accumulated in list mode, three items of information are stored for later interrogation. These are the X and Y coordinate pair. These data are then stored with a temporal accuracy of perhaps 5 ms. Once the data have been acquired and stored, a formatting subroutine can generate a dynamic study with, if necessary, different time zones. Thus, in research of physiological processes where rates of change in radioactive distribution are unknown, it is possible to store data at maximum input data rates, without presuming an image format, reflecting changes efficiently and yet retaining storage potential. For instance, if it becomes apparent that a particular renogram could be adequately expressed in two phases, the data could be formatted to reflect the changed circumstances.

While this method of acquisition does ensure maximum flexibility in data acquisition, a penalty is incurred in the additional processing time required to format image data into a form that can be viewed.

Lithium. Element symbol Li, atomic number 3, atomic weight 6.941.

L-mesons. μ-Mesons and π-mesons are sometimes collectively referred to as L-mesons in order to distinguish them from heavier K-mesons.

Load. To place a program or data in memory. To place a volume on a device unit and put the unit on line.

Loader. Program that places data into the computer from disk.

Lobe. A well-defined pendant projection or division of a body organ or part.

Lobule. Small lobe or a subdivision lobe.

Local anaphylaxis. An immediate hypersensitivity reaction that occurs in a specific target organ such as the gastrointestinal tract, nasal mucosa, or skin.

Local area network. (LAN) Combination of hardware and software that connects two or more computers, enabling them to exchange data very rapidly and to share peripherals.

Localized magnetic resonance. A particular technique for obtaining NMR spectra, for example, of phosphorus, from a limited region by by creating a sensitive volume with inhomogeneous applied gradient magnetic fields, which may be enhanced with the use of surface coils.

Local skin temperature. Measurement of the skin temperature at a specific part of the body surface. Measured by thermistors placed at the surface of the skin — infrared thermometer or thermograph.

Location. The place in or on a computer storage device where a single piece of data or a single instruction is stored.

Lock signal. The NMR signal used to control the field frequency ratio of the spectrometer generally in high-resolution NMR spectroscopy. In modern NMR high-resolution instruments, a deuterium signal from the solvent is used for lock signal.

Locus. The specific site of a gene on a chromosome.

Log amplifier. An amplifier which amplifies input signals according to a logarithmic function rather than linearly; i.e., small signals are amplified while large signals are compressed.

Logarithmic ratemeter. A counting ratemeter in which the condenser charge is allowed to leak away through a diode valve operated so that the voltage across it is proportional to the logarithm of the current flowing through it. Such an instrument enables a wide range (1 million : 1) of counting rates to be shown on one meter.

Logic. In computers, representation of quantities by the on-off positions of switches, or gates. By arranging the gates for such logic functions as and, or, and not, the computer can make decisions about data symbolized in digital form.

Logical device name. An alphanumeric name assigned by the user to represent a physical device. The name can then be used synonymously with the physical device name in all references to the device. Logical device names are used in device-independent systems to enable a program to refer to a logical device name assigned to a physical device at run time.

Logical operation. A logical operation expresses such reasoning in terms of mathematical equations and symbols. Logical operations manipulate and compare these symbols using logical operators such as AND, OR, NOT, and NAND.

Logit. Mathematical relationship defined as in

$$y/1 - y$$

Lognormal distribution. A skewed distribution which can be transformed to a normal distribution by taking the logarithms of the x values.

Long-acting thyroid stimulator. (LATS) A γ-globulin which is present in about 45% of pa-

tients with hyperthyroidism and which causes delayed uptake of iodine in an animal assay system.

Long-acting thyroid stimulator protector. An immunoglobulin that is present in the circulation of patients with hyperthyroidism and has the property of blocking the binding of LATS to human thyroid microsomes.

Longitudinal emission tomography. The acquisition of images obtained by focusing at varying depths within the organ of interest; the images maintain the same spatial orientation as conventional images (the two-dimensional images are oriented parallel to the detector). These images can be obtained with standard scintillation cameras and specially designed collimators.

Longitudinal magnetization. Component, M_z of the macroscopic magnetization vector in the direction of the static magnetic field. After excitation by a radio-frequency (rf) pulse, M_z approaches its equilibrium value M_z at a rate characterized by time constant T_1 (NMR).

Longitudinal relaxation. Return of the longitudinal magnetization, after excitation, to its equilibrium value by exchange of energy between the nuclear spins and the lattice.

Longitudinal relaxation time. Time constant, T_1, characterizing the rate at which excited nuclei reach equilibrium with the thermal or magnetic field environment (lattice). Measure of the time taken in the trend for spinning nuclei to realign with the external magnetic field. The magnetization in the Z-direction will grow after excitation from 0 to about 63% of its final thermal equilibrium value in a time of T_1.

Longitudinal resolution. Minimum reflector separation along the sound path required for separate reflections to be produced.

Longitudinal wave. Wave in which the particle motion is parallel to the direction of wave travel.

Longitudinal wave energy. Wave whose amplitude displacement is in the same or opposite direction as the motion.

Loop. A circuit, part of which may run inside a reactor, into which materials and engineering components can be put, and then subjected to radiation under variable conditions, e.g., of temperature, exposure to coolant, strain, etc. A sequence of instructions that is executed repeatedly until a terminal condition prevails.

Lorentzian line. Usual shape of the lines in an NMR spectrum, characterized by a central peak with long tails; proportional to $1/[(1/T2)^2 + (f - f_o)^2]$, where f is frequency and f_o is the frequency of the peak (i.e., central resonance frequency). The Fourier transform of the lorentzian line is an exponential function.

Loss-free counting. (LFC) Dynamic correction for pulses lost in a detector system when the electronics are busy. The technique provides proper correction for very high or changing count rates.

Loudness. The psychological response of the ear which is related to the physical quantity intensity. The loudness of a sound depends on frequency also, since the ear responds more strongly to some frequency bands than to others. The loudness is roughly related to the cube root of the intensity, and for many purposes it is convenient to represent loudness as proportional to the logarithm of the intensity.

Low-level activity counting. Both liquid scintillation counters and gas counters can be used for low-activity measurements provided great care is used to optimize the counting efficiency and reduce the background count rate. The background count is in part due to internal radioactive contamination from environmentally occurring radionuclides such as ^{40}K and members of the radium and thorium series of radionuclides. External shielding and careful selection of materials can reduce the background count considerably. The background component due to cosmic radiation is best reduced by anticoincidence shielding, with the sample counter surrounded by a ring of other counters connected in parallel with one another but in anticoincidence with the sample counter. Cosmic-ray particles such as π-mesons, which trigger the sample counter will also be registered in the ring and will therefore be recognized as being due to cosmic radiation.

Low-level language. A programming language in which the commands closely parallel those of the instruction set of the computer (machine code). Assembly language is a mnemonic code which is converted by an assembler program into machine code (ones and zeros).

Low-order byte. The least significant byte in a word. The low-order byte occupies bit positions 0 through 7 in a 16-bit word.

Low-population zone. The area immediately surrounding the exclusion area that contains residents whose total number and density are such that there is a reasonable probability that appropriate protective measures could be taken in their behalf in the event of a serious accident at a nuclear power or testing reactor.

L-shell. The second electron orbital path from the nucleus.

Lugol's solution. An iodide-saturated solution. Used in nuclear medicine in some circumstances to block the thyroid from accumulating radioactive iodine.

Lumen. The cavity or channel of a tubular device, organ, or duct.

Luminescence. Many substances emit radiation in the form of light when suitably excited; this property is known as luminescence, and can be excited by light itself, by X-rays, α-, β-, and γ-rays, cathode rays, positive rays, high-frequency radiation, etc.

Lung. The function of the lung is to supply oxygen and to remove carbon dioxide from the blood. During the pulmonary circulation the blood comes into intimate contact with the air contained in the microscopic primary units of the lung, the alveolar sacs. Through the alveolar-capillary membrane the exchange of gases takes place. Respiration is effected by changing the lungs' volume by contraction of the diaphragm and expansion of the chest mainly through elevation of the ribs. Air is sucked into the lungs during inspiration through an elaborate system of tubes. The first of these is the trachea, from where the air passes down through the primary, secondary, tertiary, and quaternary bronchi to even smaller bronchioles. These in turn branch to form alveolar ducts that lead eventually into the alveolar sacs.

Lung capacity. The maximum amount of air the lungs can inhale. Jogging and running can increase the capacity but not likely more than 10%. Smoking will decrease lung capacity.

Lutetium. Element symbol Lu, atomic number 71, atomic weight 174.967.

Lymph. Transparent slightly yellow fluid — containing cells, mostly lymphocytes — found in the lymphatic system; filtrate of plasma through capillary walls.

Lymphangiography. Lymphangiography is a study of the lymphatic vessels and their associated parenchymal components, the lymph nodes. Lymph nodes are frequently involved in malignant disease; an estimate of their size, shape, and distribution is useful prior to initiating therapy for the disease. The procedure involves the isolation of lymphatic vessels (approximately 1 mm diameter) below the region to be studied followed by an injection of an iodine-containing contrast material which is concentrated in the lymph nodes.

Lymphatic system. Comprises the lymphatics which carry the lymph and the lymph glands and associated lymphoid tissue. The lymph is derived from the cell-free fluid which filters out of the smaller blood vessels into the spaces between the cells. The lymphatics are thin-walled tubes which form a network in the vicinity of these blood vessels. They collect the lymph and pass it through a series of lymph glands until it is generally discharged into a large vein close to the heart.

The lymph glands, which are small oval bodies measuring up to 1 cm in length, are collected together in groups along the course of the lymphatics. The lymph glands and lymphoid tissue form lymphocytes, produce immunity, and contain reticuloendothelial tissue.

Lymphedema. Accumulation of interstitial lymph fluid due to obstruction of the lymphatic channels.

Lymph node. A rounded body consisting of accumulation of lymphatic tissue found at intervals in the course of lymphatic vessels. Lymph nodes vary in size from a pinhead to an olive and may occur singly or in groups. Produces lymphocytes and acts as a filter to localize bacterial and viral infections and entrap wandering malignant cells.

Lymphocyte. A mononuclear white blood cell without cytoplasmic granules, which participates in the immune response. They normally number from 20 to 50% of total white cells.

Lymphocyte activation. An *in vitro* technique in which lymphocytes are stimulated to become metabolically active by antigen or mitogen. (Also know as lymphocyte stimulation, lymphocyte transformation, or blastogenesis.)

Lymphocyte-defined antigens. A series of histocompatibility antigens that are present on the majority of mammalian cells and are detectable primarily by reactivity in the mixed lymphocyte reaction. MLR).

Lymphocyte trapping. The selective arrest of lymphocytes in lymphoid organs following the trapping of antigens or particulates.

Lymphoid cells. Cells of the lymphoid system ranging from lymphocyte precursors to mature lymphocytes.

Lymphokines. Soluble products of lymphocytes that are responsible for the multiple effects of a cellular immune reaction. Also called mediators of cellular immunity.

Lyphoscintigraphy. Functional imaging of a regional lymphatic system obtained by injecting a radioactive minicolloid into the soft tissue drained by that system.

Lymphotoxin. (LT) A multifactorial cytotoxic lymphokine that results in direct cytolysis following its release from stimulated lymphocytes.

Lyophilization. A process by which a liquid substance is rapidly frozen and then dried or dehydrated under high vacuum.

Lysis. Separation of adhesions binding different structures; destruction of a cell by a specific agent; abatement of disease symptoms.

Lysosome. Intracellular particles, particularly abundant in the liver and kidneys, which contain catabolic enzymes. Active in intracellular digestion processes.

Lysozyme. The cationic low-molecular-weight enzyme present in tears, saliva, and nasal secretions that reduces the local concentration of susceptible bacteria by attacking the mucopeptides of their cell walls. Also known as muramidase.

M

Machine code. A basic code used in computer programming in which instructions are represented by numbers in binary form, i.e., in the way in which it is executed in the central processing unit.

Machine run. A type of computing in which the operator feeds the program to the computer, after which the computer runs the program to completion. In machine run, the computer carries out all tasks without help from a human operator. The operator intervenes only if an error occurs.

Macro. The name given to a routine written in assembler and utilized as a unit by the assembly language programmer, who usually uses symbols to invoke the routine. Large.

Macroaggregated serum albumin. A particle size of 10 μm and up; this size albumin particle labeled with ^{99m}Tc is used for lung scanning.

Macro command. Program formed from a sequence of computer commands put into effect by a single command.

Macroglobulin. Protein of high molecular weight.

Macro instruction. One instruction that is equivalent to a sequence of frequently repeated machine instructions.

Macrophage. Large phagocytic cells occurring in the walls of blood vessels and connective tissue; eats foreign particles.

Macrophage activation factor. (MAF) A lymphokine that will activate macrophages to become avid phagocytic cells.

Macrophage chemotactic factor. (MCF) A lymphokine that selectively attracts monocytes or macrophages to the area of its release.

Macroscopic. Visible to the naked eye.

Macroscopic cross section. The cross section per unit volume of a given material for a specified process. It has the dimension of reciprocal length. For a pure nuclide, it is the product of the microscopic cross section and the number of target nuclei per unit volume; for a mixture of nuclides, it is the sum of such products.

Macroscopic magnetization vector. Net magnetic moment per unit volume (a vector quantity) of a sample in a given region, considered as the integrated effect of all the individual microscopic nuclear magnetic moments. Most NMR experiments actually deal with this.

Magic angle. The angle 54.7° is called the magic angle because $3 \cos^2 \Theta - 1 = 0$ for this value of Θ, e.g., the dipolar coupling contains the terms $3 \cos^2 \Theta - 1$, where Θ is the angle between the internuclear vector and the applied field. Hence for an angle $\Theta = 54.7°$, the dipolar interaction vanishes.

Magic numbers. Numbers 2, 8, 20, 28, 50, 82, and 126. Nuclei possessing these numbers of neutrons or of protons have exceptional stability (lead and helium are examples) and may have other exceptional properties, e.g., low neutron capture cross sections.

Magnesium. Element symbol Mg, atomic number, 12, atomic weight 24.305.

Magnet. Any body which has the power of attracting iron.

Magnetic anisotropy. In ferro- or ferrimagnetic crystals, it is found that the magnetization prefers to lie along certain crystal directions. There are termed easy directions of magnetization. Work must be expended to turn the magnetization away from these easy directions. That work as a function of crystal direction defines the anisotropy energy surface. Directions associated with a maximum of the anisotropy energy are termed hard directions of magnetization. In general, the energy difference between easy and hard directions decreases as the temperature is increased, and vanishes as the Curie or Neel point.

Magnetic axis. The magnetic field line enclosed by a set of nested magnetic surfaces.

Magnetic dipole. North and south poles of a magnet separated by a finite distance constitutes a magnetic dipole moment. An electrical current in a circular loop can create a magnetic dipole moment.

Magnetic disk. A plate with a magnetic surface on which data are stored in a binary arrangement.

Magnetic domains. The magnetization of a ferromagnetic or a ferrimagnetic material tends to break up into regions called domains separated by thin transition regions called domain walls. Within the volume of a domain, the magnetization has its saturation value, and is directed along a single direction. The magnetizations of other domains are directed along different directions in such a way that the net magnetization of the whole sample may be zero. The application of an external magnetic field first causes some domains to grow by the motion of their walls. At higher fields, the magnetization of the resulting domains rotate toward parallelism with the field.

Magnetic field. The region in the neighborhood of a magnetized body in which magnetic forces can be detected. Also used interchangeably to refer to magnetic induction or magnetic intensity produced by an electromagnet, permanent magnet, or a superconducting magnet. A magnet field produces a magnetizing force on a body within it.

Magnetic flux. (Φ_B) Through a closed figure (e.g., a circular or rectangular loop): the product of the area of the figure and the average component of magnetic induction normal to the area, i.e., the surface integral of the magnetic induction normal to the surface. The SI unit is the Weber (Wb) and the CGS unit, the Maxwell, is equal to 10^8 Wb : $\Phi = SBds$, where B is the magnetic induction and S is the surface area.

Magnetic flux density. May be defined as the magnetic flux per unit area at right angles to the flux or as a product of the magnetic intensity and permeability. The magnetic induction is related to the magnetic field strength H and the magnetization M through the relationship $b = \mu_0 (H + M)$, where μ_0 is the permeability of free space. The unit of B is in terms of magnetic flux density; the SI unit is the tesla (1 Wb/m^2) and the CGS unit is the gauss (1 $Maxwell/cm^2 = 10^{-4}$ T).

Magnetic gradient. Amount and direction of the rate of change of field strength in space: employed to select the imaging region and to encode the NMR response signal spatially.

Magnetic island. A filament of magnetic field lines with its own set of nested magnetic surfaces.

Magnetic lens. The ability of a magnetic field to deflect moving charged particles can be used to focus a diverging beam of particles. Many suitable magnetic field configurations have been devised and are used in nuclear particle spectrometers and spectrographs, electron microscopes, cathode ray tubes, and other devices.

Magnetic memory. Any memory device using magnetic fields as a means for storing data.

Magnetic moment. The magnetic moment associated with the nucleus is a consequence of their inherent charge and spin. It is related to the nuclear angular momentum L through the gyromagnetic ration constant ($\mu = \gamma L = \gamma I h$, where I is the spin angular momentum vector). The nucleus may be viewed as a bar magnet spinning about its north-south axis. The magnetic moment associated with the electron spin on the one hand and the orbital motion on the other. The moment of a single electron spin is 1 Bohr magneton (U_B). Electrons possess about 1000 times larger magnetic moment than the largest of the nuclear moments.

Magneticogyric ration. (γ) Also called gyromagnetic ration. A constant of each nucleus given by the ratio of the magnetic moment to the angular momentum. It is also equal to μ/Ih, where μ is the magnetic moment, I is the spin quantum number, and h is Planck's constant divided by 2π. It also appears in the Larmor equation relating the resonant frequency (Larmor frequency) to the magnetic induction field for protons $\gamma/2\pi = 4.26$ MHz/kg (or 42.6 MHz/T).

Magnetic pole. It denotes the points of a magnet from which the magnetic field appears to diverge or toward which it appears to converge. The pole strength of a magnet is the magnetic moment divided by the distance between the poles.

Magnetic resonance. Absorption or emission of electromagnetic energy by nuclei in a (static) magnetic field after excitation by suitable radio-frequency (rf) radiation: the frequency of resonance is given by the Larmor equation.

Magnetic resonance imaging. (MRI) A technique for forming tomographic images of the density or behavior of hydrogen atoms in the body.

Magnetic resonance scanner. Previously known as a nuclear magnetic resonance (NMR) scanner, the word "nuclear" has been dropped to avoid confusion with devices producing harmful radiations. This can produce images of selected planes within the body which are similar in appearance to CT scans, but the image relates to the state and content of water at each point within the scan plane. The technique has the potential to identify other aspects of the chemical structure of tissues, but at present medical imaging is limited to information derived from the spin resonance of the hydrogen nucleus. The hydrogen nucleus forms a small magnet which will absorb and emit radio-frequency energy at a resonance frequency depending on the strength of an applied magnetic field. By the application of a magnetic field gradient the resonant frequency will depend on the position in the field. An extension of this principle allows the construction of two- and three-dimensional images.

Magnetic rigidity. A charged particle (mass m, velocity v, and charge e) moving in a uniform magnetic field (H) transverses a circular path or radius r, where Hr = mv/e is the magnetic rigidity. It is momentum divided by charge.

Magnetic shield. A system employing high-intensity magnetic fields to prevent charged particles from entering a region that is to be protected.

Magnetic shielding. The reduction of the magnetic field "seen" by a nucleus in an atom or molecule due primarily to screening by the electron cloud of the molecule.

Magnetic strip card. A small card resembling a credit card to which a strip of magnetizable material is affixed. Data can be read from or written onto this magnetic strip. In medicine, these cards are useful for containing identification and/or clinical information on ambulatory patients.

Magnetic susceptibility. A characteristic quantity of a substance denoting the intensity of the magnetization produced in it by an applied magnetic field. Paramagnetic substances are characterized by positive susceptibility, while diamagnetic substances have negative susceptibilities.

Magnetization. The magnetic polarization of a material produced by a magnetic field (magnetic moment per unit volume).

Magnetogyric ratio. Of an atomic nucleus, a proportionality constant relating the magnetic moment of an isotope to the spin angular momentum.

Magnetohydrodynamics. The study of the properties of conducting fluids in motion in a magnetic field.

Magnetometer. Device used for measurement of magnetic field strength, e.g., proton magnetometer that uses proton NMR frequency for measuring the magnetic field strength.

Magnification. Enlargement of image relative to the objective plane.

Main frame. A large commercial computer. Main frames are fast, expensive, and powerful. Main frames have thousands of times more memory than personal computers.

Main program. The computer program which usually exercises primary control over the operations performed; it also calls subroutines or subprograms to perform specific functions.

Main storage. The internal memory of the computer. Main storage can be reached much faster than secondary storage devices that store information outside of the computer. (these secondary storage devices include disks, tapes, and cassettes.

Major histocompatibility complex. (MHC) An as yet undetermined number of genes located in close proximity that determine histocompatibility antigens of members of a species.

Makaton vocabulary. A method of communication used by the vocally handicapped in which arms, hands, or the movement of fingers convey words or symbols.

Malabsorption. Inadequate absorption of nutrients in the gastrointestinal tract.

Malignant. Becoming progressively worse and leading to death; invasive and metastasizing. Term used commonly when referring to terminal cancer tumors.

Malpractice. (Legal) Bad, wrong, or injudicious treatment of a patient, professionally or in respect to a particular disease or injury, resulting in injury, unnecessary suffering, or death to the patient, proceeding from ignorance, carelessness, want of proper professional skill, disregard of established rules or principles, neglect, or malicious or criminal intent.

Manganese. Element symbol Mn, atomic number 25, atomic weight 54.938.

Manipulator. A hand-operated or hand-controlled device for remotely handling an object in an environment which is too hazardous to permit direct access.

Manometer. Device used to measure the pressure of liquids.

Mantissa. The fractional part of a floating point number. For example, in the floating point number 0.1234×10^4, 0.1234 is the mantissa.

Marker. The substance used to monitor the count of a binding assay. Label, tracer.

Mask. Information in the computer exists as patterns of the digits 0 and 1 — binary digits or "bits". A mask is a special pattern of bits that alters the positions of bits in other bit patterns. The mask can be used to select, ignore, set, or clear bit patterns.

Mask-mode subtraction. Sometimes called time-mode subtraction where a "mask" X-rays image acquired before the appearance of iodinated contrast media is stored, then subtracted from each subsequent image containing iodine.

Mass. Lump or body made of cohering particles; sometimes refers to a tumor. Is a measure of an object's resistance to acceleration. Basic parameter of matter referring to the quantity of matter present. It is independent of the object's weight.

Mass and energy relation. According to the relativity theory, a body cannot acquire a velocity relative to any observer which exceeds the velocity of light. Starting from this assumption, Einstein showed that an increase in the velocity of a body (relative to an observer) was accompanied by an increase in the mass of the body (as determined by the observer). For low velocities this increase in mass is negligible, but at velocities approaching that of light the increase becomes very large. As energy is applied to the body, it is manifested as very high velocities more as an increase in mass than as an increase in velocity. This interchange between mass and energy is a general phenomenon of all processes involving a change or energy. The equivalence between mass and energy as expressed by the Einstein equation, $E = mc^2$.

Mass and weight. The kilogram is the unit of mass; it is equal to the mass of the international prototype of the kilogram. The word weight denotes a quantity of the same nature as a force; the weight of a body is the product of its mass and the acceleration due to gravity; in particular, the standard weight of a body is the product of its mass and the standard acceleration due to gravity. The value adopted in the International Service of Weights and Measures for the standard acceleration due to gravity is 9.80 m/s^2, a value already stated in the laws of some countries.

Mass attenuation coefficient. (μm) For a given indirectly ionizing beam traversing a uniform medium, the ratio of the linear radiation absorption coefficient μ_l and the density ρ of the medium (μm = μ_l/ρ). The fractional decrease in radiation intensity per unit mass of medium traversed. Mass absorption coefficient.

Mass coefficient of reactivity. The partial derivative of reactivity with respect to the mass of a given substance in a specified location.

Mass conversion factor. Any factor which converts one unit of mass into another. The term is most often used for the factor mc^2 which gives the energy equivalent, E, of a mass m.

Mass decrement. The quotient of the mass excess of a nuclide and the unified atomic mass unit. It is also the difference between the relative atomic mass and the mass number.

Mass defect. The difference between the mass of a nucleus and the sum of the masses of its constituent protons and neutrons. The energy equivalent of the mass defect must be supplied to split up the nucleus into its component parts.

Mass energy transfer coefficient. (μ_{tr}/ρ) For a given material, the mass energy transfer coefficient for indirectly ionizing particles can be written:

$$\mu_{tr}/\rho = (1/E\rho) \ (dE_{tr}/dl)$$

where E is the sum of the energies (excluding the rest energies) of the indirectly ionizing particles incident normally upon a layer of thickness dι and density ρ, and dE is the sum of the kinetic energies of all the charged particles liberated in this layer.

Mass excess. The difference between the atomic mass of a nuclide and the product of the nuclide mass number and the unified atomic mass unit, u.

Mass ionization. The ionization charge in an ionization chamber divided by the mass of the gas in the chamber.

Mass ionization conversion coefficient. The mass ionization divided by the exposure in a given gas.

Mass number. (A) The mass number of a nuclide is the nearest integer to the actual or exact mass of a nucleus in atomic mass units (a.m.u.). There can be no ambiguity in this definition because the difference between the exact mass and the nearest integer is always very small. Since the exact masses of both the neutron and the proton in a.m.u. are both very close to unity, the mass number A gives the number of nucleons (neutrons and protons) in the nucleus.

Mass separation. The separation of different isotopes of a chemical element according to their isotopic masses. In principle this separation may be achieved by the use of any physical process in which the behavior of the atoms depends on their mass.

Mass spectrometer. The mass spectrometer or spectrograph is an instrument which identifies an atom, molecule, or compound by virtue of its atomic or molecular weight. Although origi-

nally developed for identifying the isotopes of an element and measuring their relative abundance, it has since found a great application in many other fields of scientific research, e.g., nuclear mass determinations, geochemical research, analytical chemistry.

Mass stopping power. For a given material. For a given material, the mass stopping power for charged particles can be written:

$$S/\rho = (1/\rho) \ (dE_s/dl)$$

where dE is the average energy lost by a charged particle of specified energy in traversing a path length d1, and ρ is the density of the medium.

Mass storage. Pertaining to a device that can store large amounts of data that is readily accessible to the computer.

Mass velocity. The mass rate of flow per unit cross-sectional area.

Mast cell. Specialized tissue cell rich in vasoactive amines; resembled basophils in form and function. Mast cells carry receptors for IgE and together with basophils participate in anaphylactic-type reactions by releasing stored mediators on contact with antigens.

Master slave manipulators. Mechanical hands used to handle active materials. They are remotely controlled from behind a protective shield.

Master/slave system. In this type of system, a large central computer controls a number of smaller machines. Under the direction of the master, these slave computers may be assigned to carry out a variety of special tasks including the transmission, editing, and processing of information.

Mater. Mother; dura mater — hard mother; Pia mater — tender mother; membranes covering the brain.

Materials processing reactor. A reactor employed for the purpose of changing the physical characteristics of materials by utilizing the reactor-generated ionizing radiation. Such characteristics may be color, strength, elasticity, dielectric qualities, etc.

Materials testing reactor. A reactor designed to provide a flux of neutrons so that the behavior of materials and engineering components under irradiation may be determined. The more intense the flux, the shorter the period of irradiation required to determine behavior in a power-producing reactor.

Matrix. An array of numbers ordered in terms of

indices. The number of indices determines the number of dimensions in the matrix. In nuclear medicine, images are stored in two-dimensional matrices (in picture elements or pixels) in which the indices correspond to the position of an element in the image. Image sizes are often 64×64, 128×128, 256×256, or 512×512.

Matrix printer. The matrix printer forms letters by printing them as patterns of dots within an area. The area is usually 7 by 9 dots, or 5 by 7 dots. There are two types of matrix printers: impact printers — small hammers form letters by striking the paper through an inked ribbon; nonimpact printers — a spray jet of ink or a pulse of light or heat on sensitive paper forms the printing.

Matrix size. The number of pixels for data storage of one frame or image. Example: 64×64 + 4096 pixels; $128 \times 128 = 16{,}384$ elements.

Matrix storage-byte mode. A manner of image storage in which 8 b (one byte) are used to represent up to 256 (2^8) shades of gray (color) or count levels.

Matrix storage-word mode. A manner of image storage in which 16 b (one word) are used to represent up to 65,536 (2^{16}) shades of gray (color) or count levels.

Maturation. Process of coming to full development.

Maximal velocity. The highest sound velocity found within significant amplitude within the sampled area usually for the use in Bernouli-type gradient estimations.

Maximal voluntary ventilation. The volume of air that a subject can breathe with maximal effort over a given time interval.

Maximum credible accident. A hypothetical accident used for safe design of a reactor or radiochemical plant which is that sequence of plausible events that releases the largest amount of radioactivity outside the containment system.

Maximum expected heart rate. The fastest heart rate of any age group. It tends to fall with age and is independent of fitness. It can be calculated approximately by subtracting the age from 220.

Maximum expiratory flow rate. The flow rate at a particular point during forced expiration; peak flow rate.

Maximum mid-expiratory flow. The flow rate during the middle half of a forced expiration.

Maximum permissible concentration. An expected upper limit for the concentration of a specified radionuclide in a material taken into the body below which continuous exposure (or in the case of occupational maximum permissible concentration, exposure for 40 h/week) to the material is not considered biologically harmful.

Maxwell coil. A particular kind of gradient coil, commonly used to create gradient magnetic fields along the direction of the main magnetic field. (NMR.)

Maxwellian distribution. The velocity distribution of molecules in thermal equilibrium as computed on the basis of the kinetic theory.

M-capture. As an alternative to the emission of a positron, radioactive nucleus may absorb an atomic electron. If this electron belongs to the M-shell, the process is known as M-capture.

Mean. The arithmetic average.

Mean free path. The average distance that particles of a specified type travel before a specified type (or types) of interaction in a given medium. The mean free path may thus be specified for all interactions (i.e., total mean free path) or for particular types of interaction such as scattering, capture, or ionization.

Mean life. The mean life of a radioactive substance is the average time for which its nuclei exist before disintegrating. Symbol $= \tau$. It is the reciprocal of the disintegration constant (λ) and is equal to 1.442 times the half-life. $r = 1\lambda$.

Mean range. The individual ranges in matter of heavy charged particles in a monoenergetic beam are not all the same. Because of straggling, the individual ranges are spread about a mean range. Half the particles have ranges which exceed the mean range and half have ranges which fall short of it.

Mean spectral velocity of blood flow. A mathematical mean of the spectral shifts in velocity within a given sample volume.

Mean square deviation from regression. Average squared vertical deviation of the y values around the regression line: (S^2 y – x).

Mean time between failures. The average length of time that will elapse between successive failures of any device.

Mean time to repair. The average amount of time it takes to restore a failed device to functioning status.

Mean transit time. The time it takes the average indicator population to traverse a defined volume; when multiplied by the average height of the curve, it equals the area under curve generated as the indicator traverses a designated volume.

Mean velocity/time. Velocity time integral divided by the time period over which the integral was determined. (Mean temporal velocity.) (Mean velocity as a function of time as in mean systolic velocity, mean diastolic velocity, or mean velocity for the cardiac cycle.)

Measurement of radioactivity. A radioactive substance, disintegrates with the emission of nuclear particles (α particles or β particles and/or photons [usually γ-rays], and the disintegration rate, which may be determined by measuring the rate of particle (or photon) emission, is decided by the amount of radioactive material present in the sample under investigation and by its half-life. Hence measurement of the emission rate provides a convenient method for the assay of such material.

Measurement of central tendency. Average value.

Meatus. A general term for an opening or passageway into the body; acoustic meatus — opening into the ear.

Mechanical register. An electrically actuated mechanical device for recording counts or impulses.

Medial. Toward the center or middle line of the body.

Median. The middle value of data ordered from lowest to highest.

Median lethal time. (MLT) The time required for the death of 50% of the individuals of a large population or organisms of a given species that has received a specified absorbed dose.

Mediastinum. The area separating the two lungs, between the sternum in front and the vertebral column behind. It contains the heart and its great vessels in addition to the other structures and tissues.

Mediators. A general term used to designate substances that incite such reactions as inflammation, smooth muscle contraction, and lymphocyte activation.

Medical uses of radioactive isotopes. A radioactive isotope is indistinguishable chemically from its stable counterpart; it is essentially only different in that it disintegrates or decays at a constant rate (expressed in terms of its half-life), giving off radiation of α-, β-, or γ-rays. This radiation has two properties valuable in medicine. First, it can be detected and measured by extremely sensitive counters, and in addition, one of the three types of radiation, γ-rays, can be measured at a distance. Second, the radiation is ionizing and has therefore a selective destructive effect on biological tissue. These two properties lead to wide use of radioactive isotopes in medicine. In research, diagnosis, and treatment; nuclear medicine.

Medium. Any carrier on which data may be recorded, e.g., paper, disks, tapes, paper tape, punched cards. Material through which a wave travels. Plural: media.

Medulla. The innermost part of an organ; the middle.

Megakaryocyte. Giant cell of the bone marrow containing a large, irregularly lobulated nucleus; the progenitor of blood platelets.

Megaloblast. A large nucleated primitive red blood cell. Megaloblasta are not found in normal blood or normal bone marrow, but they are seen in pernicious anemia.

Megaly. Denoting great size.

Meiboom-Gill sequence. A modification of the Carr-Purcell sequence, intended to correct inaccuracies in the 180° pulse lengths. (NMR.)

Meiosis. The successive division of a diploid sex cell resulting in haploid gametes. The gametes must have their chromosome number reduced by half in order to compensate for the doubling which occurs by fertilization.

Melanin. Dark pigment of skin, hair, and various tumors; color or black moles.

Melanotropin. (MSH) Melanocyte-stimulating hormone produced by the adenohypophysis; controls skin color in lower animals.

M-electrons. One of the 18 electrons in the M-shell of the atom.

Meltdown. A condition (and it is hoped a hypothetical condition, in the sense that it should never arise) that the solid fuel in a reactor rises in temperature to such an extent that it melts. (The China Syndrome.)

Membrane. A thin layer of tissue that covers a surface or divides a space or organ. Apart from its meaning in the biological field, this term denotes a porous or permeable substance which, in sheet form, can be used to separate different substances in the liquid or gaseous phase. For instance, some semipermeable membranes will allow certain molecules in solution to pass through them, but will prevent others.

Membrane resting potential. The potential difference that exists across the membrane of the normal cell at rest. In myocardial cells, the membrane resting potential is −70 to −90 mV.

Memory. The computer has two memories, random access (RAM) and read only memory (ROM).

Random access memory — A storage device to provide memory space to retain data and the program instructions to process data. The memory contents may change while the program is running and unless the computer has a "non-volatile" memory designed to retain the contents, they will be lost when the computer is switched off.

Read only memory — The contents stored in this memory cannot be changed under normal circumstances and remain whether the computer is running or switched off. It holds the operating set of instructions needed by the computer to make it function.

Memory size. The total amount of memory of a given type in a computer system. The number of words or bytes of memory that can be used to store either programs or images. For example, a 512×512 image requires 262,144 memory locations.

Mendelevium. Element symbol Md, atomic number 101, atomic weight ~258.

Meninges. The three membranes covering the spinal cord and brain; the dura mater (external), the arachnoid (middle), and pia mater (internal).

Menses. Menstruation. Monthly flow of blood from the genital tract of women.

Menu. A computer menu is a list of program functions, each labeled with a number or letter. To select a function a number or letter is pressed on the keyboard. The computer then puts that particular sequence of instructions to work.

Mercury. Element symbol Hg (hydrargyrum), atomic number 80, atomic weight 200.59.

Mesenchyme. Primitive tissue of the embryo.

Mesoderm. Middle of three primary germinal layers of an embryo; others are ectoderm and endoderm.

Meson. Short-lived particle carrying a positive or negative charge or no charge and having a variable mass in multiples of the mass of the electron. Mesons and hyperons are unstable elementary particles which are found in cosmic radiation, especially at high altitudes, and can be produced artificially in the laboratory using machines which accelerate nuclear particles to very high energies. Mesons are subdivided into L-mesons and K-mesons. Hyperons, also called Y particles, are heavier than the proton. They are represented by capital Greek letters.

Mesonic atom. An atom in which a negatively charged π- or μ-meson is bound in an orbit around a nucleus. The mesonic orbits are similar to the electron orbits in the atom, but because the meson is much heavier than the electron they lie much closer to the nucleus; indeed, the meson may even enter the nucleus. If it is absorbed, the meson's mass or rest energy

is released, causing the nucleus to break up.

Mesonic X-rays. An X-ray is produced when a meson in a mesonic atom undergoes a transition between one allowed orbit and another. These transitions are analogous to the electron transitions responsible for the optical radiation and the characteristic X-radiation.

Messenger ribonucleic acid. (mRNA) In protein biosynthesis the genetic message is enzymatically transcribed by formation of a ribonucleic acid, called mRNA, whose nucleotide sequence is complementary to that of DNA in the gene. After transcription, the mRNA moves to the ribosomes where it serves as a template for the specific sequence of amino acids during protein biosynthesis.

Metabolic alkalosis. Alkalosis resulting from the ingestion of alkaline drugs, for example, sodium bicarbonate; potassium depletion, some diuretics, or vomiting may be other causes.

Metabolic equivalent. (MET) A term describing in terms of oxygen consumption and corrected for differences in body weight, the oxygen requirement of physical activity. One MET, the oxygen requirement at rest, equals approximately the consumption of 3.5 ml of oxygen per kilogram of body weight per minute.

Metabolic rate. Heat produced within the body associated with chemical reactions. It is usually calculated directly from the consumption of oxygen (indirect calorimetry).

Metabolism. The sum of all the physical and chemical processes by which living organized substance is produced and maintained and by which energy is made available for the uses of the organism. The processes may be either constructive (anabolism) or destructive (catabolism).

Metabolite. Any substance taking part in, or produced by, a metabolic process.

Metal. A substance possessing so-called metallic properties such as electric conductivity, heat conductivity, high reflectivity, and luster, properties due to the high degree of freedom possessed by electrons of the substance.

Metal oxide semiconductor. (MOS) A special type of high-density integrated circuit. MOS chips contain many more electronic components per area than conventional integrated circuits.

Metaphase. The stage of nuclear division when the chromosomes are much contracted and lie scattered over the equatorial plate of the spindle.

Metaphysis. Portion of a developing long bone between the diaphysis or shaft and the epiphysis; the growing portion of a bone.

Metaplasia. A change in type of adult cells to a form not natural in that particular tissue.

Metastable state. An unstable excited nuclear state having a finite and measureable half-life that decays to a more stable state by γ-emission without change in the atomic number; abbreviated by the letter m (e.g., $^{99m}Tc \rightarrow ^{99}Tc$). Also known as an isomeric state. (The prefix meta derives from the Greek word for "almost".) In a quantum mechanical system such as a nucleus, the only truly stable state is the ground state of the system where the total energy has its minimum value. Most excited states decay very rapidly to the ground state by radiation and internal conversion and are said to be unstable.

Metastasis. The transfer of a disease from its main site to another distant part of the body. It is particularly associated with the transfer of tumor cells via the lymphatic system and blood flow from a primary site, and the subsequent formation of malignant tumors.

Metathesis. Chemical process in which two compounds exchange constituents.

Meter. (m) Is the length of the path traveled by light in vacuum during a time interval of 1/299,792,458 of a second.

Methemoglobin. Hemoglobin in which the iron is in its highest state (Fe^{3+}) and is thus unable to take up oxygen.

Methylene diphosphomic acid. (MDP) A diphosphonate sterile formulation presented as a freeze-dried kit, which, when reconstituted with ^{99m}Tc produces a labeled complex suitable for skeletal imaging, or when reconstituted with sterile isotomic saline, provides a solution for *in vivo* loading of erythrocytes with stannous ions, preparatory to technetium labeling.

Micelle. Unit of living matter having power of growth and division; colloid particle.

Micro. (μ) A prefix meaning 1 millionth; very small.

Microbiologic testing. Any test for bacteria, virus, or other microorganism.

Microcode. The detailed code which controls the internal functions of a processor, i.e., how the processor responds to a given machine language instruction.

Microcomputer. A small but complete computer comprising a central processing unit (CPU), memory, and input/output. Constructed using very large-scale integration (VLSI) components.

Microdensitometer. An instrument used for determining the optical density of a specimen by measuring the absorption of light through successive small areas of the specimen.

Microdosimetry. A branch of radiological physics concerned with the pattern of energy deposition in microscopic domains within matter exposed to ionizing radiation.

Microlysis. Destruction of a substance into microscopic size.

Microprocessor. A device, usually a chip, which when combined with the memories of a computer enables a preprogrammed sequence of instructions to be carried out. Thus it controls the the task assigned to the computer; consequently, it is sometimes known as the central processing unit (CPU).

Microprogram. A program executed by the microcode interpreter inside the central processing unit. The microprogram translates machine language instructions into the actual signals which control the operation of the central processing unit. The microcode interpreter is a computer within the computer.

Microradiography. A process in which a radiograph, or photograph using X-rays instead of light, is taken on a very fine grain film. The picture is then developed and enlarged, perhaps as much as 300 times, so that very fine detail in the original radiograph is revealed. This technique is very useful in metallurgy.

Microscopic. Detectable only with the aid of a microscope.

Microscopic cross section. The cross section per target nucleus, atom, or molecule. It has the dimension of area and may be visualized as the area normal to the direction of an incident particle which has to be attributed to the target particle to account geometrically for the interaction with the incident particle.

Microsomes. Intracellular inclusions which, on escape from thyroid follicular cells, stimulate antibody production and thyroid autoimmune reactions.

Microspacing. The technique of making a printed document's right margin even by inserting equal amounts of space between all the words on a line. Microspaced output resembles typesetting in appearance.

Microsphere. A spherical particle usually 1 to 3 or 15 to 35 μm in diameter and made from heat-denatured human serum albumin. (HAM.) When labeled with suitable radionuclide, i.e., ^{99m}Tc, can be used for lung perfusion scintigraphy.

Microtome. An instrument for slicing thin sections of tissue for examination under a microscope.

Microtomography. Tomography with a fine focus tube and subsequent optical magnification of the order of 20.

Microwaves. Electromagnetic radiation with frequencies in the range of 1000MHz. For example, electron spin resonance (ESR) is observed at 10 GHz, i.e., 10^{10} KHz (~3 cm wavelength).

Microwave spectroscopy. The study of atomic and molecular energy transitions corresponding to photons in the microwave (~1 cm wavelength) region. Observations of hyperfine structure in these spectra give information about nuclear spins and quadrupole moments.

Micturition. Urination; voiding of urine; emptying of the bladder.

Midrange dose. This is a good interassay check on a kit and/or a technique. One of the controls should be run at 50% intercept or halfway on the curve, or a midrange dose can be calculated from the curve. This point should not vary by more than ±2 SDs (preferably ±1 SD. (RIA.)

Midrange slope. The midrange slope of the curve monitors interassay precision. The slope of the curve is an indication of the sensitivity of the assay. The steeper the slope, the more sensitive the assay. If the slope flattens out, this could indicate breakdown of the antibody or expiration of the kit. (RIA.)

Migrating solvent. Chromatographic solvent; used to differentially carry the unknown solute to be separated.

Migration-inhibition factor. (MIF) A lymphokine that inhibits the normal migration of microphages.

Minicolloid. Radioactive colloid with particle size averaging 10 nm in diameter, usually formulated with an antimony radionuclide and used for evaluating lymphatic drainage.

Minicomputer. Originally a computer significantly smaller in size, capacity, and software capability than the larger main-frame computers with which it is contrasted; but with the next higher class computer after the microcomputer, difference is not distinct.

Minute ventilation. (VT) The volume of air inspired or expired in 1 min.

Mirror device (mirror machine). A magnetic containment device used in plasma research. Basically a solenoid magnetic field with the field strength increased at each end. Charged particles traveling toward the ends can be reflected by these regions of stronger fields which act as magnetic mirrors.

Misregistration artifacts. Subtraction image artifacts resulting from motion between the two images being subtracted. In digital angiography common motion artifacts are caused by swallowing, bowel gas motion, and patient movement.

Mitochondria. Small organelles within the cytoplasm containing enzymes controlling oxidation; they are the site of ATP production.

Mitogens. Substances that cause DNA synthesis, blast transformation, and ultimately division of lymphocytes. Also called phytomitogens.

Mitosis. The process by which a cell nucleus divides. It is characterized by contraction of the chromosomes during prophase, breakdown of the nuclear membrane and release of the chromosomes into the cytoplasm, formation on a spindle with the chromosomes of the equatorial plate (metaphase), separation of the daughter chromosomes to opposite poles of the spindle (anaphase), and the formation of two daughter nuclei around the two groups of chromosomes (telophase).

Mitotic index. The ratio of the time taken by a cell to complete cell division to the total cell cycle time.

Mixed leukocyte culture. (MLC) An *in vitro* test for cellular immunity in which lymphocytes or leukocytes from genetically dissimilar individuals are mixed and mutually stimulate DNA synthesis.

Mixtures. Consist of two or more substances intermingled with no constant percentage composition, and with each component retaining its essential original properties.

M-mode scanning. Alternatively known as a time motion (TM), scanning time position (TP), scanning motion (M-mode), scanning echocardiography, or ultrasonic cardiography (UCG), this is an ultrasonic scanning method which traces the movements of reflecting tissue interfaces with time. It is used primarily to study the action of the heart, particularly the valves, but is also used to study the movement of blood vessels and fetal heart. The apparatus consists of an A-scanner with the hand-held transducer positioned over the heart. The A-scan signal is turned into a single-line B-scan (i.e., the intensity of the echoes is used to modulate the brightness of dots on a single line on the screen) and this line is swept slowly up or across the screen so that the movement of reflecting surfaces is seen.

Mnemonic. Abbreviation or symbol that assists the human memory. For example, mnemonics

ADD and CLR (clear) are easier to remember than instructions given in binary code.

Mobile phase. Phase in chromatography that differentially carries the unknown solutes.

Mock iodine. A mixture of isotopes having a combined γ-ray spectrum similar to ^{131}I but with a much longer half-life, used for calibration purposes.

Modal velocity. The mode in the frequency analysis of a signal is the frequency component which contains the most energy. In display of the Doppler frequency spectrum, the mode corresponds to the brightest (or darkest) display points of the individual spectra and represents the velocity component which is most commonly encountered among the various moving reflectors. (Frequency mode.)

Mode. The most frequent value (point of maximum concentration).

Model. A theory or concept.

Modem. *MO*dulator *DEM*odulator; a device that enables a computer to communicate over telephone lines. A modem works by converting data between the digital form used by a computer and an audio form (a "carrier tone") that can be transmitted over the telephone.

Moderator. The three essential materials of a thermal neutron reactor are the fuel, moderator, and coolant. The function of the moderator of a reactor is to moderate, i.e., slow down, the fast neutrons and then allow time to diffuse until they are captured by the fuel.

Modulation. To combine an analog information signal with a carrier signal. There are two methods for signal modulation. In frequency modulation the frequency of the carrier signal is altered to conform to the message signal while the strength or amplitude of the signal is kept constant. In magnetic field modulation, a time varying at a particular frequency is superimposed on the static magnetic field. Amplitude modulation — where the amplitude of the carrier signal is altered with time to conform to the message signal while the frequency of the carrier remains constant.

Modulation side bands. Bands introduced into NMR absorption spectrum by modulation of the resonance signal. This can be done either by the modulation of the static magnetic field or by the amplitude or frequency modulation of the applied radio-frequency (rf) radiation.

Modulation transfer function. (MTF) The modulation transfer function is defined as the signal-to-noise ratio of the image as compared to the signal-to-noise ratio of the source. Hence, MTF may be considered as a mathematical function describing the ability of the system to transfer modulation from a source to its image, and the value of the MTF is the fraction of source modulation which has been successfully transferred, that is, a parameter of the fidelity with which an imaging device reproduces the spatial information contained within an object.

Module. A modular system consists of many standard compatible component parts, or modules. A modular computer or other electronic system is easy to repair. If a part fails, a new modular replacement can be fitted. Modular computer programming techniques break programs into small, easy-to-write modules. Each module performs a particular function and can be treated as a separate program.

Moiré interferometry. A method of mapping the surface contours of a subject by recording photographically the interference patterns generated by superimposing a linear grid and the shadow of that grid cast on the subject.

Molal. Unit of concentration associated with molality equal to the number of moles of solute per kilogram of solvent. Molality.

Mole. The SI unit of the amount of a system which contains as many elementary entities as there are atoms in 0.012 kg of ^{12}C. When the mole is used, the elementary entities must be specified and may be atoms, molecules, ions, electrons, other particles, or specified groups of such particles.

Molecular formula. Chemical formula that states the actual number of atoms of each constituent per molecule of the compound.

Molecular orbital. Wave function of an electron in a molecule. A molecular orbital is usually a linear combination of the electron wave functions of the constituent atoms of the molecule.

Molecular volume. Volume occupied by 1 mol. Numerically equal to the molecular weight divided by the density.

Molecular weight. Weight in unified mass units of one molecule of a particular chemical compound.

Molecule. The smallest unit of a compound that can exist by itself and retain all the properties of the original substance. Basic unit of a chemical compound.

Molybdenum. Element symbol Mo, atomic number 42, atomic weight 95.94.

Molybdenum-99. The relatively long half-life parent 65 h, of ^{99m}Tc, used to make ^{99}Mo-^{99m}Tc generators.

Momentum. The product of the mass of a body and its velocity; cgs units, g-cm/s.

Monatomic. One atom per molecule, usually referring to elements (such as the noble gases) in their native state.

Monitor. Program that controls and coordinates various operations within a computer. A device similar to a television set that a computer can use to display words or images. A monitor may display color or monochrome images. A radiation detector whose purpose is to measure the level of ionizing radiation (or quantity of radioactive material) and possibly give warning when it exceeds a prescribed amount. It may also give quantitative information on dose or dose rate. The term is frequently prefixed with a word indicating the purpose of the monitor, such as: area monitor, air particle monitor.

Monitoring. Periodic or continuous determination of the amount of ionizing radiation or radioactive contamination to safeguard the health of personnel engaged on work with radioactive materials; includes the routine checking of laboratories, apparatus and equipment, etc., for alpha, beta, gamma, or neutron radiation.

Monochromatic radiation. Electromagnetic radiation of a single wavelength, or in which all the photons have the same energy.

Monoclonal antibody. A specific immunoglobulin molecule which recognizes, and binds to, a single antigenic determinant (a specific marker site on the surface of an antigen) and which can be reproduced indefinitely at will.

Monoclonal immunoglobulin molecules. Identical copies of antibody that consist of one H chain class and one L chain type.

Monoclonal protein. A protein produced from the progeny of a single cell called a clone.

Monocyte. White blood cell having one rounded nucleus that increases in number during certain types of infections.

Monoenergetic radiation. Particulate radiation of a given type in which all particles have the same energy.

Monoiodotyrosine. (MIT) The iodotyrosine formed by the incorporation of activated iodine into the 3-position of a tyrosine moiety.

Monomer. The basic unit of an immunoglobulin molecule that is comprised of 4 polypeptide chains; 2 H and 2 L.

Monte Carlo method. A general mathematical method for solving problems in which the quantities to be found are expressed as statistical averages of comparatively elementary functions of a number of randomly distributed variables; in the process the functions are evaluated many times with (different) randomly selected values of the variable — hence the name. Its main field of application is in systems with many degrees of freedom where rival analytical techniques become prohibitively complicated.

Morphogenesis. Structural changes during development of an organism.

Morphology. Study of the structure of tissues.

Mosley's law. The frequencies of the characteristic X-rays of the elements show a strict linear relationship with the square of the atomic number.

Mössbauer effect. Recoilless emission and absorption of γ-rays. In radiation absorption/scattering from a crystal, the narrowing of a spectral width of a γ emission from a crystal. The loss of recoil energy to the atom concerned in the scattering process is taken up by the whole crystal and thus movement which broadens the spectral line emitted is reduced.

Mother board. A large printed circuit board supporting wiring patterns and edge connectors. Many smaller printed circuit boards, including processing units, memories, and interfaces, may be plugged into the mother board.

Motor end plate. An accumulation of cytoplasm and nuclei of muscle fibers at the point where a motor nerve branch terminates. Also known as neuromuscular junction.

Motorized syringe. This is an automatic device for slowly discharging the contents of a syringe through a catheter into a vein. It is normally a simple electromechanical device, often employing a stepping motor to drive a gearbox coupled to a worm drive which drives the plunger of a syringe. It is often called an infusion pump or syringe pump.

Motor nerve. A nerve composed only or mainly of motor fibers.

Motor unit. One motor neuron and the skeletal muscle fibers it innervates.

Mouse. An input device that you move around on a table top or a specially ruled pad. Many application programs allow the use of a mouse to control cursor motion to represent coordinates on screen.

Moving-beam radiotherapy. A technique used to increase the radiation dose incident on the target tissue while reducing the skin dose. It involves rotating the beam in an arc with the target at the center of rotation.

Mucoid. Mucus-like substance; an animal-conjugated protein.

Mucosa. Mucous membrane lining the digestive

and respiratory tracts; consists of a superficial layer of epithelium, a supporting layer of loose connective tissue, the lamina propria, and a thin layer of muscle, the muscularis mucosa. The epithelial cells secrete a protective lubricating solution, mucus.

Mucus. Protective lubricating solution produced by epithelial cells of the digestive and respiratory tracts; contains a protein, polysaccharide, mucin.

Multiaccess computing. A technique that allows a number of people to hold a conversation with a computer at the same time. Multiaccess computing systems have anywhere from two to several hundred outlets that link the main computer to remote devices such as terminals or word processors.

Multichannel analyzer. (MCA) This could refer to any type of analyzer (e.g., chemical analyzer or frequency analyzer) and the term is sometimes applied to devices used in nuclear medicine to collect the number of counts occurring at different pulse heights (different γ-ray energies). In this latter case a graph or histogram may be plotted showing count rates resulting from different isotopes. Typically there may be 256 channels, although there may be as many as 4096. They are often small computers which can also operate on the results to subtract the counts due to the background radiation leaving only that due to radioactive isotopes in the body. They are often used on whole body scanners. In clinical chemistry this term may refer to a large analyzer (discrete or continuous flow) for performing several tests on each sample.

Multichannel scaling mode. The acquisition of time-correlated data in the multichannel analyzer. Each channel is defined as a time window, ranging from milliseconds to seconds. Data collected during each time window are stored into sequential channels, producing a record of signal strength or intensity vs. time.

Multicrystal gamma camera. The majority of gamma cameras are of the single crystal format, i.e., one scintillator embracing the field of view. However, some gamma cameras have been manufactured that consist of multicrystal detectors. The multicrystal system can function more favorably at high count rates and offers superior count rate performance over single crystal systems. However, the trade-off is generally poorer energy and intrinsic spatial resolution, as well as high cost.

Multicrystal scanner. Improvement on rectilinear scanner. Two rows of detectors (above/below) provide scanning times similar to Anger camera. Primary use is whole-body scanning.

Multifunction card. An adapter card that provides several functions, letting you add more capabilities to a personal computer without running out of system expansion slots.

Multigate Doppler. A pulse/range gated Doppler interrogation approach in which multiple range gates sample Doppler shift information from multiple, closely spaced depths along the ultrasound beam. As opposed to high pulse repetition frequency (PRF) Doppler, multigate Doppler is implemented to sample and display separately the information from the individual gates.

Multigroup model. A model which divides the neutron population into a finite number of energy groups, each group being assigned a single effective energy.

Multinomial population. Population of more than two mutually exclusive categories.

Multiple-gated acquisition. Composite study of cardiac contractility and wall motion. The blood pool is rendered radioactive; the cardiac cycle is divided into usually 16 to 32 (but can be more) equal time intervals from R to R waves, and counts from each interval are stored as they are recorded in computer frames corresponding to each interval; each R wave triggers the acquisition in a synchronized process again until sufficient data are built up in each frame to form a diagnostic image. Multiple (16 to 32) images are formed, processed, and displayed in cine format. Ejection fractions from individual cardiac chambers, as well as other indices of cardiac function, can be derived. Lung ventilation functional studies can also be acquired by synchronizing the patient's respiration movements.

Multiple line-scan imaging. (MLSI) Variation of sequential line imaging techniques that can be used if selective excitation methods that do not affect adjacent lines are employed. Adjacent lines are imaged while waiting for relaxation of the first line toward equilibrium, which may result in decreased imaging time. A different type of MLSI uses simultaneous excitation of two or more lines with different phase encoding followed by suitable decoding. (NMR.)

Multiple plane imaging. Variation of sequential plane imaging techniques that can be used with selective excitation techniques that do not affect adjacent planes. Adjacent planes are imaged while waiting for relaxation of the first plane toward equilibrium, resulting in decreased imaging time. (NMR.)

Multiple scattering. Scattering of a particle or photon in which the final displacement is the vector sum of many, usually small, displacements.

Multiple sensitive point. Sequential line imaging technique utilizing two orthogonal oscillating magnetic field gradients, a multiple sensitive point pulse sequence, and signal averaging to isolate the NMR spectrometer sensitivity to a desired line in the body.

Multiple window spatial registration. Multiple window spatial registration is a parameter of gamma cameras which characterizes positional deviations in the image at different energies.

Multiplexer. A device for mixing data coming from or going to low-speed devices and sending it along one high-speed line, or the reverse. Also refers to the device in a computer system into which terminals plug and which passes the data from many terminals onto the computer's input/output channel.

Multiplexing. A method of dividing a single channel into many channels in order to transmit a number of independent signals. Different approaches to multiplexing are based on frequency (e.g., telephone, radio, and television networks) and time (e.g., telephone channels).

Multipole moments. The electric and magnetic fields produced by a system of charges and currents (such as arise from the electrons in an atom or from the protons in a nucleus) are the same, at points outside the system, as those due to a certain combination of charges, magnetic dipoles, electric quadrupoles, etc., located at the center of the system. The strengths of these equivalent multipoles are called the multipole moments of the system.

Multipole radiation. The radiation produced in a quantum-mechanical transition between two states associated with the corresponding multipole moments.

Multiprocessing. A system that contains several central processing units. Multiprocessing has the advantage of its ability to substitute for elements which break down, increasing reliability. Parallel processing means that various central processing units all work on the same task.

Multiprogramming. In multiprogramming, the computer's main memory holds more than one program. The memory is divided into separate segments called partitions; each partition holds a program. The size and number of partitions can be varied to increase the efficiency of data processing.

Multisection screens. A series of intensifying screens with a graded sensitivity to give equal density on a series of X-ray films in one exposure.

Mu-meson. (μ) An unstable elementary particle with a mass 207 times greater than the electron. It can be positively or negatively charged and decays with a mean life of 2.2×10^{-6} s into a positron (positive muon) or electron (negative muon) and two neutrinos.

Murmur. With reference to the heart, a sound arising from turbulent blood flow and commonly associated with valvular disease.

Mutant. A strain of an organism which differs from the normal in an inherited character difference.

Mutation. A change in the characteristics of an organism produced by an alteration of the usual genetic hereditary pattern. Mutations usually occur singly and with low frequency. Mutated genes are handed down to succeeding generations and are responsible for the inheritance of the mutant character.

Myelin. The fat-like substance forming a sheath around certain nerve fibers.

Myelography. This is a general term describing a radiographic procedure in which contrast material is introduced into the spinal subarachnoid space by means of a spinal tap in order to evaluate the spinal cord and its appendages and their relationship to the body spinal canal. This is also important in the investigation of primary and secondary spinal cord tumors, spinal cord trauma, and suspected herniation of intervertebral disks. This is also a technique when a block in the flow of spinal fluid is suspected, and contrast material may be inserted either above or below the level of the block and occasionally at both sites to precisely localize the level and extent of the obstruction.

Myeloid. Referring to bone marrow; referring to the spinal cord; cell resembling a red bone marrow cell that did not originate in the bone marrow.

Myocardial blood flow. Blood flow in units of min but conventionally defined as blood flow per gram of myocardial tissue (i.e., perfusion) in units of ml/min/g.

Myocardial infarction. The death of an area of heart muscle due to the area being insufficiently supplied with blood because of coronary artery obstruction.

Myocardial ischemia. Obstruction or construction in the coronary arteries resulting in a deficiency of blood to the heart muscle.

Myocardial metabolic rate of glucose. Refers to

local value and units are μmol/min/g (units of mg/min/g are also commonly used).

Myocardial oxygen consumption. (MVO_2) The amount of oxygen required by the heart, measured in units of μmol/min/g. This is determined by four primary factors: heart rate, arterial pressure, heart size, and contractility. Interventions for reducing myocardial ischemia are aimed generally at attenuating some of these factors, so that the heart's need for oxygen will be lessened. In the treatment of patients with angina pectoris, for example, a beta blocker such as propranolol will lessen both heart rate and contractility. This reduces the amount of oxygen the heart requires, and this in turn relieves the ischemic symptoms of angina.

Myocarditis. Inflammation of the myocardium, due to such causes as infection or drug toxicity, or idiopathic in nature.

Myocardium. The muscular middle layer of the heart wall; often used to refer to the entire tissue mass of the heart. The myocardium is the tissue whose perfusion is actually distinguished by ^{201}Tl imaging.

Myofibril. Contractile element of a muscle fiber; composed of thick and thin filaments.

Myograph. An apparatus for recording the effects of muscular contraction.

Myoneural junction. Synapse between a nerve fiber and a muscle fiber. Also called neuromuscular junction.

Myoscintigraphy. A radionuclide imaging technique based on a radiolabeled monoclonal antibody (MAb) specific to cardiac myosin. Because the MAb binds solely to the intracellular myosin that is exposed on cell death, offering a high concentration only in necrotic cells, it is possible to localize precisely unsalvageable myocardium following an infarction.

Myosin. A protein found in cardiac and skeletal muscle. It interacts with actin to form actomyosin, the constituent of muscle fiber responsible for muscle contraction and relaxation.

Myxedema. A condition due to hypothyroidism and characterized by dry skin, swelling face and limbs, loss of hair, sensitivity to cold, mental dullness, and reduced metabolic rate.

N

N. Symbol for neutron number, the number of neutrons in a given nucleus.

Nadir. The lowest point, or time of greatest depression.

Nand. Stands for NOT-AND. A logical operation that is the negative or reverse of AND. A NAND gate is an electrical circuit whose output in binary code is 0 only if all inputs are 1. This is the opposite of an AND gate, where the output is 1 only if all inputs are 1.

Naperian logarithmic system. Logarithmic system using the base e, which is a mathematical constant (e = 2.71)

Narcosis. A state of deep unconsciousness produced by drugs.

Narrow beam. In beam attenuation measurements, a beam in which only the unscattered and small-angle forward-scattered radiation reach the detector.

Narrow beam absorption. In problems concerning the absorption of ionizing radiation by matter, it is convenient to distinguish between the passage of a narrow, well-collimated beam (narrow beam absorption) and that of a broad, noncollimated one (broad beam absorption). This distinction is especially useful in the case of the absorption of γ rays, due to the complexity of the formula for Compton scattering. Narrow beam absorption is much simpler to treat mathematically, because nearly all scattered particles will be lost from the beam.

National Bureau of Standards. A radioactive source standardized and/or certified by the National Bureau of Standards.

National Electrical Manufacturers Association. (NEMA) The largest trade association in the U.S, for manufacturers of electrical products. Formed by merger of several groups of electrical manufacturers in 1926, it has company members nationwide, small and giant, producing component and end-use electrical equipment.

Natural abundance. Refers to the relative fractions of each different isotope of an element normally found in nature. For example, H constitutes the fraction 0.99985 and D (or heavy hydrogen) constitutes the fraction 0.00015 of the hydrogen atoms found in nature.

Natural antibody. Antibodies that occur naturally with or without known exposure to their respective antigens. Also called physiologic antibody.

Natural killer cell. A subset of lymphocytes of the null-cell group which can act selectively to kill malignant cells in the presence of normal cells.

Natural radioactive nuclides. Radioactivity exhibited by naturally occurring substances. Natural radioactive nuclides are classified as (1) primary, (2) secondary, (3) induced, and (4) extinct. Members of the first class have lifetimes exceeding several hundred million years, and which presumably have persisted from the earliest to the present time. They include the alpha emitters ^{238}U, ^{235}U, ^{232}Th, and ^{147}Sm and the beta emitters ^{40}K, ^{87}Rb, ^{138}La, ^{115}In, ^{176}Lu,and ^{157}Re. Members of the second class have geologically short lifetimes and are decay products of members of the first class. All known members of this class belong to the uranium or radium series, the actinium series, or the thorium series. Induced natural radionuclides are products of nuclear reactions occurring currently or recently in nature. A good example of this is ^{14}C produced by cosmic-ray neutrons in the atmosphere. Extinct natural radionuclides are those which have lifetimes that are too short for survival from nucleogenesis to the present, or long enough for persistence into early geological times with measurable effects. ^{129}I is a suspected member of this class.

Natural radioactivity. The property of radioactivity exhibited by more than 50 naturally occurring isotopes (natural radioactive nuclides). These natural radioactive materials give rise to a radiation background which subjects mankind to a continuous irradiation.

Natural uranium. Natural uranium contains both the heavier uranium isotope ^{238}U, which is a not readily fissile material and is the parent material from which plutonium is created, and the lighter isotope uranium, ^{235}U, which is the fission material or fuel of most reactors. In 140 parts of natural uranium, 139 parts are of ^{238}U and one part only is ^{235}U.

Near zone. This is the part of the ultrasound beam which is predominantly parallel before it begins to diverge in the far zone.

Nebulized drugs. Drugs administered to the patient in the form of a fine spray.

Necropsy. Examination of a body after death.

Necrosis. Death of tissue as a result of loss of blood supply usually as individual cells, groups of cells, or in small localized area, generally followed by sloughing of tissue; may leave fluid-filled cavity.

Needle biopsy. A frequently used procedure for the examination of suspected abnormal tissue. The procedure involves the introduction (under local anesthesia) of a fine sterile stainless steel needle into the suspected abnormality. Cells from the suspected lesion are aspirated and sent to the pathology laboratory for examination. This diagnostic approach is often necessary in the workup of patients who are to undergo surgery, radiation therapy, or chemotherapy and may be done on an outpatient basis.

Neel point. The temperature at which ferrimagnetic and antiferromagnetic materials become paramagnetic.

Negative electron. This is a negatively charged particle (charge $e = 1.6 \times 10^{19}$ C, mass $m = 9.11 \times 10^{-28}$ g) that forms a common constituent of all atoms. A synonym for electron, also called a negatron.

Negative feedback. Process by which a substance inhibits production of itself.

Negligence. (Legal) An unintentional tort that arises when a duty of care between two parties is breached by act or omission that is at odds with what a reasonable and prudent person would do. It is necessary to prove the injury, the act, and that the act caused the injury. The act was not intended to cause the injury, but the injury was forseeable, and the act entailed an unreasonable.risk.

Neoantigens. Nonself-antigens that arise spontaneously on cell surfaces, usually during neoplasia.

Neodymium. Element symbol Nd, atomic number 60, atomic weight 144.24.

Neon. Element symbol Ne, atomic number 10, atomic weight 20.1797.

Neoplasm. A new growth of cells which is more or less unrestrained and not governed by the usual limitations of normal growth. Benign: If there is some degree of growth restraint and no spread to distant parts. Malignant: It the growth invades the tissues of the host, spreads to distant parts, or both.

Neoplastic transformation and tumor progression theory. This theory holds that neoplastic transformation occurs as multistep mutations during a long latent period during which competitive inhibition by normal cells and associated mutants favors the dominance of successive mutants of the greatest malignant potential. Thus, progression to malignancy is a gradual step-like process on a widely varying time scale.

Nephelometry. The measurement of the cloudiness or turbidity of a medium containing a suspension of small particles.

Nephrology. Study of the kidney.

Nephron. The urine-forming unit situated in the cortex of the kidney, consisting of a filtering unit (glomerulus) and a long tubule specialized in various regions to reabsorb substances from the urine that passes through it.

Neptunium. Element symbol Np, atomic number 93, atomic weight 237.048.

Nerve. A cordlike structure that conveys impulses from one part of the body to another. A nerve consists of a bundle of sensory and/or motor nerve fibers either efferent of afferent or both.

Net magnetization vector. Vector representing the magnitude and direction of the magnetization resulting from a collection of nuclei. Also referred to as the macroscopic magnetic moment.

Network. A term used to indicate the linking together of computers and terminals for inter-computer communication and sometimes an extension of computer power.

Neural crest. In mammalian embryogenesis, the ridge of cells proliferating from the lateral margin of the medullary plate; they form the nerve cells of sensory and autonomic ganglia.

Neural modeling. A branch of cybernetics in which mathematical models, developed in conjunction with microelectrode studies, are used to describe the action of single neurons or networks of neurons.

Neurohormone. Hormone stimulating the mechanism of the nerves.

Neuron. A single nerve cell; composed of a nerve cell body, short dendrite projections, and a long axon.

Neuropeptides. Hormone-like substances that are secreted from neuroendocrine cells or from some neurons.

Neurotransmitters. Substances that are released from activated axons of neurons (and from some dendrites) and communicate across synapses with other neurons.

Neutral atom. An atom with a total positive nuclear charge equal to the total negative charge of the electrons surrounding the nucleus.

Neutralization. The process by which antibody or antibody in complement neutralizes the infectivity of microorganisms, particularly viruses. Chemical reaction in which an acid and a base react to form a salt and water.

Neutrino. A particle that has no mass or electrical charge, having energy, momentum, and spin, which is emitted in β-decay and electron capture. There is evidence for an antineutrino.

Neutron. Elementary nuclear particle with a mass approximately the same as that of a hydrogen atom and electrically neutral; its mass is 1.008986 mass units. Outside a nucleus a neutron is radioactive, decaying with a half-life of about 12 min to give a proton and an electron. Neutrons are commonly divided into sub-classifications according to their energies as follows: thermal, around 0.025 eV; epithermal,

0.1 to 100 eV; slow, less than 100 eV; intermediated, 102 to 105 eV; fast, greater than 0.1 MeV. Since it has no charge it does not ionize and therefore has no fixed range in matter. It travels in straight line until it is either scattered or absorbed by a nucleus. A neutron with very little kinetic energy can interact very strongly with a nucleus since it is not repelled electrostatically by the positive nuclear charge.

Neutron absorber. A material with which neutrons interact significantly by reactions, resulting in their disappearance as free particles; an object with which neutrons interact significantly or predominantly by reactions, resulting in their disappearance as free particles without production of other neutrons.

Neutron absorption cross section. The cross section for the neutron absorption process. It is the difference between the total cross section and the scattering cross section.

Neutron activation. When certain materials are bombarded with neutrons, the nuclear reactions which take place lead to the production of radioactive nuclei. These products are frequently, but not necessarily, isotopes of the original nuclei.

Neutron activation analysis. A method of elemental trace analysis of elements based on identification of neutron-irradiation products.

Neutron activation analysis *in vivo*. The feasibility of determining the elemental composition of a living person by neutron activation analysis *in vivo* was first perceived through measurements of radioactivity in the bodies of a few people who had been accidentally exposed to high-level neutron radiation. Extrapolation of these measurements to lower neutron doses indicated that accurate measurements of the content of the major elements in the body could be made at radiation dose levels of about 0.0001 Gy (0.1 rad). The first reported neutron irradiation of a living human for the purpose of determining the body content of certain elements was carried out in 1964. Since that time numerous methods and procedures have been developed, and these have become valuable tools in medical research and in the clinical diagnosis of disease.

Neutron age. A quantity which arises in neutron transport theory, in the calculation of spatial distributions of neutrons. In the age theory, or Fermi age mode, a neutron is assumed to be slowed down continuously as a result of elastic collisions with moderator atoms, and the age represents the time taken for the neutron to slow down from its initial velocity at creation to a given velocity.

Neutron attenuation. In traversing matter neutrons are scattered and absorbed and consequently the original intensity is progressively reduced. The falloff or attenuation of the neutrons of the original energy is exponential with distance.

Neutron binding energy. The energy required to separate one neutron from a nucleus.

Neutron capture therapy. A form of cancer therapy in which the tumor is selectively loaded with a nuclide of the high neutron capture cross section and is subsequently irradiated with thermal neutrons. These neutrons interact with the nuclide, giving rise to ionizing radiation within the tumor.

Neutron collimator. Neutrons from a source are normally emitted in all directions. To obtain a neutron beam it is therefore necessary to construct a collimator through which the beam can pass. In its simplest form the collimator would be a hole in a shield surrounding the source, the shield being of sufficient thickness to attenuate the neutron intensity to negligible value. Collimator design is, however, quite complicated, and careful attention must be paid to it in practical systems.

Neutron cross section. Usually applied to the total cross section for the interaction of neutrons with nuclei. Sometimes loosely applies to any type of neutron interaction.

Neutron cycle. In a reactor assembly of critical size, for each neutron absorbed there is a chain of processes which leads to exactly one neutron available for absorption in the next generation. Such a chain is called a neutron cycle.

Neutron density. The number of free neutrons per unit volume. Partial densities may be defined for neutrons characterized by such parameters as energy and direction.

Neutron diffusion. A phenomenon in which neutrons in a medium tend, through a process of successive scattering collisions, to migrate from regions of high concentration to regions of low concentration.

Neutron economy. The extent to which neutrons are used in desired ways instead of being lost by leakage or useless absorptions.

Neutron energy. The kinetic energy of a neutron, usually expressed in electron volt units.

Neutron energy group. One of a set of groups consisting of neutrons having energies within arbitrarily chosen intervals. Each group may be assigned effective values for the characteristics of the neutrons within the group.

Neutron excess. For all nuclei, except the very light, the number of neutrons is greater than the number or protons. The difference is called the neutron excess; it increases with atomic number.

Neutron flux. A term used to express the intensity of neutron radiation. The number of neutrons passing through a unit area in unit time. For neutrons of a given energy, the product of neutron density with speed.

Neutron generator. The term is usually applied to a low energy accelerator (e.g., a Cockcroft-Walton accelerator) when used for neutron production. The accelerator charged particle beam is allowed to impinge on a suitable target such that neutrons are produced in the nuclear reactions. A typical reaction is when a deuteron reacts with a tritium nucleus to form an α-particle and a neutron.

Neutron irradiation. Material under bombardment by neutrons undergoes neutron irradiation.

Neutron monitor. A neutron detector used to measure the neutron flux

Neutron number. (N) The number of neutrons in a nucleus, equal to the difference between the mass number and the atomic number for that nuclide. (N = A − Z) Isotopes of an element have the same atomic number but different neutron numbers.

Neutron or particle current density. A vector such that its component along the normal to a surface equals the net number of particles crossing that surface in the positive direction per unit area per unit time.

Neutron source. Natural or artificial radioactive elements supply us with convenient sources of α-particles and γ-rays, but neutrons can only be produced as a result of a nuclear reaction, i.e., by the bombardment of nuclei with simple nuclear particles or γ-rays. Neutron sources fall into two main classes, those in which the bombarding particles came from a radioactive source and those in which an accelerator is used to supply them.

Neutron spectrometer. This term is applied to many different instruments used to measure the energies of neutrons.

Neutron time of flight. The time T taken for a neutron to travel a given distance D. Expressed in microseconds.

$$T = \frac{0.0723D \ (m)}{\sqrt{E \ (MeV)}}$$

where E is the neutron energy.

Neutron upscattering. Any scattering collision

in which the scattered neutron gains kinetic energy. It is important only in the thermal energy range.

Neutron wavelength. The wavelength of the de Broglie waves associated with a neutron. For a neutron of momentum p, the wavelength is equal to h/p, where h is Plank's constant. A neutron of energy 0.0253 eV has a wavelength of 1.80×10^{-8} cm.

Neutrophil. White blood cell with three to five lobes connected by chromatin and cytoplasm containing fine granules.

Nickel. Element symbol Ni, atomic number 28, atomic weight 58.69.

Niobium. Element symbol Nb, atomic number 41, atomic weight 92.906.

Nitrogen. Element symbol N, atomic number 7, atomic weight 14.0067.

Nobelium. Element symbol No, atomic number 102, atomic weight ~259.

Noble gas. Any chemical element that has a completely filled valence-shell configuration in its neutral state — helium, neon, argon, krypton, xenon, and radon.

No carrier added. (NCA) A term used to characterize the state of a radioactive material to which no stable isotope of the compound has been added purposely.

Node. A small mass of tissue as a knot or protuberance, normal or pathological. One of the computers or terminals in a network.

Noise. Unwanted signals created within the electronic circuitry of the equipment. Everything within an image not part of the structures of interest. Noise can consist of the electronic, digitization, and X-ray quantum noise, undesirable changes in the voltage, current, or frequency of an electrical signal.

Nominal frequency. Each ultrasound transducer is quoted as having a nominal frequency. It is most efficient at predicting this frequency. In fact, other frequencies are also present so each transducer really produces a limited frequency spectrum with most of the energy being transmitted as the nominal frequency. Transducers can be activated at a frequency other than their nominal one, but they will be less efficient in converting the excitation signal to the desired frequency.

Nomogram. Process of graphically changing scales using a conversion scale.

Noncentral force. A force between two particles due to a potential which depends upon the direction of their spins relative to the line joining them. The most important are the tensor force and the spin-orbit coupling.

Nondestructive measurement. A measurement that requires no change in the physical or chemical form of the material on which it is carried out (e.g., γ-ray spectroscopy).

Nonfixed radioactive contamination. Means radioactive contamination that can be readily removed from a surface by wiping with an absorbent material. Nonfixed (removable) radioactive contamination is not significant if it does not exceed the specified limits.

Nonindependent samples. Samples whose values are correlated with each other because they represent measurements on the same or related individuals and hence are not independent.

Noninterlaced readout. A special video scanning method in which the video camera viewing the output phosphor of the image intensifier is scanned only once vertically from top to bottom.

Nonisotopic labeling. A nonisotopically labeled compound is a compound which has been labeled by a procedure more complex than simple substitution of a corresponding radioisotope; it often substitutes a convenient radioisotope of an element foreign to the compound.

Nonparametric test. A test which makes no assumption about the parameters of shape of the underlying population.

Nonpolar bond. Chemical bond in which a pair of electrons is equally shared by two nuclei.

Nonresponder. An animal unable to respond to an antigen, usually because of genetic factors.

Nonspecific binding. (NSB) That portion of the tracer used in a competitive binding assay (CBA) that is found in the bound fraction, independent of the binding reaction. An assay batch control tube made up without binding agent (antibody) and treated in the same way as other assay tubes. This should not be more than 5%; it may be caused by some reaction other than the immunologic one involved in the assay, such as sticking to the tube or trapping of labeled analyte radioimmunoasssay (RIA). Also expressed as minimum binding.

Nonuniformity. Variations in image intensity observed when flooding the gamma camera crystal with a point or uniform source of radiation. Differences in γ-ray detection efficiency are a minor cause. Variations are mostly due to image nonlinearity.

Nonvolatile. Retains information after power is removed. Examples are computer magnetic memories on tape and disk.

NOR. Short for NOT-OR. A logical operation that is the negative or reverse of OR. A NOR gate is an electronic circuit whose output in binary code is 0 if any of the inputs is 1. This is the opposite of an OR gate, where the output is 1 if any of the inputs is 1.

Noradrenaline. A hormone produced in the medulla of the adrenal glands. It functions as a vasoconstrictor, thus increasing blood pressure. A hormone-transmitter substance produced in the nerve endings of the sympathetic nervous system required for the production of most of the important effects of the sympathetic nervous system. Also called norepinephrine.

Normal distribution. A bell-shaped (Gaussian) distribution of two parameters, mu, μ (mean) and sigma, σ (standard deviation). Some properties: continuous, symmetrical, both tails extend to infinity; arithmetic mean, mode, and median are identical; characteristic areas depend on distance of x from μ (in σ units); and the distance from μ to the inflection point represents σ.

Normal incidence. Sound direction is perpendicular to media boundary.

Normality. (N) A unit of concentration of a solution. A 1-N solution contains 1 g equivalent weight of solution in 1000 ml of solution (Normal solution). One equivalent weight of a substance is defined by the weight of the substance that releases or reacts with one molecule of hydrogen or hydroxilion.

Normalized plateau slope. The figure of merit for a counter tube calculated as the percentage change in counting rate divided by the percentage change in voltage, using the threshold value as a base. The slope of the straight part of the plateau of a Geiger counter divided by the ratio of the counting rate to voltage at the Geiger threshold.

NOT. A logical operator with the condition that if statement X is true, then the statement NOT X is false. If X is false, then NOT X is true. A NOT gate is an electronic circuit whose output is 1 when its input is 0 and vice versa.

Notation of atomic and nuclear composition. The notation used to summarize atomic and nuclear composition is A/Z X_N, where X represents the chemical element to which the atomic belongs; A is the mass number of the nucleus, or the total number of protons in the nucleus (this determines also the number of orbital electrons in the electrically neutral atom and therefore the chemical element to which the atom belongs; and N is the neutron number, or the difference of A — Z. For example, an atom comprised of 6 protons, 8 neutrons (and thus 14 nucleons), and 6 orbital electrons represents

the element carbon and is symbolized by $^{14}/_{6}$C-8. Since all carbon atoms have atomic number (Z) 6, either "C" or the "6" is redundant, and the "6" can be omitted. The neutron number (N), 8, can be inferred from the difference 14 - 6 and also can be omitted. Therefore, a shortened but still complete notation for this atom is ^{14}C. Acceptable alternatives in terms of medical terminology are 14-C, or the complete work, carbon-14. The notations C^{14}, 14C, and C_{14} are obsolete and therefore not acceptable. Excited states are identified by an asterisk (*) and metastable states by the letter m (^{Am}X or X-Am) such as ^{99m}Tc, Tc-99m, or technetium-99m.

Nuclear angular momentum. The concept of angular momentum is applied to a particle (nucleus) or a system of particles (atoms, molecules) that spins about an axis (or behaves as though is does) as well as a particle or system of particles that revolves in orbit.

Nuclear battery. A device in which power is continuously derived from the emission of charged particles from a radionuclide. A potential is achieved by collection of the charged particles on a suitable grid or plate.

Nuclear binding energy. For a particle in a system, the net energy required to remove it from the system; for a system, the net energy required to decompose it into its constituent particles. Some of this represents the binding energy of orbital electrons, i.e., the energy required to strip the orbital electrons away from the nucleus: however, comparison of the total binding energy of a ^{12}C atom with the K-shell binding energy of carbon indicates that most of this energy is nuclear binding energy, i.e., energy required to separate the nucleons. When the mass of an atom is compared to the sum of the masses of its individual components (protons, neutrons, and electrons), it is always found to be less by some amount Δm. This mass deficiency, expressed in energy units, is called the binding energy E_B of the atom.

$$E_B = \Delta mc^2$$

For example, consider an atom of ^{12}C. This atom is comprised of six protons, six electrons, and six neutrons, and its mass is precisely 12.0 μ (by definition of the universal mass unit u). The sum of the masses of its components is

electrons 6 × 0.000549 u = 0.003294 u
protons 6 × 1.007277 u = 6.043662 u

neutrons 6 × 1.008665 u = 6.051990 u
(total) = 12.098946 u

Thus, Δm = 0.098946 u. Since 1 u = 931.5 meV, the binding energy of a ^{12}C atom is 0.098946 × 931.5 = 92.17 meV. Nuclear processes that result in the release of energy (e.g., γ-ray emission) always increase the binding energy of the nucleus. Thus, a nucleus emitting a 1-meV γ-ray would be found to weigh less (by the mass equivalent of 1 meV) after the γ-ray was emitted than before. In essence, mass is converted to energy in the process.

Nuclear chain reaction. A process in which one nuclear transformation sets up conditions which permit a similar nuclear transformation to take place in another atom. Thus, when fission occurs in uranium atoms. neutrons are released which in turn produce fission in neighboring uranium atoms.

Nuclear charge. The positive electric charge carried by a nucleus expressed in units of the electronic charge. The nuclear charge is caused entirely by the protons present in the nucleus. Therefore, a nucleus containing Z protons carries a charge Ze.

Nuclear constants. A particular nuclear species is characterized by its mass number A and charge Z. The state of lowest energy of any species is called the ground state. This state, and likewise the excited states above it, can be characterized by a few good quantum numbers, such as spin (total angular momentum) and parity, magnetic moment, etc. These constants have been measured for many nuclei, especially for the low energy neutrons, and tend to vary in a very irregular manner from one nucleus to another.

Nuclear disintegration. Any spontaneous transformation of a nucleus.

Nuclear emulsion. A photographic emulsion specially prepared for the detection of nuclear particles. Such emulsions are generally thicker and contain a higher concentration of silver halide than those used for standard photography. The emulsion is usually deposited on a glass plate and in this form the device is known as a nuclear track plate. The ionization caused by the passage of a charged particle through the emulsion affects individual silver halide grains along its path in such a way that upon development the track of the particle is clearly recorded as a row.

Nuclear energy. The nucleons in a nucleus are bound together by strong attractive forces so that the mass of the whole is less than the sum of the masses of the constituent particles. When nuclear matter is transformed into a more tightly bound form there is a a loss of mass, which is compensated by the emission of energy. This nuclear energy appears as kinetic energy of the particles and is ultimately degraded into thermal energy.

Nuclear fission. The generation of nuclear power is based upon the fundamental process of nuclear fission. Physically the term is applied to a particular type of nuclear reaction in which a heavy nucleus is split into two nuclei of medium weight, called fission fragment, which are usually radioactive. Several neutrons and γ-rays are also emitted in the process. Some elements are known to undergo fission spontaneously, but the rates are usually very low and the process occurs much more readily when the material is bombarded with nuclear particles or γ-rays. From the practical point of view, however, fission induced by neutrons is the most important.

In each nuclear fission a large amount of energy, about 200 MeV, is released and most of this appears as kinetic energy of the fission fragments. The remainder is shared between the emitted neutrons and γ-rays and the decay particles from the fission fragments. The great importance of fission, however, is not only due to the large energy which is released, but also to the fact that more than one neutron is emitted per fission. Hence, in the case of neutron-induced fission, a chain reaction can be initiated.

Nuclear forces. These are the strong short-range forces between nucleons that bind them together into nuclei.

Nuclear fuel. The most important fissile isotopes are ^{233}U, ^{235}U, and ^{239}Pu. Of these, only ^{235}U occurs in nature, the remainder being produced by neutron capture in fertile materials.

^{235}U occurs in natural uranium to the extent of approximately 0.7 wt %, fertile ^{238}U forming the great majority of the remainder. When fission occurs in the ^{235}U fuel the ^{238}U forms ^{239}U by neutron capture; this decays by β emission to give fissile ^{239}Pu. Initially, approximately four atoms of ^{239}Pu are produced for every five ^{235}U atoms destroyed. The ^{239}Pu is extracted by chemical separation of the irradiated natural uranium.

Nuclear fusion reaction. A reaction between two light nuclei resulting in the production of at least one nuclear species heavier than either initial nucleus, together with excess energy.

Nuclear induction. A technique for measuring nuclear magnetic moments, devised by Bloch. The nuclei are placed in a magnetic field which has a constant component in the z-direction, and an oscillating one in the x-direction. When the frequency of the oscillation approaches the Larmor frequency of the nucleus a field is induced in the y-direction. Measurement of the position of the maximum determines the Larmor frequency.

Nuclear isomers. Isotopes of elements having the same mass number and atomic number but differing in radioactive properties such as half-life period.

Nuclear magnet resonance (NMR). The resonant absorption of electromagnetic energy by a system of atomic nuclei situated in a magnetic field (H_0). The frequency ω_0 of the magnetic resonance is the same as the frequency of the Larmor precession of the nuclei in the magnetic field and is proportional to the strength of the field. Thus, $\omega_0 = \gamma H_0$, where γ is a characteristic constant, called the magnetogyric ratio, for a given nucleus.

Mobile protons in molecules can be aligned by a magnetic field. If an additional high-frequency magnetic field is applied in order to disturb this condition and is then removed, the protons return to their original state and emit signals while doing this. The strength of the signal is proportional to the local concentration of the mobile protons. These signals are then used, usually with some type of computer processing, to produce an image (MRI) or for identifying the spectrum of chemical substances.

Nuclear magnetic resonance absorption band. A quantitative measure of the relative intensities of the NMR signals, defined by the areas of the spectral lines. Electromagnetic signal in the radio-frequency range produced by the precession of the transverse magnetization induces a voltage in a coil, which is amplified and demodulated by the receiver; the signal may refer only to this induced voltage.

Nuclear magnetic resonance imaging. (NMRI or MRI) Creation of tomographc images of objects such as the body of the nuclear magnetic resonance phenomenon. The immediate practical application involves imaging the distribution of hydrogen nuclei (protons) in the body. The image brightness in a given region is usually dependent jointly on the spin density

and the relaxation times, with their relative importance determined by the particular imaging technique employed. Image brightness is also affected by motion such as blood flow. Also called zeugmatography, the name given to NMR imaging by Lauterbur.

Nuclear magnetic resonance absorption line. A single transition or a set of degenerate transitions is referred to as a line. A quantitative measure of the relative intensities of NMR signals, defined by the areas of the spectral lines.

The full width, expressed in hertz (Hz), of an observed NMR line at one half maximum height (FWHM).

Electromagnetic signal in the radio-frequency range produced by the precession of the transverse magnetization induces a voltage in a coil, which is amplified and demodulated by the receiver; the signal may refer only to this indued voltage.

The width of a single line in the spectrum which is known to be sharp, such as TMS or benzene. This definition includes sample factors as well as instrumental factors.

Nuclear magnetic resonance spectroscopy. (NMRS) A means of detecting species of atomic nuclei in a sample and identifying the compounds in which they are bound. The sample may be as simple in form as a solution in a test tube or as complex as the human body itself. The technique relies upon the stimulation and detection of resonance electromagnetic radiation in the radio-frequency range emitted characteristically by certain magnetically susceptible atomic nuclei. This occurs when a sample is placed in a strong magnetic field B_0 and excited by a pulse of electromagnetic energy B_1 of appropriate frequency. The resonance frequency of the emitted radiation is characteristic of the atomic nucleus and the nature of its immediate chemical environment; its exact value is proportional to the magnetic field, B_0. NMRS in contrast to nuclear magnetic resonance imaging (NMRI) depends upon the creation of a homogeneous magnetic field (B_0) throughout the entire volume of the sample. In NMRS, small shifts in resonance frequency are observed. These chemical shifts, as they are termed, are characteristic of molecular bonding patterns adjacent to the susceptible nucleus. They also yield other information; for example, they can indicate the presence of ion complexes. Not all atoms give rise to NMR signals. Those which do and are of biological importance include ^{1}H, ^{19}F, ^{31}P, and ^{13}C, listed in order of decreasing NMR sensitivity.

Nuclear magneton. The unit of nuclear magnetic moment, given by eh/4πmc, where e is the electronic charge, h is Planck's constant, m is the rest mass of a proton, and c is the speed of light. Its value is 5.05×10^{-24} erg/G i.e., about 1/1840 that of a Bohr magneton.

Nuclear medicine. "Nuclear medicine is taken to embrace all applications of radioactive materials in diagnosis or treatment or in medical research with the exception of the use of sealed radiation sources in radiotherapy" (World Health Organization Report, Series No. 492 of 1972). "Nuclear medicine is the clinical and laboratory medical specialty that employs for diagnosis, therapy, and research the nuclear properties of radioactive and stable nuclides to evaluate metabolic, physiologic, and pathologic conditions of the body" (American Board of Nuclear Medicine). "Nuclear medicine is devoted to the diagnosis, treatment, research, and prevention of disease by making use of unsealed radioactive sources and of the properties of stable radionuclides" (Council of Europe and the Society of Nuclear Medicine Europe). It is clear and significant from the above definitions that they all include: radioactivity, diagnosis, therapy, and research.

Nuclear membrane. The membrane that separates the nuclear material of a cell from the rest of the cell.

Nuclear Nonproliferation Treaty. A treaty with the aim of preventing the diversion of nuclear materials from peaceful uses to nuclear weapons and the proliferation of nuclear explosive devices. It came into force on March 5, 1970.

Nuclear poison. A substance which, because of its high neutron absorption cross section, can reduce reactivity. Frequently a fission product, e.g., xenon. The term is commonly called "poison".

Nuclear potential. Neutrons and protons inside a nucleus or close to it move under the influence of the nuclear forces according to the laws of quantum physics. Their equation of motion is some form of the Shrödinger wave equation and this equation always involves the potential energy of the particles as a function of their coordinates. For this reason, a knowledge of the potential energy of a nucleon (called the nuclear potential) both inside and outside the nucleus is very important. As the precise nature of the nuclear forces is not known, the form of the nuclear potential used in theoretical calculations must be adjusted so that the theory fits the experimental observations.

Nuclear power stations. The present and foreseen primary commercial (as distinct from military) application of nuclear reactors is restricted to the exploitation of the energy released in fission.

A critical mass is inevitably expensive so that the energy release, if the process is to be economic, must be at least some tens of megawatts per reactor. Although applications for the direct use of this amount of power in one place do exist — for example, to process heat in the chemical industry, and for propulsion units for ships — it is usually necessary to convert the energy into electricity so that it can be transported. The use of nuclear reactors to generate electricity thus is, and is likely to remain, their most important commercial application.

Nuclear radius. The somewhat ill-defined distance from the center of a nucleus at which the density of nuclear matter drops sharply.

Nuclear reaction. A process which occurs when two nuclear particles approach closely enough to be influenced by the mutual attractive nuclear force between them. Usually, but not necessarily, one of the pair is heavier and is situated in a target material which is bombarded by a beam of the lighter particles. The bombarding particles are either accelerated in a particle accelerator or are produced as a result of other nuclear reactions. In general, an interchange of energy and angular momentum takes place and, as a result of the collision, reaction products which may differ from the original pair are observed leaving the point of collision.

Nuclear reactor. A structure in which a self-sustaining fission chain reaction can be maintained and controlled. It usually contains a fuel, coolant, moderator, and control absorbers and is most often surrounded by a concrete biological shield to absorb neutron and γ-ray emission. A nuclear reactor produces large amounts of energy as well as high neutron fluxes by nuclear fission. Radioisotopes with an excess of neutrons, and thereby exhibiting β-decay, are principally produced by reactor irradiation.

Nuclear scattering. The change of direction of particles or photons as a result of interaction or collision with a nucleus.

Nuclear spin. Intrinsic property of certain nuclei which produces an associated characteristic angular momentum and magnetic moment.

Nuclear spin quantum number. Property of all

nuclei related to the largest measurable component of the nuclear angular momentum. Nonzero values of nuclear angular momentum are quantized (fixed) as integral or half-integral multiples of $(h/2\pi)$, where h is Planck's constant. The number of possible energy states for a given nucleus in a fixed magnetic field is equal to 21 + 1.

Nuclear stability. A nucleus is stable if it retains its identity for an indefinite period of time, when not subjected to any external influences (such as bombardment of nuclear particles). Unstable nuclei are those nuclei which decay into other nuclei, the rate of decay being proportional to the number of the original species present. The decay rate varies enormously with the species and the type of decay.

Nuclear stethoscope. A simple, inexpensive nonimaging system for the nuclear cardiologic evaluation of left ventricular function made up of a scintillation probe and a microprocessor. The output from a single collimated $NaI(T_1)$ crystal is interrogated by an integrated microprocessor. Gating is accomplished by electronic identification of the R-wave on a simultaneously performed EKG. The time activity curve is displayed in real time on a cathode ray tube. The device allows choice in the manner of data acquisition. In the first-pass mode radioactivity from a bolus injection passing through the heart is recorded in 100-ms intervals. The microprocessor calculates immediately H/A (height of the equilibrium count rate divided by the integrated count data under the ventricular curve during the first pass through the heart) and displays this result as the cardiac output and ratio. Determination of blood volume allows calculation of the cardiac output. Likewise, other indices of left ventricular function: stroke volume, diastolic volume, ejection rate, rapid filling rate may be obtained and expressed in absolute physiological units, i.e., ml, ml/s, both in beat-to-beat and gated equilibrium modes. Correct positioning of the detector probe in the precordial region is indispensable to obtain reliable information.

Nuclear synthesis. The fusion of light nuclei to form more complex nuclei with an attendant release of energy resulting from a conversion of matter. An example is the reaction which occurs in the sun whereby helium is synthesized by the results in an equivalent release of energy.

Nuclear transformation. The change of one nuclide into another nuclide through some nuclear event.

Nuclear transition. For a nuclide, a change from one quantized energy state to another. It may involve the transformation from one nuclide to a different nuclide, e.g., alpha or beta decay, or a change in nuclear energy level by the emission or absorption of a photon, an orbital electron, or electron pairs.

Nuclease. An enzyme responsible for the hydrolysis of nucleic acids.

Nucleic acid. A component of the cell nucleus, comprising a union between phosphoric acid, ribose, or desoxyribose and the four bases: adenine, guanine, cystosine, and tyrosine. Polymer of nucleotides (DNA and RNA).

Nucleolus. A small, dense body, rich in RNA, found within the nucleus of a cell.

Nucleon. A common term for a constituent particle of the nucleus. This term commonly applies to protons and neutrons.

Nucleonics. The practical applications of nuclear science and the techniques associated with these applications.

Nucleon number. The number of nucleons (protons and neutrons) which a nucleus contains.

Nucleotide. Compounds formed from a pentose sugar (ribose in ribonucleotides and deoxyribose in deoxyribonucleotides), phosphoric acid, and a nitrogen-containing base (usually purines or pyrimidines). They are the building blocks of nucleic acids.

Nucleus. The positively charged central portion of an atom comprising nearly all the atomic mass and consisting of protons and neutrons, except in hydrogen which consists of only one proton. It is about 10_{-12} cm in diameter. Only nuclei with an odd number of nucleons exhibit a net spin and therefore lend themselves to NMR spectroscopy. Also a mass of gray matter in the central nervous system. The nucleus of a cell refers to an ovoid or rounded body, containing chromosomes, lying within the cytoplasm.

Nuclide. The term nuclide indicates a species of atom having specified numbers of protons and neutrons in its nucleus. Nuclides of one and the same chemical element, i.e., nuclides with the same number of protons and differing only in the number of neutrons, are known as isotopes of the element concerned. Because of this, the term is often used erroneously as a synonym for "isotope". Isotopes are the various forms of a single element and therefore are a family of nuclides with the same number of protons.

Nuclides are distinguished by their atomic mass and number as well as by energy state. Nuclides are distinct nuclear species, isotopes are nuclides of the same element. In some nuclides various energy states of the nucleus with finite lifetimes are possible. These states are called isomers of the nuclide. Isomeric nuclides have the same number of protons and neutrons and differ only in their energy content and thus their lifetime. The nature of a nuclide is indicated unambiguously by the chemical symbol of the element and the number of nucleons (sum of the protons [Z] and neutrons [N] = A, mass number) shown as an upper index to the left of the element symbol (e.g., ^{12}C, ^{32}P). Additionally, the number of protons (Z atomic number) can be given as a lower index on the left. Isomers in an excited, metastable state are indicated by a right upper index "m" (e.g., ^{99m}Tc). Approximately 1250 different nuclides are recognized at present each being a distinct species of nucleus with its own characteristic nuclear properties. Of these, 280 are naturally occurring stable nuclides, while the remainder (radionuclides) undergo spontaneous radioactive decay with half-lives which vary from a fraction of a second to greater than 10^{12} years. The only radionuclides which occur in nature are those with half-lives of the order of the age of the earth (or greater), or which are constantly being generated by natural nuclear processes.

Nude mouse. A hairless mouse that congenitally lacks a thymus and has a marked deficiency of thymus-derived lymphocytes. (T-cell deficient.)

Null cells. Cells lacking the specific identifying surface markers for either T or B lymphocytes.

Null hypothesis. The claim that two mean values are so close that, except for random errors, they represent the same true mean. This is also the claim of insignificance of difference in a comparison. Another phrasing is that two or more samples chosen for observation actually come from the same population.

Null hypothesis curve. Theoretical sampling distribution under assumption of no true difference.

Null modem cable. A RS-232C cable in which certain pairs of wires are cross-connected. A null modem cable is used to connect a personal serial interface to most serial-interface printers.

Numeric keypad. A group of keys near the right side of a computer keyboard. These keys have two functions. They can be used to enter numbers, like the keyboard of a calculator. They can also be used to perform program functions such as positioning the cursor. In the latter case, they are often called "cursor control keys".

N-Unit. That quantity of neutron radiation measured in a Victoreen condenser r-meter that will produce the same amount of ionization as 1 C/kg of X radiation.

Nutation. A displacement of the axis of a spinning body away from the simple coneshaped figure which would be traced by the axis during precession. In the rotating frame of reference, the nutation caused by a radio-frequency (rf) pulse appears as a simple precession, although the motion if more complex in the stationary frame of reference. (NMR.)

Nyquist frequency. One half the pulse repetition frequency in pulsed/range gated Doppler. Frequency shifts exceeding this limit cannot be unambiguously displayed unless other information such as the time history of a narrow band flow spectrum is available. In nuclear medicine filtering, the highest possible frequency which may be faithfully displayed (0.5 cycles/pixel) is called the Nyquist frequency. If the source image has more variations than the Nyquist frequency, it will not be faithfully reproduced and some information will be lost.

Nystagmus. Involuntary, rapid movement of the eyes, consisting of a fast forward and a slow backward movement; enables the eyes to fix on an object while the head is moving.

O

Object code. The language output from a translation process. A computer program which has not yet been linked with the computer's libraries. Also called object program.

Object size correction. It has been shown for single photon emission computerized tomography (SPECT) that even after scatter and attenuation correction, the counts recovered from reconstructed tomograms are dependent on the object size for objects smaller than two resolution elements (full width at half maximum) in any of its three dimensions. This dependence limits the accuracy with which regional radionuclide distributions are derived from these objects. For example, in a T1-201 myocardial short axis slice, if the septal wall is significantly thicker than the lateral wall and the tracer is uniformly distributed, the septum in the image will appear hot, in relation to the lateral wall. This may confuse the clinician into interpreting that the patient has a perfusion defect in the lateral wall. Correction methods to date remain experimental and depend on either measuring or calculating a recovery coefficient as a function of object size. The object size is then independently estimated. Correction consists of multiplying the pixel value by the appropriate recovery coefficient.

Oblique incidence. That incidence which occurs if the sound direction is not perpendicular to the media boundary.

Obstetric ultrasound. In a pregnant woman ultrasound analysis of the size of the fetal skull is an excellent index to the determination of fetal age and with sequential studies can establish fetal growth rate. The location of the placenta in relation to the mother's uterus has been simplified with ultrasound.

Occipital. Referring to the back part of the head.

Occlusion Act of closure; area of closure; meeting of teeth in the jaws.

Occult. Hidden or concealed, or masked by other symptoms.

Occupancy factor. The factor by which the work load should be multiplied to correct for the degree or type of occupancy of the area in question. This factor may be based in general on the degree of occupancy averaged over a year.

Occupational exposure. The exposure which is incurred as the result of a person's work with radiation sources or radioactive materials.

Octal. Pertaining to the number system with a radix of 8. Octal numbers are frequently used as a "shorthand" representation from binary numbers, with each octal digit representing a group of 3 bits (binary digits): e.g., the binary numeral 110 101 010 can be represented as octal 652.

Odd-even nuclei. Nuclei containing an odd number of protons and an even number of neutrons. The mass number is therefore odd.

Odd-odd nuclei. Nuclei containing an odd number of protons and an odd number of neutrons. The mass number is therefore even.

Off-line. A method of computer working in which programs or data input to the system are stored until the computer is free to process them and return the results to an output store. Off-line devices cannot be controlled by a computer except through human intervention.

Ohm. (Unit of electrical resistance) The electrical resistance between two points of a conductor when a constant difference of potential of 1 V, applied between these two points, produces in this conductor a current of 1 A, this conductor not being the source of any electromotive force.

Oleic acid. (Octadecanoic acid) Straight-chained organic acid with the molecular formula $C_{18}H_{36}O_2$.

Oligoclonal bands. Immunoglobulins with restricted electrophoretic mobility in agarose gels found in cerebrospinal fluid of patients with multiple sclerosis and some other central nervous system diseases.

Oligomer. A term used to describe biological macromolecules made up of more than one identical unit or protomer.

Oncogenesis. The process of producing neoplasia or malignancy.

Oncology. The study of the causes, growth, characteristics, and treatment of tumors.

One-tailed test. The alternative to the null hypothesis is that A is smaller (or larger) than B. Therefore the probability of chance events as extreme or more extreme includes the area in only one tail.

On-line. Pertaining to equipment or devices that are ready for use in direct communication with the central processor of a computer system. On-line devices are usually under the direct control of the computer with which they are in communication. Opposite of off-line.

On-line carts. An input terminal which, although mobile, functions under the control of the central processor (CPU). That is, decisions as to what is done and what happens next are made by computer as a result of predetermined steps written into the program.

Ontogeny. The developmental history of an individual organism within a group of animals.

Open ended. Open-ended computer systems are designed to expand in anticipation of future growth. Items can be added to such systems without changing those parts already in existence.

Opening burst. A complex of peaks originating at the ultrasound transducer face due to internal reverberation and ringing of the crystal. On the A-mode scope this is represented by a complex of peaks on the left of the scope; on the B-scan these are seen as a series of lines.

Open water bath. A polythene water bag with an aperture in the membrane allowing direct contact between the water and the organ of interest. Commonly used for eye and breast ultrasound scanning.

Operating frequency. Preferred frequency of operation of a transducer.

Operating system. Collection of computer programs, including a monitor or executive and system programs, that organize a central processor and peripheral devices into a coordinated working unit for the development and execution of application programs, freeing application programs to do useful work.

Operating voltage. The voltage across the electrodes in the detecting chamber required for proper detection of an ionizing event.

Operation code. Code used to start the operation of a computer program. Instructions that supervise the steps followed by a computer.

Ophthalmoscope. An optical instrument for the examination of those parts of the eye (e.g., the retina) lying behind the crystalline lens.

Opportunist. An organism that is normally nonpathogenic but which invades and produces disease when defenses are lowered.

Opsonin. A substance capable of enhancing phagocytosis. Antibodies and complement are the two main opsonins.

Optical character recognition. A device for scanning and recognizing printed characters and transforming these into computer-readable form.

Optical depth. The thickness of an optical material multiplied by its refractive index.

Optimizing compiler. A compiler that attempts to correct inefficiencies in the logic of computer programs in order to improve execution times, internal memory requirements, etc.

Option. One selection on a menu. An element of a command or command string that enables the user to select alternatives associated with the command.

OR. A logical operation that produces results depending on the pieces of information acted on. In an OR operation, the result is 1 if one or more of the bits operated on is 1. An OR gate is an electronic circuit whose output is 1 if any of the inputs is 1.

Orbital. Energy sublevels occupied by electrons in an atom.

Orbital angular momentum. That part of the total angular momentum of a particle moving about a center which is analogous to the classical angular momentum of rotation, as opposed to intrinsic angular momentum. Its quantum numbers must be integral.

Orbital electron. An orbital electron is an electron in the extranuclear structure of the atom.

Orbital electron capture. A radioactive transformation in which the nucleus captures an orbital electron.

Orbital magnetic moment. Magnetic moment of a particle which is associated with its orbiting motion. This magnetic moment is in addition to the spin magnetic moment.

Orbital particle accelerator. An accelerator in which charged particles are made to move in an orbit by the use of a magnetic field. On each revolution the particles are accelerated by an electric or magnetic field.

Ordering. In a system of a large number of particles, the order, or organization, of the particles increases as the temperature decreases. As the randomness decreases, cooperative phenomena (such as ferromagnetism) appear.

Ordinary wave. Plane polarized electromagnetic radiation propagating with the wave vector perpendicular to an externally applied magnetic field B while the electric field of the wave is parallel to B. The index of refraction of an ordinary wave is not affected by the applied magnetic field.

Organ. Organized group of tissues having one or more definite functions to perform in an animal body.

Organelle. Any specialized structure of a cell having some individual function such as movement, reproduction, or metabolism.

Organic chemistry. Branch of chemistry dealing with the study of compounds of carbon.

Organic compounds. Any of the class of chemical compounds that contain carbon.

Organ scan. The pictorial record of radionulclide distribution in an organ.

Orientation. A suggested standard orientation for the presentation of tomographic diagnostic images is (1) transverse: patient's right on the left side of the image, anterior or ventral; (2) coronal: patient's right to left side of image, superior or head to the top; (3) sagittal: patient's head to the top, anterior to the left side of image. In displaying sagittal images, it is helpful to indicate whether a slice is to the left or right of the midline. The position of substituent atoms or groups in an organic molecule, especially in a benzene nucleus. Also applied to the directions of the axis of a crystal relative to its environment.

Orthopnea. Dyspnea where the respiratory distress becomes worse when the patient lies flat; patient must sleep propped up in bed, often associated with left heart failure.

Orthotomography. Tomographic system for recording an image by means of a narrow beam of X-rays substantially perpendicular to the objective plane.

Oscilloscope. This is an instrument containing a cathode ray tube (CRT) intended for viewing signals that vary with time. There are different types of oscilloscopes, but the most common format is a short-persistence CRT with amplifiers driving the vertical (Y) deflection plates and a time base driving the horizontal (X) deflection plates. The amplifiers usually have variable gain and sometimes filtering circuits; the time base allows the horizontal sweep of the spot to be made at different speeds. Other variations are to have a storage CRT or electronic storage circuits, X and Y drive amplifiers (i.e., no time base), differential amplifiers, special time base triggering circuits, etc.

Osmium. Element symbol Os, atomic number 76, atomic weight 190.2

Osmolarity. An expression of solute concentration which takes into account the number of osmotically active particles in the solution.

Osmoreceptor. Specialized sensory nerve ending that gives rise to sense of smell and is stimulated by changes in osmotic pressures of the surrounding medium.

Osmosis. The transport of a solvent through a semipermeable membrane under the action of a concentration gradient.

Osmotic pressure. Pressure developed when a solution and its solvent component are separated by a membrane permeable to the solvent only or when two solutions of different concentration of the same solute are similarly separated.

Osmotic-pressure effect. An enhancement in the velocity of the central ion, the direction of the applied external field, as a result of more collisions on the central ion from ions behind the central ion than from ions in front of it.

Osteoblast. Cell arising from a fibroblast that, as it matures, plays a role in the production of bone.

Osteoclast. Large multinuclear cell associated with destruction of bone.

Osteogenesis. Formation and development of bone taking place in connective tissue or in cartilage.

Osteon. Basic unit of structure of compact bone; haversian canal and its concentrically arranged lamellae (4 to 20, each 3 to 7 μm thick) in a single (haversian) system. Such units are directed mainly in the long axis of the bone.

Osteoporosis. Disease of the bone, occurring chiefly in older people, characterized by loss of calcium and supporting tissues and resulting in loss of bone strength density and mass.

Otoliths. Very small crystals of calcium carbonate found in the inner ear which are responsible for sensing gravitational forces and the body's orientation relative to them.

Ouchterlony double diffusion. An immunoprecipitation technique in which antigen and antibody are allowed to diffuse toward each other and form immune complexes in agar.

Outer bremsstrahlung. The radiation produced when a charged particle is accelerated in the coulomb field of a nucleus or atom other than that in which it originated.

Output. The result of a process. To transfer data from a computer to an external device or peripheral into a form readable by people or readable by other machines (output device). A measure of radiation quantity produced by a radiation therapy unit at a specified location. The radiation quantity is usually the exposure rate or absorbed dose rate at a calibration point under specified conditions.

Overall uncertainty. Overall uncertainty, often simply called the accuracy, is an estimate of the possible divergence of the quoted result from the true value. It must allow for the uncertainty attributable to statistical variations and for the total limits of uncertainty due to the assessable systematic error.

Overflow. A condition that occurs when a mathematical operation yields a result whose magnitude is larger than the hardware register is capable of handling.

Overlay. In a computer program, a segment that is not permanently maintained in the central processor memory. The technique of repeatedly using the same areas of internal storage during different stages of a program. In the execution of a computer program, to load a segment of the computer program in a storage area hitherto occupied by parts of the computer program that are not currently needed.

Overvoltage. For a Geiger-Müller tube, the difference between the operating voltage and the threshold voltage.

Oxalation. The conversion of a bridging OH^- group to a bridging O^{-2} group with the release of hydrogen ions. This process produces insoluble forms of chromium, tin, technetium, and other metal oxides.

Oxidation. Process by which a substance loses electrons in an oxidation-reduction reaction.

Oxidation potential. The potential established at an inert electrode dipping into a solution containing equimolecular amounts of an ion or molecule in two states of oxidation, measured with a reference to some arbitrary standard electrode such as the hydrogen electrode.

Oxidizing agent. Substance in an oxidation-reduction reaction that causes another substance to lose electrons.

Oximetry. The determination of the oxygen saturation of arterial blood.

Oxygen. Element symbol O, atomic number 8, atomic weight 15.999.

Oxygen consumption. The quantity of oxygen consumed or required by the body to function at any given time. The amount of oxygen required by a given activity is a method of estimating the intensity of the activity.

Oxygen debt. The extra oxygen that must be consumed after strenuous exercise to oxidize accumulated lactic acid and to resynthesize adenosine triphosphate (ATP).

Oxygen extraction ratio. (OER) Defined as the ratio of the net oxygen equivalent of substrate extracted by tissue assuming substrate is completely oxidized to CO_2 and H_2O to the net oxygen extraction by tissue.

Oxygen saturation. The relationship between the oxygen content and the oxygen capacity of the blood. If the blood has an oxygen capacity of 20 vol % and an oxygen content of 10 vol %, the blood is 50% saturated.

Oxyhemoglobin. A compound of oxygen and hemoglobin formed in the lungs - the means whereby oxygen is carried through the arteries to the body tissues.

P

Pacemaker. The mass of tissue that rhythmically initiates the heart beat. Normally, the sinoatrial node is the heart's pacemaker. However, other cells in the cardiac conduction system may initiate impulses and act as pacemaker. An implanted device which generates a series of rhythmic electrical discharges to maintain the natural rhythm of the heart when its natural pacemaker is not functioning normally.

Package. For radioactive materials, the packaging together with its radioactive contents as presented for transport.

Package monitor. An instrument for checking that the dose rate at the surface of packages containing radioactive materials does not exceed specified levels.

Package system. The purchaser buys as a package both the hardware and the software off the shelf, complete with a commercial licensing agreement and designed to do a particular application. In the case of the mass-produced microcomputer a standard package may consist of software only. Such a system is sometimes called a "turnkey" system, should it be designed so that the operator needs no computer expertise whatsoever, beyond that of entering in a "key" to turn on the system and following the instructions displayed on screen.

Packaging. For radioactive materials, the assembly of components necessary to ensure compliance with the packaging requirements of the subpart. It may consist of one or more receptacles, absorbent materials, spacing structures, thermal insulation, radiation shielding, and devices for cooling or absorbing mechanical shocks.

Packing fraction. The ratio $(M - A)/A = \Delta/A$. This is the difference between the atomic mass M and the mass number A divided by the mass number. It is positive for most nuclides of A < 6 and A > 175, and negative for others. The mass defect Δ is equal to M − A. The packing fraction is related to the binding energy and indicates nuclear stability. The smaller the packing fraction the more stable the nucleus. The value of the packing fraction is frequently multiplied by 10,000 so that it is expressed as a number approximating unity.

Page. A subdivision of a program. Paging enables a computer's main memory to process a large program in sections.

Paired data. A set of observations where for each x value there is a corresponding (or matched) y value.

Paired electrons. Two electrons with opposing spins forming part of a covalent or coordinate bond in a molecule.

Paired production. An absorption process for X and gamma radiation in which the incident photon is annihilated in the vicinity of the nucleus of the absorbing atom with subsequent production of an electron and positron pair. This reaction only occurs for incident photon energies exceeding 1.02 MeV. This is an example of direct conversion of energy into matter according to Einstein's equation: $E = mc^2$. It only occurs when a γ-ray passes close to a nucleus which appears to act as a catalyst for the process.

Pair production attenuation coefficient. The fractional decrease in the intensity of a beam of ionizing radiation due to pair production in a medium through which it passes.

Pair spectrometer. An instrument for determining the energy of γ-radiation by observing the sum of the kinetic energies of the electron and positron in the pairs produced by the γ-radiation.

Palladium. Element symbol Pd, atomic number 46, atomic weight 106.4

Palliative treatment. Limited treatment designed in general to improve the quality of the rest of the patient's life, but not a cure, i.e., to relieve symptoms such as pain, bleeding, or cough arising from primary or secondary tumoral growth.

Pancreas. Mixed endocrine and exocrine gland in abdominal area behind and below the stomach. Exocrine secretions are the digestive juices: endocrine secretions are insulin, glucagon, and somatostatin.

Paper chromatography. When two immiscible solvents are shaken together any solute will reach equilibrium between the two phases: the ratio

$$\text{conc}^n \text{ in A} / \text{conc}^n \text{ in B}$$

is a constant, the partition coefficient. One phase may now be held stationary by absorbing onto an inert column material such as silica gel, or onto paper. The other phase is either allowed to run down the paper by gravity or up by capillary action. In either case the ratio of the distance traveled by the solvent front past the initial spot of material, to the distance traveled by the material is the R_F value (relative flow value) and will be constant for the same substance under similar conditions.

Paper tape. A continuous thin paper medium, usually about an inch wide, on which data are recorded as round punched holes. Once created, the paper cannot be altered. In most applications, this medium for storing data has become obsolete.

Papilla. Small nipple-shaped projections.

Papillary muscles. Small bundles of muscles in the ventricular septum which are attached to the chordae tendineae. They contract when the tricuspid and mitral valves close.

Paracentesis. Surgical puncture of a cavity for the aspiration of fluid.

Parallel. In parallel operations, data are transmitted several bits (pieces of information) at a time. This contrasts with serial operation, in which data are transmitted 1 bit at a time. Parallel transmission is naturally faster than serial. But it is also more expensive because it requires additional circuitry to transmit multiple bits. In computers parallel operation transmits or processes a byte, word, record, or other unit of information composed of many bits as a single unit of data.

Parallel hole collimator. The parallel hole collimator is perhaps the most basic and important gamma camera collimator used in radionuclide imaging. It is essentially a disk of lead or heavy-metal alloy in which a number of parallel holes have been drilled or cast. The cross section of the holes can be square, hexagonal, or circular. Those γ-rays which enter the collimator parallel to the holes pass through and can interact with the detector, while those traveling in any other direction hit the walls and are absorbed. The distribution of scintillations in the crystal is therefore a parallel projection of the distribution of emissions of γ-rays from the object being imaged. The area of the holes, the wall thickness, and the length of the holes are carefully chosen to obtain the best compromise between spatial resolution and sensitivity. To maintain good sensitivity it is important to achieve a high packing ratio of channels per unit area of collimator, and in this respect the cross section of the channel should be hexagonal.

Paralysis. Loss of motor function in a part due to a lesion of the neural or muscular mechanism. The pseudotolerant condition in which an ongoing immune response is masked by the presence of overwhelming amounts of antigen.

Paralyzable effect. A situation in which each event requires a deadtime for detection and processing, during which time subsequent events are ignored but introduce their own deadtime (system is paralyzed). Important at high flux rates where many sequential events are ignored.

Paramagnetic. A substance with a small but positive magnetic susceptibility (magnetizability). The addition of a small amount of paramagnetic substance may greatly reduce the relaxation time of water. Typical paramagnetic substances usually possess an unpaired electron and include atoms or ions of transition elements, rare earth elements, some metals, and some molecules including molecular oxygen and free radicals. Paramagnetic substances are considered promising for use as contrast agents in NMR imaging.

Paramagnetic materials. Those within which an applied magnetic field is slightly increased by the alignment of electron orbits. The slight diamagnetic effect in materials having magnetic dipole moments is overshadowed by this paramagnetic alignment. As the temperature increases this paramagnetism disappears leaving only diamagnetism. The permeability of paramagnetic materials is slightly greater than that of empty space.

Paramagnetism. The property shown by many substances of becoming magnetized in the direction of the applied field, but not retaining this directional magnetization when the field is removed.

Parameter. Any set of constants entering into a theory or calculation to which varying numerical values may be assigned. An argument for calls, functions, subroutines, and utilities in computer programming.

Parametric radionuclide imaging. Functional or parametric imaging has been explored to display and interpret dynamic changes in radioactive distributions. Different aspects of cardiac function have been displayed using a variety of processing and display techniques which include images depicting stroke volume, ejection fraction, phase and amplitude analysis. Another area of interest which has received much attention is the deconvolution of the program.

Parametric test. A test which assumes that the underlying population has the parameters or shape of a particular distribution.

Paraplegia. Extensive loss of neural function, both sensory and motor, below level of lesion of spinal cord at or below level of first thoracic vertebra.

Parasympathetic nervous system. The part of the autonomic nervous system that responds to rest or increase in blood volume in such a way as to increase the membrane permeability of myocardial cells to potassium, resulting in decreased heart rate and cardiac output.

Parathormone. Hormone secreted by parathyroid glands and involved in calcium and phosphorus metabolism.

Parathyroid glands. Four small endocrine glands, on the lateral aspect of the lobes of the thyroid, that control calcium and phosphorus metabolism.

Paratope. An antibody combining site for epitope, the simplest form of an antigenic determinant.

Parenchyma. The essential elements of an organ pertaining to the function of the organ.

Parent. A radionuclide that upon disintegration yields a specified nuclide, the daughter, either directly or as a later member of a radioactive series.

Parent-daughter decay. Relationship between two radionuclides, the parent and its decay product, the daughter.

Parenteral. A term indicating the route of drug administration other than oral. Examples are intrathecal, intravenous, interstitial, and intramuscular.

Parent peak. The component of mass spectrum that is caused by the undissociated molecule in mass spectroscopy.

Paresthesia. An abnormal spontaneous sensation, such as burning or prickling.

Parity. A symmetry property of a spatial wave function. The parity is said to be even (or +) if the wave function is left unchanged by reversing the sign of all the coordinates, odd (or −) if the sign of the wave function is thereby changed. A binary digit appended to an array of binary digits to make the sum of all bits always odd or always even. It is used to check the validity of data.

Parotid gland. The largest of the salivary glands, situated below the ear.

Partial backup. A backup of selected files on a computer disk. A partial backup usually includes all files changed since the most recent full backup of the disk or all files changed since the most recent backup of any sort.

Partial decay constant. For radionuclide, the probability per unit time for the spontaneous radioactive decay of a nucleus by one of two or more possible modes of decay.

Partially relaxed Fourier transform. (PRFT) A set of multiline Fourier transform spectra obtained from an inversion-recovery sequence and designed to provide information on spin-lattice relaxation times. (NMR).

Partial pressure. The pressure exerted by a single component gas in a mixture of gases.

Partial pressure of oxygen in air. The pressure of the oxygen contained in air. Since air is about 21% oxygen, partial pressure is 21% of 760 mm of mercury, or 159 mmHg. That is, oxygen needs can be supplied by pure oxygen at 159 mmHg, which is equivalent to breathing air at 760 mmHg P_{O2} (at sea level).

Partial saturation. (PS) Excitation technique applying repeated radio-frequency (rf) pulses in times on the order of or shorter than T1. In NMR imaging systems, although it results in decreased signal amplitude, there is the possibility of generating images with increased contrast between regions with different relaxation times. It does not directly produce images of T1. The change in NMR signal from a region resulting from a change in the interpulse time, TR, can be used to calculate T1 for the region. Although partial saturation is also commonly referred to as saturation recovery, that term should be properly reserved for the particular case of partial saturation in which recovery after each excitation effectively takes place from true saturation.

Partial volume effect. An effect due to the ultrasound beam width whereby a cyst that is smaller than the beam width will be seen to contain echoes which are received from the surrounding tissue.

Partial wave. An incident beam or plane wave of particles may be regarded as a coherent superposition of a number of partial waves, each having a definite angular momentum. The concept is useful in scattering because a spherically symmetric scattering center will scatter each partial wave independently, as the total angular momentum is a good quantum number.

Partial width. A nuclear energy level, above the ground state, has a width proportional to the probability of the level decaying. The level may decay in several ways, in which case each transition has a certain probability of occurring. It is then possible to define a partial width which is proportional to the probability of a particular transition. The total width is equal to the sum of all the partial widths.

Particle. This term is employed as a synonym for elementary or fundamental particles. The elementary particles are defined as those particles which are told to be simple. They are either stable (e.g., neutrino, electron, positron, proton) or disintegrate spontaneously (e.g., meson, neutron, hyperon) into two or more particles, liberating an energy which is not small compared to the rest energy of the lightest of them. In some cases, elementary particles may or may not include photons.

Particle accelerator. A machine used to accelerate charged atomic particles to high velocities (Van de Graaff generator, cyclotron, synchrotron, betatron, linear accelerator).

Particle analyzer. A term often employed for particle or radiation spectrum analyzer which is an instrument for the measurement of the α, β, and γ-ray spectra. The most usual form of this apparatus is a particle or radiation detector (e.g., a scintillation counter) in association with a pulse-amplitude analyzer.

Particle fluence. The quotient dN/da, where dN is the number of particles which enter a sphere of cross-sectional area da.

Particle flux density. The quotient $d\phi/dt$ where $d\phi$ is the particle fluence in time dt.

Particle motion. Displacement, speed, velocity, and acceleration of a particle.

Particle velocity. The velocity of a volume element of a medium due to the passage of an acoustic wave.

Particulates. Particulates are solids dispersed in a gas stream as opposed to the liquid droplets, aerosols, or vapors which it may contain.

Partition. A part of a fixed computer disk that is devoted to disk storage for a particular operating system. Each partition is visible only to the operating system it is intended for.

Partition coefficient. Synonym for distribution ratio. The ratio of the equilibrium concentrations of a given solute between two immiscible solvents.

Partition sort. A rapid sorting technique used by the computer to divide a number of items into groups or subsets. A partition sort is faster and is much more efficient for sorting a large number of items.

Pascal. An educational computer language used to teach students about programming and the elements of computer science. Pascal is designed to encourage students to form good programming habits and it is fairly easy to learn.

Passive immunity. Immunity resulting from protective agents derived from extrinsic sources, e.g., maternal antibodies acquired in utero or injected antibodies.

Password. A secret code that gives access to a computer system. Each user has his or her own special password. Passwords prevent unauthorized people from using the system.

Patch. If a computer program contains an error or weakness, a small set of instructions known as a patch can be written in to correct the deficiency.

Pathogen. An organism that can invade tissues, organs, or systems and produce disease.

Pathology. The branch of medicine dealing with the nature of disease, especially with the structural and functional changes of cells caused by disease.

Pauli exclusion principle. Two electrons in the same atom cannot have the exact same set of quantum numbers.

Peak scatter factor. The tissue/air ratio at the point within an irradiated object along the beam axis at which the absorbed dose rate is a maximum.

Peak systolic pressure. The pressure (or tension) of blood within the arteries at the moment of end ventricular systole.

Pedicle. The stalk of an organ or mass; peduncle.

Pellet. Small pill; a granule.

Pelvis. The lower portion of the trunk of the body, bounded anteriorly and laterally by the two hip bones and posteriorly by the sacrum and coccyx, and anteriorly by the symphysis pubis.

Penetrating shower. A group of particles in the cosmic radiation which are observed to pass through a few centimeters of lead without appreciable deflection or multiplication.

Penetration. The depth an ultrasound beam will pass into a tissue before its echoes become too feeble to be detected by the receiving system. Penetration is inversely proportional to the frequency of the transducer. Passage of γ-rays through septa or other shielding components. This radiation, from other than the geometrically defined field of view, contributes to image degradation.

Peptic. Pertaining to pepsin or digestion; peptic ulcer of the stomach.

Peptide. A unit in the structure of proteins composed of two or more amino acids.

Peptide bond. The bond which links amino acids together to form proteins.

Peptide hormone. Hormones excreted by the pituitary, parathyroid, and pancreas.

Percentage forced expiratory volume. The forced expiratory volume expressed as percentage of the vital capacity: $100 \, FEV_t/VC$.

Percentiles. Values that divide a distribution of ordered data into 100 equal parts.

Percent trace binding. The amount of radioactivity bound by specific reactor substance in a solution containing the substance of interest, divided by the amount of radioactivity bound by the same amount of specific reactor substance in a solution where the substance of interest is undetectable, times 100. Mathematically:

$$100 \times \frac{\text{counts bound}}{\text{counts bound in absence of substance}}$$

often written as $\% \, B/B_0$

Perchlorate. Any chemical compound that contains the ClO_4 group.

Percutaneous. Performed through the skin, as by needle.

Perfusion. The passing of a fluid through the vessels of a specific organ; perfusion of the liver.

Perineum. The space between the anus and the scrotum; the pelvic floor and the associated structures occupying the pelvic outlet, bounded anteriorly by the pubic symphysis, laterally by the ischial tuberosities, and posteriorly by the coccyx.

Period. In wave motion phenomena, it is the time required to complete one cyclic motion, equalizing the reciprocal of frequency; element in a horizontal line on the periodic chart. In a nuclear reactor, in which the neutron flux is rising or falling exponentially, the time required for it to change by a factor of e (2.718). The constant asymptote to the reciprocal of the derivative of the natural logarithm of the reactor power. The reciprocal of the time derivative of the natural logarithm of the reactor power.

Periodic law. Elements, when arranged in the order of their atomic weights or atomic numbers, show regular variations in most of their physical and chemical properties.

Periodic table. An arrangement of chemical elements in order of increasing atomic number. Elements of similar properties are placed one under the other, yielding groups and families of elements. Within each group there is a gradation of chemical and physical properties, but in general a similarity of chemical behavior. From group to group, however, there is a progressive shift of chemical behavior from one end of the table to the other.

Periosteum. The fibrous membrane that forms the investing covering of the bones except at their articular surfaces.

Peripheral. Near the surface, distant; distal, opposite of proximal. Any device distinct from the central processor that can provide input or accept output from the computer, e.g., input and output devices, printer, plotter, disk units.

Peripheral blood. Blood that circulates in the vessels that are remote from the heart.

Peripheral resistance. Frictional resistance to the flow of blood, especially in the arterioles.

Peristalsis. A progressive wavelike movement that occurs involuntarily in hollow tubes of the body, especially the alimentary canal, by which the contents are moved forward. It is characteristic of tubes contracting and relaxing longitudinally and circular layers of smooth muscle fibers.

Peritoneoscopy. An endoscopic examination of the peritoneum through an incision in the abdominal wall.

Peritoneum. The serous membrane reflected over the viscera and lining the abdominal cavity.

Permanent magnet. A magnet whose magnetic

field originates from permanently magnetized material.

Permeability. (μ) Tendency of a substance to concentrate magnetic field $\mu = B/H$.

Permeable. Affording passage or penetration.

Permeate. To pass through the pores or interstices.

Permissible dose. The amount of radiation which may be received by an individual within a specified period with expectation of no significantly harmful result to himself.

Permutation. A selection of terms (objects) arranged in a specified order.

Personal dosimeter. An integrating dosimeter that is not direct-reading and from which the dose equivalent is determined after a fixed wearing period.

Personnel monitoring. Periodic or continuous determination of the amount of radiation or radioactive contamination present in or on an individual. Includes monitoring of the individual's breath, excretions, clothing, or body tissues.

Pertechnetate. ($^{99m}TcO_4$) The form in which ^{99m}Tc is obtained from commonly available generators; the technetium in this molecule may be reduced and made reactive to label a variety of other compounds.

Petechiae. Small pinpoints of red hemorrhagic spots in the skin.

pH. The unit of hydrogen ion concentration. It is given by the negative common logarithm of the hydrogen ion concentration in a solution: $pH = \log_{10}[H^+]$. It expresses the acidity or alkalinity of a solution, a pH of 7 being neutral. Acid <7; alkaline >7.

Phagocyte. A cell with the ability to ingest and destroy particulate substances, such as bacteria, protozoa, cells and cell debris, dust particles, and colloids. Phagocytosis, the engulfing of particles by cells.

Phagolysosome. A cellular organelle that is the product of the fusion of a phagosome and a lysosome.

Phagosome. A phogocytic vesicle bounded by inverted plasma membrane.

Phantom. Performance evaluation of radiotherapy apparatus may be conducted using a model known as a phantom, which has properties similar to human tissue. Water demonstrates similar absorbing properties to normal tissue, and a water-filled phantom may be constructed in which a radiation sensor (e.g., a small ionization chamber) may be moved to map the level of radiation at each point in the phantom.

In this way the distribution of radiotherapy dose can be calculated for real treatment situations. Phantoms are also used as teaching aids, to simulate real conditions with X-ray or ultrasonic machines. Such phantoms are also useful when setting up or calibrating imaging equipment. In nuclear medicine, phantoms are containers of radioactivity often made of perspex in the shape of an organ of flat drums used for making absolute activity measurements and control of instrumentation performance.

Pharmacokinetics. Study of the activity of drugs and medicines.

Pharmacology. Study of drugs and medicine.

Phase. If the peaks of the signal waves coincide (in position and in time), then the two are exactly in phase. If the peak of one coincides with the trough of the other, then the signals are exactly out of phase. Phase is the fractional part of a period through which the quantity has advanced from an arbitrary origin, the position relative to a particular segment of the cycle; angular difference between timing of two sine waves of the same frequency.

Phase angle. The phase difference of two periodically recurring phenomena of the same frequency, expressed in angular measure.

Phased array scanning. Moving-picture ultrasonic B-scanning can be produced by a variety of methods including rotating or rocking transducers, electronic switching of the transducer elements (linear array scanners), or by electronic steering of the ultrasound beam to produce a sector scan. Phased array scanners use a transducer with a small contact area with the skin (e.g., 1×3 cm) which can project and receive the ultrasound in a number of directions to produce a triangular image diverging from the point of contact. Inside the transducer the piezoelectric element (crystal) is divided into several parallel strips (typically 16) which are connected to the transmit pulse generator and to the receiving amplifier via a set of delay lines. If all the elements are subject to the same time delays on transmit and receive then the ultrasound beam is projected straight ahead and echoes are received from the same direction. If the left-hand end of the transducer is subject to less delay then the beam will be deflected toward the right. By progressively changing the time delay the beam may be switched or steered from the left to right and back again. The electronic control over the delay lines can be improved to effect focusing of the beam on transmit, and dynamic focusing (focal length changes with time) on receive. Such scanners are useful where the ultrasound beam must be transmitted through a small "window" to the tissue being studied. This is particularly useful in cardiology where the heart may be viewed through a space between the ribs.

Phase sensitive detector. A filter which allows only those signals modulated at a certain frequency to pass by comparing the phase of the signal with that of the modulated source.

Phenols. Organic compounds with the functional group OH⁻ attached to an aromatic ring.

Phenotype. Entire physical, biochemical, and physiological, as opposed to genetic, constitution of an individual.

pH meter. Device used to measure the pH of a solution based on the potential difference between the solution and a standard calomel electrode.

Phoneme. A quantum of sound with given frequency, timing, etc., characteristics that, when concatenated with other such quanta of different characteristics, can be used to generate a reasonable facsimile of human speech.

Phonocardiogram. A graphic display of the sounds generated by the heart and picked up by a microphone at the surface of the body. Frequency response required is 5 to 2000 Hz. Measured by special crystal transducer or microphone.

Phosphene. A subjective sensation of light due to nonluminous stimulation of the retina.

Phosphocreatine. An energy-rich compound found in muscle.

Phospholipid. A fatty substance important in membrane construction.

Phosphonates. Phosphate analogs with a P-C-P linkage replacing the P-O-P linkage; they may be labeled with ^{99m}Tc and serve as bone-imaging agents.

Phosphor. Chemical compound that upon photonic absorption will deexcite slowly by emitting light.

Phosphorescence. Emission of radiation by a substance as a result of previous absorption of radiation of shorter wavelength. In contrast to fluorescence, the emission may continue for a considerable time after cessation of the exciting irradiation.

Phosphorus. Element symbol P, atomic number 15, atomic weight 30.974.

Phosphorylation. Addition of phosphate to a molecule.

Photocathode. Negative electrode of a photomultiplier tube.

Photodiode. Device that converts light into electrical signals, used to sense visual information.

Photoeffect. This is the interaction of a photon with a nucleus, and the consequent emission of one or more nucleons. The process may also be referred to as photodisintegration or photonuclear reaction. The term photoeffect is sometimes used synonymously with photoelectric effect.

Photoelectric absorption. The absorption of gamma radiation as a result of the photoelectric effect.

Photoelectric effect. A process by which a photon ejects an electron from an atom. All the energy of the photon is absorbed in ejecting the electron and in imparting kinetic energy to it; a characteristic X-ray (or Auger electron) is subsequently produced when the vacated shell is filled by another orbital electron.

Photoelectric effect attenuation coefficient. That fractional decrease in the intensity of a beam of ionizing radiation due to photoelectric effect in a medium through which it is passing.

Photoelectric threshold. The quantum of energy hv_0 that is just sufficient to release an electron from a given system in the photoelectric effect. The corresponding frequency, v_0, and wavelength, γ_0, are the threshold frequency and wavelength, respectively. For example, in the surface photoelectric effect, the threshold hv_0 for a particular surface is the energy of a photon which, when incident on the surface, causes the electron to emerge with zero kinetic energy.

Photoelectron. The electron ejected in the photoelectric effect. Electrons ejected from the photocathode surface of the photomultiplier tube when struck by the light photons from the NaI crystal.

Photofission. Nuclear fission induced by γ-rays. In the case of the heaviest nuclei the γ-quantum may induce the nucleus to break into two nearly equal parts.

Photofluorography. The process of combining X-ray and photographic apparatus for the purpose of producing miniature films, as of the chest.

Photofraction. The fraction of detected γ-rays that produce output signals in the photopeak region.

Photogrammetry. The process of obtaining accurate and precise measurements from conventional photographs taken under strictly controlled conditions.

Photographic dosimetry. The determination of

the accumulative radiation dosage by use of photographic film.

Photoluminescence. Refers to fluorescence of phosphorescence shown by certain substances when excited by light. The emitted light is normally of longer wavelength than the exciting light. Many organic compounds show this effect, which is also shown by uranium compounds, molybdates, tungstates, rare earths, zinc sulfide, cadmium sulfide, etc.

Photomeson. A meson produced by the interaction of very high energy γ-rays with nucleons.

Photometer. An instrument for the measurement of light, usually the luminous flux or the luminous intensity. It is mainly used for comparing two sources.

Photomultiplication. Multiplication of the signal given off by the interaction of a photon in a scintillation detector.

Photomultiplier tube. (PMT) Photomultiplier tubes produce electric currents which are proportional to light intensity, and can detect extremely low levels of light. An important use is in scintillation counters. In this application they detect the flashes of light occurring in a scintillation crystal due to ionizing radiation. These flashes cause the release of one or more electrons at the tube cathode and these are drawn toward the next electrode (dynode) by a high positive voltage. When these electrons strike the dynode more electrons are displaced by "secondary emission" and they are attracted to the next dynode, and so on. By the time this sequence has been repeated several times the number of electrons is large enough to be measured. The construction of a photomultiplier tube is a series of curved dynodes (sometimes called venetian blind construction) in an evacuated glass envelope. They require a very stable high voltage supply since the output pulse height is dependent on the energy of the original radiation and on the voltage applied to the tube.

Photon. A quantum of electromagnetic energy having no charge and characterized by its wavelength or frequency. Its energy content is the product of its frequency and Plank's constant, the equation for which is E = hv.

Photoneutron. A neutron ejected from a nucleus by a (γ, n) reaction, i.e., by a photonuclear reaction.

Photo propulsion. Use of the directional emission of photons for propulsion. The "exhaust" velocity is the velocity of light.

Photonuclear reaction. When an energetic γ-quantum interacts with a nucleus it is either scattered by the nucleus or a photonuclear reaction takes place. If the effect of the γ-quantum is to cause the nucleus to break up, this is referred to as photodisintegration. Frequently the effect of the γ-quantum is to cause the nucleus to emit one or more neutrons or protons (photoneutron, photoproton).

Photopeak. The energy of the predominant gamma spectrum released during decay of the radionuclide as measured by a scintillation detector. (^{99m}Tc = 140 keV)

Photopigment. A photolabile pigment, the structure of which changes on absorption of light.

Photoproton. A proton released from a nucleus by a photonuclear reaction.

Photo scan. A display on X-ray film of variable density dots in a manner that reproduces the spatial distribution of radioactivity in the area desired to be visualized as produced by a rectilinear scanner.

Phylogenetic. Referring to the development history of an organism or race.

Physical half-life. ($T_{1/2}$, T_p) The amount of time required for a radionuclide to reduce its radioactivity to one half of its original value.

Physical quantities. Quantities are characterized as fundamental or derived. A fundamental quantity is one that "stands alone", i.e., no reference is made to other quantities for its definition. Usually, fundamental quantities ant their units are defined with reference to standards kept at national or international laboratories. Time, distance, and mass are examples of fundamental quantities (units: second, meter, and kilogram). Derived quantities are defined in terms of combinations of fundamental quantities. Energy is an example of a derived quantity; its unit (the joule) is equal to kg^2/s^2.

Physical tracer. A foreign substance attached by purely physical means to a given substance in order to determine the subsequent distribution or location of the latter.

Physiology. The science of the function of living organisms and its parts; physio — pertaining to life.

Pia mater. The innermost of the three membranes (meninges) of the brain and spinal cord.

Piezoelectric effect. The property, exhibited by all asymmetrical crystals, of generating electrical potentials when mechanically stressed. Conversely, these crystals generate mechanical strains when electrically stressed. This effect is the basis of electromechanical transduction of energy in transducers.

Piezoelectricity. Piezoelectricity is the physical phenomenon by which the sound waves used in medical imaging are generated. "Piézein" is a Greek word meaning "to squeeze". Piezoelectricity is only possible in materials, usually crystals or composites of crystals that are anisotropic, with properties that are different in different directions. When a voltage is applied to a piezoelectric element, it will either expand or compress, according to the polarity of the voltage. If the element is in contact with material, a sound waves will be generated. Conversely, when the element is mechanically compressed or expanded, as when a sound wave strikes it, a voltage will be produced. The same element can therefore generate and receive sound waves. Some naturally occurring piezoelectric materials used to generate sound are quartz, lithium sulfate, and Rochelle salt. Although quartz is often still used above 20 MHz, most piezoelectric elements used for medical diagnosis (1- to 10-MHz frequencies) are synthetic ceramics.

Pig. A container used to store or ship radioactive substances usually made of lead.

Pile. Obsolete term for nuclear reactor.

Pi-meson. An unstable elementary particle which can be either charged or neutral. The positively and negatively charged mesons have a mass equal to 273 electron masses, m, and decay into mumeson and neutrino with a mean life of 2.5×10^{-8} s. The neutral π-meson has a mass of 264 m and decays into two γ-rays with a mean life of about 10^{-15} s. Synonym of pion.

Pinch effect. The effect of the associated magnetic field on the ions and electrons carrying an electric current in a plasma. The current channel is constricted (or pinched in) towards its central axis. The effect also causes heating of the plasma.

Pin-feed paper. Paper with a row of sprocket holes along each edge. Also called "continuous forms". It is usually sold in cartons of several thousand sheets, with the sheets joined end to end in a continuous folded strip.

Pinhole collimator. This collimator has a small circular aperture at the end of a conical lead shield and it projects an inverted image of the distribution of activity on the detector. The field of view in this case can be varied by changing the distance between the area to be scanned and the collimator hole. Geometric efficiency increases with increases in the area of the hole, whereas resolution decreases. As the image is a conical projection of the distribution of activity viewed, the magnification, the spatial resolution, and the geometric efficiency all vary markedly with the distance between the radiation source and the collimator.

Pinocytosis. The intake of fluid droplets or small particulates within fluid droplets by cells in which small invaginations of the cell membrane pinch off and become internalized as cytoplasmic vesicles.

Pipelining. A scheme which chains multiple processing steps to improve a computer system throughput. Like an assembly line, all operations performed are conducted simultaneously.

Pipet. (Or pipette) Device used to deliver a precise amount of a liquid; the act of using such a device.

Pitchblende. A rich uranium ore, consisting largely of uranium oxide.

Pituitary gland. An endocrine gland lying below the hypothalamus of the brain and divided into two lobes, anterior and posterior, separated by a cleft. It secretes hormones affecting skeletal growth, the development of the sex glands, and the functioning of the other endocrine glands.

Pixel. Acronym for a picture element; the smallest discrete part of a digital image display. Digital images are composed of a grid of picture elements (pixels). Each pixel is characterized by its position in the grid and by the density or color it will display.

Placebo. A pharmacologically inert substance which is administered either to satisfy a patient's wish for medication or for use in clinical trials as a reference material.

Placebo effect. Even in patients with typical symptoms a definite, if less pronounced, effect can be produced by administration of a placebo. This phenomenon has been observed in all placebo-controlled studies.

Placenta. The complex structure joining the umbilical cord of the fetus to the walls of the uterus. The respiratory, excretory, and nutritional functions of the uterus are carried out through this structure.

Placental barrier. Term used to describe the semipermeable barrier interposed between the maternal and fetal blood by the placental membrane.

Planar imaging. Imaging technique in which image of a plane is built up from signals received from the whole plane.

Planar spin imaging. One particular technique of planar imaging that creates an NMR image of a plane from one excitation sequence by selectively exciting a grid of points within the plane and then applying a gradient magnetic field so that each point has a different Larmor frequency. Fourier transformation of the FID can then be used to separate the signals from each selected point and create the image.

Planck's constant. (h) A universal constant of nature which relates the energy of a quantum of radiation to the frequency of the oscillator which emitted it. It has the dimensions of action (energy × time). Expressed by $E = h\nu$, where E is the energy of the quantum and ν is its frequency. Its numerical value is $6.626176(36) \times 10^{-27}$ erg s.

Planes of the body. The median of sagittal plane passes longitudinally through the body from front to back and divides it into right and left halves; the transverse plane passes horizontally through the body at right angles to the median plane and divides the body into upper and lower portions; the coronal or frontal plane passes longitudinally through the body from side to side, at right angles to the median plane, and divides the body into front and back parts.

Planimetry. The measurement of level surfaces; plane geometry.

Plaque. Any patch or flat area.

Plasma. A plasma is a sample of ionized gas which behaves in its interaction with external forces as a body and not as a system of individual particles. In this sense it is similar to a fluid. This definition requires that the linear dimensions of the plasma are greater than the distance over which interparticle forces act. These forces are coulomb forces and therefore are infinite in range. Pale-yellow fluid component of blood, containing proteins and mineral salts in which the blood cells are suspended.

Plasma cells. Fully differentiated antibody-synthesizing cells that are derived from B lymphocytes.

Plasma membrane. The membrane enclosing the cytoplasm of a cell, through which nutrients enter the cell and waste products leave. Also known as the cell membrane.

Plateau. The plot of counting rate against voltage applied to a Geiger counter in the presence of a constant source of radiation. As the voltage is increased from zero, this counting rate first rises sharply to a plateau several hundred volts long. Over the plateau the counting rate rises very slowly, and at the end it increases rapidly as instability sets in.

Platelet. A minute, irregularly disk-shaped structure found in circulating blood that assists in blood clotting. Also called thrombocytes.

Platinum. Element symbol Pt, atomic number 78, atomic weight 195.08.

Pleomorphic. Widely different forms of the same species.

Pleura. The serous membrane investing the lungs and lining the thoracic cavity, completely enclosing a potential space known as the pleural cavity.

Plexus. A term for a network where nerves or blood vessels are interwoven together.

Plica. A general term for a ridge or fold.

Plotter. Automatic output device for drawing graphs and other images on paper. The graphs are produced by moving a pen according to coordinates supplied by a computer.

Plume. The stream of gas, warm air, or smoke leaving a stack or chimney.

Plural scattering. Scattering of a particle of a photon in which the final deflection is the vector sum of a small number of displacements.

Plutonium. Element symbol Pu, atomic number 94, atomic weight ~244.

Pneumotachograph. An instrument which measures the volume of pulmonary ventilation during respiration.

Pocket dosimeter. A small ionization chamber, having a physical appearance similar to a fountain pen, used to monitor the amount of radiation to which an individual is exposed.

Pointer. A word or number that indicates an address or location in a computer memory.

Point scanned radiography. A radiographic system in which the image is created by scanning a microbeam of X-rays over the patient.

Point scanning. A type of NMR imaging method in which information is interrogated one point at a time. A complete image is obtained by sequentially scanning throughout the sample. (Also called "sensitive point" imaging.)

Poiseuille equation. For liquid flow in a capillary, $V = \pi r^4 p / 8\eta l$, where V is the volume of liquid flowing per second through a capillary of length l and radius r under the influence of pressure difference p, and η is the coefficient of viscosity.

Poisson distribution. If random discrete events occur over a long period of time, then the relative frequency or probability of a particular number of events N happening in a given short interval is given by the Poisson distribution, viz., $P(N) = a^N e^{-a} / N!$, where a is the most probable value. The standard deviation is $N^{1/2}$. For large positive values of N and a, the Poisson and Gaussian distribution refers to the random fluctuations that, e.g., an item of equipment introduces into measurement due to imperfections in performance, some measurements in the physical sense are inherently random. Radioactivity is one such phenomenon in which either an event occurs or it does not. Therefore, there is a bias in the distribution that does not allow negative values and as a consequence, the distribution is not symmetrical. This type of distribution is known as the Poisson distribution and is relatively complex. However, the distribution can be completely described in terms of a single parameter (N). It is usual to let this parameter increase such that the Poisson distribution becomes more symmetrical and approaches a Gaussian form.

Poisson noise. One of the primary reasons for applying low-pass (smoothing) filters is to reduce the high-frequency random noise associated with Poisson noise (statistical count fluctuations). The Hann filter appears to be better suited for studies where higher statistical accuracy is needed at the expense of a loss in spatial resolution. (SPECT.)

Polar covalent bond. Covalent bond formed by the unequal sharing of a pair of electrons between two atoms.

Polarity. Direction of electrical flow, positive or negative.

Polarization. Recovery of potential difference across cell membrane.

Polling. The process whereby a computer indicates to a terminal that holds data that the terminal can transmit its data to the computer.

Polonium. Element symbol Po, atomic number 84, atomic weight ~209.

Polyatomic ion. Ion composed of more than one atom.

Polyclonal antibodies. Antibodies directed to multiple epitopes on the surface of the same antigens.

Polyclonal B-cell activators. (PBAs) Substances that indiscriminately activate a large population of virgin B cells for antibody production.

Polyclonal mitogens. Mitogens that activate large subpopulations of lymphocytes.

Polyclonal proteins. A group of molecules derived from multiple clones of cells.

Polyclonal T-cell activators. (PTAs) Substances that indiscriminately activate a large population of TE-cell precursors.

Polymer. Compound formed of simpler molecules usually of high molecular weight. Immunoglobulins composed of more than a single basic monomeric unit, e.g., an IgA dimer consists of two units.

Polymorphonuclear neutrophil. A highly motile phagocyte of the granulocytic series of white blood cells characterized by fine neutrophilic cytoplasmic granules.

Polypeptide. Compound containing two or more amino acids linked by a peptide bond.

Polyphosphate. Any molecule containing the $(PO_3)_n$ group. Labeled with ^{99m}Tc it is used for bone scintigraphy.

Polyribosome. A group of ribosomes held together by a strand of messenger RNA.

Polysaccharides. A group of complex carbohydrates which contain five or more monosaccharide residues. Important examples include starch, cellulose, and glycogen.

Pons. Slip of tissue connecting two parts of an organ; a bridge; part of the base of the brain.

Pooled variance. Estimate of the population variance (σ^2) obtained by pooling the sample variance estimates (s^2). Each s^2 value is weighted by the $n-1$ terms which enter into its calculation.

Pool reactor. A reactor whose fuel elements are immersed in a pool of water which serves as moderator, coolant, and biological shield. (Also called "swimming pool reactor".)

Population. The entire group about which information is desired.

Population center distance. The distance from a power or testing reactor to the nearest boundary of a densely populated center containing more than 25,000 residents.

Port. Access or connection to a device, frequently memory. There is usually only one port of each device; however, when access from multiple components is required, more than one port to the device can improve the speed of access.

Porta hepatis. Part of the liver receiving the major blood vessels.

Positive rays. A stream of positive ions or particles produced in a potential gradient by ionizing agents.

Positron. A transitory nuclear particle similar to the electron, but positively charged. The rest masses of the electron and positron are equal, and their electric charges are equal in magnitude but opposite in sign.

Positron decay. Accelerator-produced radionuclides have an excess of protons and achieve stability by the conversion of a proton to a neutron. A positron (e^+) and a neutrino v are emitted during the process, i.e.,

$$p \rightarrow n + e^+ + v$$

As in beta decay the positrons have a range of energies up to a maximum energy, the balance at energies below the maximum being imparted to the neutrino. An example of positron decay is the decay of ^{11}C:

$$11/6C \rightarrow 11/5B + e^+ + \nu$$

The positron loses its energy by excitation and ionization interactions along its path. When its energy is dissipated, it is annihilated by combination with an electron. The mass of the two particles is converted to electromagnetic radiation and two photons (annihilation radiation) are produced:

$$e^+ + e^- \rightarrow 2\gamma$$

The photons each have an energy of 0.51 MeV and travel in diametrically opposite directions (to conserve the zero momentum of the system).

Positron emission tomography. (PET) A non-invasive, investigative procedure used in clinical research for the study of regional tissue physiology and biochemistry and pharmacology. It is based on the *in vivo* detection and imaging of positron-emitting radioisotopes that are introduced as tracer elements into the physiological systems of interest. A positron is a positively charged but otherwise "beta-like" particle which travels, in tissue, no more than a few millimeters from its source atomic nucleus. Within this distance it is captured by an electron, whereupon both particles are annihilated. Two photons, each of 511 keV energy, are emitted which leave the point of capture in approximately opposite directions. It is these simultaneously emitted γ-rays that make PET feasible, the γ radiation being detected outside the body by suitably mounted radioactivity counter. The use of positron emitters is the only means of labeling a biomolecule with a γ-ray emitting isotopes of one of its natural, constituent elements; this is an important consideration because the tracer tag should not perturb the behavior of the molecule. Suitable radioisotopes of oxygen, nitrogen, and carbon are ^{15}O ($t_{1/2}$ = 2.1 min), ^{13}N ($t_{1/2}$ = 10 min), and ^{11}C ($t_{1/2}$ = 20.1 min), respectively. There is no suitable γ-ray emitting radioactive form of hydrogen. However, the positron emitter ^{18}F ($t_{1/2}$ = 110 min) can be substituted for hydrogen in certain circumstances.

Positronium. A system consisting of a positron and an electron in which the positron is bound

to the otherwise free electron. Except for the effect of the lower mass of the positron the system behaves exactly like a hydrogen atom. It has a mean life of about 10^{-7} s. It is destroyed by electron-positron annihilation.

Postcapillary venules. Specialized blood vessels line with cuboid ephthelium located in paracortical region of lymph nodes through which lymphocytes traverse.

Posterior. Toward the rear or back.

Potassium. Element symbol K (kalium), atomic number 19, atomic weight 39.0983.

Potassium-40. A radioactive isotope which emits a beta particle and γ-rays. It has a half-life of 1.3×10^9 years. Since the naturally occurring radioactive isotope of potassium, ^{40}K, is present in quantities capable of precise measurement, and since the isotopic composition of potassium throughout nature is the same irrespective of its source, the total-body content of potassium can be calculated.

Potential difference. Work required to carry a unit positive charge from one point to another.

Potential energy. Energy of a particle by virtue of its position, e.g., orientation within a magnetic field.

Potential gradient. The rate of change of potential with distance. Unit = V/cm.

Potential scattering. The scattering of a particle, especially a neutron, by a nucleus due to the mean potential of the nucleus, as opposed to resonance scattering due to compound nucleus formation. It provides the background of scattering between resonance peaks.

Potential well. A simple model of the interaction between two particles or between a nucleon and a nucleus etc., described by an attractive potential with a short range. If the potential is sufficiently strong, bound states will exist. A simple model of the nucleus is provided by a deep well in which there are many bound states, which are occupied by the nucleons in accordance with the exclusion principle.

Potentiometer. A variable resistor for control of current or voltage.

Power. The rate at which work is done or the rate at which energy is transferred. It is equal to the work done divided by the time required to do the work. It is also equal to energy transferred divided by the time required to transfer the energy.

$$\text{power (W)} = \frac{\text{work (J)}}{\text{time (s)}} = \frac{\text{energy (J)}}{\text{time (s)}}$$

The quantity of energy flow per unit time, expressed in joules per second.

Power breeder. A nuclear reactor designed to produce both useful power and fuel.

Power conditioner. A device that protects a computer and peripherals from certain types of electrical damage by filtering the line power that runs them.

Power-on diagnostics. Checkout procedures that the personal computer (PC) runs automatically when it is turned on. These checkout procedures verify that all the PC's hardware is functioning properly. If the diagnostics detect problems, the PC displays error codes before for (or instead of) booting the disk operating system (DOS). The error codes can help a service person determine what is wrong with a PC.

Power output in Doppler mode. Power output in Doppler mode, as defined in the American Institute of Ultrasound in Medicine and national Electrical Manufacturers Association Standards may be defined as a spatial peak intensity averaged over time.

Power reactor. A reactor capable of providing useful mechanical power. In reactors planned at the present time, this is done by generating energy in the form of heat conveyed at a temperature high enough for reasonably efficient conversion to mechanical work.

Praesodymium. Element symbol Pr. atomic number 59, atomic weight 140.907.

Precission. Comparatively slow gyration of the axis of a spinning body so as to trace out a cone; caused by the application of a torque tending to change the direction of the rotation axis, and continuously directed at right angles to the plane of the torque. The magnetic moment of a nucleus with spin will experience such a torque when inclined at an angle to the magnetic field, resulting in precession at the Larmor frequency. A familiar example is the effect of gravity on the motion of a spinning top or gyroscope. (NMR.)

Precipitate. Solid compound that is produced in a chemical reaction between two soluble compounds in a solution. A reaction between a soluble antigen and soluble antibody in which a complex lattice of interlocking aggregates forms.

Precipitin. An antibody which reacts specifically with soluble antigen to form a precipitate.

Precision. A term used to indicate the reproducibility of the measurement of a quantity when determined repeatedly, usually stated as a coefficient of variation, or confidence limits.

Precordium. The area of the chest overlying the heart.

Precursor. A forerunner; something that goes before. Of a nuclide, any radioactive nuclide which precedes that nuclide in a decay chain. The term is often restricted to the immediately preceding nuclide, e.g., ^{133}I is the precursor of the radioactive gaseous species xenon ^{133}Xe, which is formed from ^{133}I by beta decay.

Predefined sequence. A series of computer commands which can be defined, saved, and used repeatedly for specific procedures.

Preload. A term describing the initial stretch of the left ventricle just prior to contraction. Normally, the ventricle can increase its stroke volume by increasing its preload over a moderate range (this is the ascending limb of the Frank-Starling mechanism, in which the heart output per beat is related to the diastolic filling pressure).

Preneoplastic. Before the appearance of a tumor, but with potential to become malignant in a certain percentages of cases.

Preparation gradient. Gradient used to produce spatial encoding by phase in 2DF and 3DF imaging methods. (NMR.)

Pressoreceptors. Baroreceptors; receptors sensitive to pressure.

Pressure. The force divided by the area over which the force is applied is a useful quantity. This is called pressure. It is force per unit area (the concentration of force).

$$\text{pressure (N/m}^2\text{)} = \frac{\text{force (N)}}{\text{area (m}^2\text{)}}$$

SI unit, the pascal (Pa).

Pressure gradient. When blood passes through a stenotic site, the pressure proximal to the stenosis will be greater than the pressure distal to the stenosis. The difference between the proximal and distal pressures is termed the pressure gradient. In contrast to the pressure changes, the velocity of blood flow distal to the stenosis is greater than the velocity proximally, because blood flow is accelerated across the stenosis. The velocity distal to stenosis can be measured by Doppler and the pressure gradient across the stenosis can then be calculated according to the modified Bernoulli equation.

Pressure transducer. The electrical versions of this transducer usually work by allowing the pressure to bend a diaphragm in the transducer and measure the bending by resistance strain gauges arranged into a bridge circuit which may be attached to the diaphragm (as in the case of most semiconductor gauges) or metallic film gauges. Such device is used extensively for recording of blood pressure (via intraarterial or intravenous cannulas), bladder pressure, etc.

Pressure vessel. The container for the reactor core. It serves to contain the coolant which passes through the channel inside the core to transfer the heat to the exchanger.

Pressurized water reactor. Reactor in which the water coolant and moderator are kept at a high pressure to prevent it readily boiling and hence to keep it liquid. This type requires enriched fuel. The water is taken out to a heat exchanger to generate steam which can run through a turbo-alternator to give electricity.

Primary. The initial site of a malignancy, used to differentiate this site from sites of subsequent spread, or metastasis.

Primary cosmic rays. Those particles which enter the earth's atmosphere from outer space. They consist mainly (90%) of protons, the remainder being α particles and a few (1%) heavier nuclei.

Primary ionization. The ionization produced directly by the interaction of an energetic charged primary particle with the atoms of the matter through which it is passing, as contrasted to the "total ionization" which includes the "secondary ionization" produced by Δ-rays. In counter tubes: the total ionization produced by incident radiation without gas amplification.

Primary protective barrier. Barrier sufficient to attenuate the useful beam to the required degree.

Primary radiation. All radiation coming directly from the target of an X-ray tube or other ionizing radiation source.

Principal quantum number. (n or ni) Relative distance from the nucleus at which the electron will be found and also its relative energy.

Printed circuit board. (PCB) Also known as printed circuit card. The PCB is a thin insulating board. Integrated circuits, resistors, capacitors, and other electronic components are mounted on the board and interconnected as a circuit by a pattern of conductive lines etched onto the board's surface. This etched circuit pattern eliminates the need to connect components with wire, clips, and solder.

Printer. A typewriter-like device controlled by a computer. The printer prints results of programs, information retrieved from memory, and other computer output on either individual sheets or continuous strips of paper.

Printer-plotter. Typically refers to an elec-

trostatic output device that is capable of producing both characters (for text) and graphical output. These devices are also available for producing characters only or for graphic output only.

Printout. The output of a printer is also called "hard copy" as it can be handled as opposed to the "soft" data displayed on a visual display screen.

Prinzmetal angina. In 1947 Prinzmetal described for the first time a type of pain which occurs mostly during the night, is unrelated to effort, lasts longer than the typical anginal attack, and produces ST segment elevations in the electrocardiogram. The findings made today through coronary angiography suggest that this type of pain is due to a reversible coronary vasospasm which is usually caused by a preexisting atheromatosis of the coronaries but which occasionally occurs also when the coronary vessels are anatomically normal.

Priority. A number associated with a task that determines the order in which the monitor will process the request for services by that task relative to other tasks requesting service.

Private antigen. A type of tumor antigen that is expressed on a particular type of chemically induced tumor.

Probability. Probability measures the odds of a given event taking place. In a mathematical sense, probability is defined as the number of ways an event can happen divided by the number of possible happenings. Calculating the probabilities of complex events can be a long, tedious process. And that is where the computer's high-speed data processing capabilities are most useful.

Probability distribution. A distribution which indicates the probability of all possible outcomes; the total area under the curve adds to one. May be a sampling distribution.

Probability of an event. Proportion of all possible events that are of the specified type.

Probe. The portion of an NMR spectrometer comprising the sample container and the radio-frequency (rf) coils, with some associated electronics. The rf coils may consist of separate receiver and transmitter coils in a crossed-coil configuration, or alternatively, a single coil to perform both functions. Transducer assembly. Detector.

Problem-orientated medical record. Structured medical record form, so designed to represent the process of problem solving followed by a physician during the consultation. It captures the various elements of this process as they are encountered.

Process. A set of related procedures and data that are executed and manipulated by a computer. The chemical processing of radioactive materials.

Process-heat reactor. A reactor for the production of heat for utilization in space heating, industrial processing, or other processes where conversion to other energy forms is not desireed.

Processor. A data processing term for the hardware computer unit used in the execution of instructions, reduction, and storage of data. In software, a computer program that includes the compiler, assembler, translator, and related functions for a specific programing language (e.g., FORTRAN IV processor).

Production reactor. A nuclear reactor designed primarily for large-scale production of transmutation products (e.g., plutonium).

Profile slice. A slice through an image by one of two lines generating a histogram curve which shows count values along the line or between the two lines.

Prognosis. A prediction of the probable course of a disease and the chances of recovery.

Program. A set of instructions to the computer, designed to achieve a particular end. The instructions may be written in machine code or a high-level language such as basic. Programs written in machine code are generally to make the hardware work and are sets of operating instructions for the central processing unit (CPU), the storage device, the input/output devices, as well as the communication devices. Programs written in the high-level languages are to instruct the computer to operate the various applications.

Program counter. A register in the central processing unit (CPU) that specifies the address of the next instruction. After each instruction is executed, the program counter increments one step.

Program development. Process of writing, entering, translating, and debugging source computer programs.

Program function keys. Ten keys at the left end of the personal computer keyboard. Many application programs let you use the program function keys to perform control operations. For example, a word processor might let you use them to move the cursor around, insert or delete text, and search the text for words or phrases.

Program listing. Sequence of program instructions.

Programmer. The person who creates logical and error-free lists of instructions in a programming language for the solution of a problem. Some programmers are also responsible for definition of the program itself.

Programming language. A set of instructions or symbols, and syntactical rules for using and combining them, for the writing of programs. There is a continuous evolution of high-level programming languages toward the point where the instructions (words) and the syntax (grammar) are as close to natural language as possible.

Projection. The result of summing the activity along lines (rays) through the object. The usual gamma camera image is a two-dimensional projection of activity through the body. One-dimensional projections are formed by summing the activity or density along parallel lines through a plane or transverse section. A projection is a count profile of the rays that compose it. There is one projection for each angular position of the detector during data collection and a complete set of projections for each tomogram to be reconstructed.

Projection profile. Spectrum of NMR signal whose frequency components are broadened by a gradient magnetic field. In the simplest case (negligible line width, no relaxation effects, and no effects of prior gradients), it corresponds to a one-dimensional projection of the spin density along the direction of the gradient; in this form it is used in reconstruction from projections imaging.

Projection reconstruction. Method of (planar) imaging employing a magnetic gradient, for spatial encoding in one direction which is rotated successively until sufficient data are obtained for contraction of an image by back-projection. (NMR.)

Proliferation. The spread of nuclear weapons into countries that did not previously possess them.

Promethium. Element symbol Pm, atomic number 61, atomic weight ~ 145

Prompt. Any chosen symbol (usually a keyboard character) that lets the user know at which level the computer is operating and also lets the user know it is waiting for an input.

Prompt critical. Capable of sustaining a chain reaction on the prompt neutrons alone, without contribution from delayed neutrons.

Prompt neutrons. Those fission neutrons which are emitted in the fission process, or from the freshly formed fission fragments, without measurable delay, i.e., in less than a millionth of a second.

Prone. Lying face downward.

Proof. (Legal) The conviction or persuasion of the mind of a judge or jury by the exhibition of evidence and the presentation of argument, of the reality of a fact alleged. (Anything you can get a judge or jury to believe.)

Propagation. Progression or travel.

Propagation speed. Speed with which a wave moves through a medium.

Prophase. The first stage of mitosis or meiosis in which the nuclear membrane disappears and the nuclear material resolves itself into chromosomes.

Prophylactic. Preventing the spread of disease not yet detectable, such as prophylactic radiation designed to prevent the spread of a malignancy along the route of lymphatic drainage.

Proportional counter. A gas-filled radiation detector in which the pulse produced is proportional to the number of ions formed in the gas by the incident radiation.

Proportional region. That region of operation of a gas counter wherein the gas amplification is greater than unity and the output pulse height is proportional to the initial ionization.

Proprioception. Process of receiving stimulation that signals spatial and motor information from the joints, tendons, and muscles.

Proptosis. Forward displacement of any organ.

Prostaglandins. A variety of naturally occurring aliphatic acids with various biologic activities, including increased vascular permeability, smooth muscle contraction, bronchial constriction, and alteration in the pain threshold.

Prosthesis. An artificial substitute for a missing or diseased limb or organ.

Protactinium. Element symbol Pa, atomic number 91, atomic weight 231.0359.

Protease. An enzyme that catalyzes the digestion of proteins.

Protection survey. A survey made to measure the level of radiation or radioactive contamination in a laboratory or other area so as to ensure the protection of its occupants.

Protective clothing. Worn by personnel handling radioactive material for two reasons: (1) to protect the wearer, and (2) to prevent the spread of radioactive contamination.

Protective source housing. Enclosure for one or more sealed sources, which limits the leakage of radiation to a specified level.

Protective tube housing. Housing which surrounds the X-ray tube itself, or the tube and other parts of the X-ray apparatus (for example, transformer) and limits the major portion of the radiation emerging from the tube to the "useful beam". Each protective tube housing shall have its type marked upon it.

Protein. Complex organic nitrogenous molecule composed of amino acids linked in a specific sequence by peptide bounds. Proteins are essential constituents of the cells of all living organisms.

Protein-bound iodine. (PBI) A laboratory test for thyroid function involving the determination of serum total hormonal iodine bound to serum proteins. (Now considered obsolete because of nonspecificity.)

Proteolysis. Enzymatic or hydrolytic conversion of proteins into simple substances.

Prothrombin. A plasma protein precursor of thrombin, which, in turn, converts fibrinogen to fibrin in the process of blood coagulation.

Protium. A name sometimes applied to the hydrogen isotope of mass 1 ($_1H^1$) in contradistinction to deuterium ($_1H^2$) and tritium ($_1H^3$).

Protocol. A format set of conventions governing the format and relative timing of information exchange between two communicating processes. A step-by-step acquisition or processing sequence that prompts the operator for input every step of the way, or detailed description of the exact manner in which an assay is to be performed.

Proton. Elementary nuclear particle of unit mass number having a positive electric charge equal numerically and opposite to that of an electron (i.e., 1.6×10^{-19} C) and having a mass of 1.0079 a.m.u. The proton is the nucleus of the atom of a protium, i.e., the isotope of hydrogen of mass number unity.

Proton density. In the context of NMR, the number of hydrogen atoms per unit volume.

Proton-induced X-ray emission. (PIXIE) The emission of X-rays when a sample is bombarded by protons. The X-rays emitted are characteristic of the elements present in the sample. Used for trace analysis.

Proton-proton reaction. A thermonuclear reaction in which two protons collide at very high velocities and combine to form a deuteron. The resultant deuteron may capture another proton to form tritium and the latter may undergo proton capture to form helium.

Protoplasm. The viscous, translucent, polyphasic water colloid that makes up the material of all plant and animal cells.

Protraction dose. A method of administration of radiation by delivering it continuously over a relatively long period at a low dosage rate.

Proximal. Nearest the point of attachment, center of the body, or point of reference.

Prozone. The precipitin-free zone preceding the zone of precipitation in a precipitin test; the prozone occurs because antigen-antibody (Ag-Ab) complexes remain soluble in the region of extreme Ag excess.

Pseudo-random access memory. Memory in which it is possible to skip over most, but not all, locations in order to access any one desired location. For example, disks are said to be "pseudo-random access devices" since one can skip rapidly to the desired track. It is then necessary to wait until data on that track moves sequentially into place for reading.

Psychosis. A general term for any kind of mental disorder, particularly those characterized by lack of insight.

Psychosomatic. Pertaining to the mind-body relationship; having bodily symptoms of psychic, emotional, or mental origin.

Pterygium. Anything like a wing; disease of the eye in which a membrane grows over it from the inner corner.

Ptosis. A drooping or falling down of a part or organ, such as the eyelid, the kidney, stomach, and intestine.

Pulmonary angiography. Selective examination of the left and right pulmonary arteries is occasionally used to document or further clarify suspected pulmonary embolism (blood clots to the lungs).

Pulmonary arterial pressure. (PAP) The blood pressure in the pulmonary artery, generated mainly by the repetitive contractions of the right ventricle and therefore varying over the heart cycle. Higher than normal PAP in indicative of raised pulmonary vascular resistance. It may also be indicative of pulmonary edema, and of pulmonary embolism if pulmonary capillary wedge pressure is normal.

Pulmonary arterial wedge pressure. (PAWP) The arterial pressure measurement obtained by wedging a catheter in one of the branches of the pulmonary arterial system.

Pulmonary artery. The artery taking blood pumped from the heart's right ventricle. It branches into right and left pulmonary arteries, taking blood to the right and left pulmonary vasculatures, respectively, to be oxygenated.

Pulmonary atelectasis. Lung collapse.

Pulmonary capillary wedge pressure. (PCWP) The blood pressure measured in the pulmonary artery when the pressure sensor lodged in the artery is shielded from the pressure generated by the ventricle of the heart (as by the inflated balloon of a Swan-Ganz catheter "wedged" within the pulmonary artery). It represents the pressure in the left atrium. It gives, too, some indication of left ventricular function, the mitral valve between the left heart chambers being open during diastole. Higher than normal PCWP can be indicative of hyperbolemia (high blood volume), of cardiac insufficiency, or of pulmonary congestion. Low PCWP is indicative of hypovolemia (low blood volume) and noncardiac edema.

Pulmonary circulation. The circulation that carries venous blood from the right ventricle of the heart to the lungs and returns oxygenated blood to the left atrium.

Pulmonary edema. Effusion of fluid into the air sacs and tissues of the lungs, most commonly due to left heart failure.

Pulmonary embolism. Obstruction of one or more of the pulmonary arteries, usually caused by fragments of a thrombus from a leg vein. Pulmonary embolism is a common complication of long confinement to bed, abdomino-pelvic surgery, diabetes, obesity, hypertension, cigarette smoking.

Pulmonary gas exchange. The transfer of oxygen from atmosphere to blood and of carbon dioxide from blood to atmosphere.

Pulmonary minute volume. Volume of air respired per minute = tidal volume × breaths/minute; pulmonary ventilation.

Pulmonary stenosis. Narrowing of the opening into the pulmonary artery from the right cardiac ventricle.

Pulmonary tissue resistance. Frictional and deformational resistance of the pulmonary tissue.

Pulmonary valve. The valve that guards the pulmonary orifice in the right ventricle of the heart. The pulmonary valve prevents backflow into the right ventricle.

Pulmonary veins. Four large veins (two from each lung) through which oxygenated blood passes from the lungs to the heart.

Pulse. A brief increase in intensity. Principally used in connection with electronic circuits in which electric pulses are generated, shaped, or amplified. Most particle detectors give rise to electronic pulses when traversed by an ionizing particle. A brief burst of ultrasound, normally about 1μs in duration. The rhythmic expansion of an artery which may be felt with the finger and corresponds to the beating of the heart and pulsatile blood flow.

Pulse amplifier. An amplifier, designed specifically to amplify intermittent signals of a nuclear detector, incorporating appropriate pulse-shaping characteristics.

Pulse amplitude. The radio-frequency field, H_1, in gauss.

Pulse average intensity. The ratio of the time integral of pulse intensity to the pulse duration.

Pulsed mode. Digital fluoroscopic images created using short pulses of X-rays at high currents. Video readout of the image is synchronized to follow the X-ray pulse. Short pulses minimize patient motion.

Pulsed ultrasound. Diagnostic ultrasound, other than Doppler, consists of short bursts (pulses) with long silent periods between them when the transducer acts as a receiver.

Pulsed-wave Doppler. In pulsed-wave Doppler examination single crystal is used to transmit short bursts of ultrasound and to receive the reflected signal in the interval between transmissions. By using a process called range gating, it is possible to analyze only those signals emanating from a small area within the heart, or blood vessels. This small area (sample volume) can be positioned anywhere along the path of the ultrasound beam. When pulsed-wave Doppler is combined with two-dimensional echocardiography, the site of abnormal blood flow can be localized. The major limitation of this technique is the inability to record high velocity signals.

Pulse-echo imaging. Most diagnostic applications are based on the pulse-echo method which gives information about the positions of interfaces within the body, which act as reflectors and scatters; to a lesser extent, this technique also gives clues about their characteristics. Pulses of ultrasonic energy, typically 1000 s^{-1} and each of a few microseconds duration, are generated by a transducer. These pulses are directed along a narrow beam into the patient. Echoes which return from characteristic impedance discontinuities within the patient may be detected by the transducer, delayed (following the transmission of each pulse) by times corresponding to depths along the ultrasonic beam. Pulse-echo methods depend on the satisfactory detection of ultrasonic signals. This requirement often prevents their application in the examination of structures surrounded by, or containing, gas or bone. This is because both gas and bone present large mismatches in characteristic impedance (and hence large reflections) at interfaces with soft tissues, and they also have relatively high attenuations and dissimilar propagation speeds. In soft tissues, compensation for attenuation may be provided by swept (time-varied) gain in the receiver amplifier.

Pulse flip angle. The angle (in degrees or in radians) through which the magnetization is rotated by a specific pulse.

Pulse height analyzer. The amplitudes of pulses from a scintillation detector used in nuclear medicine vary according to the energy of the incident rays. A pulse height analyzer is an electronic device employed to identify and select those pulses falling between two preset amplitude levels which may relate only to the product of a single isotope photopeak and rejects pulses due to scattered radiation above and below the photopeak; the range of energies which are accepted constitutes the window of the analyzer or discriminator. A number of pulse height analyzers may be operated in parallel and the results collected by a multichannel analyzer show count rates from a number of isotopes simultaneously.

Pulse interval. The time between two pulses of a sequence.

Pulse ionization chamber. The pulse ionization chamber is similar to the current ionization chamber but records, instead of the current flowing, a discrete pulse arising from the passage of each charged particle through the filling gas. Under the influence of the electric field the ions acquire a drift velocity in the direction of the appropriate electrodes which, in the case of heavy positive ions, is approximately proportional to the electric field strength and inversely proportional to the gas pressure.

Pulse length. Time duration of a pulse. For a radio-frequency (rf) pulse near the Larmor frequency, the longer the pulse length, the greater the angle of rotation of macroscopic magnetization vector will be (greater than 180° can bring it back toward its original orientation). (NMR.)

Pulse phase. The phase of the radio-frequency field as measured relative to a chosen axis in the rotating coordinate frame.

Pulse pileup. Occurs at high counting rates when two γ-rays are detected within the resolving time of the system. The resultant pulses sum, and both may be rejected if the sum is outside the selected energy window.

Pulse pressure. Pressure variations at the surface of the body due to arterial blood pulsations. Used for timing of pulse waves, pulse-wave velocity measurement, and as an indicator of arterial blood pressure variations. Required frequency response: 0.1 to 40 Hz. Measured by a low-frequency microphone or crystal pressure pickup. The difference between systolic and diastolic pressures.

Pulse programer. Part of the spectrometer or interface that controls the timing, duration, and amplitude of the pulses (radio frequency or gradient). (NMR.)

Pulse rate. Number of pulsations per minute measured in an artery in responses to the contraction of the heart; usually measured in the wrist, where the radial artery pulsates against the radius. Equivalent to the heart rate.

Pulse repetition frequency. The rate at which pulses of acoustic energy are transmitted in a pulsed ultrasound beam or range-gated Doppler system. This is usually a function of the depth of the (first) sample volume and determines peak velocity limit which can be unambiguously detected by range gated or pulsed Doppler systems.

Pulse repetition period. The time between corresponding parts in the waveform of successive pulses from a transmitter. The pulse repetition period is equal to the reciprocal of the pulse repetition frequency.

Pulse sequence. Set of radio-frequency (rf) (and/or gradient) magnetic field pulses and time spacings between these pulses; used in conjunction with gradient magnetic fields and NMR signal reception to produce NMR images.

Pulse 180° (π pulse). Radio-frequency (rf) pulse designed to rotate the macroscopic magnetization vector 180° in space as referred to the rotating frame of reference, usually about an axis at right angles to the main magnetic field. If the spins are initially aligned with the magnetic field, this pulse will produce inversion. (NMR.)

Pulse 90° (π/2 pulse). Radio-frequency (rf) pulse designed to rotate the macroscopic magnetization vector 90° in space as referred to the rotating frame of reference, usually about an axis at right angles to the main magnetic field. If the spins are initially aligned with the magnetic field, this pulse will produce transverse magnetization and a free induction decay (FID). (NMR.)

Punch card. A card containing data represented by holes punched out in a particular way and able to be read by a "card reader". The cards, together with the card reader, represent an input to the computer (obsolete).

Purkinje effect. The shift in the maximum spectral sensitive of the eye from the yellow-green, at a good level illumination, towards the blue, as the illumination is reduced.

Purkinje fibers. The treelike terminal brachings of the right and left bundle branches that carry the excitation impulse to the myocardial fibers.

Pus. Liquid composed of white blood cells and the decomposition of tissue in a wound.

P wave. A low-amplitude, broad deflection on an electrocardiogram due to atrial depolarization.

Pyelogram. A roetgenogram of the kidney and ureter, especially showing the pelvis of the kidney.

Pyknosis. Thickening; especially degeneration of a cell in which the nucleus decreases in size and the chromatin condenses.

Pyogenic microorganisms. Microorganisms whose presence in tissues stimulates an outpouring of polymorphonuclear leukocytes.

Pyrogen. The metabolic product of bacteria, yeasts, and fungi and can therefore be present as a result of actual, recent, or past microbiological contamination. Sterility is not an indication of freedom from pyrogen. When given a injection, pyrogens is achieved by using pyrogen-free containers, sterile materials, and aseptic procedures throughout the production process.

Pyrophosphate. Chemical compound containing a $P_2O_7^{-4}$. Labeled with ^{99m}T it is used for bone scintigraphy, recent myocardial infarction detection, and tagging of pre-primed red blood cells for blood pool imaging.

Q

Q factor. Coil quality factor. A measure of energy loss described as the ratio of energy in the system to energy that is lost in one oscillating cycle. (NMR.)

QRS wave. The waveform consisting of the Q wave, R wave, and S wave, produced by an electrocardiograph recording ventricular depolarization. The Q wave is the initial downward deflection, the R wave is the initial upward deflection, and the S wave is the downward deflection following the R wave.

Quadrature detector. A phase-sensitive detector or demodulator that detects the components of the signal in phase with a reference oscillator and 90° out of phase with the reference oscillator. (NMR.)

Qualitative. Relating to, or involving quality of kind. Q analysis: chemical analysis designed to identify the components of a substance or mixture.

Qualitative data. Data based on the categorization and enumeration of individuals according to some characteristic which they either have or do not have, such as living or dead. Such data are always discrete.

Quality assurance. The term "quality assurance" refers to all of those aspects (including administrative techniques and training) of a diagnostic program that contribute directly or indirectly to the quality of the imaging procedure in any of its final or user-oriented forms. It also comprises the total process whereby a manufacturer ensures that a product meets the quality required for its intended use. It covers the design and development stages through to manufacturing, quality control, and delivery processes to final storage and use by customers. The quality assurance process must be directed to the final product and regulatory needs which will include the establishment of documented support for product claims, testing, specifications, and validation of quality control as well as extensive clinical trial and safety support investigations.

Quality control. The set of operations (programming coordinating, carrying out) intended to maintain or to improve quality. As applied to a diagnostic procedure, it covers monitoring, evaluation, and maintenance at optimum levels of all characteristics of performance that can be defined, measured, and controlled. Quality control is a fundamental part of the quality assurance process and focuses on the testing and approval of raw materials, bulk stocks, final pack batches, and manufacturing equipment and facilities. It cannot be part of the manufacturing function: quality cannot be controlled into a product after it is made. It is essential to design in the right qualities, including robustness, at the development phase so that manufacture, quality control, and use by customers are easy and uncomplicated. Quality control constitutes a variety of tests and approvals which contribute toward the total quality assurance situation.

Quality control serum. A serum sample that is analyzed many times to yield data about the statistical reproducibility of a radioassay.

Quality factor. (Q) In radiation, a dimensionless variable weighting factor to be applied to the absorbed dose to provide an estimate of the relative human hazard of different types and energies of ionizing radiations. Values of Q are selected from experimental values of the relative biological effectiveness (RBE), which is the ratio of X- or γ-ray dose to that of the radiation in question giving the same kind and degree of biological effect. Q is chosen by the International Commission on Radiological Protection (ICRP) to be a smooth function of the unrestricted linear energy transfer (L∞) of the radiation. It is also called the collision stopping power. In electronics it applies to any electrical circuit component; most often the coil quality factor is limiting. Inversely related to the fraction of the energy in an oscillating system lost in one oscillation cycle. Q is inversely related to the range of frequency over which the system will exhibit resonance. It affects the signal-to-noise ratio, because the detected signal increases proportionally to Q while the noise is proportional to the square root of Q. The Q of a coil will depend on whether it is unloaded (no patient) or loaded (patient).

Quality of radiation. Penetration of radiation: frequently measured by its half-value layer (HVL). The HVL is the thickness of some standard material which transmits 50% of the incident radiation.

Quantitative. Relating to, or involving the measurement of quantity or amount.

Quantitative chemical analysis. Branch of chemical analysis dealing with the determination of how much of a constituent there is in a chemical compound.

Quantities and units. Physical properties and processes are described in terms of quantities such as time and energy. These quantities are measured in units such as seconds and joules. Thus, a quantity describes what is measured whereas a unit describes how much.

Quantum. In 1901 Planck introduced the idea that electromagnetic radiation could only be emitted or absorbed in discrete quanta, which for radiation of frequency v contained an amount hv of energy, with h a universal constant, Planck's constant. The quantum of the radiation field is called the photon, and this term is generally used when it is desired to emphasize the particle nature rather than the wave nature of radiation.

Quantum efficiency of fluorescence. The number of molecules which fluoresce per quantum of incident exciting radiation of a given wavelength.

Quantum mechanics. The set of physical laws which universally apply to certain microsystems and predict that their properties (such as magnetic moment, energy) cannot have a continuous set of values, but must have a set of discrete, discontinuous values.

Quantum number. Value describing the location of an electron in the electronic configuration of an atom.

Quantum theory. This name is often reserved

for the older theory of Planck, Einstein, and Bohr, while the term quantum mechanics is used for the later developments of the theory by Schrödinger, Heisenberg, Dirac, and others. The theory, in both its original and modern forms, was developed to explain many phenomena inexplicable by classical physics. The theory applies to all phenomena on any scale, but for macroscopic events it becomes indistinguishable from classical physics, so that in a sense it can be said to be a theory of the behavior of systems on the atomic and subatomic scale. The main prediction of the theory is that certain physical quantities may only have certain definite values, and that the measurement of a quantity will, in general, change the state of the system that is being investigated.

Quarks. Particles, whose existence is not established, which have fractional electric charge. Elementary particles are conjectured to be built up of various combinations of two or three quarks and antiquarks.

Quartiles. Values that divide a distribution of ordered data into four equal parts.

Quartz fiber electroscope. An electroscope used for continual personal monitoring of integrated radiation dose. A gold-plated quartz fiber is the flexible member and behaves like the gold leaf in the familiar electroscope, its elasticity providing the restoring force. The motion of the fiber is observed with a low-power microscope against an eyepiece scale calibrated in roentgens, milliroentgens or C/kg.

Quench corrections. In liquid scintillation counting a number of substances may absorb radiation energy before they are transferred to the scintillator. This phenomenon is known as chemical quenching and it is important for aqueous samples. It is particularly noticeable if oxygen is present. Oxygen can be removed by bubbling an inert gas such as nitrogen through the scintillator solution. Color quenching can also occur. Here, the overall light transmission of the system is reduced. Decoloration may be possible. If the count rate is adequate it is often useful to dilute the sample. Both chemical and color quenching reduce the voltage pulse output of the counter (a function of the β-energy dissipated) causing an apparent downward shift in the pulse-height spectrum or, in the case of tritium, an actual reduction in the number of β-particles detected. Since quenching is normally present, and may well vary between individual samples, it is necessary to determine the amount of quenching present and correct for its effects. The two main methods of quench correction

are based on internal and external standards.

1. The internal-standard method. The sample is first counted on its own and then re-counted following the addition of a known activity of the radionuclide. The difference between the two counts enables the counting efficiency (and therefore the degree of quenching) to be determined. This is in turn used to correct the initial reading obtained with the sample alone. This method is capable of high accuracy, but is tedious.
2. The external-standard method. The measured spectrum is divided into two counting channels, covering different ranges of pulse height. Quenching causes a shift in pulse height and therefore alters the ratio of counts in the two channels. A calibration curve can thus be prepared of channel ratio vs. counting efficiency provided a set of samples is available which is of known activity but exhibits different degrees of quenching.

Quenching. Loss of superconductivity of the current-carrying coil that may occur unexpectedly in a superconducting magnet. As the magnet becomes resistive, heat will be released that can result in rapid evaporation of liquid helium in the cryostat. This may present a hazard if not properly planned for. (NMR.) In liquid scintillation counting, a decrease in counting efficiency resulting from physicochemical interferences in the scintillation process of attenuation of the photons produced. It can also be the process of limiting the discharge of an ionization detector (such as a Geiger counter), either externally by a momentary reduction in applied potential to the tube through suitable electronic circuitry, or internally by the introduction of a quenching agent, such as butane or chlorine.

Quenching gas. A polyatomic gas used in Geiger-Müller counters to quench or extinguish avalanche ionization.

Queue. Any dynamic list of items waiting to be scheduled or computer processed according to system- or user-assigned priorities.

Q value. The energy in MeV that is emitted or absorbed in a nuclear reaction.

R

Rabbit. A small container propelled, usually pneumatically or hydraulically, through a tube in a nuclear reactor or near an accelerator for exposing substances experimentally to the radiation and neutron flux of the active section; used for rapid removal of samples with very short half-lives.

Radial immunodiffusion. Immunochemical method used for the determination of serum concentrations of physiologically important substances.

Radian. (rad) Is the supplementary SI unit of plane angle between two radii of a circle which cut off on the circumference an arc equal in length to the radius.

Radiant energy. (R) Defined as the energy of particles (excluding rest energy) emitted, transferred, or received. The energy of electromagnetic waves, such as radio waves, visible light, X-rays, and γ-rays.

Radiation. The emission and propagation of energy through space or through a material medium in the form of waves; for instance, the emission and propagation of electromagnetic waves, or of sound and elastic waves. Briefly, the term radiation refers to "energy in transit". In nuclear medicine, two specific forms of radiation are of interest: (1) particulate radiation, consisting of atomic or subatomic particles (electrons, protons, etc.) which carry energy in the form of kinetic energy of mass in motion; and (2) electromagnetic radiation, in which energy is carried by oscillating electrical magnetic fields traveling through space at the speed of light. In cardiology, the angina pain that frequently, though not necessarily, radiates to other regions such as the mandibular angles on both sides, the area between the shoulder blades, the left arm, and, occasionally, both arms.

Radiation burns. If radiation is sufficiently intense or prolonged it causes surface burns on the skin which redden and blister, not unlike heat burns or severe sunburn. These are called radiation burns. Patients subject to intense irradiation, e.g., in cancer therapy by X- or γ-rays, sometimes get surface or skin radiation burns.

Radiation chemistry. A branch of chemistry concerned with the gross chemical effects of ionizing radiation and energetic particles on chemical substances and on chemical reactions.

Radiation cross-sectional area. The beam cross-sectional area at the surface of the ultrasound transducer assembly.

Radiation damage. Deleterious changes in the physical or chemical properties of a material as a result of exposure to ionizing radiation. This term does not apply to biological systems.

Radiation detector. An instrument or a material which measures or indicates the presence of ionizing radiation.

Radiation dose. A general form denoting the quantity of radiation or energy absorbed; for special purposes, it must be appropriately qualified; if unqualified, it refers to an absorbed dose.

Radiation exposure. Exposure to ionizing radiation.

Radiation force. Steady force exerted on an object on which a sound beam is incident.

Radiation frequency. (ν) Number of complete phase cycles per second of an electromagnetic radiation treated as a wave function, which is related directly to the photon's energy by Planck's constant, h, in the formula $E = h\nu$.

Radiation hazard. A condition due to which persons might receive radiation in excess of the relevant recommended dose-equivalent limit or from which material damage might result.

Radiation hygiene. Synonymous with radiological health.

Radiation length. When a fast electron is traversing matter it loses energy mainly by radiation and the logarithm of the energy decreases linearly with the distance traveled. The radiation length is the distance traveled by the electron in having its energy decreased by a factor of e (2.718...).

Radiation level. The intensity of radiation at the point in question.

Radiation loss. When a charged particle passes through matter it loses energy partly by producing ionization and partly by producing bremsstrahlung (radiation). At low energies the former process, ionization loss, predominates, while at high (relativistic) energies, the latter process, radiation loss, is more important.

Radiation maze. A maze designed to allow access to an enclosure which may contain a very high radiation level, but without permitting the escape of direct radiation.

Radiation measurement. As is well known, elementary particles and high-energy quanta are not directly perceptible by man in sublethal doses, and instruments are therefore necessary to detect their presence and provide quantitative information. There are two main types of detecting instruments: (1) passive elements, which store up the information so long as they are exposed to the radiation, and which have to be inspected in order to extract the information; (2) active elements, which produce an electrical signal indicating the presence of the radiation.

Radiation monitoring. The continuing collection and assessment of the pertinent information to determine the adequacy of radiation protection practices and to alert to potentially significant changes in conditions or protection performance.

Radiation oncology. Specialty of medicine in which radiation is administered by a treatment machine (^{60}Co, linear accelerator, neutron generator, etc.) or by intracavitary or interstitial applicators to treat malignant disease (radiotherapy).

Radiation physics. That field of physics that deals with the properties and physical effects of ionizing radiation. It may also refer to nonionizing radiation.

Radiation polymerization. Under the influence of ionizing radiation many organic compounds form quantities of material of substantially higher molecular weight than the initial substance. These products are usually loosely termed polymers and may or may not consist of the monomer units combined in a chain, sheets, or a network. Compounds which are particularly noteworthy for this behavior include the aromatic hydrocarbons, the unsaturated aliphatic hydrocarbons, dienes, and especially the vinyl compounds.

Radiation potentiator. Any agent such as a drug which increases the sensitivity of the cells or tissues to the radiation.

Radiation protection. All measures concerned with reducing deleterious effect of radiation to persons or materials.

Radiation risk. The risk, if any, to health from exposure to ionizing radiation.

Radiation safety. Methods of protecting workers and the general population from the deleterious effects of radiation.

Radiation sensor. The component of a radiation detector which responds directly to ionizing radiation. It may indicate this response itself or may induce a response in other components.

Radiation sickness. Part of the radiation syndrome following intense, acute exposure to ionizing radiation. A few hours after such exposure nausea and vomiting appear, which last a few hours and subside after a variable period.

Radiation source. An apparatus or a material emitting or capable of emitting ionizing radiation. In nuclear medicine often used to designate a quantity of radioactive material used as a source of ionizing radiation, used for calibration, as a marker, etc.

Radiation spectrum. When a beam of radiation is analyzed according to the energies of its constituent particles or photons, the curve of numbers of particles or photons as a function of their energy is called the energy spectrum, or simply the spectrum, of the radiation.

Radiation stability. The stability of materials toward high energy radiation.

Radiation survey. An evaluation of the radiation hazard potential associated with a specified set of conditions incident to the production, use, release, storage, or presence of radiation sources. Such evaluation customarily includes a physical survey of the disposition of materials and equipment, measurements or estimates of the levels of radiation that may be involved, and a sufficient knowledge of processes using or affecting these materials to predict hazards resulting from expected or possible changes in materials or equipment.

Radiation worker. Any person who is potentially exposed to ionizing radiation as a result of his occupation and who is designated as such in the register by the holder of the authority.

Radiative capture. When a nucleus captures or absorbs a particle (for example, a neutron), the resultant compound nucleus is highly excited. When the compound nucleus becomes de-excited by the emission of electromagnetic radiation only, the process is known as radiative capture.

Radiative collision. A collision between two particles in which part of their combined kinetic energy is converted to electromagnetic radiation.

Radiative energy loss. The conversion of charged-particle kinetic energy to photon energy, through either bremsstrahlung X-ray production or in flight annihilation of positrons. In the latter case only the kinetic energy possessed by the positron at the instant of annihilation (which is carried away by the resulting photons along with 1.022 MeV of rest-mass energy) is classified as radiative energy loss.

Radical treatment. Treatment designed with the aim of removing or destroying all the malignancy present.

Radioactive. Possessing or pertaining to radioactivity. The term "radio" is used as an abbreviation of radioactive.

Radioactive chain. A succession of nuclides, each of which transforms by radioactive decay into the next nuclide until a stable nuclide results.

Radioactive contamination. The deposition of radioactive material in any place where it is not desired, and (particularly) in any place where its presence can be harmful.

Radioactive decay. This is the spontaneous transformation with a measurable half-life of a nuclide into one or more different nuclides. The process involves the emission from the nucleus of alpha particles, electrons, positrons, γ-rays or the nuclear capture or ejection of orbital electrons, or fission. To be considered as radioactive, a process must have a measurable life-time between about 10^{-10} s and about 10^{17} years.

Radioactive effluent. A term often used to denote radioactive liquid or gaseous wastes.

Radioactive equilibrium. The condition in which the activities of the members of a radioactive chain decrease exponentially in time with the half-life of the chain precursor. Such radioactive equilibrium is only possible when the half-life of the precursor is longer than that of any other chain member. If the precursor half-life is so long that the change in the precursor population during the period of interest can be ignored, all the activities become sensibly equal, and the equilibrium is said to be secular; otherwise it is said to be transient.

Radioactive family. A number of radioactive nuclides, each, except the first, being the daughter product of the previous one. The final member, the end product, although stable, is included in the family. Thus, ^{238}U decays by α-emission to thorium, $_{90}$TH^{234}. This daughter is itself radioactive and decays to protactinium $_{91}$Pa^{234}, which is again radioactive and is the precursor of a chain of daughter products ending in an isotope of lead $_{82}$Pb^{206}. $_{82}$Pb^{206} is referred to as the end product.

Radioactive growth. When a radionuclide has a radioactive daughter whose half-life is short compared with the parent, the quantity of daughter product present will gradually grow until it is equal, when measured in becquerel units, to that of the parent. They are then in equilibrium and this equilibrium will continue so long as the daughter is not removed. Until this state of equilibrium is reached the phenomenon of radioactive growth is present.

Radioactive heat. Radioactive heat is a secondary effect, for it is a measure of energy of radiation which is absorbed in the active substance or the envelope containing it. All radioactive substances exhibit this heating effect.

Radioactive iodine uptake. A thyroid function test based on the gland's ability to take up an administered tracer dose of iodice as ^{131}I, ^{123}I. This is expressed as percentage of total administered radioactivity. A 24-h interval is most commonly used because of its convenience and because, except in severe abnormal states, the uptake value is at or near its peak at this time.

Radioactive material. Any substance which consists of or contains any radionuclide, whether natural or artificial, and whose specific activity exceeds 74 kBq kg^{-1} (0.002 µCi g^{-1}) or 3.7 kBq (0.1 µCi). (Materials such as uranium and thorium that are defined as source materials are excluded from this definition.)

Radioactive period. Synonymous with mean life, which is the average time for which its nuclei exist before disintegration. It is the reciprocal of the disintegration constant, equal to 1.442 times the half-life.

Radioactive purity. Fraction of an isotope in the total activity of a labeled compound.

Radioactive series. A succession of radioactive nuclides, one decaying to the next until a stable nucleus is formed. There are three natural radioactive decay series known, respectively, as the uranium-radium series, the actinium series, and the thorium series. These series are comprised, respectively, of uranium, actinium, and thorium together with their decay products. The end product of each series is inactive lead, The uranium-radium series giving ^{206}Pb, the actinium series ^{207}Pb, and throrium series ^{208}Pb.

Radioactive source. Any quantity of radioactive material which is intended for use as a source of ionizing radiation.

Radioactive standard. A specimen of a radioactive nuclide, the activity of which in the specimen is known, having been determined at a specified time to a specified accuracy by a recognized standardizing organization. Such specimens are used for the assay of samples of the same nuclide, or for the calibration of equipment.

Radioactive tracer. A material recognizable by its radioactivity which is introduced into a physical, chemical, or biological system in order to trace the behavior of some component of that system.

Radioactive uptake. The process in which the amount or the rate of appearance of a radioactive substance in tissue is determined.

Radioactive waste. Unusable radioactive materials obtained in the processing or handling of radioactive materials.

Radioactive waste incinerator. Combustible low-activity solid waste materials may be burnt in incinerators as a means of reducing their bulk. Gases and fumes from the combustion must be scrubbed and filtered to remove radioactive matter before discharge into the atmosphere, and the radioactive ash must be handled in such a way as to avoid dispersion.

Radioactivity. Radioactivity is the property of certain nuclides of spontaneously emitting either particles or γ-rays from the nucleus (nuclear radiation) or X-rays from the shell after capture of an electron from the shell by the nucleus (characteristic X radiation). Except for isomeric transitions, this process always results in a change in the nature of the nuclide (radioactive transformation or radioactive disintegration). Nuclides possessing this property are known as radionuclides, often colloquially termed "activity".

Radioactivity standard. A radioactive source whose nature and activity at a precise time are known and which can be used as a reference radiation source.

Radioaerosol. Radioactive compound nebulized into an aerosol for inhalation.

Radioallergosorbent test. (RAST) A radioimmunoassay capable of detecting IgE antibody directed at specific allergens.

Radioassay. The *in vitro* use of radionuclides to detect and quantitate a physiologic substance.

Radiobinding assay. A general method of analysis in which the concentration of a ligand (L) is measured by allowing L and a fixed amount of a similar radiolabeled ligand (L*) to react with a given amount of receptor reagent (R), resulting in a distribution of L* into two separable compartments (bound and unbound). The distribution of L*, which varies as function of the total concentration of a ligand (L + L*) present, is estimated by the magnitude that the dilution L exerts on the label in the bound or free compartment or on some function of bound and free.

Radiobiology. That branch of biology which deals with the effects of ionizing radiation upon biological material. Research in this field is usually relevant to two important practical issues, the improved use of radiation in the treatment of cancer, and the safeguarding of the health of the community from the hazards that may arise from the increasing use of radiation and radioactive materials.

Radiochemical. A compound labeled by one or more radionuclides, This is usually used to indicate a substance that is not sterile or pyrogenfree, in contrast to a radiopharmaceutical.

Radiochemical preparation. The designation refers to a chemical product with one or more radionuclides. Although this product may be sterilized, it cannot be administered to humans.

Radiochemical purity. Radiochemical purity of a radiopharmaceutical has been defined as the fraction of the stated radionuclide present in the stated chemical form. The diagnostic value of the radiopharmaceutical depends on the differences in their kinetic and metabolic behavior in normal and diseased conditions; the radiochemical impurities in the compound, either present in the beginning or generated due to storage, might interfere significantly with the results. Diverse methods have been used for the detection and estimation of impurities; the most commonly used procedure is based on chromatography and gel-filtration techniques.

Radiochemistry. The branch of chemistry con cerned with the chemical and nuclear behavior of the radioactive elements (production to ap plication), including fission products and other radioisotopes. It is to be distinguished from ra diation chemistry, which is concerned with the effects of high-energy particles and radiation on solids, liquids, and gases.

Radiochromatography. Chromatography using a NaI crystal for detection of substances labeled with a radioisotope.

Radiocolloid. Radioactive material in a true or apparent colloidal condition.

Radioelement. An element which is naturally radioactive.

Radio frequency. (rf) Wave frequency intermediate between auditory and infrared. The rf used in NMR studies is commonly in the megahertz (MHz) range. The principal effect of rf magnetic fields on the body is power deposition in the form of heating, mainly at the surface; this is a principal area of concern for safety limits.

Radio-frequency bandwidth. The range of radio frequency within which the performance with respect to a given characteristic falls between specified limits.

Radio-frequency coil. Coils of a resonant circuit serving to detect the magnetic resonance signal or to apply excitation pulses. (NMR.)

Radio-frequency modulator. A device that adapts a television set for use as a computer display.

Radio-frequency pulse. A short burst of radiofrequency electromagnetic radiation. Rotation of the magnetization vector can be caused by controlling the duration and amplitude of the rf pulse.

Radiogenic. Resulting from radioactive decay; usually refers to natural products, e.g., radiogenic helium.

Radiograph. A processed photographic film which has been exposed to X-rays after their passage through tissues as part of a diagnostic examination; roentgenogram.

Radiography. The process of generating shadow images on photographic emulsion by the action of ionizing radiation. The image is the result of the differential attenuation of the radiation in its passage through the object being radiographed.

Radioimmunoassay. (RIA) An assay using competition between a radiolabeled antigen and the same antigen in the serum for antibody binding sites; during equilibrium, the less radiolabeled serum antigen present, the less radiolabeled antigen will be bound to the antibody; the serum level is measured by determining the bound/free ratio it produces compared with known standards in the same system.

Radioimmunodiffusion. A method by which a radioactive antibody is incorporated in order to increase the sensitivity by means of autoradiography.

Radioimmunosorbent test. (RIST) A solid phase radioimmunoassay that can detect approximately 1 ng of IgE.

Radioimmunotherapy. The ability to treat certain types of tumors using B-emitting radiolabeled monoclonal antibodies directed against tumor antigens.

Radioisotope. Synonym for radioactive isotope. Any isotope which is unstable, thus undergoing decay with the emission of a characteristic radiation.

Radiolesion. Damage to a living organism due to ionizing radiation. This can range from the severe burns which may be caused by high dose irradiation of the skin, to the breakage of a chromosome within a living cell by the passage of one ionizing particle.

Radiological health. The art and science of protecting human beings from injury by radiation.

Radiologic survey. A physical survey of the disposition of materials and equipment, measurements or estimates of the levels of radiation that may be involved incident to the production or use of radioactive materials, or other source of radiation under a specific set of conditions. This will include prediction of possible hazards and means suggested for correcting them.

Radiologist. A physician with specialized training in the diagnosis, and in some instances treatment, of disease by the use of ionizing radiation (X-rays, radium, and radioactive isotopes).

Radiology. The medical specialty which deals with the application of X-rays, γ-rays, or other penetrating ionizing radiations for the diagno-sis and, in some instances, the treatment of disease.

Radioluminescence. Light emissions caused by radiations from radioactive materials.

Radiolysis. The chemical decomposition of materials by ionizing particles or radiation. The normal chemical and pharmaceutical stability is usually altered by radiation, hence the radiopharmaceutical stability is always lower than the chemical and pharmaceutical stability; the substances with high specific activity show autodecomposition due to direct radiation damage, which becomes significant with time.

Radiometric analysis. An analytical technique of quantitative chemical analysis that includes procedures for measuring by radioactive tracer methods elements which themselves are not radioactive.

Radionuclide. A nuclide of artificial or natural origin that exhibits radioactivity. For example, ^{131}I is a radionuclide, whereas ^{127}I is a stable nuclide. Radionuclides are radioactive nuclides.

Radionuclide generators. A radionuclide generator is a device which permits ready separation of a daughter radionuclide from its parent. In generator systems of practical importance the parent has a relatively long half-life compared with the daughter, and the device (often referred as a "cow") permits repeated elutions ("milkings") at suitable intervals. Generators make possible the routine use of certain short-lived radionuclides at locations remote from centers of radionuclide production. The example of outstanding importance is that of the ^{99}Mo-^{99m}Tc generator. ^{99m}Tc is widely used in diagnostic medicine, as it emits as γ photon or ideal energy (140 keV) for imaging, and its half-life (6.02 h) and freedom of β radiation lead to low radiological doses to the patient.

Radionuclide purity. Radionuclide purity is defined as the percentage of the total radioactivity present as the stated radionuclide. This is not a constant value, but will depend on the relative half-lives of the stated nuclide and any contaminant nuclides. Contaminants with longer half-lives than the stated nuclides are potentially more hazardous because they will increase the radiation dose to the patient. They must therefore be reduced to an acceptable level at the time of production. Contaminants with a shorter half-life than the stated nuclide are less of a problem because storage will reduce the contaminant to a level acceptable for clinical use. For radionuclides produced by generators, the most probable contaminant is the parent nuclide. The generator manufacturer has to ensure that the level of the parent nuclide is below the acceptable limit in normal usage throughout the generator's working life. Detection of small quantities of impurities may be difficult in the presence of larger activities of the stated nuclide and the sample may have to be chemically separated or allowed to decay before spectral analysis can proceed.

Radionuclide therapy. Therapy of diseases by the intracavitary, intravenous, oral, or other routes of administration of sealed and unsealed radiopharmaceuticals emitting electrons, γ-rays, or X-rays.

Radiopaque. Material that absorbs most of incident X radiation.

Radiopharmaceutical. A sterile, pyrogen-free radionuclide or radioactively tagged compound administered to a patient for diagnostic or therapeutic purposes. A radiopharmaceutical has no pharmacological effect because of the small amount of material administered.

Radiopharmaceutical preparation. The designation refers to a substance of a component with one or more radionuclides, which can be administered to humans for diagnosis or therapy.

Radiopharmacology. Study of the properties of radioactive drugs and their therapeutic and diagnostic uses.

Radiopharmacy. Laboratory preparation and dispensing of solutions labeled with radioisotopes for therapeutic and diagnostic purposes.

Radioreceptor assay. A type of radiobinding assay in which the receptor is a structural component of a tissue.

Radioresistance. Relative resistance of cells, tissues, organs, or organisms to the injurious action of radiation. The opposite of radiosensitivity. The term may also be applied to chemical compounds or to any substances.

Radiosensitivity. The relative susceptibility of cells, tissues organs, organisms, and any substances to the injurious action of ionizing radiation. Radioresistance and radiosensitivity are usually employed in a comparative sense, rather than in an absolute one.

Radiosensitizers. All forms of cancer treatment depend for their effectiveness on eliminating cancer cells without causing excessive injury to the surrounding normal tissues because intrinsically, malignant cells are no more radiosensitive than normal cells. Much research effort has been used on designing drugs that will sensitize tumor cells to radiation (radiosensitizers), and on drugs that will protect the normal tissues (radioprotectors). Fully hypoxic cells are some three times more resistant to radiation than well-oxygenated cells. Thus, tumors with such cells are difficult to destroy without causing excessive damage to surrounding well-vascularized, well-oxygenated, and hence radiosensitive normal tissue.

In 1963, Adams and Dewey put forward the hypothesis that the sensitizing action of oxygen was a result of its electron-affinity properties and that its action could be mimicked by other electron-affinic compounds which could substitute for oxygen as electron acceptors at the site of an ionizing event, thus preventing chemical repair of the radical ions produced by the radiation. Many electron-affinic compounds have now been characterized, such as quinones, benzenes, furans, and imidazoles, but the nitroimidazoles, particularly with the nitro group at the 2-position, have proved to be the most effective. Metronidazole and its 2-nitro equivalent Misonidazole radiosensitize hypoxic cells in a wide range of animal tumors and have no effect on well-oxygenated cells.

Radiotherapy. Radiotherapy is that specialty of medicine that uses ionizing radiation and radioactive substances for the treatment of disease. Although ionizing radiations are used to a limited and decreasing extent in the treatment of a number of nonmalignant conditions, their main use in medical treatment is for cancer and allied disease.

Radiothermoluminescence. The reappearance of luminescence in radioluminescent materials brought about by heating. Quartz and certain types of glass show the effect.

Radiotoxicity. The ability of a substance to give rise to adverse biological toxic effects as a result of the ionizing radiation it emits.

Radio wave. Electromagnetic waves of frequencies between 30 kHz and 3 THz propagated without guide in free space.

Radium. Element symbol Ra, atomic number 88, atomic weight 226.025.

Radix. The base of a number system; the number of digit symbols required by a number system. For example, in decimal notation the radix of each place is 10.

Radon. Element symbol Rn, atomic number 86, atomic weight ~222.

Rales. Abnormal breathing sounds heard (usually with a stethoscope) in certain disorders of the lung: rattling, bubbling, whistling, or crackling sounds heard in the chest.

Raman scattering. The appearance of additional weak lines in the spectrum of the light scattered by a substance illuminated by monochromatic light. These lines arise from the increase or decrease of frequency when the incident light quanta lose energy to, or gain energy from, the molecular vibrations of the substance concerned.

Raman spectroscopy. The study of the Raman lines or spectra to gain information on the scattering substance. The lines are characteristic of the molecular species present.

Ramp. The display of all 256 translation table levels in a fixed portion of the video screen; i.e., shows screen contrast and visual levels (color or black and white). A filter function that resembles an incline plane in frequency space.

Ramp filter. A high-pass filter that enchances the edges of the radioactive distribution in the image. Intuitively, the reconstruction process known as filtered backprojection may be thought of as first extracting the edges of a three-dimensional radioactive source from different angles and, second, backprojecting the edges from the different angles to generate the count distribution in a transaxial tomogram. The Ramp filter, being a high-pass filter that linearly enhances higher frequencies, yields the highest resolution possible in a reconstruction but also propagates the high frequency noise associated with low count statistics. This propagation of noise often results in images which are difficult to interpret clinically.

Random access. Access to data in which the next location from which data are to be obtained is not dependent on the location of previously obtained data.

Random access memory. (RAM) A kind of internal memory whose locations can be accessed and the contents retrieved with the same access time for all locations. Usually refers to electronic (as opposed to magnetic) internal memory.

Random coincidence. When two or more counters are connected in coincidence an output signal is obtained when each counter records an event within a certain time interval. The system is designed to record real or true coincidences due to related events; e.g., when one particle passes through each counter in turn. A certain number of coincidences are recorded, however, due to unrelated events. These are called random coincidences.

Random sampling. A method of selecting a sample which gives every element in the population a known opportunity (probability) of being selected for the sample.

Range. When an energetic, charged, nuclear particle passes through matter it loses energy and eventually stops. The energy is lost mainly by the ionization and excitation of the atoms and molecules in the absorbing material. For charged particles heavier than the electron the particle undergoes a very large number of collisions with the atoms or molecules, in each of which a small amount of energy is lost and in which the particle is not appreciably deflected. Hence most of the charged particles of a given energy travel approximately the same distance and so have a fairly well-defined range.

Range-energy relation. An expression giving the range of an energetic particle in matter as a function of the energy of the particle.

Range equation. Relationship between round-trip wound pulse travel time and distance to a reflector.

Range resolution of ultrasound. The smallest separation of two objects that can be distinguished along the axis of the ultrasound beam. It is roughly twice the wavelength of the ultrasound.

Rare earth. Any of the series of very similar metals ranging in atomic number from 57 through 71.

Raster effect. An effect arising from the construction of an image by a series of many closely paced parallel lines. The resolution of such an image can be altered by the discrete thickness and separation of these lines.

Raster graphics. The technique of constructing a picture out of a pattern of parallel scan lines. This technique is used by television sets and most computer display screens.

Raster scanning. The scanning of a plane by repetitive parallel movements of a probe in the same direction across the plane.

Ratemeter. An instrument that detects and displays a time-averaged count rate of radioactivity viewed by a detector.

Raw data. Information waiting to be processed by a computer. Before they can be processed, raw data are first converted to punch cards, magnetic tape, disk, or some other form a computer can accept.

Ray. A narrow band of radioisotopic activity extending outward from, and perpendicular to, the axis of rotation. The width of this band is determined by how well the object is digitized. If the effects of attenuation are ignored, the count rate at any point on the camera face will be proportional to the amount of activity along the ray originating at that point.

Rayleigh scattering. Scattering of a photon or

particle in which no energy is transferred. An elastic collision sometimes referred to as coherent or unmodified scattering.

Reaction. Any process resulting in a net change to the constituents of the system.

Reaction energy. (Q_0) In the disintegration of a nuclear reaction, the reaction energy is equal to the sum of the kinetic or radiant energies of the reactants minus the sum of the kinetic or radiant energies of the products. (If any product of a specified reaction is in an excited nuclear state, the energy of subsequently emitted gamma radiation is not included in the sum.) The ground-state nuclear reaction energy is the reaction energy when all reactant and product nuclei are in their ground states.

Reaction rate. In a nuclear reactor the number of nuclei undergoing fission per unit time.

Reactivity. A parameter, ρ, giving the deviation from criticality of a nuclear chain reacting medium such that positive values correspond to a supercritical state and negative values to a subcritical state. Quantitatively, $\rho = 1 - 1/k_{eff}$, where k_{eff} is the effective multiplication factor.

Reactor core. The central portion of a nuclear reactor containing the nuclear fuel, such as uranium or plutonium, and the moderator, if any.

Reactor fuel. The fissionable material employed as the source of energy in a reactor. It consists of a fissionable isotope of uranium or plutonium.

Reactor fuel elements. Heterogeneous reactor fuel elements consist of a core of fissionable material contained in a diluent and cladded in a suitable container to protect the fuel from corrosion and prevent the fission products from contaminating the coolant.

Reactor moderator coolants. In most nuclear reactors separate moderators and coolants are employed, but in some designs it is convenient to use the same material both as moderator and coolant. An example is the water-moderated reactor, where the water is employed both as the moderator and coolant. This is possible because both kinds of water (light water and heavy water) are both good moderators as well as good coolants.

Reactor safety considerations. Because of the great potential hazard associated with the operation of nuclear reactors it is not feasible to base considerations of reactor safety upon an analysis of failures and accidents. Instead, it is necessary to deduce the likely behavior of the system under fault conditions by extrapolation from current engineering knowledge supported by theoretical analysis experimental investiga-

tion, and by a study of the available operating experience.

Such work has led to the following objectives in safe design. First, it is necessary to reduce the radiation exposure to individuals during the normal operation; second, it is necessary to reduce the probability that the reactor gets accidentally into a condition outside its safe operating range; third, the design should be such as to reduce the effect of any fault condition on the reactor and its operators; and finally, if an uncontrollable accident occurs the containment building design should be capable of limiting any leakage of radioactivity.

Reactor safety fuse. A self-contained device designed to respond to excessive temperature or flux in a reactor and to act to reduce the reaction rate to a safe level. The device may or may not contain stored energy to facilitate its operation.

Reactor vessel. The container of a reactor and its moderator, if any, and coolant.

Read. To retrieve data or an instruction from some computer storage location or medium.

Read-only input. (ROI) Input only from the memory or from an internal source.

Read-only memory. (ROM) A form of computer memory which holds information that cannot be changed under computer operation, and which can only be read by a computer. In other words, it is the memory from which it is possible to read information but onto which data cannot be written.

Readout. A method of presenting a total count or rate of detected radiation events.

Read/write. The venetian blind effect produced on an analog scan converter image to enable the image to be visualized while it is being written.

Read/write head. Electromagnetic device that reads, records, or erases information on magnetic tape, disk, or drum.

Read/write memory. A type of computer memory in which the contents can be erased and changed. Random access memory (RAM), magnetic tapes, and floppy disks are all examples of read/write memory.

Reagent. Any chemical used in a process.

Reagin. Antibodies of the class IgE which are responsible for allergies and anaphylaxis.

Real image. Image formed by converging rays which form a focused image in space.

Real space. The three-dimensional space we know naturally, when described by the mathematician, is called real space, configuration space, or Cartesian space, and describes the object density or activity in terms of x, y, z coordinates or in terms of a radius (r), elevation or height, and azimuthal angle.

Real time. Time scale determined by the environment in which the computer operates. In real time working the computer accepts and processes data at effectively the same rate as they are generated. Frequently, the computer is interacting with a human; as long as the computer responds at a rate of about 10 Hz, it will appear instantaneous to the user.

Real-time display. A device whose image is continuously renewed so that it keeps space with changes in the object, and in which storage or processing time does not delay the image presentation appreciably.

Real-time subtraction. Digital subtraction of images as they are generated; i.e., no delay between image production and the display of the subtracted image.

Real-time ultrasonic scanning. This is an ultrasound technique which produces a moving picture at the time of scanning. The expression "real time" is an unfortunate use of a computer term which relates to the immediate processing and presentation of information. Real-time scanners include linear array scanners, electronic sector scanners, rocking and rotating transducer types, and moving mirror scanners. Most impact has been made by those with no moving parts. The picture quality with most real-time scanners appears inferior to the classical hand-operated b-scanner. However, it now seems as if the overall information gained by the operator is greater using the new types of scanner, partly due to the more positive appreciation of the scanning plane, but mostly due to the extra prompts and landmarks provided by moving structures which enable better identification of organs.

Reasonableness checks. A means of protecting systems by testing the data or signals that enter or exit the system for conformity to ranges or tables of acceptable values.

Receive only. (RO) A computer terminal with a page printer only and no keyboard or transmission capability.

Receiver. Portion of the NMR apparatus that detects and amplifies radio-frequency (rf) signals picked up by the receiving coil. Includes a preamplifier, amplifier, and demodulator.

Receiver coil. Coil, or antenna, positioned within the magnet bore to detect the NMR signal: sometimes also used for excitation.

Receptor. A chemical compound on a cell mem-

brane or in a cell that binds other chemicals, e.g., hormones: neurotransmitter anatomical structures that respond to stimuli such as heat, touch pressure, pain.

Receptor modulation. The patching, capping, and endocytosis of cell surface receptors induced by treatment with excess ligand.

Recessive. A term applied to genes which have relatively little phenotypic effect.

Recipe. (Rx, symbol for latin recipe) Used as a symbol for therapy; also used to indicate a therapeutically useful radiopharmaceutical.

Receiver operating characteristic analysis. (ROC) A graph illustrating the correctness of decisions as a function of the criteria used to make the decision. Used for choosing the best criteria and indicating the value of additional diagnostic information.

Recoil. The motion imparted to a particle as a result of interaction with radiation or as a result of a nuclear transformation.

Recoil electron. An electron that has acquired its motion through a collision with another particle or through the emission of radiation.

Recoil nucleus. A nucleus that has acquired its motion either through being struck by a nuclear particle or through the emission of radiation.

Recoil particle. A particle that has acquired its motion through a collision with another particle or through the emission of radiation.

Recoil proton. The predominant method of energy loss of fast neutrons up to 20 MeV in tissue is by elastic collision with the nuclei of hydrogen atoms. In such a collision an average of half the neutron energy is given to the nucleus, which is referred to as a recoil or knock-on proton.

Recombination. The rearrangement process which brings about combinations of genes in an offspring not present in the parents, usually due to gene or chromosome crossover at meiosis. The disappearance of positive and negative ions by mutual neutralization.

Recombination coefficient. The recombination coefficient of an ionized material is the coefficient A in the expression An + n – for the rate at which pairs of positive and negative ions present at densities n+ and n–, respectively, neutralize each other.

Reconstructed system spatial resolution. The spatial resolution of a single photon emission computerized tomography (SPECT) system is measured for reconstructed slices transverse to three-line source, located in a cylindrical, water-filled phantom.

Reconstruction from projections imaging.
NMR imaging technique in which a set of projection profiles of the body is obtained by observing NMR signals in the presence of a suitable corresponding set of gradient magnetic fields. Images can then be reconstructed using techniques analogous to those used in conventional computed tomography (CT), such as filtered backprojection. It can be used for volume imaging, or with plane selection techniques, for sequential plane imaging.

Reconstruction image. An image representing a two-dimensional slice of a structure, reconstructed from data obtained via any of the tomographic techniques.

Record. A collection of related items of data treated as a unit; for example, a line of source code or a person's name, rank, and serial number.

Recording density. The density of magnetized spots (each representing a single piece of information or "bit") on the surface of magnetic storage media such as tapes, disks, and drums. The rate at which data can be recorded on the tape depends on the recording density and the speed of the tape drive.

Recovery. (Radiobiology) The return toward normal of a particular cell, tissue, or organism, after radiation injury. Restoration of a computer system to its former condition after it has switched to a fallback mode of operation when the cause of the fallback has been removed. The recovery process can involve updating information in the files to produce two copies of the file.

Recovery rate. The rate at which recovery takes place following radiation injury. It may proceed at different rates for different tissues. Differential recovery rate: among tissues recovering at different rates those having slower rates will ultimately suffer greater damage from a series of successive irradiations. This differential effect is taken advantage of in fractionated radiation therapy if the neoplastic tissues have a slower recovery rate than surrounding normal structures.

Recovery time. The time, following detection of a pulse, which must elapse before a second pulse can be detected. Also called resolving time or coincidence time.

Rectilinear scanner. The rectilinear scanner is a moving detector imaging system that produces a two-dimensional image, which represents the three-dimensional distribution of radioactivity within an organ structure. The image is a pattern of dots on film, the density of which corresponds to the relative concentration of the radionuclide in the organ of interest. The rectilinear scanner can have either a single probe or a dual probe. While dual-probe scanners have synchronously moving but axially opposed detectors designed so that a patient can be placed between the two detectors, the single-probe unit has but one detector that scans the organ structure of interest. In the conventional mechanical scanner, a system of motors and controls moves the detector mechanically on a boustrophedonic raster (i.e., in a rectilinear fashion). The shielded crystal mechanically advances across the field of interest, increments a specific but constant distance (line spacing) down the patient, and then moves back across the patient. During this process, the readout system moves in synchrony with the detector. The pattern is repeated until the small focal region of the collimator has swept across the entire field of interest. While the focusing collimator scans the distribution of radioactivity, the detector converts the radiation transmitted by the collimator into electrical pulses, which can be further amplified and treated by the electronic components of the scanner. The readout system presents the processed information in a form suitable for visual interpretation. Although the rectilinear scanners have been superseded by an array of sophisticated gamma cameras, the term "scan" which was coined during its use remains as a synonym of scintigraphy or image (i.e., scan, NMR scan, bone scan, etc.).

Recycle. Any material or stream returned to an operation for further processing.

Red blood cell. (RBC) Blood cell containing hemoglobin; erythrocyte.

Red-green-blue (RGB) interface. A kind of interface used between computers and certain color monitors. It uses a separate wire to send image information for each color (red, green, and blue). It tends to produce a higher quality image than a composite video interface.

Redox. Abbreviation for an oxidation-reduction reaction.

Reducing agent. Substance that donates electrons in an oxidation-reduction reaction.

Reduction. Decrease in positive oxidation number; gain in number of electrons by an atom or group of atoms. The opposite of oxidation.

Redundancy. In data transmission, the portion

of characters and bits that can be eliminated without losing information.

Redundancy check. A hardware or software check based on the systematic insertion of components or characters used especially for checking purposes.

Redundant shadows. Unwanted images of planes above and below the objective plane.

Reference source. A radioactive source used as a reference for setting up assay equipment.

Reference test. A test of an instrument whose results provide a measure against which future performance of the instrument may be comprehensively assessed.

Reflection. Partition of the energy of an ultrasound beam incident on an interface accompanied by reversal of the normal (to the interface) component of the incident wave vector. Acoustic energy is reflected from a structure where there is a discontinuity in the characteristic acoustic impedance along the propagation path. The intensity of the reflection is related to the ratio of the characteristic acoustic impedances across the interface. The angle of the reflection from a plane interface which is largely compared to the acoustic wavelength is equal to the angle (between the wave vector and normal to the interface) of the incident wave in accordance with Snell's Law.

Reflection angle. Angle between reflected sound direction and line perpendicular to media boundary.

Reflector. An extra layer of moderator or other material outside the reactor core which acts as a reflector for some of the neutrons which would otherwise escape. Media boundary that produces a reflection; reflecting surface.

Reflex. Sum total of any involuntary activity in response to particular stimuli; often a jerk of muscles.

Reflex arc. The pathway involved in a reflex and consisting of a receptor, an afferent nerve, a center, an efferent nerve, and an effector.

Reflux. A backward or return flow.

Reflux study. In gastroenterology, a study done to document reflux of gastric contents into the esophagus; in urology, a study done to document reflux of a substance instilled in the bladder that goes back into the upper urinary tract; in cisternography, a study done to demonstrate cerebrospinal fluid reflux into the ventricular system of the brain.

Reformatting. The retrospective rearrangement of a study's data; the conversion of list mode data to matrix mode.

Refraction. The bending of light rays when passing from one medium into another, e.g., from air into water, from air into the eye. Change of sound direction on passing from one medium to another.

Refractory. Not responding readily to treatment.

Refractory period. The time lapse after the response of a neuron or muscle fiber to an impulse before it can respond again.

Regenerative process. A biological term for the process whereby damaged cells are replaced by new ones of the same type.

Region of interest. (ROI) Outlined area on a computer-processed image, defined automatically or manually with a joystick or light pen to obtain the accepted events in that area. Time-activity curves result when the ROI is sequentially measured in multiple images of a study.

Register. A temporary electronic storage location in which instructions or data are placed while being subject to some arithmetic or other operation. Usually a register has the same bit length as a standard computer word.

Registration. Process by which a given point in tissue is represented as a point at exactly the same depth from the ultrasound transducer face despite different angulation and position of the probe.

Registration error. The misrepresentation of an echo point in a subject which is interpreted as being at different depths when viewed from different angles, caused by: poor scanning motion with uneven pressure, instability of the probe mount, grossly different thicknesses of tissues with different acoustic properties, temperature of transmitting medium, and incorrect system velocity.

Regression. Return to former state; for tumors, a loss in size and return to normal appearance. A form of analysis which expresses the dependence of one variable on other variables.

Regression coefficient. Represents the average unit change of one variable on another variable.

Regression curve. The curve which is the best fit to experimental measurements of two interdependent variables. The best fit means that curve for which the sum of the squares of the deviations of the experimental points from the values predicted by the curve is a minimum.

Regression line. An equation which relates the average y (the dependent variable) to the associated value for x (the independent variable). For linear regression the equation is

$$y_c = a + bx$$

Regulating rod. A control rod intended to accomplish rapid, fine adjustment of the radioactivity of a nuclear reactor. It usually is capable of moving much more rapidly than a shim rod but of making a smaller change in the reactor's reactivity. Its rapid and sometimes continuous readjustment may be accomplished by a servo system.

Regurgitant fraction. A quantitative measure of the severity of the valvular lesion in patients with mitral or aortic regurgitation (backflow of blood into the heart or between the chambers of the heart). The regurgitant fraction equals the amount of blood regurgitated divided by the total stroke output of the left ventricle. In normal subjects this is zero, but in patients with severe mitral insufficiency or aortic regurgitation, it can approach 80%.

Regurgitation. The flow in the opposite direction to normal of a substance such as food or blood; for example, the backward flow of blood through a defective valve.

Rejection. A technique to improve the apparent signal-to-noise ratio by eliminating low amplitude signals from a display. This technique emphasizes strong echoes at the expense of weaker echoes. Eliminating smaller-amplitude voltage pulses. Immune reaction against transplanted tissue.

Rejection region. α region or tail(s) of the null hypothesis curve.

Rejection response. An immune response with both humoral and cellular components directed against transplanted tissue.

Relative address. Computer memory location found by searching in the vicinity of an instruction.

Relative biological effectiveness. (RBE) An expression of the effectiveness of absorbed doses of different types of radiation, e.g., X-rays, neutrons, alpha particles. In general, the RBE may vary with the kind and degree of biologic effect considered, the duration of the exposure, and other factors. In general the higher the linear energy transfer (LET) of the radiation, i.e., the energy dissipated per unit distance along the track of an ionizing particle, the greater is the biological effect produced by a dose of 1 gray. Dense ionization, and hence LET, is associated with heavy particles (i.e., protons, deuterons, α-particles, etc.), and these therefore tend to produce more biological ef-

fect per gray than X- and γ-rays, or electrons. The relative biological effectiveness of an ionizing radiation is defined as the dose of 250 kV X radiation which will produce the same biological effect as 1 gray of the radiation in question. It should be emphasized that the RBE may have different values for the same radiation depending on the type of biological effect used as the criterion. In clinical radiotherapy it has been found that the RBE for X- or γ-rays above 0.4 MeV lies between 0.8 and 0.9. For neutrons and other heavy particles it may be as high as 10 or 20.

Relative flow value. A term used in paper chromatography to express the relative speeds of migration of the individual components of mixtures through the chromatographic paper-separating medium.

Relative humidity. The ratio of the quantity of water vapor present in the atmosphere to the quantity which would saturate at the existing temperature. It is also the ratio of the pressure of water vapor present to the pressure of saturated water vapor at the same temperature.

Relative refractory period. The brief portion of the depolarization-repolarization cycle during which the membrane potential is approaching the threshold level, and myocardial fibers may respond to a stronger-than-normal stimulus.

Relative sensitivity. Relative sensitivity refers to the ability of a scintigraphic instrument with a given collimator to register a certain fraction of the γ-rays emitted from a radioactive source.

Relativistic mass. The increased mass associated with a particle when its velocity is increased. The increase in mass becomes appreciable only at velocities approaching the velocity of light, 3×10^{10} cm/s.

Relativistic particle. A particle having a speed comparable to that of light so that the relativistic mass is substantially greater than the rest mass.

Relativistic velocity. A speed, approaching that of light, for which relativistic effects are important.

Relativity. The theory of relativity, introduced by Einstein in 1905, allows for the effect of the velocity of light in assessing the size and motion of fast-moving objects.
The special theory of relativity deals with objects moving at constant relative velocity and shows that the effect is apparently to foreshorten bodies that are moving with a speed, relative to the observer, comparable with that of light. Also, there is an increase of apparent

mass of the object and the time scale is different from that observed on the moving body. The effects are not apparent to observers moving with the object but are a result of the finite time taken for light to travel through space.

Relaxation. A process by which atoms or molecules in an excited state return to their ground state (or lower energy state).

Relaxation rates. Spin-lattice relaxation rate $R_2 = (1/T_1)$. Spin-spin relaxation rate $R_1 = (1/T_2)$. Inverse of relaxation times. (NMR.)

Relaxation times. After excitation, nuclei tend to return to their equilibrium distribution in which the longitudinal magnetization is at its maximum value and oriented in the direction of the static magnetic field, the value of the transverse magnetization being zero. On cessation of the radio-frequency (rf) excitation pulse, the longitudinal magnetization Mz return toward the equilibrium value M_0 at a rate characterized by the time constant T_1, and any transverse magnetization decays towards zero with a time constant T_2 (or T_2^* in the real situation). (NMR.)

Relay. Electromechanical switch.

Reliability. The extent to which a system yields the same results on repeated trials.

Relocate. In computer programming, to move a routine from one portion of storage to another and to adjust the necessary address references so that the routine, in its new location, can be executed.

Remission. A diminution or abatement of symptoms; temporary or permanent.

Remote job entry. A process for permitting batch input of programs and/or data to a computer system in situations in which the user is distant from the computer. Data or programs to be transmitted are assembled into messages following one or another industry-standard format and are transmitted according to a standard protocol. Usually methods are employed for detecting errors and initiating retransmission when errors are detected. Ordinarily, at least a small processor and local storage devices (internal memory and/or small secondary memory devices) are employed to optimally use the long-distance communications link.

Remote maintenance. Maintenance of radioactive or contaminated equipment by means of a manipulator operated from a shielded position.

Remote processing. The use of a computer for processing data transmitted from remote locations.

Remote sequelae. Effects which occur after an extended period of time and are very slow in occurrence.

Renal clearance. The rate of removal by the kidneys of a substance from the plasma per unit of concentration of the substance.

Renal threshold. The plasma concentration at which a substance is excreted in the urine.

Renin. An enzyme-like substance secreted by the kidney.

Renogram. Plot of radioactivity measured by an external detector vs. time as a radiotracer transits through the kidneys; although ^{131}I-hippuran was the tracer originally used, a number of other radiopharmaceuticals, such as ^{123}I-hippuran and ^{99m}Tc-DTPA, may be used.

Repeated free induction decay. Another term for saturation recovery. A sequence in which 90° pulses are repeated for excitation and measurement. It results in partial saturation if the period between the 90° pulses is of the order of T_1 or less and gives a T_1 weighted signal. Generally the term is only applied where the signal is detected as an free induction decay (FID) (and not as an echo). (NMR.)

Repeater. A device that amplifies, reconstitutes, or reshapes signals to acceptable levels for retransmission.

Repetition time. Period between the beginning of a pulse sequence and the start of the succeeding sequence.

Rephasing gradient. Gradient magnetic field applied for a brief period after a selective excitation pulse, in the opposite direction to the gradient used for the selective excitation. The result of the gradient reversal is a rephasing of the spins (which will have gotten out of phase with each other along the direction of the selection gradient), forming an echo by "time reversal", and improving the sensitivity of imaging after the selective excitation process. (NMR.)

Replacement reaction. Chemical process in which an ion is replaced by another species in a compound.

Replicate. Identical sample.

Repolarization. The return of the cell membrane potential to the negative resting potential following depolarization; recharging of myocardial cells so they may again respond to stimulation.

Reprocessing. The procedure of removing fission products from fuel before reusing it. One main aim is to remove poisons which would absorb and waste neutrons; another is to remove mechanical stresses due to irradiation especially in the case of metallic fuels.

Research reactor. A reactor whose primary purpose is use as a research tool, for which it may supply neutrons, other particles, and gamma radiation. It will include special provision for exposing samples (which may include living organisms) to these fluxes and may have provision for the production of transmutation products as well as various special experimental facilities.

Resection. Excision or removal of a portion of an organ or structure.

Reset. To return a computer storage device or register to zero.

Resident. Any program permanently stored in the main memory of the computer. Some resident programs include: the editor, a program designed to handle test; the assembler, a program that converts programming language into binary code; the debugger, a program that eliminates software errors.

Residual dose equivalent. The dose equivalent remaining after correction for such physiological recovery as has occurred at a specific time. It is based on the ability of the body to recover to some degree from radiation injury following exposure. It is used only to predict immediate effects.

Residual nucleus. According to Nils Bohr's theory of nuclear reactions, when a particle strikes a target nucleus it fuses with it to form an excited compound nucleus which exists for some time before decaying by the emission of a second particle. The nucleus remaining finally is called the residual nucleus.

Residual range. The range of an energetic charged heavy nuclear particle that has already lost some of its energy in passing through matter.

Residual volume. The volume of air remaining in the lungs after a maximum expiration (about 1.2 l) of urine in the bladder, etc.

Resistive magnet. An electromagnet that uses wires with sufficient electrical resistance so that there is considerable loss of power in terms of generation of heat in the conduction wires rather than conversion into magnetic field.

Resolution. Ability of a detection system to separate, or discriminate, quantities very close to each other. Example: a γ-ray spectrometer separating energy levels (lines); an optical system or radioisotope imaging system distinguishing between a single source and two neighboring sources. Resolution is a measure of how much detail a graphics device can print or display.

Resolution recovery. Data manipulation technique involving subtraction of a highly smoothed image from the original image, itself perhaps slightly smoothed.

Resolving power. Resolving power refers to the ability of the imaging device to produce and display images, discernible as separate entities, from an array of radioactive sources. Resolving power is expressed as the maximum spatial frequency, in line pairs per cm (cm^{-1}), which may be discerned on the image of a bar phantom.

Resolving time. The smallest time interval which must elapse between the occurrence of two consecutive ionizing events or signal pulses in order that the measuring device be capable of producing an identical response to each of them separately.

Resonance. A vibration of large amplitude caused by a relatively small periodic stimulus of the same or nearly the same period as the natural vibration period of the system. In NMR experiments, the frequency of the radio-frequency (rf) waves have to match the Larmor frequency of the nuclei in the magnetic field to create resonance phenomenon. Energy is then transferred from the rf field to the nucleus.

Resonance capture. A nuclear reaction involving the capture of a particle of specific energy by a resonance level of a nucleus. The nucleus presents a very large cross section to particles possessing this particular energy.

Resonance energy. The kinetic energy (measured with respect to the laboratory system) of a particle that makes the total energy of the system composed of the incident particle and the target nucleus close to the energy of a resonance level of the compound nucleus.

Resonance neutron. Neutrons having kinetic energy in the resonance energy range, that is, in the range for which the resonance level structure is evident from the variations in cross sections with energy.

Resonance region. A neutron energy region in which the neutron cross sections of many nuclides exhibit successive maxima due to resonance energy levels for neutron interactions.

Resonance scattering. The reemission of a neutron after it has formed a compound nucleus at a resonance level. If, following reemission, the residual nucleus is not in an excited state, the process is energetically identical to elastic scattering.

Resonance strength function. For resonance

levels excited in a specified nuclide by neutrons, the average reduced neutron width of the resonances divided by the mean level spacing.

Resonance width. Level width, measured in energy units, with reference to a nuclear state only.

Resonant frequency. Frequency at which resonance phenomenon occurs; given by the Larmor equation for NMR; determined by inductance and capacitance for radio-frequency (rf) circuits.

Resource. Any hardware or software capabilities offered by a computer system. For example, file management problems, the central processing unit, and the line printer are all resources. The major concerns with resources are that they be available and that they be utilized as completely as possible so that one can get the maximum amount of work out of them.

Respiration. The exchange of oxygen and carbon dioxide between the air and the cells of the body.

Respiration flow measurements. A measurement of the rate at which air is inspired or expired. Range: 250 to 3000 ml/s, peak. Frequency response: 0 to 20 Hz. Used to determine breathing rate, minute volume, depth of respiration. Measured by pneumotachometer or as the derivative of volume measurement.

Respiration volume. Measurement of quantity of air breathed in or out during a single breathing cycle or over a given period of time. Frequency response required: 0 to 10 Hz. Used for determination of various respiration functions. Measure by integration of respiration flow-rate measurements or by collection of expired air over a given period. Indirect measurement by belt transducer, impedance pneumograph, or whole-body plethysmograph.

Respiratory alkalosis. Alkalosis resulting from hyperventilation that results in depletion of carbon dioxide dissolved in the blood.

Respiratory center. The center in the medulla oblongata that controls breathing.

Respiratory quotient. Ratio of volume of exhaled CO_2 to the volume of consumed O_2 (0.85).

Respiratory system. The group of organs concerned with the exchange of oxygen and carbon dioxide in organisms. In higher animals this consists successively of the air passages through the mouth, nose, and throat, the trachea, the bronchi, the bronchioles, and the alveoli of the lungs.

Respiratory time quotient. Ratio of the time of expiration to the time of inspiration.

Response time. The system reaction time to given input. The time interval between pressing the send key of a computer terminal and the display of the first character of the system's reply.

Responsible person. A suitably qualified and acceptable person, designated by the holder of the authority and directly responsible for radiation protection.

Resting potential. The potential difference across the membrane of a resting cell due to an excess of positive ions outside and negative ions inside.

Rest mass. The mass m_0 of a particle at rest. It represents the Newtonian mass and does not include the additional mass acquired by a particle in motion by the relativistic effect.

Restricted area. Place in which there is a possibility of radiation or contamination at a level exceeding that which is permissible for exposure of the general public.

Retention. In nuclear terminology that fraction of atoms undergoing a nuclear transformation which remains in, or reverts to, its initial chemical condition.

Reticulocyte. A nonnucleated, immature red blood cell (erythrocyte), normally making up 0.5 to 2.0% of red blood cells in peripheral blood.

Reticuloendothelial system. A mononuclear phagocytic system located primarily in the reticular connective tissue framework of the spleen, liver, and lymphoid tissues.

Reticulum. A fine network of filaments or fibrils either within a cell in the intracellular matrix.

Retina. A layer of photosensitive receptor cells and associated neurons, in which the incident patterns of light are encoded into nerve pulses for onward transmission along the optic nerves to the visual areas of the brain.

Reverberation. The phenomenon of multiple reflections caused by the re-echoing of signals within a closed system, thereby presenting false information. Multiple reflections may be identified in an image by moving the ultrasound transducer relative to the object. The multiple reflections will move a distance on the display which is equivalent to twice the incremental distance, while the first multiple reflection moves a distance equivalent to four times the increment. Artefact usually best seen in cystic spaces.

Reynold's number. A dimensionless parameter

of importance in fluid flow, given by $\rho ul/\mu$, where u is the fluid speed, ρ the fluid density, l a characteristic length, and μ the viscosity. It is an expression of the ratio of the inertial forces to the viscous forces governing fluid flow.

Rhenium. Element symbol Re, atomic number 75, atomic weight 186.2.

Rhodium. Element symbol Rh, atomic number 45, atomic weight 102.905.

Ribonucleic acid. (RNA) A complex, usually threadlike polymer composed of repeating units of adenine, guanine, cytosine, and uracil. Several types of RNA are known, all essential to the production of proteins. These are messenger RNA, ribosomal RNA, and transfer or soluble RNA. Responsible for transmission of inherited traits.

Ribosomes. Minute particles found in the cytoplasm of cells. They are composed of ribonucleic acid (RNA) and protein, and are the intracellular site for protein synthesis.

Rig. Colloquial term for an experimental assembly into which material specimens can be placed and then subjected to irradiation under selected and controlled environments of temperature, pressure, type of coolant, stress, etc.

Right. (Legal) That which a man is entitled to have, or to do, or to receive from others, by custom, by law, or by agreement. There is no right unless there is an identifiable person with a duty to satisfy the desire.

Ring topology. A configuration of computers connected by one circular communications link.

Rise time. The time taken for an electronic impulse to reach some specified fractions of its maximum amplitude.

Risk. (Legal) The probability of injury. It is in the power of the physician to decrease or increase this probability by care, or lack of it, in a given circumstance. This is the basis for liability.

Risk factor. A factor statistically linked to some event such that the presence of the factor can be said to increase the risk that the event will occur.

Rocket electrophoresis. An electroimmunodiffusion technique in which antigen is electrophoresed into agar containing specific antibody and precipitates in a tapered rocket-shaped pattern (Laurell technique). This technique is used for quantitation of antigens.

Rod. A relatively long and slender body of material used in or in conjunction with a nuclear reactor. It may contain fuel, absorber, or fertile materials or other material in which activation or transmutation is desired.

Rod-type fuel elements. Solid rods containing fuel which are employed in heterogeneous reactors; they are arranged in lattice formation and separated by a moderator.

Roentgen. (R) A non-SI unit of radiation exposure. Defined as that quantity of X or gamma radiation such that the associated corpuscular emission per 0.001293 g of air produces in air ions carrying 1 ESU of quantity of electricity of either sign. For a wide range of radiation energies, 1 R will result in an absorbed dose in soft tissue of approximately 1 rad. The roentgen is equivalent to 2.58×10^{-4} C/kg air.

Roentgen equivalent man. (REM) Non-SI unit of dose equivalent. The dose in rems is equal to the absorbed dose in rads multiplied by appropriate modifying factors aimed at expressing different types of radiation and different distributions to absorbed dose on a common scale related to the possible long-term radiation risks. For many radiations, including X-, gamma, and beta radiation, and for most dose distributions, the modifying factor is unity and rems and rads are numerically equal. 1 rem = 0.01 sievert (Sv).

Roentgen equivalent physical. (REP) The amount of ionizing radiation which is capable of producing 1.615×10^{12} ion pairs per gram of tissue or that amount which will be absorbed by tissue to the extent of 93 ergs/g. This obsolete non-SI unit was used to measure beta radiation.

Roentgenogram. A processed photographic film which has been exposed to X-rays after their passage through tissues as part of the diagnostic examination.

Roentgenography. Radiography by means of X-rays.

Roentgenology. That part of radiology which pertains to X-rays.

Roentgen ray. Electromagnetic radiation produced when a beam of high-speed electrons collides with a solid metal target, as in an X-ray tube; includes both characteristic X-rays and bremsstrahlung. Synonym for X-ray.

Roll in, roll out. To roll in is to carry out a process in a computer by bringing parts of the process into main memory in sequence. To roll out is to remove a process from main memory. This technique is used when computers have to shift quickly from one process to another.

Root directory. The first directory defined on a computer disk. All files and subdirectories on a disk must be stored in the root directory or in subdirectories that can be traced back to the root directory.

Rotate. A computer instruction that causes the "bits" in a word to shift a certain number of places to the left or to the right. If a word is shifted to the right, for example, the bits at the right end of the word get pushed off and reappear at the other end.

Rotating frame. In NMR experiments, the effects of external radio-frequency (rf) field on the precessing nuclear magnetic moments are studies in detail. As a reference, a coordinate system is chosen with its Z axis in the same direction as the applied magnetic field. If the motion of the precessing moments is viewed from the coordinate system which is also rotating around the magnetic field at the same Larmor frequency and in the same direction as the precessing nuclear moments, the motion is much simpler.

Rotating frame of reference. A frame of reference (with corresponding coordinate systems) that is rotating about the axis of the static magnetic field B_0 (with respect to a stationary ["laboratory"] frame of reference) at a frequence equal to that of the applied radio-frequency (rf) magnetic field, B_1. Although B_1 is a rotating vector, it appears stationary in the rotating frame, leading to simpler mathematical formulations. (NMR.)

Rotating frame zeugmatography. Technique of NMR imaging that uses a gradient of the radio-frequency (rf) excitation field (to give a corresponding variation of the flip angle along the gradient as a means of encoding the spatial location of spins in the direction of the rf field gradient) in conjunction with a static gradient magnetic field (to give spatial encoding in an orthogonal direction). It can be considered to be a form of Fourier transform imaging.

Rotating slant hole collimator. All holes oriented 60° with crystal. Multiple static images are obtained as the collimator is rotated 360° in 60° increments. Subsequent computer reconstruction produces tomographic images.

Rotation therapy. Radiation therapy during which either the patient is rotated before the source or radiation is revolved around the patient. In this way, a larger dose is built up at the center of rotation within the patient's body than on any area of the skin.

Route. The process of directing a data message to the appropriate line and terminal, based on information contained in the message header.

Routine. A self-contained collection of program statements that perform some very specific subsection of an overall program. The same routine may be invoked numerous times within the same program. Thus it is useful to separate routines from the main body of a program, so that routines can be invoked many times without the necessity of repeating their statements many times.

Routine/subroutine. A section or subsection of program which carries out one part of a given task; e.g., a routine may be written to regulate the input of data with a subroutine to check the values for consistency.

Routine test. A procedure, to be carried out at regular intervals, whereby a few attributes of an instrument or of a radiopharmaceutical are checked to ensure that the performance of the instrument has not altered or that the radiopharmaceuticals can be expected to meet given specifications.

RS-232C interface. A kind of serial interface used by many peripherals and computers. The terms "RS-232C interface" and "serial interface" are often used interchangeably, although an RS-232C interface is actually a specific type of serial interface.

Rubidium. Element symbol Rb, atomic number 37, atomic weight 85.4678.

Run. A single, continuous execution of a computer program.

Runaway reactor. An increase in power or reactivity of such a nature that it cannot be controlled by the normal control system (although it may be terminated safely by the emergency shutdown system). Usually the term implies the presence of an autocatalytic effect, i.e., a positive power coefficient of reactivity.

Ruthenium. Element symbol Ru, atomic number 44, atomic weight 101.07.

Rutherford. An obsolete unit of radioactivity equivalent to 10^6 disintegrations per second. A quantity of a nuclide having an activity of one rutherford.

Rutherford backscattering spectroscopy. A materials analysis technique used to obtain depth profiling information about chemical elements in a sample.

Rydberg constant. A fundamental constant (R) which enters into the wave-number formula for all atomic spectra, and equal to $2\pi me^4/ch^3$ for a hypothetical atom of infinite mass, where m is the rest mass of the electron, e is the electronic charge, c is the velocity of light, and h is Planck's constant.

S

Sac. Pouch, bag-like structure; sacculus — little bag.

Saddle coil. Radio-frequency (rf) coil configuration design commonly used when the static magnetic field is coaxial with the axis of the coil along the long axis of the body (e.g., superconducting magnets and most resistive magnets) as opposed to solenoid or surface coil. (NMR.)

Safety rod. A neutron-absorbing rod which, in an emergency, can in a fraction of a second be put into and shut down a nuclear reactor. It is normally operated by gravity so as to be independent of power supply.

Sagittal. Plane or section parallel to the long axis of the body, arrowlike shape; in an anteroposterior direction.

Saline solution. Consisting of, or containing salt, NACl. Physiologic saline is 0.9% NaCl by weight.

Salt. Any substance that yields ions, other than hydogen or hydroxyl ions. A salt is obtained by displacing the hydrogen of an acid by a metal.

Samarium. Element symbol Sm, atomic number 62, atomic weight 150.36.

Sample. That portion of a population about which information is actually obtained.

Sample preparation. A colloquial phrase to denote any of the steps required to convert specimen material to samples appropriate for a given analytic protocol.

Sample volume. The region in space from which Doppler data are collected for analysis in pulsed/range gated Doppler systems. The size of the sample volume is axially determined by the length of the transmitted acoustic pulse and the length of the range gate. The width is determined by the lateral width of the ultrasound beam.

Sampling angle. The angle of incidence between the direction of flow and the direction of sampling within the imaged plane. This angle may be estimated during the Doppler examination.

Sampling distribution. Frequency distribution of all possible sampling outcomes indicating relative proportion of each.

Sarcolemma. The delicate sheath surrounding a muscle fiber.

Saturation. After exposure to a single radio-frequency (rf) pulse, if T_2 is much shorter than T_1 then the net transverse magnetization will disappear before significant repolarization of the spins occurs. During this time the sample is said to be saturated (NMR). The rate of containing or exhibiting the maximum amount of substance, energy, field, etc., or the action of bringing about that state, e.g., if the rates of upward and downward energy-level transitions are equal, no net energy can be absorbed and the system is said to be saturated.

Saturation activity. The amount of an active isotope present in a given sample after irradiation (e.g., in a nuclear reactor) for an infinite time, when its rate of decay becomes equal to its rate of production.

Saturation analysis. A type of competitive-binding assay where the specific reactor substance-binding sites are all occupied (saturated) with ligand radioimmunoassay (RIA).

Saturation current. If a current ionization chamber is placed near a constant source of radiation (so that ions are produced in the chamber at a constant rate), then as the potential applied between the electrodes is increased from zero a current begins to flow and this rises to a steady value, the saturation current.

Saturation recovery. The repeated free induction decay in NMR sequence using images whose pixel values are proportional to nuclear density and have a T_1 dependence that varies with the repetition time of the sequence.

Saturation transfer. Nuclei can retain their magnetic orientation through a chemical reaction. Thus, if UHF radiation is supplied to the spins at a frequency corresponding to the chemical shift of the nuclei in one chemical state so as to produce saturation or inversion, and chemical reactions transform the nuclei into another chemical state with a different chemical shift in a time short compared to the relaxation time, the NMR spectrum may show the effects of the saturation or inversion on the corresponding, unirradiated line in the spectrum. This technique can be used to study reaction kinetics of suitable molecules, also called inversion transfer.

Saturation voltage. The potential that must be applied between the electrodes of an ionization chamber to achieve saturation.

Scaler. An electronic device which produces an output voltage pulse for a given number of input pulses received. Term generally applied to a device for indicating the total number of observed pulses or events. An instrument that records detected radioactivity as counts.

Scaling circuit. An electronic circuit for counting purposes, e.g., of the number of particles detected.

Scan. Term originally referring to images made of radionuclide distribution obtained with a moving detector that scanned the area of interest by moving back and forth over the area (scanning) in a pattern like mowing a lawn; now refers in general to represent any type of imaging procedure in which anatomic or physiologic information is determined by the use of X-ray or γ photons, ultrasound, or magnetic fields.

Scan converter. Apparatus that stores the Z axis enabling the different amplitudes of the echo signals to be reinterpreted electronically and represented as proportionally different shades of gray on a television monitor.

Scan cross-sectional area. For ultrasound autoscanning systems, means the area on the surface considered, consisting of all points occurring within the beam cross-sectional area of any beam passing through the surface during these scans.

Scandium. Element symbol Sc, atomic number 21, atomic weight 44.956.

Scan line. A line produced on a display by moving a spot (produced by an electron beam) across the face (of the display) at constant speed.

Scanning. The sequential measurement of some quantity at a number of positions on an area, or in a volume either (1) continously, by mechanical movement of the detector, or (2) discontinuously, by means of systematic electrical or mechanical switching.

Scanning camera. An arrangement where a gamma camera and a patient bed move relative to each other, obtaining a whole-body image on a single sheet of film.

Scan projection radiography. A general category of digital radiography including line scanning and point scanning systems.

Scan repetition frequency. The repetition rate of a complete frame, sector, or scan. The term only applies to automatic scanning systems.

Scan repetition period. The inverse of the scan repetition frequency.

Scan speed. The rate of travel of the scanner detector as it traverses the area being visualized.

Scatter correction. Scatter correction is the ability to compensate for photons which have undergone a Compton scattering event in the patient and have continued on to be recorded by the detector. These accepted scattered photons significantly degrade the image during the reconstruction process since they are backprojected along lines different from the original path.

Scattered radiation. Radiation that, through its interaction with matter, has undergone a change or changes in direction. In most cases radiation that has been scattered will have had its energy diminished.

Scatter factor. The ratio of the exposure at a reference point in a phantom to the exposure at the same point in space under similar conditions of irradiation in the absence of the phantom. For radiation up to 400 keV the reference point is taken at the intersection of the central ray with the surface, and the scatter factor is usually called "backscatter factor", while for radiation above 400 keV, the reference point is taken at the position of the peak dose. In measuring the scatter factor the phantom should have a cross section of 30×30 cm and extend at least 10 cm beyond the depth at which the factor is being measured.

Scattering. In nuclear physics the term scattering is applied to any process in which a particle collides with a nucleus and the same kind of particle emerges after the encounter. The definition also requires that no other particles are emitted at the time of the collision, for this would change the nuclear species and the process would then be a nuclear disintegration.

The diffuse reflection, refraction, or diffraction of ultrasound in many directions from irregular surfaces or inhomogeneities within a medium. The discontinuities are dimensionally comparable to or smaller than an acoustic wavelength; e.g., small spheres in the path of a plane wave give rise to complex reflection, refraction, and diffraction behavior called scattering. In an ultrasonic visualization system, by far the largest number of reflective objects in a specimen are scattered. Visualization of scattering sources provides a much more complete picture than visualization of specular reflections. For this reason, images based on scattered acoustic energy are easier to interpret, but systems with higher sensitivity and greater dynamic range (gray scale) are required to display the weak scattered signals.

Scattering coefficient. A measure of the attenuation due to scattering of radiation as it traverses a medium containing scattering particles. Also called total scattering coefficient.

Scattering cross section. The hypothetical area

normal to the incident radiation that would geometrically intercept the total amount of radiation actually scattered by a scattering particle. It is also defined, equivalently, as the cross-section area of an isotropic scatterer (a sphere) which would scatter the same amount of radiation as the actual amount. Also called extinction cross section, effective area.

Scavenger. A substance added to a system to remove or inactivate another substance.

Scavenging. The use of a precipitate to remove from solution by absorption or coprecipitation, a large fraction of one or more radionuclides. In radiation chemistry, the process of capturing and removing free radicals.

Schilling test. Test for measuring the gastrointestinal absorption of vitamin B_{12} done by administering radiolabeled vitamin B_{12}, giving a loading dose of nonradioactive vitamin B_{12}, then measuring the radioactivity in a 24-h urine collection, if the test is done with concomitant administration of intrinsic factor, it is called a second-stage Schilling test and is used to distinguish malabsorption attributable to intrinsic factor deficit from other causes.

Schlieren. An acousto-optic system that displays a cross section of beam shape.

Scintigram. An image of the distribution of activity obtained with a scintillation camera following the internal administration of a radionuclide.

Scintigraphy. The process of obtaining an image or series of sequential images of the distribution of a radionuclide in tissues, organs, or body systems using a scintillation γ camera, i.e., hepatic scintigraphy. Also known as radionuclide scintigraphy.

Scintillation. Name given to the production of light flashes emitted by luminescent substances when excited by high-energy radiation. The flashes can in turn liberate photoelectrons from photosensitive substances (for instance, cesium/antimony phosphors or some type of inorganic salt crystal such as NaI) (Tl activated); the photoelectrons are amplified by means of a photomultiplier tube before being converted into current pulses. The pulse height depends on the energy or the original γ- or corpuscular radiation, and the pulses can thus be sorted by means of a discriminator (pulse height analyzer). By using different discriminator channels the different nuclides in a mixture of isotopes can be determined either successively or simultaneously.

Scintillation camera. This is another name for a γ-camera. It usually consists of a large sodium iodide crystal and a collimator arranged so that radioactivity within an organ causes scintillations within the crystal at points corresponding to the position of radionuclides within the organs. The positions are calculated by computer from the light flashes (scintillations) detected by an array of photomultiplier (PM) tubes positioned above the crystal. The device is used in nuclear medicine for producing images of the distribution of radionuclides in the organs under investigation. A variation, the multicrystal scintillation camera, records high count rates.

Scintillation crystal. A crystalline solid, such as sodium iodide containing trace amounts of thallium activator NaI(Tl), which emits light scintillation when it absorbs ionizing radiation; essentially transforms invisible electromagnetic radiation or particles into visible photons.

Scintillation detector. The ionizing radiation detection system used in gamma cameras, rectilinear scanners, and gamma counters. It consists of a scintillator (usually a sodium iodide crystal, thallium activated), a photomultiplier (PM) tube, and supporting electronics. Scintillators glow when exposed to X-rays and small flashes occur in response to γ-rays. Thus an elecric pulse can be genereated by the photomultiplier tube for each γ-ray interaction. This system is employed in the gamma camera and rectilinear scanner, to produce a map of radionuclide distribution within the body. In a well-scintillation counter the count rate indicates the quantity of a radionuclide and the intensity of the scintillation indicates the energy of the γ-rays.

Scintillation image. A display obtained from any one of several rectilinear scanner or gamma camera systems. The image obtained from a moving detector is called a scan, while the image obtained from stationary camera device is called a scintiphotograph or scintigram.

Scintillation spectrometer. A scintillation counter designed to permit the measurement of the energy distribution of radiation.

Scintiphotograph. photographic recording of the isotope distribution within an organ, obtained from the visual display unit (VDU) or multiformatter of a scintillation gamma camera.

Sclerosis. A hardening of an interstitial surface; arterial sclerosis.

Scram. Sudden shutting down of a nuclear reactor, usually by dropping of safety rods. This may be arranged to occur automatically at a predetermined neutron flux or under other dangerous conditions, the reaching of which causes the monitors and associated equipment to generate a scram signal. To shut down a reactor by causing a scram.

Scrambler device. A chip that converts plaintext from ciphertext.

Screen. A term applied to both a flouroscopic screen or an intensifying screen. In the case of the former, a thin sheet of radiolucent material is coated with calcium tungstate crystals and mounted beneath a sheet of lead protective glass. An X-ray beam directed through a patient placed behind this screen produces light and shadows on the flouroscent screen by flourescence of the crystal coating. In the case of the latter, the flouroscent screens are mounted inside of a cassette and intensify the effect of X-rays on the film by giving off visible light, thus requiring less radiation for a given exposure.

Screening. The reduction of the electric field about a nucleus by the space charge of the surrounding electrons. The screening constant of an element for a given process is the atomic number minus the apparent atomic number which is effective for the purpose.

Scrubbing. A chemical operation in which a fluid is purified by contact with an immiscible liquid phase which preferentially removes the contaminants.

Sealed source. A radioactive source sealed in a container or having a bonded cover, where the container or cover has sufficient mechanical strength to prevent contact with and dispersion of the radioactive material under the conditions of use and wear for which it was designed.

Second. (s) The duration of 9 192 631 770 periods of the radiation corresponding to the transition between the two hyperfine levels of the ground state of the ^{133}Cs atom.

Secondary cosmic rays. These particles are found in the earth's atmosphere and originate, either directly or indirectly, from collisions between the primary cosmic rays which come from outer space and the molecules of the earth's atomosphere.

Secondary electron. An electron ejected from an atom, molecule, or surface as a result of a collision with a charged particle or photon. Such electrons are called secondary electrons, and their emission is called secondary emission. The fact that more than one secondary electron can be released for each incident electron is utilized in electron multiplying tubes, such as photomultipliers.

Secondary memory device. Those computer devices (excluding internal memory) that are used for storage of programs and data. One can usually write data onto these devices and read from them, although some secondary memory devices are read-only.

Secondary radiation. When a beam of radiation passes through matter and interacts with it, some of the energy of the incident beam is converted to other forms. For example, a beam of energetic X-rays will eject electron-positron pairs, Compton electrons, and photoelectrons from the material. These particles would be secondary radiations caused by the passage of the primary X-rays through the material.

Secondary slices. If a series of adjacent transverse slices is performed during computerized tomographic imaging, the column created by stacking the individual slices on top of each other represents a body volume gridded continuously in volume elements. The analogous picture element of the adjacent slice can be located and reproduced on the monitor for every diameter and every row and column of the image matrix. This results in the production of secondary coronal or sagittal slices which can only be assessed visually if thin slices are chosen. Complicated interpolation programs are required if slice planes are chosen which deviate from the orthogonal coordinates (x,y,z) (multiplanner reconstruction in the narrow sense).

Second-set graft rejection. Commonly used to designate accelerated rejection of a secondary allograft due to immunity developed to a preceding primary graft.

Second-wind angina. This term describes a phenomenon in which an exertion that initially provoked pain is tolerated later on. The pathophysiological explanation must be that at the beginning of the effort the tachycardia and the blood pressure rise produce an oxygen debt which causes pain. Diminution of the peripheral resistance with continuing exertion results in a decrease of cardiac work so that the stress is subsequently tolerated.

Secretin. A hormone secreted by the epithelial cells of the duodenum in response to the passage of food from the stomach, stimulating the secretion of pancreatic juice and bile.

Secretion. The process of production of a substance by a gland; the substance produced.

Secretory immune system. A distinct immune system that is common to external secretions and consists predominantly of IgA.

Section scanning. This is an ultrasonic B-scanning procedure which presents echo amplitude as brightness on the screen and related the point of origin of the echo to the correct point on the screeen of a cathode ray tube (CRT). There are many types of section scanners including static B-scanners on which the ultrasonic transducer is moved over the skin by hand, its position and orientation being related to the CRT by a set of potentiometers mounted on an articulated connecting arm between the transducer and the scanner. In the case of moving picture scanners the orientation and position of the transducer, or active element on a multielement transducer, are related to the display by a complex electronic mechanism.

Sector. A unit of storage of a computer magnetic disk of n words (n varies with disk models): HELP sector, a single set of decision criteria.

Sector scan. A system of ultrasound scanning in which the transducer or transmitted beam is rotated through an angle, the center of rotation being near or behind the surface of the transducer.

Secular radioactive equilibrium. In many cases a radioactive nucleus is produced as a result of the decay of another and it is thus possible to have a chain of decay processes leading to sucessive radioactive products. When the life of the parent is very much longer than any of the products, an equilibrium is reached which is called secular radioactive equilibrium, in which case the number of atoms disintegrated per unit time is the same for all products. Otherwise the equilibrium is referred to as transient.

Security. Prevention of unauthorized access to or use of data, programs, equipment, or installations.

Selection. A term to indicate a means of getting from one place to another in a computer program by selecting a particular option from a display list contained within the program called a "menu".

Selection gradient. Magnetic gradient, applied perpendicularly to the plane to be imaged, which limits excitation by the radio-frequency (rf) pulse to the plane. (NMR.)

Selection rule. The energy of atomic or molecular systems, or energy of systems of their constituent nuclei, is quantized. The transition between these energy levels is governed by certain rules called selection rules.

Selective absorption. Absorption that varies with the frequency of the incident radiation. The variation may be due to the presence of a resonance at a particular frequency.

Selective calling. The ability of a transmitting device to specify which of several devices on the same line is to receive a message.

Selective excitation. Controlling the frequency spectrum of an irradiating radio-frequency (rf) pulse (via tailoring) while imposing a gradient magnetic field on spins, such that only a desired region will have a suitable resonant frequency to be excited. Originally used to excite all but a desired region, such as a plane, for excitation. (NMR.)

Selective irradiation. Radio-frequency (rf) excitation so designed that only a limited spatial region of the sample is excited. (NMR.)

Selective localization. The accumulation of a particular isotope to a significantly greater degree in certain cells or tissues than in others. In general, the greater the degree of selective localization, the higher the target/nontarget ratio.

Selenium. Element symbol Se, atomic number 34, atomic weight 78.96.

Selenomethionine. An analogue of the amino acid methionine in which the sulfur atom is replaced by a selenium atom. The radiolabeled (^{75}Se) selenenomethionine is used for pancreatic imaging.

Self-absorption. The absorption of radiation by the radioactive substance itself. This phenomenon presents a particular problem in the measurement of weak radiation in a bulky sample. This process tends to decrease the observed activity of a sample.

Self-quenched counter tube. A Geiger tube which is quenched internally by incorporation of a quenching gas (isobutane, cholorine, etc.) with the counting gas.

Self-radiolysis. A process in which a compound is damaged by radioactive decay products originating from an atom within the compound.

Self-scattering. The scattering of radiation by the body of the substance that emits it. It may be greater than the self-absorption, in which case the total radiation from the body will be increased, and additional shielding will be required.

Self-shielding. Shielding of the inner parts of a body through absorption of radiation in its outer parts.

Self-shielding factor. The factor by which the value of a radiation quantity inside an irradiated body is reduced by self-shielding.

Semiconductor. The crystalline substance used to make chips and transistors — the circuits in computers. Silicon is the material most often used as a semiconductor. The silicon used in chips is grown in a laboratory. It is 99.9% pure. By adding slight chemical impurities to the silicon, scientists are able to change its electrical characteristics. Silicon crystals used in semiconductors are sliced into wafers as thin as this page and cut into tiny chips.

Semiconductor detector. The semiconductor detector behaves much like an ionization chamber, but because solids are about 10^3 times denser than gases, its volume can be considerably smaller. Furthermore, because the ionization produced for a given incident energy is greater, the electrical pulses are large enough to be detected individually with good statistical accuracy. Semiconductor materials commonly used are silicon and germanium, but because both elements have relatively low atomic numbers, the absorption of γ radiation is not as high as is desirable. Owing to difficulties in producing high-purity materials it is usually necessary to introduce another element, lithium, by a special technique known as drifting. This introduction has the effect of canceling out the impurities and reducing the leakage current measured when no radiation is present. The two commonly used materials are hence designated Si(Li) and Ge(Li). More recently the production of high-purity germanium has become possible. This may prove particularly useful as, of the two elements, it has the higher atomic number and density.

Semiconductor memory. Electronic memory whose individual memory cells (each storing a binary bit) are made up of transistorlike devices.

Semigraphics. The technique of constructing a picture out of characters, often utilizing special symbols such as boxes and triangles.

Semipermeable. Refers to a membrane that permits passage of some molecules but not of others.

Senescence. The clearing of old red blood cells by the spleen. Growing old; characteristic of old age.

Sensitive line imaging. An imaging method in which a given characteristic, such as spin density, is determined along a line and then the procedure is repeated sequentially throughout the sample. (NMR.)

Sensitive plane. Technique of selecting a plane for sequential plane imaging by using an oscil-

lating gradient magnetic field and filtering out the corresponding time-dependent part of the NMR signal. The gradient used is at right angles to the desired plane and the magnitude of the oscillating gradient magnetic field is equal to zero only in the desired plane.

Sensitive point. Technique of selecting out a point for sequential point imaging by applying three orthogonal oscillating gradient magnetic fields such that the local magnetic field is time-dependent everywhere except at the desired point, and then filtering out the corresponding time-dependent portion of the NMR signal.

Sensitive volume. Region of the object from which NMR signal will preferentially be acquired becasuse of strong magnetic field inhomogeneity elsewhere. Effect can be enhanced by use of a shaped radio-frequency (rf) field that is strongest in the sensitive region. That portion of a structure (counter tube, ionization chamber, or living system) which responds to radiation.

Sensitivity. In diagnostic tests, the number of test results registered as true positives in relation to the actual number of positives in the group tested. The minimum signal that can be detected satisfactorily. Measure of the NMR signal strength obtained from a number of nuclei of a particular isotope relative to that from an equal number of ^1H nuclei. The lowest concentration of test substance measurable in an assay, or the minimal difference in test substance concentrations distinguishable by a given assay, usually a function of the steepness of the assay curve.

Sensitize. To increase the specific sensitivity of an individual or a cell to an antigen (Ag) or hapten. Sensitization commonly occurs as the result of natural or artificial exposure to the Ag or hapten.

Sentinel. A group of "bits" that indicates a specific condition such as the end of a reel, a computer tape, or the end of a record.

Separation. The technique used in recovering ligand-binding agent complex to measure the extent of tracer bound during radioimmunoassay (RIA).

Separation agent. Reagent used to effect or to aid in the separation of bound and free tracer in radioassay (for example, heterologous antibody, solid-phase antibody, protein precipitating agent, or adsorbent).

Separation energy. The energy per unit mass required to achieve a specified degree of separation of a given mixture of two or more isotopic species. It can be either the theoretical minimum (thermodynamic) value or the actual value for a given process.

Septa. Those thicknesses of lead or other photon-absorbing material in a collimator that separate the holes and define the field of view of the crystal detector.

Septicemia. A severe type of infection in which large numbers of the causal bacteria circulate and multiply in the bloodstream.

Septum. Anatomically, a thin partition between two body cavities.

Sequelae. Diseases or morbid conditions resulting from or dependent upon a former illness.

Sequence delay time. It is the time between the last pulse of a pulse sequence and the beginning of the next identical pulse sequence. It is the time allowed for the nuclear spin system to recover its magnetization and is equal to the sum of the acquisition delay time, data acquisition time, and the waiting time. (NMR.)

Sequence repetition time. This is the time between the beginning of a pulse sequence and the beginning of the succeeding identical pulse sequence.

Sequential access. A method of data access computer processing in which the next location from which data is to be obtained immediately follows the location of the previously obtained data.

Sequential determinants. Determinants whose specificity is dictated by the sequence of subunits within the determinant rather than by the molecular structure of the antigen molecule.

Sequential imaging. A series of closely timed images, usually performed on a rapidly changing distribution of radioactivity.

Sequential line imaging. NMR imaging techniques in which the image is built up from successive lines through the object (line scanning). In various schemes, the lines are isolated by oscillating gradient magnetic fields or selective excitation, and then the NMR signals from the selected line are encoded for position by detecting the free induction decay (FID) or spin echo in the presence of a gradient magnetic field along the line; the Fourier transform of the detected signal then yields the distribution of emitted NMR signals along the line.

Sequential logic. A circuit arrangement in which an output is determined by the state of the previous input.

Sequential plane imaging. NMR imaging technique in which the image of an object is built up from successive planes in the object. In various schemes, the planes are selected by oscillating gradient magnetic fields or selective excitation.

Sequential point imaging. NMR imaging techniques in which the image is built from successive point positions in the object (point scanning). In various schemes, the points are isolated by oscillating gradient magnetic fields (sensitive points) or shaped magnetic fields.

Sequential saturation. Modification of saturation assays in which the forward reaction is significantly favored so that, theoretically, the binding of ligand to binding reagent is irreversible.

Sequestering agents. Or sequestrants, are compounds capable of binding metal ions so that they no longer exhibit their normal reactions in the presence of precipitating agents. Thus, in the presence of a polyphosphate sequestrant, a solution containing calcium ions no longer precipitates calcium sulfate on addition of sulfate. Most sequestrants owe their action to the formation, with the metal ion, of stable coordination compounds of chelates. Sequestering agents may be inorganic or organic. The former are typified by the condensed polyphosphates and the latter by the well-known ethylenediaminetetracetic acid (EDTA).

Sequestration. A process of separation of cells, such as removal of aged red blood cells by the spleen.

Sequestrum. Fragment of a necrosed bone that has become separated from surrounding tissue.

Serial. Consecutive, one-by-one processing.

Serial dilution. The progressive dilution of standard or sample in a row of tubes so that the first tube contains the highest concentration of test substance.

Serial interface. An input or output device for a computer system that effects data transmission or reception. For output it transforms parallel data into a sequential train of pulses. For input it transforms data from a sequential train of pulses into parallel binary words.

Serial mode. Or list mode acquisition, storage, or operation upon data is a sequential string of words (x/y pairs, time markers, and trigger events). This mode is in contrast to frame mode operations in which an entire segment of data becomes an image.

Serial transmission. Transmission of data in which each unit of data being transferred travels in sequence.

Series effect. Extension or propagation of turbulent flow within the circulatory system downstream from an abnormal flow area.

Serologically defined antigens. Antigens that are present on membranes of nearly all mammalian cells and are controlled by genes present in the major histocompatibility complex. They can be easily detected with antibodies.

Serology. Literally, the study of serum. Refers to the determination of antibodies to infectious agents important in clinical medicine.

Serous. Pertaining to or resembling serum; producing or containing serum, as a serous gland or cyst.

Serum. The fluid part of the blood which remains after the red and white cells, platelets, and fibrinogen have been removed by allowing the blood to clot.

Serum albumin. The major protein constituent of blood serum, usually found in concentrations of 35 to 50 g/l of serum.

Serum glutamic oxaloacetic transaminase. (SGOT) An enzyme normally present in various body tissues — especially the heart and liver — which is released into the serum as the result of tissue injury.

Serum sickness. An adverse immunologic response to a foreign antigen, usually a heterologous protein.

Servo systems. Servo systems are used extensively in automatic plant systems to obtain precise control over position, speed, temperature, pressure, chemical constituents in a mixture, etc.

Seven-pinhole tomography. Employs a collimator with seven pinholes, producing seven independent nonoverlapping images. These images are processed to yield multiple two-dimensional images from different depths.

Sex chromosomes. The chromosomes, X and Y, associated with the determination of sex. In humans, female somatic cells carry a pair of X chromosomes while male somatic cells each carry an X chromosome and a Y chromosome. Every female gamete carries an X chromosome, while 50% of male gametes carry and X chromosome and 50% a Y chromosome.

Shadowing. A technique in electron microscopy in which heavy metals are evaporated at low angles onto a specimen. This emphasizes surface topography and increases surface contrast. Reduction in sound reflection amplitude from reflectors that lie behind a strongly reflecting or attenuating structure.

Shadow shield. A barrier of material placed between the region to be protected and the source in order to reduce the intensity of direct (unscattered) radiation entering the region.

Shared electrons. Electrons forming a covalent bond between atoms. For each bond, one electron is contributed by each atom, so that the electrons in the immediate vicinity of either nucleus form complete shells.

Shear wave. Wave motion with particle movements perpendicular to the propagation direction. Shear waves propagate in solids but are highly attenuated in liquid systems. One of the mechanisms of absorption of longitudinal waves involves mode conversion from longitudinal to shear waves with the attendant high absorption rate of shear waves. Shear waves are generated when a longitudinal ultrasound wave impinges obliquely on soft tissue-bone interfaces and partially account for the heating of the periosteum and bone at this location.

Sheath. Tubular structure of membranes.

Shell. According to Pauli's exclusion principle the extranuclear electrons do not circle around the nucleus all in orbits of the same radium but are arranged in orbits at various distance from the nucleus. The extranuclear orbital electrons are thus assumed to be arranged in a series of concentric spheres, called shells, which are designated, in the order of increasing distance from the nucleus, as K, L, M, N, O, P, and Q shells. The number of the electrons which each of these shells can contain is limited. All electrons arranged in the same shell have the same principal quantum number. The electrons in the same shell are grouped into various subshells and all the electrons in the same subshell have the same orbital angular momentum.

Shell model. A concept that neutrons and protons in a nucleus may be arranged in shells or layers somewhat similar to the electron shells in an atom.

Shield. A body or material used to prevent or reduce the passage of particles or radiation. A shield may be designated according to what it is intended to absorb, as a γ-ray shield or neutron shield, or according to the kind of protection it is intended to give, as a background, biological, or thermal shield.

Shielding. The use of shields. Also the material of which a shield is composed.

Shift register. A register in which data can be moved right or left a desired number of places.

Shim coils. Coils carrying a relatively small current that are used to provide auxiliary magnetic fields in order to compensate for inhomogeneities in the main magnetic field of an NMR system.

Shimming. Correction of inhomogeneity of the magnetic field produced by the main magnet of an NMR system due to imperfections in the magnet or to the presence of external ferromagnetic objects. May involve changing the configuration of the magnet or the addition of shim coils or small pieces of steel.

Shim rod. A control rod used for making occasional coarse adjustments in the reactivity of a nuclear reactor. It commonly moves more slowly than a regulating rod and, singly or as one of a group, is capable of making a greater total change in the reactivity. Its name is derived from analogy to a mechanical shim; a shim rod commonly is positioned so that the reactor will be just critical (reactivity = 0, effective multiplication constant = 1) when the regulating rod is near the middle of its range of travel.

Shock. A term applied to a number of several different, often unrelated conditions, associated with a state of distress or collapse, e.g., traumatic shock, anaphylactic shock, hemorrhagic shock.

Shock excitation. Short, electrical impluses to the transducer crystal to cause it to ring.

Shower. The practically simultaneous appearance of several or many fast particles originating from one high-energy particle (from cosmic radiation or particles from a high-energy accelerator).

Shunt. A diversion or bypass of blood or cerebrospinal fluid from its normal path. May be caused by congenital defects, pathological processes, or surgical procedures.

Shunt study. Study using a radionuclide to detect abnormal shunting of blood in the cardiopulmonary circulation, either from the left (systemic) side of the circulation to the right (pulmonary) side of the circulation or from right to left; also refers to study of a shunt placed surgically in order to divert body fluids (for example, a ventriculoperitoneal cerebrospinal fluid shunt).

Shutdown. The state of a reactor when its effective multiplication constant is less than unity. To stop the chain reaction in a reactor by making it subcritical.

Shutter. Lead shields operated as a variable diaphragm to narrow a beam of X-rays emerging from a fluoroscopic tube.

Sialogram. Sialography involves the introduction of contrast material into the ducts of the major salivary glands, usually the paratid or submandibular gland. Evaluation for the presence of small stones (calculi), recurrent inflammatory disease, or tumor is the primary indication for this examination.

Sideband. The frequency band higher and/or lower than the carrier frequency that is produced as a result of modulation.

Side chain theory. A theory of antibody synthesis proposed by Ehrlich in 1896 suggesting that specific side chains that form antigen receptors are present on the surface membranes of antibody-producing cells.

Side lobe. A characteristic of an acoustic beam in which secondary, off-axis maxima occur in the near or far acoustic field, or in the focal zone. The presence of side lobes tends to cause target ambiguity and limit the resolution.

Side-scattered radiation. Radiation which is scattered in directions approximately at right angles to the direction of the primary beam.

Sidestream network management. A computerized method of controlling and diagnosing networks that rely on the modems and multiplexors to monitor the various components in the analog portion of the network. Some can also check the digital facilities.

Sievert. (Sv) The SI unit of dose equivalent (J/kg). The absorbed dose in grays multiplied by the quality factor of the type of radiation. One Sievert equals 100 rem.

Sigmoid. The sigmoid flexure is the S-shaped portion of the colon extending from the descending colon, downward to the anus.

Sigmoid curve. S-shaped curve, approaching linearity in the middle and curved at either end, which is characteristic of the cumulative normal distribution.

Signal. Aggregate of waves propagated along a transmission channel and intended to act on a receiving unit.

Signal averaging. Technique of improving signal-to-noise ratio by adding up repeated scans through the same region of interest. The noise tends to average because of its random nature, whereas the signal reinforces itself.

Signal element. Each part of a digital signal, distinguished from others by its duration, position, and/or sense; can be a start, information, or stop element.

Signal-to-noise-ratio. In general, the ratio of the value of the signal to that of the noise. This ratio is usually in terms of peak values in the case of impulse noise and in terms of root-mean-square values in the case of random noise. Where there is a possibility of ambiguity, suitable definitions of the signal and noise should be associated with the term: e.g., peak-signal/peak-noise ratio, root-mean-square signal/root-mean-square noise ratio, peak-to-peak signal/peak-to-peak noise ratio, etc.

Sign test. A nonparametric test based on the number of positive and negative differences between pairs. Under the null hypothesis, the number of + and − signs should be binomially distributed with $p = 0.5$.

SI international system of units. In 1948, the General Conference on Weights and Measures, a diplomatic conference responsible for the "international unification and development of the metric system", instructed its International Committee for Weights and Measures to develop a set of rules for the units of measurement. The "International System of Units" (Le Système International d'Unités, SI) was developed under this charge, adopted by the CGPM (Conference General des Poids et Measures) in 1960, and accepted by all signatories to the Meter Convention in 1977.

Silicon. Element symbol Si, atomic number 14, atomic weight 28.0855.

Silver. Element symbol Ag (argentum), atomic number 47, atomic weight 107.8682.

Simple diffusion. The process by which radioactive material enters a cell membrane that has lost its integrity because of a disease process. Brain scanning presumably makes use of breakdowns in the blood-brain barrier.

Simulation. A technique through which a model of the working system is built in the form of a computer program. Special computer languages are available for producing this model, and the program is run on a separate computer.

Single-channel pulse height analyzer. A pulse height selector is an electronic circuit which permits only those voltage pulses which have amplitudes between predetermined levels to be passed to the succeeding circuits. The difference between these two levels is referred to as the window or channel width. The lower reference level is called the threshold. A single-channel pulse height analyzer is an instrument incorporating a pulse height selector in which the channel width is preset and the threshold varied, either manually or automatically, to scan the amplitude spectrum of the incoming pulses.

Single photon emission computerized tomography. (SPECT) Technique that uses a computer for tomographic reconstruction (in a variety of planes, transaxial, coronal, sagittal) of the distribution of a single photon γ-emitting radionuclide detected by a rotating scintillation camera. (The widely used ^{99m}Tc, which emits single 140-keV γ photons, is an example.) Its essential goal is enhancement of the image detectability and the extraction of quantitative data from a true three-dimensional distribution of structure (or radioactivity) in space. The title SPECT excludes positron emission tomography (PET) from the discussion, as PET is based on the detection, by means of opposed detectors and coincidence counting techniques, of the two 511-keV photons which are simultaneously emitted in almost opposite directions by a positron-emitting radionuclide. Any conventional (planar) imaging technique is restricted mainly to the visualization of objects in three-dimensional space by means of two-dimensional projections. Multiple views of an object from different angles are required to appreciate its three-dimensional structure. These separate views are usually called projections. A complete set of projections potentially permits a complete reconstruction of object structures in three dimensions.

Single radial diffusion. A technique for quantitating antigens by immunodiffusion in which an antigen is allowed to diffuse radially into agar containing antibody. The resultant precipitation ring reflects the concentration of the antigen. Also known as radioimmunodiffusion.

Single scattering. If a particle in passing through matter, say a thin metal foil, makes only one collision with an atom or nucleus before emerging again, it is said to have suffered single scattering.

Sinoatrial node. A mass of specialized muscle fibers in the wall of the right atrium near the entrance of the superior vena cava. The pacemaker of the heart, giving rise to the electrical impulses that initiate contractions of the heart.

Sinus. A cavity or channel in an organ; fluid and air spaces in the cranium; cavity within a bone; dilated channel for venous blood.

Sinusoid. Beginning of the venous system in the spleen, liver, bone marrow, and so on, that has an irregularly shaped, thin-walled space.

Size of field of view. The size of field of view is the maximum area from which a scintigraphic instrument can collect useful information. This area may vary with the type of collimator and also with the distance of the source from the collimator.

Skiagraph. Early name for an X-ray radiograph.

Skin. The skin covers the entire body, providing containment for the body fluids and protection for the muscles, bones, and viscera beneath its surface. An actively growing organ, richly endowed with capillary blood vessels, it is waterproof, elastic, and self-repairing. It carries myriads of sensory nerve endings which keep the body in touch with its environment, and innumerable sweat glands which pour out perspiration to cool the body by evaporation whenever there is danger of overheating. Also very numerous in the skin are the sebaceous glands secreting a fatty substance, sebum, which is water repellant, lubricant, and has bactericidal and fungicidal properties. Except on the palms and soles, the skin carries hairs, thick and strong on the scalp, armpits, and pubis and small and downy elsewhere as a rule. Another type of skin appendage are the nails of the fingers and toes.

Skin depth. Time-dependent electromagnetic fields are significantly attenuated by conducting media (including the human body); the skin depth gives a measure of the average depth of penetration of the radio-frequency (rf) field. It may be a limiting factor in NMR imaging at very high frequencies (high magnetic fields). The skin depth also affects the Q of the coils.

Skin dose. The dose of radiation measured on the skin, representing the sum of the air dose and the X-rays scattered back from the internal body tissues.

Skin effect. The decrease in the depth of penetration of an electrical current in a conductor as the frequency of the current increases. The skin depth is the depth below the surface at which the current density has decreased to $1/e$ of its value at the surface.

Slant hole collimator. The slant hold collimator was designed principally to achieve emission computed tomography without rotating the complete gamma camera head about the patient. Although this form of tomography appears useful when imaging the head and heart, the rotating slant hole collimator can be used to obtain complex views of various organs. The slant hole collimator can be thought of as similar to the parallel hole collimator, except that images are formed from objects shifted from the gamma camera head axis. The field of view is symmetrical about the central channel axis and spatial resolution at depth is variable.

Slave. The processor computer which acts on commands from a master processor or computer.

Slaving. Making an operating system copy its display output to a printer is called "slaving the printer to the display".

Slit radiography. A special case of scan projection radiography using a slit to create a collimated beam of X-rays which is scanned over the patient.

Slope. Electronic boosting or bias given to sound echoes returning from depth to compensate for their weakening by attenuation in tissue.

Slope of a line. Change in y value (ordinate) per unit change in the x value (abscissa).

Slowing-down area. One sixth of the mean square distance traveled by neutrons in an infinite homogeneous medium from their points of origin to the points where they have been slowed down from the initial energy to a specified energy.

Slowing-down density. The number of neutrons per unit volume and unit time which, in slowing down, pass a given energy value.

Slow neutrons. Neutrons of kinetic energy less than some specified value. This value may vary over a wide range and depends on the application, such as reactor physics, shielding, or dosimetry. In reactor physics the value is frequently chosen to be 1 eV; in dosimetry the cadmium cutoff energy is used.

Slug. A bar-shaped piece of material prepared especially for insertion in a nuclear reactor. The term often refers to the fuel unit of a natural uranium-graphite reactor.

Small bowel series. The small bowel consists of the duodenum, jejenum, and ileum. Collectively these are known as the small bowel (as opposed to the colon or large bowel). Barium is used to further outline radiologically the gut to look for evidence of inflammation, neoplastic disease, or obstruction.

Small parts scanner. High-resolution (10 MHz) real-time ultrasound scanners to visualize carotid arteries, thyroid, etc.

Smear test. The object of smear testing, or wipe testing as it is sometimes called, is to estimate the amount of loose radioacitivity or contamination which is present on surfaces such as benches, floors, equipment, and the like, which might become airborne or be transferred to hands.

Smoothing. The term "smoothing" has often fallen into disrepute, although the use of this technique is still widely used in radionuclide imaging, even if not directly or intentionally. The aim of smoothing data has been to remove statistical irregularities which would otherwise hinder the interpretation of results. Smoothing can be applied to both images and curves from radionuclide images with good effect. For instance, in many "dynamic" studies temporal (i.e., between corresponding pixels in several frames) or spatial (i.e., between adjacent pixels within a frame) smoothing is usually implemented prior to viewing the data in cine mode. It is important to understand that if the image data have been smoothed, then subsequent data extraction or display may be modified by the smoothing algorithm. The purpose of smoothing is to enhance an image by reducing high-frequency phenomena, such as statistical noise, while preserving the overall form of the data. However, since edges within an image or large gradients in a curve are dominated by high-frequency components, the effect of smoothing is to reduce or "average out" such features.

Snell's law. Relates incidence and transmission angles of refraction.

Snow. Term for an electronic artefact consisting of small amplitude noise seen on the ultrasound B scan.

Sodium. Element symbol Na (natrium), atomic number 11, atomic weight 22.9898.

Sodium-potassium pump. The mechanism of active transport by which sodium is extruded from the interior of cells in order to maintain the normal higher extracellular concentration of sodium and higher intracellular concentraion of potassium.

Soft data. ubjective data, often difficult to reproduce or reduce to numbers.

Soft radiation. Ionizing radiation of such low energy that is has low penetrating ability. In general, the longer the wavelength the softer the radiation.

Software. The set of instructions (algorithms), or programs, which the computer follows in order to carry its own functions. Programs may be written in machine language (sequence of numbers directly interpretable by the computer), assembly language, or higher level languages such as Fortran or Basic. The software includes overall supervising "executive" programs, data acquisition programs, data processing programs (including image reconstruction), and display programs.

Software-compatible. If two computers are software-compatible, the software designed for one will also work with the second computer. Software-compatible computers "speak" the same machine language.

Software documentation. Instruction manuals that tell programmers, operators, and users what a computer program does, how it is written, and how to use it.

Software engineering. A relatively new field that addresses the efficient development of reliable and error-free computer software.

Software maintenance. The ongoing process of detecting and removing errors from existing computer programs. Commercially, this usually refers to the process of the manufacturer's supplying and installing new versions or corrections to old versions of software products such as operating systems, programming languages, and applications packages.

Software package. Usually refers to an applications package, but could refer to all the software in a computer system.

Software transportability. The ability to take a program written and working on one computer and to run it without modification on a different computer.

Sol. Liquid colloid solution.

Solenoid coil. A coil of wire wound in the form of a long cylinder. When a current is passed through the coil, the magnetic field within the coil is relatively uniform. Solenoid radio-frequency (rf) coils are commonly used when the static magnetic field is perpendicular to the long axis of the body.

Solid. A state of matter in which the relative motion of the molecules is restricted and they tend to retain a definite fixed position relative to each other, giving rise to crystal structure. A solid may be said to have a definite shape and volume.

Solid phase. Separation method in which the binding reagent is immobilized by coupling to an insoluble material (coated tubes, polymers, etc.).

Solid phase radioimmunoassay. A modification of radioimmunoassay in which an antibody is absorbed onto solid particles or tubes.

Solid scintillators. The most common type in use in nuclear medicine consists of single crystals of thallium-activated sodium iodide. Since the decay time of the fluorescence is only 0.25 μs the scintillation crystals have a resolving power about a thousand times greater than gas-filled counters. Moreover, the pulse yield for X- and γ-rays is 10 to 1000 times greater — depending on the crystal volume and surface — as a result of the higher density of the material. Since there is no dissipation of the crystals the lifetime of these scintillation detectors is limited only by that of the replaceable multiplier and its semipermanent photosensitive layer. The wavelength of the luminescent radiation is about 410 nm. Organic scintillators and plastic scintillators have a decay time of 5 to 24 ns, their secondary luminescence a wavelenght of 410 to 440 nm.

Solid solution. If, in a crystal structure, certain atoms can be replaced by chemically different ones without changing the structure, the result is a solid solution.

Solid state. Electronic components, like transistors and integrated circuits, that depend on a flow of electricity in solid materials. The material is usually a semiconductor substance made from silicon or germanium.

Solute. The constituent of a solution that is considered to be dissolved in the other, the solvent. The solvent is usually present in larger amount than the solute.

Solution. Physical system consisting of one or more substances dissolved in another substance.

Solvates. Complexes formed between inorganic compounds and organic solvents in solvent extraction.

Solvent. The constituent of a solution that is present in larger amount and acts as the dissolving agent, or constituent that is liquid in the pure state, in the case of solutions of solids or gases in liquids.

Solvent extraction. A method of separating one or more substances from a mixture, by treating a solution of the mixture with a solvent that will dissolve the required substances and leave the others.

Somatic. Pertaining to the body as distinguished from the mind. Related to the framework of the body and not to the viscera, such as the somatic musculature (the muscles of the body wall or somatopleure) as distinguished from the splanchnic musculature (the splanchnopleure).

Somatic cells. Body cells, usually having two sets of chromosomes. Germ cells have only one set.

Sonar. Applied to medical ultrasound, the term sonar is the generic term for echo ranging. From the acronym sound navigation ranging.

Sorenson method for attenuation precorrection. This method uses modified projection values based on the geometric mean of opposing raysums and a hyperbolic sine corrector:

$$P_{new} = x \cdot e^x \sqrt{P_a \cdot P_b} / \sin(x)$$

where x - μL/2, P_{new} is the modified projection, μ the attenuation coefficient for correction, L the path length through the attenuating me-

dium, P_a one projection bin value, and P_b the opposite projection bin value.

Sorption. A general term used in chemistry for the processes of absorption, adsorption, and persorption.

Sort. To arrange a group of items according to size, number, alphabetical order, or some other organizational scheme. Computer sorting techniques include bubble sorts, partition sorts, and selection sorts.

Sound. Traveling wave of acoustic variables.

Sound absorption. Absorption, results in the dissipation of sound into heat. The absorption process is poorly understood in tissue, although it has been studied extensively in blood where it is related to relaxation phenomena in the protein constituent of the blood. The resulting decrease in beam intensity is exponential and increases with frequency. In most biological soft tissues, the absorption is approximately proportional to frequency, whereas in bone it is a function of the frequency squared. Absorption is the most important determinant of the depth of penetration of the sound beam into the body.

Sound beam. The region of a medium that contains virtually all the sound produced by a transducer.

Sound waves. Unlike the electromagnetic waves responsible for most imaging systems, sound waves are mechanical phenomena that require an elastic, deformable medium for their propagation. Sound can be envisioned as a displacement or pressure wave with the particles of the medium oscillating about their average positions. This vibration produces localized changes in the density of the medium. Sound waves are longitudinal or transverse vibrations, or they are combinations of both. In water and soft biological tissue, pure longitudinal waves predominate, with particle motion along the direction of propagation. In such solids as bone, transverse or shear waves also may be generated and have a particle motion normal (90°) to the wave propagation.

Source. Concentrated radioactive matter used as a source of radiation.

Source code. The computer program in its original programming language, before it is translated into machine language.

Source organs. Organs containing concentrations of radioactivity exceeding the average concentration in the body. Used to calculate radiation dose to the target organ.

Source strength. The strength of a radioactive

source, meaning the amount of radioactive material contained in it, is expressed in curies or becquerels.

Source-surface distance. The distance measured along the radiation beam axis from the front surface of the source to the nearest surface of the irradiated object in radiation therapy.

Space. An impulse that, in a neutral circuit, causes the loop to open or causes absence of signal. In a polar circuit, space causes the loop current to flow in a direction opposite to that for a mark impulse. A space impulse is equivalent to a binary 0. In some computer codes, a character that causes a printer to leave a character width with no printed symbol.

Space charge. The electric charge carried by a cloud or stream of electrons or ions in a vacuum or a region of low gas pressure, when the charge is sufficient to produce local charges in the potential distribution. It is of importance in thermionic tubes, photoelectric cells, ion accelerators, etc.

Spallation. A nuclear reaction induced by high-energy bombardment in which several particles or nuclei are ejected from a target nucleus, the nucleus being appreciably reduced in consequence both in mass number and atomic number.

Sparging. The introduction of a gas or vapor below the surface of a liquid for agitation, heat transfer, or stripping a volatile solute, especially an organic solvent.

Spatial average intensity. The spatial average of any intensity distribution is calculated within the contour for 95% of the maximum intensity.

Spatial average pulse average intensity. The pulse average instensity averaged over the beam cross-sectional area. (May be calculated as the ratio of ultrasonic power to the product of duty cycle and beam cross-sectional area.)

Spatial average temporal average intensity. The temporal average intensity averaged over the beam cross-sectional area. (May be calculated as the ratio of ultrasonic power to the product of duty cycle and beam cross-sectional area.)

Spatial distortion. Spatial distortion refers to the ability of a scintigraphic instrument to reproduce planar arrays of linear source of radioactivity in a manner which conserves all the spatial and geometric relationships of the array.

Spatial frequency. Sine wave representation of a light intensity function along a line through a picture.

Spatial frequency filtering. Technique for eliminating the higher spatial frequencies, assumed to be noise, in a image. Employs Fourier transform analysis.

Spatial peak-pulse average intensity. The value of the pulse average intensity at the point in space where the pulse average intensity is a maximum, or is a local maximum within a specified region.

Spatial peak temporal average intensity. The value of the temporal average intensity at the point in the acoustic field where the temporal average intensity is a maximum, or is a local maximum within a specified region.

Spatial peak temporal peak intensity. The value of the temporal peak intensity at the point in the acoustic field where the temporal peak intensity is a maximum, or is a local maximum within a specified region.

Spatial resolution. Spatial resolution refers to the ability of an instrument to image two separate line or point sources of radioactivity as separate entities. The smaller the distance between the two sources that can be imagined, the better the spatial resolution. A measure of spatial resolution is the point spread function (PSF) or the line spread function (LSF) and the derived system transfer function (STF). Although generally referring to the ability of the imaging process to distinguish adjacent structures in the object, the specific criterion of resolution to be used depends on the type of test used (e.g., bar pattern or contrast-detail phantom). As the ability to separate or detect objects depends on their contrast, and the different NMR parameters of objects will affect differently image constrast imaging techniques, care must be taken in comparing the results of resolution phantom tests of different machines and no single simple measure of resolution can be specified.

Spatial velocity profile. Plot of velocity distribution across a vessel diameter which may be described as irregular, parabolic, or flat, "flat" suggesting that approximately 80 to 90% of the flow cross section of the vessel has the same velocity.

Species specificity. Situation in which the same antigen from two different animal species exhibits different reactivity toward an antibody. Hormones exhibit species specificity to a high degree. When assaying these hormones, it is often necessary to use the same antigen for the preparation of tracer and standards and the production of antibodies. In these cases, of course, all the antiserum must be obtained from the same species.

Specific activity. The activity per unit mass of an element or compound containing a radioactive nuclide. The SI unit of specific activity is the becquerel per kilogram (Bq kg^{-1}) or becquerel per mole (Bq mol^{-1}). The non-SI unit is the curie per kilogram, mole (Ci kg^{-1}) Ci mol^{-1}).

Specific compliance. The ratio of compliance to functional residual capacity.

Specific energy. The energy imparted by ionizing radiation to matter, given by a $= \varepsilon/m$, where ε is energy and m is the mass of the irradiated matter.

Specific gamma-ray constant. For a nuclide emitting γ-rays: the product of exposure rate at a given distance from a point source of that nuclide and the square of that distance divided by the activity of the source, neglecting attenuation; it is expressed as in units of C kg^{-1} m^2/ MBq s (R cm^2/mCi h).

Specific gravity. Measured mass of a substance with that of an equal volume of another taken as a standard. For gases, hydrogen or air may be the standard; for liquids and solids, distilled water at a specified temperature is the standard.

Specific ionization. When an energetic charged particle passes through a gas, the gas becomes ionized, i.e., an electron becomes detached from an atom or molecule of the gas. The electron may remain free or it may attach itself to another atom or molecule to form a negative ion. In either case two charges of opposite sign are formed and these are called an ion pair. The specific ionization is the number of ion pairs formed per unit path length.

Specificity. In diagnostic tests, the number of true-negative detections divided by the total number of negatives in the group tested. Ability of a substance to recognize and bind to only one other molecule.

Specific label. A compound which contains a radioactive atom only at a single specifc position in the molecule.

Specific reactor substance. Material capable of specifically and reversibly reacting with another molecule.

SPECT elliptical rotation. Single photon emission computerized tomography (SPECT) elliptical rotation data acquisition, by allowing the detector head to move in a noncircular orbit around the patient, such that the patient's con-

tour can be followed much more closely with a significant improvement in uniformity. Usually the elliptical motion is obtained by combining the detector's head rotation with a lateral displacement of the gantry along a rail or track. The lateral shift of the center of rotation moves the detector's head away from the center of the patient, thus allowing the detector to follow an elliptical path. The shift from the detector center results from the lateral translation of the gantry and this must be compensated before reconstruction in order to realign the central pixel with the ellipse center of rotation. In order to be able to perform this correciton, the lateral displacement of the gantry and the angular position of the detector's head should be recorded throughout the acquisition.

Spectral analysis. A method of analyzing waveforms derived from Doppler shift information by separating the waveform into its frequency velocity components. Multiple frequency components may be derived from a single waveform. A common technique for spectral analysis is the fast Fourier transform.

Spectral purity. The extent to which an atomic or nuclear process or set of processes gives rise to monochromatic electromagnetic radiation.

Spectral shift reactor. A water reactor, which is initially undermoderated and in which the ratio of heavy to light water in the moderator is reduced as burn-up proceeds.

Spectral width. The spectral width can be defined by a variety of statistical terms including: the standard deviation, full width to half-maximal amplitude, or 6dB falloff from the model velocity within the spectrum. In NMR, the frequency range represented without foldover.

Spectrometer. The portions of the NMR apparatus that actually produce the NMR phenomenon and acquire the signals, including the magnet, the probe, the radio-frequency (rf) circuitry, etc. The spectrometer is controlled by the computer via the interface under the direction of the software. A device used to count an emission of radiation of a specific energy or range of energies to the exclusion of all other energies.

Spectrophotometry. Use of an instrument that measures light or color by photonic transmission.

Spectrum. A visual display, a photographic record, or a plot of the distribution of the intensity of radiation of a given kind as a function of its wave-length, energy, frequency, momentum, mass, or any related quantity. In NMR, the display of absorption peaks in the frequency domain, plotted as function of their resonant frequency.

Speed. The rate at which position is changing. It is the distance moved divided by the time over which the movement occurs.

$$\text{speed (m/s)} = \frac{\text{displacement (m)}}{\text{time (s)}}$$

Spent fuel. Nuclear fuel removed from a reactor following irradiation, or which is no longer usable because of depletion of fissile material, poison buildup, or radiation damage.

Sphincter. A circular muscle which controls the opening and closing of the natural orifice of an organ.

Sphygmomanometer. An instrument used to measure of systolic and diastolic arterial blood pressure noninvasively. The values of these parameters, usually expressed as a ratio, are a good indication of healthy or otherwise cardiovascular function.

Spin. (I) The intrinsic angular momentum of an elementary particle, or system or particles such as a nucleus, that is also responsible for the magnetic moment; or, a particle or nucleus possessing such a spin. The spins of nuclei have characteristic fixed values. Pairs of neutrons and protons align to cancel out their spins, so that nuclei with an odd number of neutrons and/or protons will have a net nonzero rotational component characterized by an integer or half-integer quantum "nuclear spin number".

Spin coupling. The interaction between the magnetic moments of two neighboring nuclei.

Spin density. The density of resonating spins in a given region; one of the principal determinants of the strength of the NMR signal from the region. The SI units would be mol/m^3. For water, there are about 1.1×10^5 mol of hydrogen per m^3, or 0.11 moles of hydrogen/cm^3. True spin density is not imaged directly, but must be calculated from signals received with different interpulse times.

Spin diffusion. The diffusion of magnetic moments due to actual movement of the associated molecule and/or chemical exchange.

Spin echo. The reappearance of an NMR signal, arising from refocusing or rephasing of the various components of magnetization in the x, y plane. This usually results from the application of the 180° pulse after decay of the initial free induction decay (FID). It can be used to determine T$_2$ without contamination from in-

homogeneous effects of the magnetic field. The Carr-Purcell sequence may be used, applying a series of 180° pulses for more accurate T$_2$ measurement.

Spin-echo imaging. Any of many NMR imaging techniques in which the spin-echo NMR signal rather than the free induction decay (FID) is used. Can be used to create images that depend strongly on T$_2$. Note that spin echoes do not directly produce an image of T$_2$.

Spin-echo sequence. An NMR experiment used to produce images with a strong T$_2$ dependence.

Spin-lattice relaxation time. (T$_1$) The exponential time constant that characterizes the growth or decay of the component of magnetization parallel to the external field. The physical mechanism involed in this process is the interaction of the nucleus with its entire surroundings (lattice). Also called the longitudinal relaxation time. (NMR.)

Spinning sidebands. Bands, paired symmetrically about a principal band, arising from spinning of the sample in a field that is inhomogeneous at the sample position. (NMR.)

Spin-spin broadening. Increased line width due to interactions between neighboring dipoles. (NMR.)

Spin-spin relaxation time. (T$_2$) The exponential time constant that characterizes the decay of confinement of magnetization perpendicular to the external field. This decay results from interaction at the nuclei with its immediate neighboring nuclei. Also called transverse relaxation time. (NMR.)

Spin-spin splitting. Splittings in the lines of an NMR spectrum arising from the interaction of the nuclear magnetic moment with those of neighboring nuclei.

Spin tagging. Nuclei will retain their magnetic orientation for a time on the order of T$_1$ even in the presence of motion. Thus, if the nuclei in a given region have their spin orientation changed, the altered spins will serve as a "tag" to trace the motion of any fluid that may have been in the tagged region for a time on the order of T$_1$. (NMR.)

Spinthariscope. An early detector of radiation in which alpha particles from a radioactive source struck a zinc sulfide screen and produced individual light flashes which were observed through a lens.

Spin-warp imaging. A form of Fourier transform (FT) imaging in which phase encoding gradient pulses are applied for a constant duration but with varying amplitude. This is distinct from the original FT imaging methods in which phase encoding is performed by applying gradient pulses of constant amplitude but varying duration. The spin-warp method, as other Fourier imaging techniques, is relatively tolerant of nonuniformities (inhomogeneities) in the static or gradient magnetic fields. (NMR.)

Spiral ridged accelerator. A cyclotron or synchrotron which uses spiral ridges on the surface of the magnet pole tips to improve beam focusing and enable radical redesign of the accelerator.

Spirometer. An instrument for measuring the air capacity of the lungs.

Splanchnic. Pertaining to the interior organs in any of the four great body cavities.

Spontaneous reaction. The spontaneous decay of a nucleus into other nuclei and elementary particles.

Spooling. The process of sending computer text files to a queue, from which they may then be printed. The wood "spool" is an acronym for "system peripheral output, on-line".

Spread spectrum communications. The process of modulating a signal over a significantly larger bandwidth than is necessary for the given data rate for the purpose of lowering the bit error rate (BER) in the presence of strong interference signals.

Spurious count. Recorded counts which are due neither to the process under observation nor to background from other genuine nuclear effects. They may be due to electrical breakdown in the counter or associated apparatus, failure of quenching (Geiger counter), or pickup of stray electromagnetic radiation.

Sputum. Mucus ejected from the lungs upon deep coughing.

Squamous cells. Plate-like cells composing the outer layer of the skin or lining of a body cavity.

Stability. Stability of a pharmaceutical has been defined as the extent to which a product retains, within a specified limit and throughout its period of storage and use, the same properties and characteristics that are possessed at the time of its manufacture; during the period of stability, physical, chemical, radiochemical, microbiological, toxicological, and clinical value should not change to any significant extent.

Stabilizer. A normal conductor adjacent to and in electrical contact with a superconductor to provide a low-resistance current path during normal transitions of the superconductors.

Stable. A nuclide is said to be stable if it will not change its composition without the introduction of energy to the system. That is, the atom will not lose electrons, protons, or neutrons spontaneously, as does a radioactive nuclide.

Stable electron configurations. Configuration of electrons about an atom in the atom's lowest energy state.

Stable isotope. An isotope of an atom incapable of spontaneous disintegration; hence, not radioactive.

Stack. Portion of a computer memory for temporary storage. New words are stored and removed from the stack in "last in, first out" fashion.

Stage. The section of an isotope separation cascade in which a single separation process is performed. It may consist of a number of elements in parallel handling material of the same isotopic abundance. A theoretical stage is that section of a separation system over which there is a separation factor equal to the simple process factor.

Standard. In general standard defines a product, process, or procedure with reference to one or more of the following: nomenclature, composition, construction, dimensions, tolerance, safety, operating characteristics, performance, quality, rating, testing, and the service for which designed. Specifically, a comparison source of radioactivity. It may represent an aliquot of the amount given to a patient, a known amount of radioactivity to standardize or calibrate the detection device, or a known amount of the substance to be tested in a radioassay. A solution of a pure substance of known concentration to which unknown substances may be compared.

Standard curve. A plot of tracer binding vs. the known concentrations of test substance in a set of standards, usually prepared by serial dilution or incremental addition.

Standard deviation. The statistical variation observed in a population or series of measurements determined by the population distribution.

Standard deviation from regression. The square root of the average squared vertical deviation of the y values around the regression line: (S_{y-x}).

Standard error of the difference. Standard deviation of the distribution of chance differences between two sample means ($X_1 - X_2$). Hence the standard error of the difference.

Formula varies depending upon (1) whether the population variance (σ^2) is known or (2) whether the sample sizes are equal or unequal.

Standardization. The process of ensuring that established criteria, codes, standards, and guides are satisfied; the process whereby a specific component, system, or facility, having the established criteria, codes, standards, and guides, can be utilized without further design, development, or license review.

Standard normal deviate. (Z test) Any significance test using the standard normal curve. The critical ratio is

$$a = x - \mu/\sigma$$

where x = observed outcome, μ = center of normal curve, and σ = standard deviation of normal curve. The specific interpretation of x, μ, and σ depends upon the specific normal distribution and test.

Standard normal distribution. The normal distribution of the variate z with a mean (μ) of zero (0), and a standard deviation (σ) of 1.

Standard views of the chest. The most common examination performed in a radiology department is a frontal view of the chest. This is often combined with a lateral projection for evaluation of the lungs, heart, and central mediastinal structures. Typical indications for examination of the chest would be suspected pneumonia, tumoral masses, a history of chest injury, obstructive airways disease, inflammatory or parenchymal pulmonary disorders.

Standby power system. A device that protects a computer or other electrical device from blackouts. It is similar to an uninterruptible power supply but does not provide protection against such power disturbances as spikes and surges.

Stannous ion. Ion of tin in the +2 valence state.

Star. A nuclear event, recorded in photographic emulsion, in which the tracks of three or more charged particles radiate from a single point, is called a star.

Star formation. The emission of protons, neutrons, deuteron, and other charged particles occurring when negatively charge pions are stopped in tissue and the atomic nuclei in the tissue disintegrate.

Start bit. In a serial computer transmission, the first bit (a space bit) that provides synchronization for the asynchronously transmitted character(s) that follow.

Starting voltage. A term applied particularly to Geiger counters. It is the minimum voltage which must be applied to the counter to cause it to count with the particular recording which may be attached.

Star topology. A computer network configuration with all remote nodes directly linked to a central host computer. Sometimes referred to as a radial network.

Stasis. A slowing down or stopping, usually applied to blood lymph, cerebrospinal fluid, or urine flow.

Statcoulomb. (ESU) The electrostatic unit of charge: that quantity of electrical charge which, when placed in a vacuum 1 cm distant from an equal and like charge, will repel it with a force of 1 dyne.

Static radionuclide image acquisition. A static acquisition implies that, within the bounds of the time required to acquire an image, the radioacive distribution in the organ is essentially constant both in radioactivity and spatial location, or has reached a state of dynamic equilibrium. Radionuclide imaging of static distributions usually entails acquiring several views of an organ and includes anterior, posterior, and lateral projections. In some instances, oblique views can reveal lesions that would otherwise be obscured by over- or underlying radioactivity. Variations in organ size, magnification due to selection of different collimators, image format size, or patient/detector geometry can affect the quality of an image. In general, as the size of the organ increases, so an adjustment of either total counts acquired or of the intensity setting should be made. To maintain similar count statistics and local count density, it is preferable to increase the total counts acquired at the expense of increase imaging time.

The same methods and effects of static acquisition apply to images obtained using data processors. The main advantage of acquiring images using a data processor is the ability to store the image data and then decide on the format size and the consequent image intensity to highlight relevant features. However, despite postprocessing capabilities, there is no substitute for acquiring sufficient events from the area of interest.

Stationary phase. Chromatographic phase that does not move with the solvent front.

Statistical error. The random error involved in any measurement. For example, if particles emitted from a nuclear reaction are being counted, the number counted per second will fluctuate in a random fashion, because the process of emission is not a continuous process, but a discrete, statistical one. In general, the statistical error will decrease as the number of events observed increases.

Statistical fluctuations. Variation in count rate arising from the statistical, probabilistic character of radioactive decay.

Statistical straggling. If a measurable effect is brought about by a number of individual processes which are subject to statistical fluctuations, then the magnitude of the effect is not perfectly defined; there is a spread or straggling and the energy straggling which occur when a charged particle loses energy passing through matter.

Status anginosus. Persistent pain of varying severity which occurs at rest and is only briefly and incompletely suppressed by nitrates.

Steady-state free precession. Method of NMR excitation in which strings of radio-frequency (rf) pulses are applied rapidly and repeatedly with interpulse intervals short compared to both T_1 and T_2. Alternating the phases of the (rf) pulses by 180° can be useful in obtaining maximal signal strength.

Steaming. The production of nonphysiological movement in tissue or cellular fluids during ultrasound exposure.

Stellarator. A toroidal plasma confinement system, formed by a combination of magnetic fields, all of which are produced by currents flowing in conductors wound outside the plasma chamber.

Stellate. Star shaped.

Stem radiation. X-rays given off from parts of the anode other than the target; in particular, from the target support.

Stenosis. The constriction of narrowing of a canal or orifice usually as a result of a disease process.

Step and shoot acquisition. A mode of acquisition in single photon emission computerized tomography (SPECT), where the motion of the rotating gantry is discontinuous, that is, it acquires (shoots) data at predefined angular stops. The dwell time at each stop is determined by the frame time parameter.

Steradian. (sr) SI unit defined as the solid angle which, having its vertex in the center of a sphere, cuts off an area of the surface of the sphere equal to that of a square with sides of length equal to the radius of the sphere.

Stereopsis. The phenomenon of perceiving depth, arising from the fact that the image of an object formed on the retina is different for each eye, the eyes seeing objects in space from two different directions.

Stereosynthesis. Reconstruction of the third dimension by the superposition of a series of tomograms.

Stereotomography. Process of taking a pair of stereographic tomograms.

Sterility. Sterility has been defined as "the state of having been sufficiently freed from microorganisms to be deemed safe for some special purpose by some competent body"; the choice of method for radiopharmaceutical sterilization is determined largely by the character of the product and a prescribed method, such as that followed by the U.S. Pharmacopeia; steam sterilization (autoclaving) and membrane filtration (usually 0.22 μm) are commonly used for radiopharmaceuticals. Compounds which cannot be sterilized either by autoclaving or the filtration method, such as aggregated human serum albumin, must be prepared from previously sterile starting materials. Temporary or permanent incapability to reproduce.

Sterilization by radiation. At present the most important application of gamma radiation is the destruction of microorganisms such as bacteria and viruses. This property, coupled with the ability of γ-rays to penetrate bulk materials, makes it invaluable for carrying out sterilization on a large scale. The γ-rays from ^{60}Co and ^{137}Cs do not induce any radioactivity in the treated material.

Steroid. A type of hormone with a complex molecular structure containing four interlocking rings — three contain six carbon atoms each and the fourth contains five carbon atoms.

Stiffness. A description of the resistance of a material to compression. It is equal to the applied pressure divided by the fractional change in volume resulting from the pressure.

$$\text{stiffness (N/m}^2) = \frac{\text{pressure (N/m}^2)}{\text{fractional volume change}}$$

Stimulus. A change in the environment which modifies the activity of cells.

Stochastic. Based on probabilistic or statistical considerations.

Stoichiometry. Study of numerical interrelationships between chemical elements and compounds and the mathematical laws governing such relationships.

Stop-action scanning. Stop-action scanning may be used to provide a frozen ultrasonic B-scan corresponding to a particular time in the cardiac cycle to identify the positions of the valve leaflets. It can be applied to a hand-operated static B-scanner by using the EKG R wave to trigger the mechanism so that the image contains only lines corresponding to a particular time. Thus images of "valves open" or "valves closed" positions may be built up. The same principle may be employed with a real-time scanner in which the frame freeze facility is invoked at the desired time in the cardiac cycle.

Stopping cross section. The linear stopping power (energy loss per unit thickness, dE/dx) divided by the number of atoms per unit volume of the stopping material.

Stopping power. A measure of the effect of a substance upon the kinetic energy of a charged particle passing through it.

Storage. Pertaining to a computer device into which data can be entered, in which it can be held, and from which it can be retrieved at a later time.

Storage capacity. The quantity of data that can be stored in a computer memory (expressed in multiples of 1K bytes where K is a symbol for 1024).

Storage of radioactive materials. All radioactive material that is not actually in use should be kept in a proper storage place and should not be allowed to lie about in laboratories or workshops. The storage place may be a special locker in the laboratory for small quantities or may be a separate building designed to keep larger quantities under safe conditions. (Certain compounds also require refrigeration.)

In either case the store should give protection to people in the vicinity; this may be merely simple ventilation for α- or low-energy β-emitting materials or may involve considerable amounts of lead, concrete, or water for high-activity γ-emitters. Small γ-emitting sources used in the laboratory can be adequately shielded by a few inches of lead.

Storage protection. Protection against unauthorized writing in and/or reading from all or part of a computer storage device. This may be implemented by manually set switches or by automatic hardward facilities, usually in connection with an operating system.

Straggling. A term used to express the fact that the ranges of charged particles of a given energy in matter are not constant but show a small spread about the mean range. This uncertainty in the range occurs because the loss of energy by charged particles is not a continuous process, but one in which energy is transferred in discrete amounts to the electrons in the matter through which the particle is passing.

Stratum. A layer; sheetlike mass of uniform thickness.

Stray radiation. Radiation not serving any useful purpose. It includes direct leakage radiation and secondary radiation from irradiated objects.

Streaming. The increased transmission of electromagnetic or particulate radiation through a medium resulting from the presence of extended voids or other regions of low attenuation. (Also called channeling effect.)

Streamline flow. A type of fluid flow in which there is a continuous steady motion of the particles, the motion at a fixed point always remaining constant. It is also called viscous flow and laminar flow.

Strength. Nonspecific term referring to amplitude or intensity.

Stress. If the patient's environment imposes an undue strain, he reacts with tenseness and anxiousness. Under these conditions minor exertions and excitements can lead to higher secretion of epinephrine and severe circulatory stress, provoking an anginal attack. Outside of their stressful environment, these patients frequently show a much higher exercise tolerance.

Stress test. Measurement of cardiac reserve, heart rate, blood pressure, EKG, oxygen comsumption during strenuous exercise or myocardial perfusion using ^{201}Tl usually measured with the subject being stressed on a treadmill or exercise bicycle.

Stria. A streak or line.

String. A sequence of characters. Many computer programs can search files for occurrences of a string in one manner or another.

Stringer. A long structure occupying a hole through the shield and sometimes into the active section of a nuclear reactor, whose removal permits access to the core for inserting experimental materials. If it is part of a large graphite reactor, for instance, part of its length may consist of graphite blocks keyed together so as to be withdrawn as a unit.

Strip chart recorder. A device for recording the movement of certain structures (usually cardiac) on a long strip of moving paper.

Stroke. Abnormal function in one or more parts of the brain owing to interference with its blood supply. Symptoms may include paralysis, altered sensation, inability to speak, or many others. The blood supply may be reduced by narrowing or blockage of the arteries by atherosclerosis, rupture of the artery (ruptured aneurysm), or a blood clot formed in the heart or large arteries and carried to the brain in the bloodstream (embolus).

Stroke volume. Amount of blood pumped during each heartbeat (diastolic volume of the ventricle minus the volume of blood in the ventricle at the end of systole).

Stroke work index. A measure of the work done by the heart with each contraction, adjusted for body surface area. One determines the stroke work index by multiplying the stroke volume of the heart by the arterial pressure and then dividing this product by the patient's body surface area (as obtained from a nomogram). A normal stroke work index is > 40 g-m/m^2.

Stroma. The structure elements or an organ, a general term to designate the tissue that forms the framework or matrix of an organ, as distinguished from the functioning elements, or parenchyma.

Strontium. Element symbol Sr, atomic number 38, atomic weight 87.62.

Strontium unit. A measure of the concentration of ^{90}Sr in food and in the body (i.e., in bone). It is measured as the ratio of strontium to calcium, with which strontium becomes mixed in soil and living tissue. One strontium unit is 1 millibecquerel (mBq) of ^{90}Sr per gram of calcium.

Structured programming. An attempt to achieve better organization of computer programs and better program documentation in order to make program more understandable, more error free, and more efficient. This also involves the stepwise refinement of the problem itself, until a stage is reached where there is a simple correspondence between the logic of the program solution and the instructions or routines available in some programming language.

Subarachnoid. Below the membrane between the dura mater and pia mater.

Subassembly. A discrete, functional, and essential unit for any computer, excluding the central processing unit (CPU) and CPU memory, but including any devices or boards necessary for acquiring or processing/displaying data. Subsystem.

Subcritical. The state of a reactor in which a self-sustaining chain reaction cannot occur.

Subendocardial infarction. Infarction that involves only the layer of muscle beneath the endocardium, and thus not the entire thickness of the myocardial wall.

Subendothelial. Situated beneath the innermost layer of cells lining the cavities of the heart and blood vessels.

Sublimation. Passing from the solid to the vapor state by heating.

Subphrenic. Below the diaphragm.

Subroutine. A small computer program or section of a program which performs a specific operation with information given or passed to it. May be stored separately and called by several programs when needed. Used to break larger programs up into smaller segments thus aiding in program coding and eliminating errors.

Subshell. The electrons within the same shell (energy level) of the atom are characterized by the same principal quantum number (n), and are further divided into groups according to the value of their azimuthal quantum number (1); the electrons which possess the same azimuthal quantum number for the same principal quantum number are considered to occupy the same subshell (or sublevel). The individual subshells are designated with the letters s, p, d, f, g, and h, as follows:

1 value	designation of subshell
0	s
1	p
2	d
3	f
4	g
5	h

An electron assigned to the s subshell is called an s electron, one assigned to the p subshell is referred to as p electron, etc. In formulas of electron structure, the value of the principal quantum number (n) is prefixed to the letter indicating the azimuthal quantum number (1) of the electron; thus, e.g. an f4 electron is an electron which has the principal quantum number 4 (i.e., assigned to the N shell) and the orbital angular momentum 3 (f subshell).

Substrate. A substance on which an enzyme acts.

Subtraction image. An image produced by adding a reversed baseline mask to a positive image. In radiology, usually with contrast media injected, to bring out the differences between the images, for example, the contrast media distribution.

Sucrose. A double sugar composed of one molecule of glucose and one molecule of fructose. Ordinary sugar.

Sulcus. A furrow, groove, slight depression, or fissure, especially of the brain.

Sulfhydryl. A chemical radical (SH) constituting an important component of many tissue enzymes.

Sulfur. Element symbol S, atomic number 16, atomic weight 32.066.

Sum of squares. Sum of squared deviations around the population mean, $\sum (x - \mu)^2$, or sample mean $\sum (x - X)^2$. The numerator of the variance term.

Superconductive magnet. Magnet whose field is generated by current in wires made of a material, such as niobium-titanium, that has no resistance at temperatures near absolute zero. Such magnets must be cooled by, for example, liquid helium.

Superconductor. A substance whose electrical resistance essentially disappears at temperatures near absolute zero. A commonly used superconductor in NMR imaging system magnets is niobium-titanium , embedded in a copper matrix to help protect the superconductor from quenching.

Supercritical. A reactor, in which the multiplication constant is greater than unity, is called supercritical.

Superior vena cava. The large blood vessel through which venous blood from the head, upper extremities, and chest enters the right atrium of the heart.

Supernatant. Liquid lying above or floating on a precipitated material.

Supine. Lying on back with face upward.

Support programs. A set of computer programs (for example, diagnostics, testing aids, data generator programs, terminal simulators) required to install an operating system.

Suppression. The elimination of selected signals. Logarithmic amplification suppresses large signals relative to weak ones. Squaring the signals suppresses weak signals relative to strong ones.

Suppressor T cells. A subset of T lymphocytes that suppresses antibody synthesis by B cells or inhibits other cellular immune reactions by effector T cells.

Supraclavicular. Situated above the clavicle.

Surface coil NMR. A simple, flat, radio-frequency (rf) receiver coil placed over a region of interest will have an effective selectivity for a volume approximately subtended by the coil circumference and one radius deep from the coil center. Such a coil can be used for simple localization of sites for measurement of chemical shift spectra, especially of phosphorus, and blood flow studies. Some additional spatial selectivity can be achieved with gradient magnetic fields.

Surface phagocytosis. The enhancement of phagocytosis by entrapment of organisms on surfaces such as leukocytes, fibrin clots, or other tissue surfaces.

Surfactant. A substance that lowers surface tension, e.g., in the lung alveoli.

Survey meter. A battery-powered portable device containing a gas ionization chamber for monitoring radiation levels.

Survival curve. When a group of living organisms are all given the same dose of radiation a certain fraction of the organisms will be killed. This fraction will be small for small doses and will increase as the dose increases, while for very high doses none of the organisms will survive. If a number of groups are each given different doses, then the dose-effect relation may be shown by plotting the fraction of each group surviving against the dose received.

Suture. A type of closely knit joint as in the skull; or a material used in sewing up a wound.

Swan-Ganz catheter. A multilumen (usually four), flow-directed, balloon-tip catheter which may be passed along a vein through the right heart chambers into the pulmonary artery. Its passage and placement facilitate the measurement of central venous pressure, pulmonary arterial pressure, and pulmonary capillary wedge pressure. It may also be used in the measurement of cardiac output (thermodilution method).

Sweep rate. The rate, in hertz per second (Hz s^{-1}), at which the applied radio frequency is varied to produce an NMR spectrum.

Swept gain. The process by which the gain of a pulse-echo system is varied with time to compensate for the effects of absorption.

Switching center. A center that stores and processes messages for transmission to intended destinations. Computers provide the communications functions of routing, priority processing, code and speed conversion, and transmission in addition to their other functions.

Switchover. When equipment fails, an automatic or manual switch can be made to an alternate component (for example, file unit, communications line, computer).

Sympathetic nervous system. That part of the autonomic nervous system that originates in the thoracolumbar region of the spinal cord, synapses in the chain of sympathetic ganglia with neurons that release norepinephrine in the organs they innervate; in general, the sympathetic nervous system prepares the body for activity in emergency.

Synapse. The point at which a nervous impulse passes from one neuron to another.

Synchro-cyclotron. A cyclotron in which the radio frequency of the electric field is frequency modulated to permit acceleration of particles to relativistic energies.

Synchronizing pulses. Timing pulses used to assure that X-ray production, video scanning, digitization, and data storage are coordinated.

Synchronous. Pertaining to one or more processes that depend upon the occurrences of specific events, such as common timing signals. Occurring with a regular or predictable time relationship. Generally supports higher baud rates/bandwidths than asynchronous transmission.

Synchronous transfer. Sequenced computer program operated by an external clock that does not permit a step to proceed until the previous step is completed.

Synchrony. Simultaneous occurrence. Specifically that characteristic of the healthy heartbeat whereby the entire mass of myocardial fibers contracts more or less simultaneously.

Synchroton. A machine for accelerating electrons to high speeds; the electrons are kept in a circular path by a guiding magnetic field and are accelerated in this path by synchronous electric impulses. Proton synchrotrons have been developed on the same principle to accelerate protons.

Syncope. A mild and transient form of shock with a short period of unconsciousness from which rapid recovery is made upon assuming a horizontal position (fainting); in the emotional or psychogenic type, vasovagal reflexes slow the heart and bring on peripheral vasodilation, thereby diminishing cardiac output.

Syndrome. The complex of symptoms associated with any disease.

Synergism. A characteristic exhibited when two separate agents in combination produce an effect greater than that produced by each agent separately.

Syngeneic. Denotes the relationship that exists between genetically identical members of the same species.

Syngraft. A graft derived from a syngeneic donor.

Synovia. Transparent fluid found in joint cavities.

Synovial membrane. A layer of connective tissue lining the cavity of a joint, but not covering the articular surfaces.

Syntax. The structure of expressions in a language and the rules governing the structure of a language. Rules governing the expression of a computer language.

Synthesis. A process in which a new chemical compound is formed in a reaction.

System. Embraces all the objects that relate or interact to form a whole. In computer terms it is understood to include such things as hardware, software of all levels, input/output devices, communication pathways in networks, and all other machines making up the functional unit. Synonym — "configuration".

System board. The large printed circuit board inside the system unit with many electronic components mounted on it. It contains most of the electronics at the heart of the computer's operations.

System count rate performance with scatter. Count rate performance with scatter characterizes a system's ability to accurately function at high count rates and under conditions where a high fraction of scattered radiation is present, which more accurately reflects the clinical imaging conditions than does the intrinsic count rate procedure.

System expansion slot. A socket for holding an adapter card in a computer crate. The system unit and system expansion unit both have system expansion slots.

System expansion unit. A component that attaches to the computer system unit through a data cable. It provides slots for additional adapter cards and room for additional disk drives.

Systemic. Pertaining to or affecting the body as a whole.

Systemic circulation. The circulation of blood through all parts of the body other than the lungs.

Systemic temperature. A measure of the basic temperature of the complete organism. Measured by thermometer, rectal or oral, or by rectal or oral thermistor probe.

Systemic vascular resistance. An index of arteriolar constriction throughout the body. It is obtained by dividing the blood pressure by the cardiac output.

Systems analysis. Refers to analyzing a functional area with a view to specifying a particular computing "configuration". In this case the individuals and their particular behaviors in relation to data manipulation are considered part of the system to be analyzed. Systems analysis can be applied as a rigorous discipline, through no unique method is generally accepted to date.

System sensitivity. System sensitivity is a parameter of a scintillation camera with its collimator in place, which characterizes its ability to efficiently detect incident γ-rays.

System spatial resolution with and without scatter. System spatial resolution with and without scatter is a parameter of a scintillation camera and collimator which characterizes its ability to accurately determine the original location of a γ-ray on an X-Y plane.

System velocity. Assumed velocity of sound as applied in the apparatus in order to translate the speed of return of echoes into depth. Conventionally 1540 m s^{-1}.

Systole. The stage of the cardiac cycle at which contraction of a cardiac chamber occurs and blood is expelled. In the cardiac cycle, atrial systole precedes ventricular systole.

Systolic blood pressure. The pressure of blood in the arteries during systole. The average systolic pressure in the brachial artery of a young adult is 110 to 130 mm Hg.

Systolic sound. A heart sound formed during systole.

Szilard-Chalmers reaction. A chemical change caused by a nuclear transformation in which there is no change in atomic number. The term is most commonly used for a reaction in which a radiotactive isotope is obtained from an (n, γ) reaction in a chemically different form from the isotopic target, due to recoil of the new nucleus breaking chemical bonds.

T

Tachycardia. Rapid heart rate; usually applied to rates over 100 beats per minute.

Tachypnea. Very rapid breathing.

Tagged atom. Or labeled atom, is that atomic position in a molecular formula which is occupied by an isotopic tracer.

Tailored excitation. Radio-frequency (rf) excitation designed to excite only a selected region of the sample.

Tailored pulse. Shaped pulse whose magnitude is varied with time in a predetermined manner. Affects the frequency components of a radio-frequency (rf) pulse in a manner determined by the Fourier transform of the pulse. (NMR.)

Tailored system. Following the rigors of sys-

tems analysis a system is designed to meet the needs of a particular user and that user only.

Tanaka method for weighted backprojection. This method is basically an image reconstruction filtered backprojection with some modifications. The algorithm consists of three steps: normalization of observed projections, modified convolution operation, and weighted backprojection. In this study, the reconstruction index which controls the relative contributions of two conjugate projections to the image was zero.

Tantalum. Element symbol Ta, atomic number 73, atomic weight 180.948.

T antigens. Tumor antigens, probably protein products of the viral genome present only on infected neoplastic cells.

Tapetum. A covering layer of cells; a part of the brain.

Target. The material subjected to bombardment by radiation, high-energy particles, or high-energy nuclei for the purpose of producing a nuclear reaction.

Target heart rate. Generally, that heart rate which defines activity intense enough to produce a training effect. Specifically, between 70 and 85% of the age-corrected maximum expected heart rate. (220 — age in years.)

Target organ. For imaging, the organ intended to receive the greatest concentration of a radioactive tracer; for dosimetry, the organ receiving the largest cumulated radioactivity or the organ for which the dose is being calculated.

Target theory. Theory explaining some biologic effects of radiation on basis of ionization occurring in a very small, sensitive region within the cell. One, two, or more "hits" (hit theory): i.e., ionizing events within the sensitive volume may be necessary to bring about the effect.

Task. Work to be accomplished by a computer. The task is usually specified to a control program in a multiprogramming or multiprocessing environment.

T cell (T lymphocyte). A thymus-derived cell that participates in a variety of cell-mediated immune reactions.

Technetium. Element symbol Tc, atomic number 43, atomic weight 98.

Technetium-99m. (^{99m}Tc) Metastable form of technetium widely used as a label in nuclear medicine. Decays with a 6-h half-life with emission of a monoenergetic 140-keV γ-ray.

Telangiectasia. Chronic dilatation of capillaries and small arterial branches producing small, reddish tumors in the skin, as of the face.

Telecommunications. Any system in which electric or electromagnetic signals transmit information between two or more separate locations. Telecommunications systems link computers to each other and to remote computer terminals.

Telecommunications access method. A method used to transfer data between main storage and remote or local terminals, eliminating terminal input/output delays.

Teleconferencing. The process of conferring between multiple groups in separate geographic areas by using telephonic means. Also refers to a type of communication (for example, electronic mail) conducted by computers.

Teleprinter. A combination of a printer and typewriter-style keyboard used to send and receive data in a telegraph system.

Teleprocessing. A form of information handling in which a data processing system uses communications facilities.

Teletherapy. A radiotherapy method of using a radiation source in which the radioelement is shielded on all sides except one, thus giving a directional beam of radiation which is directed at a distant area to be treated.

Tellurium. Element symbol Te, atomic number 52, atomic weight 127.60.

Telophase. The final stage of mitosis or meiosis in cell division.

Temperature. The condition of a body that determines transfer of heat to or from other bodies. No heat flows when two bodies of equal temperatures come in contact with each other. Heat flows from a body of higher temperature to one of lower temperature when they come in contact.

Temperature transducer. The thermoelectric potential between two dissimilar metals (thermocouple), or the change in resistance due to temperature (thermistor) may be used to measure and record temperatures.

Template. A line of text that disk operation system's (DOS's) line editing feature uses as the basis for creating a new or modified line of text. By using the program function keys, the INS key, and the DEL key, it is possible to copy characters from the template to the new line, skip over template characters, and insert new characters in the new line.

Temporal average intensity. The time average of intensity at a point in space. For a nonautoscanning ultrasound system, the average is taken over one or more pulse repetition periods. For autoscanning ultrasound systems, the intensity may be averaged over one or more scan repetition periods for a specified operating mode.

Temporal filter. Method for smoothing computer images from a dynamic study by averaging each image with the preceding and following images.

Temporal peak intensity. The peak instantaneous value of the intensity at the point considered.

Temporal resolution. Temporal resolution refers to the ability of an instrument, e.g., scintillation camera, to register events occurring within a very small time interval as separate events.

Tendon. Fibrous cord by which a muscle is attached to a bone.

Tenth-value layer. (TVL) The thickness of a specified absorbing material which, when introduced into the path of a beam of radiation, reduces the dose rate to one tenth of its original value.

Tentorium. Fibrous tissue shelf separating the cerebrum from the cerebellum.

Terbium. Element symbol Tb, atomic number 65, atomic weight 158.925.

Terminal. End; or leading to death. Any device that sends and/or receives information over a communications channel, enters data into a computer, and communicates system decisions.

Tesla. The preferred (SI) unit of magnetic flux density. One tesla is equal to 10,000 g, the older (CGS) unit.

Testimony. (Legal) Information presented orally by a competent witness under oath, sometimes used synonymously with the broader term evidence which includes all testimony.

Testing. The process of subjecting a program to the conditions under which it must normally function in order to see if it works correctly.

Tetrahedron. Molecular geometry in which the central atom is attached to four other atoms and the bond axes are directed along the diagonals of a cube.

Tetralogy of fallot. A congenital disease of the heart involving four defects: (1) an abnormal opening in the interventricular septum, (2) misplacement of the aorta such that it receives blood from both ventricles, (3) a narrowing of the pulmonary artery, and (4) an enlargement of the right ventricle.

Text display. The display of alphanumeric text or special characters on the video screen for photographic and viewing purposes.

Text editor. Program that enables an operator to alter a text by adding or deleting words, changing sentences, making corrections, etc.

Thalamus. A large mass of gray matter located on the sides of the third ventricle of the brain, serving as a major coordinating region for sensory information.

Thallium. Element symbol T1, atomic number 81, atomic weight 204.3833.

T_1. ("T-one") Spin-lattice or longitudinal relaxation time; the characteristic time constant for spins to tend to align themselves with the external magnetic field. Starting from zero magnetization in the z direction, the z magnetization will grow to 63% of its final maximum value in a time T_1 (NMR).

T_1 relaxation time. Time constant for the longitudinal magnetization to reach its equilibrium value. (NMR.)

T_2. ("T-two") Spin-spin or transverse relaxation time; the characteristic time constant for loss of phase coherence among spins oriented at an angle to the static magnetic field, due to interactions between the spins, with the resulting loss of transverse magnetization and NMR signal. Starting from a nonzero value of the magnetization in the xy plane, the xy magnetization will decay so that it loses 63% of its initial value in a time T_2.

T_2^*. ("T-two-star") The characteristic time constant for loss of phase coherence among spins oriented at an angle to the static magnetic field to a combination of magnetic field inhomogeneities, ΔB, and spin-spin transverse relaxation with resultant more rapid loss in transverse magnetization and NMR signal. NMR signal can still be recovered as a spin echo in times less than or on the order of T_2. 1/R2* + $1/T_2$ + $\Delta\omega/2$; $\Delta\omega = \gamma\Delta B$.

T_2 relaxation time. Time constant for the transverse magnetization to reach its equilibrium value in a magnetic field. Also denoted effective transverse relaxation time ($T_2^* < T_2$). (NMR.)

Therapeutic embolization. The purposeful administration of intravascular foreign bodies (emboli) aimed at the termination of bleeding when surgical interruption might not be feasible, occlusion of blood supply to large vascular tumors, or the obstruction of arteriovenous malformations is termed therapeutic embolization. The foreign material introduced may be in the form of silastic beads, bits of preclotted blood, as well as numerous other approved and sterile foreign material. The primary purpose

of this procedure is to diminish the blood supply to a potentially surgically correctable abnormality by reducing the blood loss at the time of operation.

Therapeutic-type protective tube housing. Housing so constructed that at every specified rating of the X-ray tube the leakage radiation at a focal distance of 1 m does not exceed 2.58 × 10^{-4} kg^{-1} h^{-1}, 77.4 × 10^{-4} kg^{-1} h^{-1} at any point accessible to the patient at a distance of 5 cm from the surface of the housing or its accessory equipment.

Therapy. The medical treatment of any disease.

Thermal column. A column or large body of moderator, such as graphite, extending away from the active section of a nuclear reactor to provide near its other end, for experimental purposes, a flux of thermal neutrons of high cadmium ratio, i.e., containing few virgin and epithermal neutrons.

Thermal equlibrium. A state in which all parts of a system are at the same effective temperature, in particular where the relative alignment of the spins with the magnetic field is determined solely by the thermal energy of the system (in which case the relative numbers of spins with different alignments will be given by the Boltzmann distribution). (NMR.)

Thermal leakage factor. The fraction of neutrons in a chain-reacting system which leak out of the system after they have been thermalized and before they are absorbed by the system.

Thermal neutron. Neutrons in approximately thermal equilibrium with their surroundings. At room temperature their mean energy is about 0.025 eV. Neutrons of higher energies are referred to as fast neutrons.

Thermal reactor. A nuclear reactor in which fission is induced primarily by neutrons of such energy that they are in substantial termal equilibrium with the material of the core. A representative energy for thermal neutrons often is taken as 0.025 (2200 m/s), which corresponds to the mean energy of neutrons in a Maxwellian distribution at 293 K, although most thermal reactors actually operate at a higher temperature.

Thermal shield. A shield intended to reduce heat generation by ionizing radiation in, and heat transfer to, exterior regions.

Thermocouple. A device that converts temperature to a voltage.

Thermodilution technique. A technique used to measure cardiac output. Using a multichannel catheter, a solution, cooled to less than body temperature, is injected into the venous system. A thermistor, incorporated into the distal end of a catheter positioned in the pulmonary artery, detects the resultant blood temperature change, which is proportional to blood flow.

Thermodynamics. Study of processes based on energy changes in the system.

Thermogenesis. The production of heat in the body.

Thermography. There is a known relationship between the surface temperature of an object and its radiant power. This principle makes it possible to measure the temperature of a body without physical contact with it. Medical thermography is a technique whereby the temperature distribution on the surface of the body is mapped within a few tenths of a degree Kelvin. The detector in a radiation thermometer is typically arsenic trisulfide, indium antimonide, lead sulfide, or thallium bromide iodine. Most thermography apparatuses employ a mirror-type focusing device and the radiation beam is fed to the detector through a chopping disk which has a slot in it to interrupt the beam at a frequency of several hundred hertz so that an AC amplifier and phase-sensitive detector can be used to amplify without the drift associated with DC amplifiers. The best-known use of the heat camera or thermograph is in breast scanning, where irregularities in the temperature distribution may indicate underlying disease.

Thermoluminescence. Luminescence produced in certain substances by heating. Many minerals show the effect: fluorite and quartz are examples. The effect if often shown more strongly after excitation by nuclear radiation (α-, β-, and γ-rays).

Thermoluminescent detector. (TLD) Type of crystal used to monitor radiation exposure by emitting light; used in a film badge, or ring badge.

Thermoluminescent dosimetry. A method of monitoring radiation exposure. Thermoluminescent materials, particularly lithium fluoride, are exposed to the radiation. Such materials emit light when heated after being exposed to the radiation. The light output measured is dependent on exposure dose.

Thermonuclear reaction. A nuclear reaction in which the energy necessary for the reaction is provided by colliding particles that have kinetic energy by virtue of their thermal agitation. Such reactions occur at appreciable rates only for temperatures of millions of degrees

and higher, the rate increasing enormously with the temperature.

Thetatron. A device for producing hot, dense plasma. A large electric current is rapidly developed around a single turn coil wound (in the theta direction) on a cylinder and compresses the plasma toward the axis.

Thick source. This is a radioactive source in which self-absorption or scattering is important.

Thimble ionization chamber. A small, cylindrical, spherical ionization chamber, usually with walls of organic material.

Thin-film memory. An extremely fast, extremely compact type of magnetic storage medium. To construct such a memory, a layer of magnetic substance only a few millionths of a centimeter thick is deposited on a plate of glass or other nonmagnetic material. Then, microscopic areas on the film are polarized (electrically charged) to store digital information. A single binary digit can be retrieved from thin-film memory in about a billionth of a second.

Thinking. The exercising of powers of judgment, conception, or inference as distinguised from simple sensory perception.

Thin source. A radioactive source in which self-absorption or scattering is not important.

Thin window. Part of a wall of a radiation detector is often made especially thin to enable weakly penetrating particles to get inside and be counted, e.g., for alpha and beta particles.

Thin-window counter tube. In order that radiation may be detected it must pass into the sensitive volume of the counter tube and produce ionization. In the case of short-range radiation it is usual to provide the counter tube with a window through which the radiation may pass to penetrate into the sensitive volume. For the detection of alpha particles and soft beta particles it is essential to use a thin window; counter tubes designed for this purpose are often referred to as thin-window counter tubes.

Thiols. Family of organic compounds containing the functional group — SH.

Thoracentesis. Puncture of the wall of the thorax for the withdrawal of fluid.

Thoracic aortography. An arterial catheter is placed into the ascending aorta above the aortic valve. Contrast material is then injected to evaluate the origins of the great vessels supplying the cerebral circulation or to look for evidence of abnormality of the aortic wall (e.g., aneurysm or dissection).

Thoracotomy. The surgical opening of the chest wall.

Thorax. The part of the body of man and other mammals between the neck and the abdomen.

Thorium. Element symbol Th, atomic number 90, atomic weight 232.038.

Threshold. Lower limit of stimulus capable of producing an impression on consciousness or of evoking a response in an irritable tissue. Entrance of a canal. That level of radiation dose below which there may be no permanent injury to the organisms. Contrast enhancement technique where intensities less than a specified lower level are black and those above an upper threshold level are saturated, i.e., white.

Threshold energy. The energy of an incident particle or photon below which a particular endothermic reaction will not occur.

Thrill. A fine vibration felt by the hand or fingertips on the surface of the body, associated in some instances with disease in underlying organs, such as a septal defect following myocardial infarction.

Thrombin. An enzyme which converts fibrinogen to fibrin in the blood-clotting process.

Thrombogenicity. The ability of a material to activate the clotting of blood.

Thrombosis. The formation of a blood clot in a blood vessel or cavity of the heart.

Thrombus. A blood clot that forms gradually at an area of blood vessel wall damage or over an atherosclerotic lesion. Thrombi may be occlusive or may remain attached to the vessel or heart wall without obstructing blood flow. (An embolus is a clot that breaks away and travels through the circulation to lodge distally.)

Throughput. Decay events actually stored in the multichannel analyzer. The total amount of useful work performed by a data processing system during a given period of time.

Thulium. Element symbol Tm, atomic number 69, atomic weight 168.934.

Thymus. A primary lymphoid organ in the upper thorax where T cells mature.

Thymus-dependent antigen. Antigen that depends on T-cell interaction with B cells for antibody synthesis, e.g., erythrocytes, serum proteins, and hapten-carrier complexes.

Thymus-independent antigen. Antigen that can induce an immune response without the apparent participation of T lymphocytes.

Thyroglobulin. A glycoprotein stored in thyroid-gland acini which contains T_4, T_3, and iodotyrosines (diiodotyrosine and moniodotyrosine). Thyroglobulin is the principal iodoprotein of the thyroid gland. As a result of proteolysis, thyroglobulin is broken down so efficiently that normally no iodoproteins pass into the circulation. Abnormal circulating iodoproteins may be present in the serum of patients with Hashimoto's thyroiditis. It is believed that this compound is related to thyroglobulin "leaking" from the thyroid as part of the autoimmunizing process.

Thyroid gland. An endocrine gland lying in front of the trachea. It secretes the thyroid hormones that control the rate of metabolism, growth, and development.

Thyroid-stimulating hormone. (TSH, thyrotropin, thyrotropic hormone) A hormone released by the anterior pituitary under thyroid hormone servomechanism which stimulates thyroid activity and elevates the level of circulating thyroid hormones. The concentration of TSH, expressed as microunits/milliliter (μU/ml), is determined by radioimmunoassay (designated TSH-RIA). Used in differentiating pituitary or hypothalamus-related hypothyroid states from a primary deficiency in thyroid-gland secretion.

Thyroid uptake study. (RAIU, radioactive iodine uptake) Measurement of percentage of administered radioiodine (^{131}I, ^{123}I) taken up in the thyroid gland at a particular time interval.

Thyrotropin-releasing hormone. (TRH) A neurohumoral factor from the hypothalamus which helps regulate the release of thyroid-stimulating hormone (TSH) from the anterior pituitary.

Thyroxine. (3,5,3′,5′-L-tetraiodothyronine, T4, or levothyroxine) The more abundant of the two natural thyroid hormones. It differs from T_3 by having an iodine atom in the 5′-position.

Thyroxine-binding globulin. (TBG) A serum protein which is the major binding protein of thyroxine (T-4). It also binds triiodothyronine (T-3). TBG is an interalphaglobulin, being the primary agent for transport of thyroid hormone.

Tidal volume. Volume of gas inspired or expired during each quiet respiration cycle.

Time-activity curve. A histogram of the change in the count rate as a function of time.

Time base. The (real or virtual) trace on a display representing the time coordinate. The distance of a displayed echo from the time origin is proprotional to the distance of the echo source from the transducer. (The electronic circuits which produce the trace on the display are also called the time base.)

Time coincidence. The occurrence of counts in

two or more detectors simultaneously or within a fixed short time interval. A true coincidence is one due to the incidence of a single particle or of several genetically related particles. An accidental or chance coincidence is one due to the fortuitous occurrence of unrelated counts in separate detectors.

Time compression analyzer. Frequency analysis of ultrasonic Doppler blood flow signals can be achieved using a bank of electronic filters, but a more modern method is to use a computer to perform fast Fourier transform (FFT) analysis. Doppler blood flow signals may contain frequency components from (say) 200 Hz to 15 kHz. This wide range of frequencies cannot be analyzed quickly enough in a sequential mode. This problem is solved by dividing the signal into short periods (e.g., 10 ms) and reading these into a computer memory. These are then read out at a much faster rate (e.g., 250 times faster) and rapid analysis applied to the time compressed signal. The flow pattern is then displayed on a strip chart usually produced on a fiber-optic recorder with the frequency components (velocity components) displayed across the strip. By using the amplitude of these components as well as the frequency, the rate of blood flow may also be calculated.

Time constant. Characteristic response time of a system. The longer the time constant, the longer it takes for the system to respond. (The response is usually exponential in time.)

Time gain compensation. Change in gain with time to compensate for loss in echo amplitude, usually due to attenuation, with depth.

Time-interval difference. A real-time digital difference imaging in which temporally adjacent video images are subtracted and displayed. This mode of imaging presents a continuous display of the difference between adjacent video frames.

Time-motion scanning. This is a special ultrasonic scanning used for tracing the motion of structures within the body, particularly the walls and valves of the heart. It is commonly called an M-mode (motion) scanner or an echocardiograph. In effect it is a single-line B-scanner presenting the echoes immediately beneath the ultrasonic transducer and moving this line slowly across a cathode ray tube screen so that static structures draw straight lines, whereas moving structures have characteristic movement patterns.

Time-of-flight detection. (TOF) Time-of-flight coincidence detection involves measuring the time difference between the coincident events being registered in the two detectors concerned. It is therefore possible to determine directly where the annihilation events occurred. Plastic scintillator detectors are traditionally used for TOF measurement, but the poor stopping power of plastic for 511-keV photons prohibits their use in PET scanners. Using cesium fluoride (CsF) detectors or barium fluoride (BaF_2) detectors, coincidence resolving times of some 400 ps are achievable — giving a positional resolution. This means, for a whole-body PET scanner, a fourfold statistical improvement (in relation to the number of counts recorded).

Time-of-flight measurements. Time-of-flight measurements are usually made by using a time-to-amplitude converter in association with a pulse-amplitude analyzer. By plotting the time distribution of the neutrons it is possible to investigate the velocity distribution, i.e., the energy distribution of the neutrons admitted into the apparatus.

Time position scan. Ultrasound M-mode. Representation of motion within the organs being studies by causing a B-mode to travel along the X or Y axis of the cathode ray tube (CRT). Echoes from stationary area remain straight lines. Those from moving areas will be wavy or zig-zag lines depending on the regularity and amplitude of the motion.

Time reversal. Technique of producing a spin echo by subjecting excited spins to a gradient magnetic field, and then reversing the direction of the gradient field. All methods of spin-echo production can be viewed as effective time reversal. (NMR.)

Time sharing. The use of a given device by a number of other devices, programs, or human users, one at a time and in rapid succession. A technique or system for furnishing computing services to multiple users, providing rapid responses to each of the users. Time-sharing computer systems usually employ multiprocessing techniques and are often capable of serving users at remote locations via a data communications network.

Time sorter. An apparatus for sorting pulses according to the time at which they occur in relation to some standard time. It comprises a number of gates which open at defined times, the pulses being fed to a selection of channels according to the times at which they occur.

Timing unit. A device that controls the operation of different parts of an experimental setup, switching on and off the equipment and taking readings at predetermined times. A device for measuring the time delay between two events.

Tin. Element symbol Sn (stannum), atomic number 50, atomic weight 118.71.

Tissue. An aggregation of similarly specialized cells united in the performance of a particular function.

Tissue/air ratio. The ratio of the absorbed dose rate at a given point in a phantom to the absorbed dose rate at the same point, but at the center of a small amount of phantom material of mass just large enough the provide electronic equilibrium at the point of measurement. (Radiation therapy.)

Tissue dose. Radiation dose received by a tissue in the region of interest. In the case of X-rays and γ-rays, tissue doses are expressed in gray.

Tissue equivalent ionization chamber. Ionization chamber in which the material of the walls, electrodes, and gas are so selected as to produce ionization essentially equivalent to that characteristic of the tissue under consideration. In some cases it is sufficient to have only tissue equivalent walls, and the gas may be air, provided the air volume is very small. The essential requisite in such a case is that the contribution by ionizating particles originating in the air is negligible compared to that produced by ionizing particles characteristic of the wall material.

Tissue equivalent material. Material which has the same reaction to radiation (e.g., absorption) as living tissue and so can be used in models to study probable doses, radiation scatter, etc. Since soft tissue contains about 80% of water, water itself is a very convenient tissue equivalent material for many purposes, e.g., phantoms in which to measure isodose curves. But for other purposes such as the estimation of doses in irregular-shaped body sections a solid material is more convenient. The main requirement is that the material shall have the same atomic number as soft tissue.

Titanium. Element symbol Ti, atomic number 22, atomic weight 47.88.

Titer. The amount of a substance (standard) needed to react with a volume of another substance. A measure of antibody concentration in an antiserum. In radioimmunoassay (RIA), that dilution of an antiserum that binds a predetermined precentage (usually 50%) of tracer antigen in the absence of unlabeled antigen.

Titration. Method of quantitative analysis in which one substance is volumetrically added to another substance with which it quantitatively reacts.

Tokamak. A toroidal plasma confinement system formed by a combination of magnetic fields, one of which is produced by current flowing through the plasma.

Tolerance. Traditionally denotes that condition in which responsive cell clones have been eliminated or inactivated by prior contact with antigen, with the result that no immune response occurs on administration of antigen.

Tolerance dose. Synonym for "permissible dose". The latter is generally considered the preferrable term.

Tomogram. The resultant picture from a tomographic reconstruction of a slice taken through a series of images. These images, e.g., in transaxial tomography, are taken at different angles or views of the particular object of intest, about a single axis or center of rotation.

Tomographic section thickness. The effective thickness of a section determined by an absolute or an arbitrary factor. The term thickness alone is not recommended.

Tomography. The term that describes all types of body section techniques, since all these are bound by the same principles, that is, a visual representation restricted to a specified section or "cut" of tissue within an organ or part of the body produced by an X-ray (transmission), photon (emission), or magnetic field technique. Computer processing of the data may or may not be employed in order to assist in generating the image. The term tomography is now so universally used and established that it has been chosen, although planigraphy and stratigraphy have priority, chronologically and historically.

Topical nuclear magnetic resonance. *In vivo* NMR spectroscopic technique using gradient fields to localize a volume for excitation.

Topology. The way in which computers and terminals are linked together to form a network. Common network topologies include the star, tree, fully-linked, and ring configurations.

Torcula. Hollow, expanded area.

Toroidal experiment. One in which the plasma is confined within a tube bent into a circle (like a tire's inner tube).

Torque. The effectiveness of a force in setting a body into rotation. It is a vector quantity given by the vector product of the force and the position vector where the force is applied; for a rotation body, the torque is the product of the moment of inertia and the resulting angular acceleration.

Tort. (Legal) This is the offense. It has four essential components. A legal injury must be proven. There must be a duty which one party owes another. There must be a violation of this duty. The injury must result from such violation.

Torts. (Legal) This is the study of a continuously evolving area of law which has to do with the rights, wants, and desires of the individual. When these are recognized in law (and this is a state of mind, restrained by the past, and urged by the future), one who interferes with his realization will be liable.

Total attenuation of sound in tissue. The reduction of the intensity of a sound beam as it passes through biological tissues, the result of scattering and absorption, is known as attenuation. Attenuation is conveniently expressed as a rate of decrease of intensity in decibels per centimeter depth of tissue and is found to increase linearly with frequency in most tissues.

Total-body dose. Average radiation dose to the entire body obtained by averaging the dose to different tissues and organs.

Total count tube. A tube in a radioimmunoassay (RIA) to which an aliquot of radiolabeled ligand only has been added to serve as a check on the delivery of that material.

Total cross section. The sum of the cross sections for all the separate interactions between the incident radiation and a specified target.

Total ionization. The total electric charge of one sign on the ions produced by radiation in the process of losing all of its kinetic energy. For a given gas, the total ionization is closely proportional to the initial ionization and is nearly independent of the nature of ionizing radiation; the total number of ion pairs produced by the ionizing particle along its entire length. It is frequently used as a measure of radiation energy.

Total lung capacity. The volume of air contained in the lungs after a maximum inspiration.

Total mass stopping power. The average energy lost by a charged particle of ionizing radiation traversing a tissue of given thickness and mass density.

Total (nonelastic) respiratory resistance. Total pulmonary resistance plus thoracic tissue resistance.

Total-performance phantom. A device that permits the evaluation of an imaging procedure, including the performance of the equipment and of the nuclear medicine personnel.

Total-performance test. An uncomplicated test for verifying the overall performance of a nuclear medicine procedure without separately testing each individual factor involved in the procedure.

Tourniquet. A simple tourniquet is a strapping or bandage wound tightly around a limb so that it prevents blood flow. It can be used to prevent bleeding during surgery on the extremities or to prevent blood loss from a wound (for a short period). Automatic tourniquets exist which have inflatable cuffs, similar to blood pressure cuffs applied around the upper part of each limb, and they are inflated to reduce the return of venous blood from the limbs (i.e., to a pressure of about 50 mmHg).

Toxicity. The quality of being poisonous, especially the degree of virulence of a toxic microbe or of a poison. It is expressed by a fraction indicating the ratio between the smallest amount that will cause an animal's death and the weight of that animal.

Toxicology. The sudy of poisons.

Toxoids. Antigenic but nontoxic derivatives of toxins.

Trabeculae. Fibrous tissue supporting the structure of an organ.

Trace. A small quantity of material measurable only by special techniques.

Trace analysis. The analysis of very small quantities of material or of material found in extremely low concentrations.

Tracer. An element or compound used to trace the handling and distribution of the same substance from which it differs physically but not chemically. It should be readily detected and should not affect the process it is used to measure. A usually radioactive substance introduced into the body, the progress of which may be followed by means of an external radioactive detector.

Tracer study. Radioactive materials can be used as tracers or indicators because: (1) they emit a characteristic radiation, which allows their presence to be detected even when present in very minute quantities; (2) living organism and chemical reactions, as well as many physical processes, are largely insensitive to the small differences in mass which exist between the radioisotope and the corresponding stable material. It is therefore possible to mix a small quantity of the radioisotope in question with the stable material; it will then follow this material and behave in every way as it does in biological processes, chemical reactions, etc., except in one respect — it will emit radiation, thus permitting its presence to be detected and, if necessary, located.

Track. The visible record of the passage of a charged particle in a cloud chamber, bubble chamber, or photographic emulsion. In cloud chambers the tracks consist of closely spaced liquid droplets suspended in a gas, and in bubble chambers the tracks are formed from bubbles of gas suspended in a liquid. In photographic emulsions it is the developed silver grains suspended in the gelatin of the emulsion that form the track. A term that applies to magnetic storage media — disk or tape. Refers to the area that can be magnetized by a magnetic recording head. On a tape drive there are normally seven or nine heads that record seven or nine linear tracks on the tape. On a spinning disk, a single track is a circle. There are several hundred concentric circular tracks on a disk, and all can contain the same number of pieces of data.

Tractor. A mechanism that pulls pin-feed paper through a printer. It engages the paper's sprocket holes with a pair of sprocketed wheels or belts. A tractor may be built into a printer or may be added as an accessory.

Transaction logging. The process of reduntantly recording everything that users input to a computer. Used in conjunction with a backup copy of system data for restoring data stored on the computer system to its original condition in cases in which data base is inadvertently destroyed.

Transaxial emission tomography. Transverse section reconstruction of the radionuclide distribution obtained by acquiring slices (about 1 to 2 cm in thickness) of the head or body. Coincidence detection (with positrons) or single photon detection (with nuclides such as ^{99m}Tc or ^{201}Tl) is used.

Transcobalamin. Derivative of the cobalt-containing complex common to all members of the vitamin B_{12} group.

Transcribe. To copy information stored on one storage medium onto another storage medium (e.g., from punched cards to paper tape; from bubble memory to thin film; from disk to tape). This can be done by computers or by a special off-line device.

Transducer. This is a device for the conversion of one form of energy to another. In medical work the best-known examples are temperature, pressure, sound, ion concentration, force, and displacement transducers. The term could

be applied to any energy-converting device such as a motor or light bulb, but it is usually reserved for an electrically operated measuring device or actuator.

Transducer array. Transducer assembly containing more than one transducer element.

Transducer attenuation. A control whereby the intensity of the sound beam that is being transmitted by the transducer can be varied to provide a quantitative control of insonation.

Transducer element. Piece of piezoelectric material in a transducer assembly.

Transfer factor. A dialyzable extract of immune lymphocytes that is capable of transferring cell-mediated immunity in humans and possibly in other animal species.

Transferrin. Serum β-globulin that serves as a transport of metals (iron, indium, and gallium) in blood.

Transformation. A term used in connection with radioactive transformation, which is the change of one nuclide into another. Thus the alpha decay of ^{238}U to give ^{234}Th is an example of a radioactive transformation: $_{92}U^{238} \rightarrow {}_{90}Th^{234}$. Mathematical operation which changes the algebraic expression of a set of values.

Transformation constant. As used in radioactivity, this is synonymous with decay constant or disintegration constant.

Transhepatic cholangiography and biliary drainage. Under local anesthesia a percutaneous transhepatic cholangiogram is performed. The site of obstruction in the biliary tract and the cause of the obstructive jaundice are localized. The slender cholangiographic needle is replaced by a larger diameter catheter with multiple side holes. This catheter is then advanced under fluoroscopic visualization across the area of obstruction thereby allowing normal egress of bile from the biliary tract into and through the duodenum. This is termed "internal biliary drainage". It is currently used in certain patients to decompress the biliary tree before a definitive surgical procedure is accomplished.

Transhepatic portography. Under local anesthesia, a fine-gauge needle and catheter are inserted through the skin, across the hepatic tissue into the major venous components of the liver (portal veins) for the purposes of outlining the direction of flow in the portal vein and its tributaries. This is of primary importance in the evaluation of patients with nutritional or alcoholic liver disease (cirrhosis). It is also occasionally used as a means to enter the venous system to purposely obstruct bleeding esophageal varices (veins) which frequently accompany severe end-stage liver disease.

Transient equilibrium. If the half-life of the parent is sufficiently short, so that the quantity present decreases appreciably during the period under consideration, but is still longer than that of successive members of the series, a stage of equilibrium will be reached after which all members of the series decrease in amount exponentially with the period of the parent.

Transistor. A small solid-state semiconductor used as a switch or amplifier. Transistors consist of three electrodes attached to a wafer of silicon or germanium. The material is treated so its electrical properties vary at each of the places where an electrode touches the wafer. Transistors are small, light, and can switch at high speed.

Transition metals. The metallic elements in the center of the periodic chart.

Translation (color) tables. A set of tables that allow flexible specifications of the intensity to be used for the display of each count value.

Translator. A device or computer program that performs translations from one language or code to another; e.g., an assembler or compiler.

Translumbar aortography. Under local anesthesia and fluoroscopic guidance a steel needle is then inserted directly into the aorta for the purposes of examining the blood vessels in the abdomen. This approach is frequently used when the femoral arteries are not available for entrance either due to disease or previous surgery.

Transluminal angioplasty. Certain forms of arteriosclerosis are associated with localized rather than diffuse areas of narrowing. It is currently possible to percutaneously introduce a balloon-tipped catheter, advance it to the area of narrowing, inflate the balloon under fluoroscopic visualization, and dilate the area of narrowing. The catheter is subsequently removed.

Transmission. A general term used to apply to the movement of X-rays from the X-ray-producing machine through body tissues and onto a recording medium.

Transmission angle. Angle between transmitted sound direction and line perpendicular to media boundary.

Transmission media. Twisted-pair wire, fiber-optic cable, microwaves, radio, and broadband or baseband coaxial cable.

Transmission-mode scanning. Just as an X-ray computerized tomography (CT) scanner can produce a map of the X-ray absorption in a tissue section the same principle can be applied to some organs using ultrasound. The method is not widely applicable since there are few places where ultrasound can be transmitted right through the body without encountering total reflection or high attenuation in bone or air-filled spaces. However, the breasts and testes can be scanned by this method to produce a map of ultrasound absorption for the various tissues involved.

Transmission scan. Detection of radiation transmitted through the body from a source on one side of the body to the detector on the opposite side, which provides an image of body absorption densities much like a radiograph but generally lacking the detailed resolution.

Transmittance. For a parallel beam of light, the ratio of the transmitted to the incident luminous flux.

Transmitter. Portion of the NMR apparatus that produces radio-frequency (rf) current and delivers it to the transmitting coil.

Transmural infarction. Infarction that involves the entire thickness of myocardium.

Transmural pressure. The difference between the blood pressure in the vessel and the external pressure on the vessel.

Transmutation. The name given to the transformation of one element into another. Transmutation takes place spontaneously with some of the radioactive elements; with others it can be induced by bombardment of the element with nuclear particles.

Transonic. An area of tissue or organ which transmits ultrasound with little attenuation.

Transplantation antigens. Those antigens which are expressed on the surface of virtually all cells and which induce rejection of tissues transplanted from one individual to a genetically disparate individual.

Transponder. A combination receiver/transmitter that retransmits the received signal at a greater amplification and different frequency.

Transuranic elements. The artificial elements no. 93 and higher which have heavier and more complex nuclei than uranium. They can be made by neutron bombardment of uranium.

Transverse. Lying at right angles to the long axis of the body; crosswise.

Transverse magnetization. Component (M_{xy}) of the net magnetization vector orthogonal to the direction of the main field, the precession of which, at the Larmor frequency, generates the NMR response signal. In the absence of externally applied radio-frequency (rf) energy. M_{xy} decays to zero with a characteristic time constant T_2, or more strictly T_2^*.

Transverse relaxation time. Time constant, T_2, characterizing the rate at which nuclei reach equilibrium, or go out of phase, with each other: a measure of the rate at which phase coherence among nuclei spinning at an angle to the static magnetic field is lost due to interaction between spins, resulting in a reduction in the transverse magnetization. (NMR.)

Transverse tomography. Tangential scanning of a cross section of an organ, done from multiple directions, and then superimposed in a specific manner.

Trauma. A wound or injury; sometimes caused by a physical blow.

Traveling-wave linear accelerator. The principal type of high-energy electron-beam generator used in radiotherapy. Electrons are injected into an evacuated tube (waveguide) along which a magnetron-generated radio-frequency wave is traveling. Irises distributed along the length of the waveguide control the velocity of the wave so that the injected electrons are continuously accelerated as they travel along the guide. The resulting beam of high-energy electrons (4, 6, or 8 MeV, etc.) may be used in electron beam therapy or, more commonly, it is made to strike a tungsten target to generate high-energy X-rays.

Treadmill. A treadmill consists of a wide belt on which the patient walks against the resistance to the movement of the belt. The device includes circuits to measure the work being done in moving the belt. Patients with heart diesease may undergo changes in the EKG along with blood pressure changes during physical stress.

Trephine. A surgical saw with a circular cutting edge that is rotated by means of an attached handle. The saw is used, for example, in removing segments of bone from the skull.

Triad. A group of three similar elements.

Trial. Experimental or sample of specified size n.

Tribo-luminescence. The luminescence shown by certain substances on being rubbed or otherwise exposed to friction.

Tricuspid valve. The right atrioventricular valve, between the right atrium and right ventricle of the heart. The tricuspid valve has three cusps.

Triggering. (Gating) In a triggered image process, the measurements are performed at identical moments during the heart or respiratory cycle in order to minimize motion artefacts. The physiologic process within the patient determines ("trigger") the pulse sequence repetition rate.

Triglycerides. Important fats (lipids) that constitute a major source and storage form of energy. Each triglyceride molecule is made up of three fatty acid molecules attached to a compound called glycerol.

Triiodothyronine. (3,5,3′,-L-triiodothyronine, T_3, or liothyronine) The more calorigenically potent of the two major natural thyroid hormones. It is synthesized and secreted in part by the thyroid gland, and is also derived in part from tissue deiodination of T_4 (thyroxine).

Trilinear chart of the nuclides. A trilinear coordinate grid on which the nuclides have been plotted according to their mass, atomic, and neutron numbers.

Tripalmitin fat utilization study. Procedure using ^{14}C-labeled tripalmitin at the C-1 position to measure absorption and hepatic metabolism of tripalmitin to CO_2 and H_2O; requires CO_2 collection from breath.

Tritium. (^3H or ^3T) The isotope of hydrogen of mass 3 (consisting of one proton and two neutrons). It is very rare, naturally radioactive, but can be made by neutron absorption in lithium and in deuterium or heavy water, and is present in fallout. Exhibiting beta decay, with a half-life of 12.3 years.

Triton. The nucleus of tritium, the hydrogen isotope of mass number 3, in its use as a nuclear projectile or as a product of a nuclear reaction.

Trocar. A sharp instrument used to puncture a body part so that access can be gained, e.g., to withdraw fluid.

Troposphere. The lower part of the earth's atmosphere, containing our weather.

Trouble-shooting. Trouble-shooting is a search for errors in a computer program or mechanical failures in the hardware.

True coincidence. The recording in coincidence of two or more pulses, from independent detector circuits, due to related nuclear events occurring within a time less than the resolving time of the coincidence circuit.

***t*-test for paired data**. (Difference method) A *t* test which treats the difference, d, between a pair of data (i.e., x − y) as the variable.

Tumor. A mass of new tissue growth independent of its surrounding structures, having no physiological function; neoplasm: tumors are classified as benign or malignant.

Tumor-associated antigen. (TAA) Cell surface antigens that are expressed on malignant but not normal cells.

Tumor-associated rejection antigens. TARA) Antigens on tumor cells that result in initiation of immune rejection when the tumor is transplanted.

Tumor-specific antigens. Antigens unique to tumors, including antigens (Ags) that are unique to the individual tumor, common to tumors of the same cell type or to tumors induced by the same virus; they include internal as well as cell surface Ags.

Tumor-specific transplantation antigens. Unique antigens of tumors that are involved in tumor rejection, i.e., they are true immunogens.

Tumor staging. The practice of dividing malignancies into groups according to the extent or spread of the disease. Staging is useful both in prognosis and in planning of treatment.

Tungsten. Element symbol W (wolfram), atomic number 74, atomic weight 183.85.

Tuning. Process of adjusting the resonant frequency, e.g., of the radio-frequency circuit, to a desired value, e.g., the Larmor frequency. More generally, the process of adjusting the components of the spectrometer for optimal NMR signal strength.

Tunnel. Opening into NMR imaging machine to place patient into imaging region. Gantry.

Turbidimetry. The measurement of the cloudiness of a medium containing a suspension of small particles by determining the decrease in intensity of a light beam passed through the medium.

Turnaround time. Can be measured in many ways, but nominally is the elapsed time from submission of a job to a computer system until all output has been produced.

T wave. A low-amplitude, broad defection of an electrocardiogram arising from ventricular repolarization.

Two-dimensional Fourier. Planar method using Fourier imaging technique.

Two-dimensional scanning. A two-dimensional scan can be generated by viewing a B-scope display while the ultrasonic beam is scanned through a plane within the patient, if the direction and position of the time base are linked to those of the ultrasonic beam. If the scanning sequence is sufficiently rapid, as with real-time systems, the image is flicker free and movements can be followed. Slower scanners, in which the transducer is moved by hand in contact with the patient, or in which water bath coupling is used with automatic movement of the transducer, require the image to be stored. This storage can be done photographically, or (as is usual with modern instruments) by means of an analog or a digital scan converter. Real-time scanning may be done either by fast mechanical movement of one or more single-element transducers, or by electronically addressed and controlled arrays of transducers. Linear arrays have rectangular scan formats; electronically steered arrays have sector scan formats. Synthetic swept (time-varied) focusing can be applied during reception to improve resolution in azimuth. Also called compound B-scanning: static and real time.

Two's complement. In some computers, a positive or negative number used to represent a given value. This number is formed from the given binary value by changing all ones to zeros and all zeros to ones and then adding one.

Two-tailed test. he alternative to the null hypothesis is a nondirectional difference $(A \neq B)$. Therefore the probability of chance events as extreme or more extreme includes the area in both tails.

Tyndall effect. Light reflected or dispersed by particles suspended in a gas or liquid.

Type I (α) error. The null hypothesis is true (the true difference is zero) but is rejected because the observed result falls in the α (alpha) or rejection region of the null hypothesis curve. The error risk is therefore α, the arbitrary level of significance, and is predetermined.

Type II (β) error. The null hypothesis is false (a true difference does exist) but is accepted because the observed result falls within the $1 - \alpha$ region (acceptance region) of the null hypothesis curve. Error risk cannot be readily determined. Also called the β error.

Tyrosine. Amino acid present in proteins that are susceptible to radioiodination.

U

Ultimate waste disposal. A two-step operation that comprises the preparation of radioactive waste for final and permanent disposal and the actual placing of the product at the final site. The term commonly applies to the disposal of waste of high activity.

Ultracentrifugation. A high-speed centrifugation technique that can be used for the analytic identification of proteins of various sedimentation coefficients or as a preparative technique for separating proteins of different shapes and densities.

Ultrafiltration. The separation under pressure of colloids and certain viruses from their dispersion media by the use of filters with very small pore sizes.

Ultra high frequency. (UHF) Between 3×10^8 and 3×10^9 Hz.

Ultrasonic nebulizer. Device used for dispersing liquids in a fine mist through the use of sound waves.

Ultrasonic power. Usually, the temporal average power emitted in the form of ultrasonic radiation by a transducer assembly.

Ultrasonic transducer. Sound or ultrasound may be produced by an inductive device such as the loudspeaker or magnetostrictive transducer, or be a piezoelectric element which expands or contracts according to the applied voltage. The advantage of the later for medical applications is that it can work at high frequencies (e.g., 5 MHz) and is reciprocal in that it can convert acoustic energy into electrical signals as well as the reverse.

Ultrasound. The use of ultrahigh-frequency sound waves to generate anatomic images based upon the reflection of the sound waves at different tissue interfaces. Acoustic radiation at frequencies above the range of human hearing; sound of frequency greater than 20 kHz.

Ultrasound coupling medium. The coupling medium between the patient and the transducer is an important part of the diagnostic system. In practice, one of the most common causes of decreased sensitivity and poor results is insufficient coupling material. An adequate amount of coupling medium eliminates an air gap or air bubbles that have a reflection coefficient approaching 100%, thus decreasing the transmitted sound to practically zero. Either mineral oil or water-soluble gels are used as coupling agents for contact B-scan systems. Both materials have good acoustic properties.

Ultrasound display modes. Echo signals from a transducer can be displayed in a number of formats, depending upon whether amplitudes, time, or spatial distribution are of interest. In the A-mode, or amplitude mode, the target depth and amplitude are displayed either on the horizontal and vertical scales or on a cathode ray tube (CRT), respectively. The anatomical origin of the signal being displayed is difficult to determine, since only the depth information is present on the horizontal axis. The A-mode display is commonly used in ophthalmology,

echoencephalography, echocardiology, and as an adjunct to B-mode displays for more accurate measurement.

In the M-mode, or motion-mode display, the position and pattern of movement of reflecting surfaces are displayed. Depth information is displayed vertically, with a slow horizontal sweep tracing out the motional pattern of the target. Amplitude information is encoded into the shades of gray on the display. The M-mode display is used primarily in echocardiology and as an adjunct to B-mode displays to determine the pulsatile nature of a mass or the fetal heart motion.

The B-mode, or brightness-mode display, gives a two-dimensional cross-sectional spatial representation of the examined tissue on the horizontal and vertical axes while encoding echo amplitude information in gray levels. It is the primary display mode of noncardiac ultrasound.

Ultrasound scanning arm. Beam positioning information is generated by an articulated scanning arm. The transducer is attached by this arm to a support which in turn is attached to a mobile base on the floor next to the patient. The scanning arm serves two critical functions: it determines the spatial orientation of the sound beam, so that the origin of a reflection from within the patient is correctly placed into the electronic memory; and it constrains the scanning to a plane, so that a meaningful "cut" can be made. The X and Y coordinates of the sound beam are determined by the angles at the joints of the arm which are measured by potentiometers or optical digital encoders.

Unattended operation. The ability of communications devices to automatically perform functions without human intervention.

Unbiased estimate. A sample estimate which has the property that the average of all possible sample estimates obtained in the specified manner equals exactly the population parameter.

Uncertainty principle. The indeterminancy principle of Heisenberg which postulates that any physical measurement disturbs the system being measured, thus limiting the accuracy of measurements, especially at the atomic, nuclear, and particulate levels of magnitude.

Underflow. A condition that occurs when a mathematical operation yields a result whose magnitude is smaller than the smallest amount the hardware can handle.

Uniformity. Uniformity refers to the ability of a scintigraphic instrument to reproduce with fidelity an image of a uniformly distributed radioactive source. When registered photographically, deviations from uniform count density across the field of view of less than 10% should generally not be discernible.

Uniformity correction. Adding or subtracting counts from an image to correct for blood field irregularities. Present methods correct by repositioning incoming events according to a prerecorded image map.

Uniform label. A compound where the radioactive atoms appear in statistical uniformity at each available site within the molecule.

Uniform (rectangular) distribution. A distribution with equal frequency for all X values.

Unintentional tort. (Legal) This is negligence.

Uninterruptible power supply. (UPS) A device that protects a computer or other electrical device from all types of electric power disturbances, including blackouts. When the voltage in the power main drops below an acceptable level, the UPS automatically provides AC power generated from a battery. Most UPS for small computers deliver power only long enough to halt the work and turn off the computer system in an orderly way.

Unit. Specific magnitude of a quantity, set apart by appropriate definition, which is to serve as a basis of comparison or measurement for other quantities of the same nature.

United States Pharmacopeia. (USP) Official listing of all drugs and medications.

Univalent antibodies. Hypothetial antibodies (Abs) with but one valence; the only univalent Abs are artificial Abs produced by splitting Ab molecules with papain to produce the univalent fragment, Fab.

Universal asynchronous receiver/transmitter. A circuit that converts data between serial and parallel form.

Universal mass unit. (u) The basic unit of mass. One u is defined as being equal to exactly 1/12 the mass of a single carbon atom of the type that contains 12 particles in its nucleus (^{12}C). A slightly different unit, commonly used in chemistry, is the atomic mass unit (amu), based on the average weight of oxygen isotopes in their natural abundance (^{16}O). One u $12/12 \times 6.02 \times 10^{23} = 1.66 \times 10^{-24}$ g.

Unpaired electron. An atomic or molecular electron whose spin is not paired with the oppositely directed spin of another electron in the atom or molecule.

Unrestricted area. An area to which access is not controlled for the purpose of protecting individuals from exposure to radiation and radioactive materials.

Unsaturated iron-binding capacity. Amount of serum transferrin that is not saturated with iron.

Unsealed source. Any radioactive source which is not a sealed source.

Unstable. The products of many nuclear reactions are nuclei which are not found in nature. The number of neutrons and protons in these nuclides is out of stable balance. The nuclides proceed to adjust this by those nucleons which are in excess changing, by a decay process, to the type in which the nuclide is deficient. Hence, if the nuclide has more neutrons than its stable isobars, this is corrected by the neutrons changing to protons until the nuclide becomes stable.

Update. A colloquial expression implying the bringing up-to-date of data stored in the computer memory, or programs.

Uranium. Element symbol U, atomic number 92, atomic weight 238.0289.

Uranium hexafluoride. A gaseous compound of uranium with fluorine used in the gaseous diffusion process for separating the uranium isotopes (commonly called Hex).

Urea. A nitrogen-containing waste product formed from amino acids and excreted in the urine.

Uric acid. A nitrogen-containing waste product formed from nucleic acids.

Urine. Filtrate of the blood excreted by the kidneys.

Useful beam. Ionizing radiation that, having passed through an aperture, cone, or other collimating device, can be employed for the purpose intended.

User friendly. Anybody who uses a computer is a user. User friendly means the computer system is easy to use. User friendly systems check errors, display information in easy-to-read formats, and tell the user what to do next.

User program. An application program, written by a system user.

Utility. The probability of a given outcome times the difference between benefit and cost of that outcome.

Utility program. Any general-purpose program included in an operating system to perform common functions.

V

Vacancy. A vacancy (or defect) results when a site normally occupied by an ion or an atom is left unoccupied.

Vagus nerve. Parasympathetic pneumogastric nerve; the tenth cranial nerve, composed of both motor and sensory fibers. It has a wide distribution in the neck, thorax, and abdomen and sends important branches to the heart, lungs, stomach, and so on.

Valence. Number representing the combining or displacing power of an atom; number of electrons lost, gained, or shared by an atom in a compound; numbers of hydrogen atoms with which an atom will combine, or which it will displace.

Valence electrons. Of the atom are electrons which are gained, lost, or shared in chemical reactions.

Valence of antibodies and antigens. The respective numbers of antigen (Ag) determinants on an Ag molecule and Ag-binding sites on an antibody (Ab) molecule. Although most Ags possess numerous Ag determinants, all monomeric Abs except IgM are bivalent; IgM Abs have a theoretic valence of 10.

Valence state. Ionization state of an element in an ionic compound.

Valva. Valve; one-way passage.

Vanadium. Element symbol V, atomic number 23, atomic weight 50.9415.

Van de Graaff generator. This electrostatic generator, first described in a practical form by Van de Graaff in 1931, is a generator in which a high potential is produced by the accumulation of electric charge conveyed to an insulated conductor by a continuously moving belt. The potential generated is used for accelerating charged particles.

Van der Waals bond. Attraction between the charged portions of two molecules, known as dipoles.

Vapor. The words vapor and gas are often used interchangeably. Vapor is more frequently used for a substance which, though present in the gaseous phase, generally exists as a liquid or solid at room temperature. Gas is more frequently used for a substance that generally exists in the gaseous phase at room temperature. Thus one would speak of iodine or carbon tetrachloride vapors and of oxygen gas.

Vapor pressure. The pressure exerted when a solid or liquid is in equilibrium with its own vapor. The vapor pressure is a function of the substance and of the temperature.

Variance. A measure of variability represented by the average squared deviation around the mean.

Variate Z. A new unit, the scale of the standard normal curve; it is created by transforming the distance any observation, x, is from the mean (or center) μ, of the normal curve, into multiples of the standard deviation, σ, of that curve; thus, if $x - \mu$ is 10, and σ is 2, x is 5 multiples of σ from μ. In this case,

$$z = \frac{x - \mu}{\sigma} = \frac{10}{2} = 5$$

Vas. A vessel, a canal for carrying fluid such as blood, lymph, or spermatozoa.

Vascular. Referring to the blood vessels, arteries, capillaries, and veins.

Vascular bed. Entire blood supply of an organ or structure.

Vascularization. The development of new blood vessels in a part of the body.

Vascular resistance. Ratio of the driving pressure in the pulmonary circulation to the minute volume.

Vasoactive drug. An agent that affects the caliber of blood vessels, especially one that increases or decreases arterial caliber to correspondingly decrease or increase blood pressure.

Vasoconstriction. Narrowing of the lumen of blood vessels, especially as a result of vasomotor action.

Vasodilation. Dilation or opening of blood vessel by vasomotor action.

Vasodilator. A drug that causes the blood vessels to dilate, used to treat both acute and chronic heart failure. Drugs that dilate arterioles reduce the workload of the left ventricle by decreasing afterload, impedance, and systemic vascular resistance. Hence, the left ventricle can pump more blood in a forward direction. Some vasodilators (e.g., nitroprusside) affect the arterioles and the veins equally, thereby increasing stroke volume and cardiac output, while reducing pulmonary capillary wedge pressure.

Vasomotor. Having to do with the musculature that affects the caliber of a blood vessel, or changing the internal diameter of a blood vessel brought about by constrictor or dilator nerves acting on the muscle of the vessel walls.

Vasopressor. Any substance that causes contraction of blood vessel smooth muscle, thus diminishing the vessels' cross-sectional area and increasing the intravascular blood pressure.

Vasospastic. Characterized by, or causing, vasospasm, i.e., the spasmodic construction of the small arteries resulting in cramp and difficulty in walking.

Vector. A quantity having both magnitude and direction, frequently represented by an arrow whose length is proportional to the magnitude and with an arrowhead at one end to indicate the direction. Living agent that transmits microbial pathogens.

Vectorcardiography. A technique of recording the magnitude and direction of the P-, QRS-, and T-wave vectors of the heart, with each of the vectors displayed as a continuous loop on an oscilloscope.

Veiling glare. Nonzero light levels detected under radiopaque objects with an image intensifier due to lateral dark areas. Veiling glare makes quantitative imaging difficult in digital radiography.

Veins. Vessels which return the circulating blood to the heart, typically having thin walls and valves that prevent the reverse flow of blood.

Velocity. The rate of change of position with time. The term velocity implies both direction and speed; the term speed of sound should be used where direction is not important.

Velocity of sound. The velocity (c) of sound waves is a constant of a medium and is dependent upon the inertial (density, ζ) and elastic (bulk modulus of elasticity, E) characteristics of the medium. The unit of the velocity of sound is meter per second (m/s).

$$c = \frac{E}{\zeta} \text{ m/s}$$

For soft, living tissues in which the propagation of sound is longitudinal, there is essentially no dependence of the velocity of sound on frequency, at least not in the frequency ranges normally used in diagnostic ultrasound. With the exception of air, bone, fat, water, and the lens of the eye, the velocity of sound is very similar in most biological tissues, averaging 1540 m/s.

Velocity profile. The variation of flow velocity across a blood vessel.

Velocity (Q)-mode. A display of Doppler velocities as a function of time (or waveform display), usually with an accompanying EKG.

Velocity time integral. Calculated area under the Doppler curve over a specified period of time. Flow velocity.

Venipuncture. Placement of a needle within a vein.

Venocavagraphy. Evaluation of the inferior (lower half of the body) or superior (upper half of the body) vena cava is frequently done by administration of i.v. contrast material through a periferal vein. Obstruction of the superior/inferior vena cava is frequently due to malignant neoplasm but may also be associated with inflammatory disease and clot formation.

Venogram. Radionuclide delineation of a portion of the venous system after downstream injection of an appropiate radiopharmeceutical. Radiography of the veins using a contrast medium; phlebography.

Venous blood. Blood returning to the heart — usually contains less O_2 and more CO_2 than arterial blood.

Venous blood pressure. Pressure variations from 0 to 15 mmHg. An almost static pressure with some variations with each heart beat. Frequency-response requirements: 0 to 30 Hz. Measured at various points in the venous circulatory system by manometer, implanted pressure tranducer, or external transducer connected to catheter.

Venous stasis. The slowing down of the flow of blood in the veins.

Venous trombi. Blood clots within the veins.

Ventilation. Process of supplying fresh air.

Ventilation/perfusion ratio. (V/Q or V_A/Q_C) Comparison of functioning ventilatory space and perfused tissue within the lung; ratio of minute flow of air through alveoli to minute flow of blood through pulmonary capillaries.

Ventral. Front aspect of the human body, or the underside of a quadruped; opposed to dorsal.

Ventricle. A small cavity or chamber, particularly of the heart or brain. The ventricles of the heart form the lower part of the heart, the right ventricle receiving venous blood and pumping it to the lungs, and the left ventricle receiving oxygenated blood from the lungs and pumping it to the body.

Ventricular fibrillation. A condition similar to atrial fibrillation resulting in rapid, tremulous, and ineffectual contraction of the ventricles. May result from mechanical injury to the heart, occlusion of coronary vessels, effects of certain drugs such as excess of digitalis or chloroform, and electrical stimuli.

Ventricular septum. The partition that separates the ventricles of the heart.

Ventricular tachycardia. An abnormally rapid ventricular rhythm, usually over 150 beats per minute, that may easily convert to ventricular fibrillation.

Venule. A small vein; especially one of the minute veins connecting the capillary bed with the larger systemic veins.

Verification. The process, in a computer, of reading back disk data after writing it to be sure it was written correctly.

Vesicle. Any small sac or cavity formed by the accumulation of serous fluid.

Vibrating-reed electrometer. An extremely sensitive instrument used to measure very small potentials. At converts the small DC potential to AC by means of a small vibrating capacitor; the AC is then amplified and reconverted, if desired, back to DC.

Vibrocardiogram. A measure of the movement of the chest due to the heart beat. Frequency response required: 0.1 to 50 Hz. Special pressure or displacement transducer placed on the appropriate point on the chest.

Video disk. An analog storage device used to store video frames or fields in real time. Images stored on video disk or video tape must be redigitized for postprocessing operations.

Vidicon. A type of television camera tube in which a low-velocity electron beam scans a photoconducting mosaic on which the optical image is projected. Different photoconductive materials are available that are sensitive to X-rays, ultraviolet radiation, and infrared radiation as well as visible light, so that the "optical" image may arise from any of these radiations.

Viewdata. A generic term for systems permitting users to access data banks via the telephone network or some other communication pathway and display their choices on a video monitor.

Villus. Finger-like projections, e.g., villi in the small intestine.

Virgin medium. Any computer storage medium totally devoid of information — a paper tape with no holes, a bubble memory with no charges, a magnetic tape with no magnetized areas.

Virgin neutrons. Neutrons from any source, before they make a collision.

Virtual circuit. A connection between two points in the computer data network that uses different circuits during a transmission but behaves as a dedicated path.

Virtual image. An image that cannot be shown on a surface but is visible, as in a mirror.

Virtual memory. A scheme of memory management used to map a theoretically infinite memory space into a smaller physical space

(central processing unit main memory). With no memory limit on programs, programming becomes much easier.

Virtual storage. A store managment system enables a user to use the storage resources of a computer without regard to contraints imposed by a limited main store.

Virulence. A term used to designate the degrees of pathogenicity of various strains of organisms within a species: hence, respective strains of a pathogen may be of high virulence, low virulence, or without virulence (avirulent).

Virus. A type of microorganism consisting of a single nucleic acid (DNA or RNA) surrounded by a layer of protein. They are 20 to 250 nm in diameter, and are capable of replication only within cells of plants and animals. Viruses are the cause of many infectious diseases in man.

Viscera. Internal organs enclosed within a cavity, especially the abdominal organs.

Viscosity. The resistance to fluid flow set up by sheer stresses within the flowing liquid. The physical property of serum that is determined by the size, shape, and deformability of serum molecules. The hydrostatic state, molecular charge, and temperature sensitivity of proteins.

Viscous flow. The type of flow in which the viscosity of the fluid is the dominating factor. The term is practically synonymous with laminar flow.

Visual display unit. (VDU) A terminal designed to display computer-generated data on a cathode ray tube. It enables the user to put data into the computer using an imput device and acts as an output, too. Television screens are an example of cathode ray tubes but are usually called "raster-scan" devices. VDUs are also known as video monitors or video display tubes.

Vital capacity. Volume of air that can be exhaled after the deepest possible inhalation.

Vitamin. Organic compound necessary to maintain normal growth of function; found in small amounts in plants and animals, e.g., vitamin B_{12} is needed for the normal maturation of cells of the erythrocytic series and for normal neurologic function. When given parenterally, it corrects both the hematologic and neurologic symptoms of pernicious anemia.

VO$_2$max (maximal oxygen consumption). The maximum amount of oxygen the body can use; that is, the amount of oxygen consumed during maximal physical activity. Also called maximal aerobic power or capacity.

Volatile memory. Storage device that loses information when power is turned off. A computer's main, or RAM, memory is usually volatile.

Volt. The fundamental unit of measurement of difference in potential or pressure between two points in a electric circuit, usually connected across the circuit. Equal to 1 J/C.

Voltage pulse. Brief excursion of voltage from its normal value.

Voltmeter. Device used to measure potential difference in electric circuits; potentiometer.

Volume. Amount of space occupied in three dimensions; a mass storage medium that can be treated as file-structured data storage.

Volume dilution. Dilution of a solution by addition of pure liquid solvent.

Volume imaging. Imaging techniques in which NMR signals are gathered from the whole object volume to be imaged at once, with appropriate encoding pulse/gradient sequences to encode positions of the spins. Many sequential plane imaging techniques can be generalized to volume imaging, at least in principle. Advantages include potential improvement in signal-to-noise ratio by including signal from the whole volume at once; disadvantages include a bigger computational task for image reconstruction and longer image acquisition times (although the entire volume can be imaged from the one set of data). Imaging technique in which the NMR signal is collected simultaneously from the whole object volume. Known as 3DF, or three-dimensional Fourier imaging when both frequency and phase are used for spatial encoding.

Volume ionization. Average ionization density in a given volume, irrespective of the specific ionization of the ionizing particles.

Volume velocity. Volume velocity is that rate of alternating flow of the medium through a specified surface due to a sound wave.

Vortex shed distance. The distance distal to a jet orifice after which laminar flow becomes disturbed.

Voxel. A volume element of a specimen being imaged. The element of 3-D space corresponding to a pixel, for a given slice thickness.

V wave. A large pressure wave on the pulmonary artery pressure trace that is characteristic of mitral regurgitation and occurs when blood is pumped back into the left atrium during systole. V waves can be detected in a pulmonary capillary wedge pressure tracing. Such pressure tracings supply one means of detecting mitral regurgitation in critically ill patients.

W

Wafer. Thin disk sliced from silicon rod during the manufacture of integrated circuits.

Waiting time. The time between the end of data acquisition after the last pulse of a sequence and the initiation of a new sequence. (Some NMR systems place the waiting time prior to the initiation of the first pulse of the sequence in order to ensure equilibrium at the beginning of the first sequence.) Synonym for latency.

Wall filter. A filter in a Doppler system which rejects echo information from low-velocity reflectors such as stationary or slow-moving tissue. This filtering is needed to keep high-amplitude tissue echos from saturating the Doppler receiver, masking very low-amplitude echoes from flowing blood. Synonym: thump filter.

Wand. An input device used to read optical bar code labels by sensing the optical pattern of the light and dark areas.

Waste. The waste from a nuclear power installation is predominantly in liquid or solid form and, because it is often associated with radioactivity, must be disposed of under safe and controlled conditions.

Watchdog timer. A timer set by a program to interrupt the processor after a given period, ensuring that a system does not lose track of buffers and communication lines because of a hardware error.

Watt. A metric unit of power; the rate of energy consumption or conversion when 1 J of energy is consumed or converted per second.

Wave. A disturbance propagated in a medium in such a manner that at any point in the medium, the displacement is a function of time, while at any instant, the displacement at a point is a function of the positions of the point.

Waveform. The representation of an acoustic or electrical parameter as a function of time in a rectangular coordinate system.

Wave function. A function giving the probability distribution of electric charge (e.g., electron) in space. For atoms, it is a wave-mechanical description of their stationary states.

Wave guide. A hollow conductor used to efficiently transmit high-energy, high-frequency waves in the centimeter to micrometer range. Fiber-optic cables are one form of solid conductors for micrometric and smaller frequencies.

Wavelength. Distance between any two similar points of two consecutive waves; for electromagnetic radiation the wavelength is equal to the velocity of light (c) divided by the frequency of the wave (ν). The acoustic wavelength is the distance between two adjacent, equivalent points of the waveform, such as two adjacent crests, and corresponds to the distance traveled by the wave during one cycle; $\lambda = c/f$, where λ is the wavelength, c is the speed of sound, and f is the frequency. For water or tissue at 1 MHz, the wavelength is approximately 1.5 mm.

Wave motion. The transmission of a periodic motion or vibration through a medium or empty space. Transverse wave motion is that in which the vibration is perpendicular to the direction of propagation. Longitudinal wave motion is that in which the vibration is parallel to the direction of propagation.

Wave number. The reciprocal of the wavelength in a harmonic wave $(1/\lambda)$.

Wave variables. Things that are functions of space and time in a wave.

Weak interaction. The interaction that is responsible for beta decay and the decay of some mesons and hyperons.

Weber. (Unit of magnetic flux, Wb.) The magnetic flux which, linking a circuit of one turn, produces in it an electromotive force of 1 V as it is reduced to zero at a uniform rate in 1 s. (Symbol Wb.)

Wedge filter. Used in radiotherapy, a wedge-shaped radiation filter placed in the radiation beam so that the beam's rays pass through different thicknesses of metal before impinging on the patient.

Weight. The gravitational force between two bodies attracting each other. The mass of a body is the same whether it is on the earth or on the moon, but the weights of the body in the two places are quite different.

Well counter. This is a special type of scintillation counter in which the scintillation crystal is shaped in the form of a well to receive a small vial containing the sample whose radioactivity is to be counted. The crystal must be covered in a thin aluminum can to exclude light, and so it is only suitable for counting relatively high radiation energy (greater than 20 keV of γ-rays). It is used in an autogamma counter in conjunction with an automatic sample changer.

White blood cell. (WBC) Type of blood cell (leukocyte) whose nucleus determines the type of cell; lymphocyte, monocyte, neutrophil, eosinophil, basophil.

White blood cell study. Procedure using ^{111}In oxine-labeled polymorphonuclear leukocytes to track their accumulation and thereby identify sites of pyogenic infection.

White matter. Tissue of the central nervous system, consisting mainly of nerve fibers, although glia and blood vessels are also present.

Whole-body counter. The whole-body counter, also known as a low-level radiation counter, is an elaborate instrument assembly which has been designed to measure minute quantities of radioactivity in human subjects. The sensitivity, precision, and accuracy of such instruments permit the measurement of radioactive contamination at levels greatly below the maximum permissible body burdens of most gamma-emitting nuclides. Although the whole-body counter was originally developed to resolve the problems of health physics, this instrument has important clinical application in the measurement of body potassium and in long-term tracer studies with many radioisotopes at levels for below those required by conventional instrumentation.

Wigner effect. Displacements of atoms from their positions in a crystal structure by radiation. In graphite, for example, neutron bombardment causes changes in physical shape, e.g., swelling in one direction and contraction in the perpendicular one. If and when the atoms return to their normal position they give off energy which appears as heat.

Wild card operation. A shorthand method of referring to all computer files with a specific characteristic in their name.

Winchester disk. A special high-speed, sealed, large-capacity fixed disk used in most systems for digital image storage, and smaller personal computers.

Window. A term which describes the upper and lower limits of radiation energy accepted for counting by a spectrometer; also termed "window width".

Wipe test. Testing for removable contamination.

Wolfram. (Tungsten) Element symbol W, atomic number 74, atomic weight 183.85.

Word. In computing, group of bites or characters treated as a basic unit and capable of being stored in one storage location. Note: Within a word, each location that may be occupied by a bit or character is called a position.

Word length. The number of bits or characters in a word.

Word mode. In this mode the depth of each

pixel is 16 bits; i.e., it can hold 16 binary digits or a decimal count of 65536.

Word processor. A computer text editor designed expecially for editing documents like letters, memos, and manuscripts, as distinguished from data files like mailing lists and financial records.

Work. Done when a force acts against a resistance to produce motion of a body. It is equal to the applied net force multiplied by the distance the body moves (displacement).

$$\text{work (J)} = \text{force (N)} \times \text{displacement (m)}$$

If there is no motion, no work is done. If a body is in motion but no force is being applied, again, no work is done.

Work load. A quantity indicating the average output of a radiation source over a specified period of time.

Wound. Body injury caused by physical means.

Write. To record data on a computer memory device.

Write-enabled. The condition of a volume that allows information to be written on it.

Write-protected. The condition of a volume that protects the volume against information being written on it.

Write-protect notch. A notch in the right edge of diskette's plastic jacket. If the notch is covered by a piece of tape, any attempt to write on the diskette will fail.

W-value. The amount of energy which a nuclear particle loses on the average to form one ion pair (W electronvolts). The value for fast electrons is usually taken as 32 eV.

X

x. Dimension in the stationary (laboratory) frame of reference in the plane orthogonal (at right angles) to the direction of the static magnetic field (B_o), z, and orthogonal to y, the other dimension in this plane. (NMR.)

Xenogeneic. Denotes the relationship that exists between members of genetically different species.

Xenograft. A tissue or organ graft between members of two distinct or different species.

Xenon. Element symbol Xe, atomic number 54, atomic weight 131.29.

Xenon equilibrium. In a reactor, the condition in which the production of the neutron absorber ^{135}Xe as fission product is exactly balanced by its destruction by neutron capture and radioac-

tive decay.

X-ray diffraction. Spectroscopic method for determining crystal structure by the interaction of X-rays with the atoms involved in the crystalline structure.

X-ray fluorescence analysis. The X-ray emission may be excited not only by direct electron bombardment, but also by a fluorescent mechanism when harder X-rays than those to be excited impinge on the target. The radiation excited in this way is then analyzed in a crystal spectrometer generally using proportional counter detectors. This method of analysis is nondestructive. It is not well suited to the lightest elements, say with Z < 10.

X-rays. Penetrating electromagnetic radiation of wavelength shorter than those of visible light (less than 10^{-7} cm). They were also called Roentgen rays, being first observed by Roentgen in Wurzburg in 1895 when he discovered that a fluorescent screen placed near a low pressure discharge tube was excited to emit visible light whenever the discharge tube was operated. Furthermore, the fluorescent screen continued to glow even when the discharge tube was surrounded with black cardboard, thereby showing that the new radiation was of a penetrating nature.

X-rays are produced when fast electrons are suddenly retarded on striking a metallic target. The X-rays produced in this way consist of a white or continuous spectrum extending downward in wavelength to a limit which depends on the energy of the electrons, with a set of discrete lines superposed on it. The white spectrum is produced by the fast electrons on being retarded by the coulomb field of the target atoms, while the sharp lines, or characteristic X-rays, are due to the target material itself and are emitted when holes in the electronic structure of the target atoms are reoccupied by other electrons.

Because of their penetrating nature, X-rays have been used for many years in medical diagnosis (radiology). The transparency of various materials to X-rays depends strongly on their atomic number and density: thus bone and other regions of high density or atomic number are readily observed through the relatively transparent flesh. In X-ray therapy, diseased regions are destroyed by a carefully controlled beam of X-rays in such a manner as to do the minimum amount of damage to the surrounding healthy tissue. Penetrating X-rays are also of great value in detecting flaws in solid objects, and with the use of microradiography they are used to study such things as the structure of metallic alloys.

X-ray spectrometer. An instrument which measures the intensity of a beam of X-rays as a function of their wavelength or energy. This may be done, for example, by causing the X-rays to be diffracted by a crystal so that the energy of the X-rays which strike a detector is determined by the Bragg condition.

X-ray tube. X-rays are produced by two processes. Electrons may collide with the nuclear field around an atom, losing part of their energy, producing X-ray energies up to the maximum energy of the incident electrons, or electrons are ejected from the target atom which, when replaced, release energy dependent upon the atomic structure of that atom. Thus the energy spectrum produced will contain both continuous and line spectra. The X-ray tube as used in diagnostic X-ray apparatus consists of an evacuated envelope containing a source of focused electrons (cathode) directed onto an anode which has a very high melting point and a high atomic number. The anode becomes very hot and so for all but the lowest power units this problem is dealt with by rotating the anode at high speed (3000 to 10,000 rpm) to distribute the heat. The target material on the anode is usually tungsten (melting point 3370°C, atomic number 74), but molybdenum is also used for low power (e.g., mammography) sets. The assembly, which one sees containing the tube, also contains terminals for the very high voltages applied between anode and cathode (up to 150 kV), and an air or oil-cooling system on high-power sets. There is also the rotating mechanism for the anode and special filters, cones or collimators, and diaphragms, making up the X-ray window.

x^1. Dimension in the rotating frame of reference in the plane at right angles to the direction of the static magnetic field (B_o), z; defined to be in the direction of the magnetic vector of the radio-frequency (rf) field (B_1). (NMR.)

X unit. (Xu) The unit used in expressing the wavelength of X-rays and γ-rays. It is about 10^{-11} cm, or 10^{-3}Å.

$$1 \text{ Xu} = 1.00202 \pm 0.00003 \times 10\text{--}3\text{Å}$$

X-Y digitizer. An input device that allows the motion of a pen or cursor to be transduced and fed to the computer as a series of X-Y coordinates.

Y

y. Dimension in the stationary (laboratory) frame of reference in the plane orthogonal to the direction of the static magnetic field (B_o and H_o), z, and orthogonal to x, the other dimension in this plane. (NMR.)

Yates' correction. A correction for continuity, to compensate for the application of a continuous distribution to discrete (qualitative) data, used in chi-square tests with 1 df. The correction is to subtract $1/2$ from each (observed – expected) difference before squaring

$$\chi^2_c = \Sigma \frac{(|O - E| - 1/2)^2}{E}$$

Yellowcake. A uranium-oxide concentrate that results from milling (concentrating) uranium ore. It typically contains 80 to 90% U_3O_8.

y^1. Dimension in the rotating frame of reference in the plane orthogonal (at right angles) to the direction of the static magnetic field (B_o and H_o), z, and orthogonal to the other dimension in this plane, x^1. (NMR.)

Ytterbium. Element symbol Yb, atomic number 70, atomic weight 173.04.

Yttrium. Element symbol Y, atomic number 39, atomic weight 88.905.

Z

z. Dimension in the direction of the static magnetic field (B_o and H_o), in both the stationary and rotating frames of reference. (NMR.)

Z axis. The amplitude of the echo signal at any given point. This can be made to control the number of electrons leaving the electron gun on a conventional cathode ray tube (CRT) and hence the brightness of a particular spot on the display phosphor, or the amplitude of the stored charge on the storage face of a scan converter. A coordinate vertical to the slice plane which usually runs parallel to the body axis.

Zeeman effect. Quantization of orbital angular momentum of atoms can be observed experimentally by placing atoms in a uniform magnetic field. The normal energy levels of the atom, i.e., in the absence of magnetic field, are split into multiple levels in the presence of magnetic field, since each slightly different quantized angular momentum state has a different energy associated with it in the presence of the magnetic field. One can "observe" such splitting by looking at transitions between the shift levels. Such quantization of orbital angular momentum in the presence of a uniform magnetic field and its observation by looking at transitions between different energy states are called normal Zeeman effect.

Zero-area tissue/air ratio. The tissue/air ratio for zero area at a given depth. This is obtained by extrapolating the ratio from a finite-sized area to zero area (radiation therapy).

Zero-bit insertion. A computer technique used to achieve transparency in bit-oriented protocols. A zero is inserted into sequences on one bit that would cause false flag detection. Also called bit stuffing.

Zero dose. The absence of added ligand, synonymous with B_o.

Zero field splitting. Refers to the removal of degeneracy, i.e., an energy level is further split, in the absence of an applied magnetic field. This is due to the presence of the internal crystalline electric field. (NMR.)

Zero-power reactor. A research reactor which operates at a very low power level in order to check reactor theory, but gives little trouble with cooling problems or residual radioactivity and needs relatively little shielding.

Zeta potential. The potential at the interface of two electrostatically attracted surfaces that separates the immobile compact part of the double layer from the diffuse part; e.g., a colloid particle with a negative surface charge attracts both a strong adherent inner layer of positive charge from the surrounding suspension and a more diffuse outer layer that is needed to completely neutralize the negative colloid charge. Zeta potential exists between these two positively charged layers. It is intimately related to the force with which and the

distance over which particle can influence one another.

Zeugmatography. The name given to NMR imaging by Lauterbur. Taken from the Greek zeugma, to join together, referrring to the coupling of the static B field and the radiofrequency (rf) field by the tissue nuclei.

Zinc. Element symbol Zn, atomic number 30, atomic weight 65.39.

Zipper effect. Overlap of two or more images.

Zirconium. Element symbol Zr, atomic number 40, atomic weight 91.22.

Zone electrophoresis. Electrophoresis performed on paper or cellulose acetate in which proteins are separated almost exclusively on the basis of charge.

Zonography. Tomography with a very small exposure angle.

Zoom. During acquisition, a method for image modification which amplified the X and Y camera-positioning signals. This allows the entire image matrix to represent a center portion of the detector field. Rescaling of image dimensions either in whole or in part.

Z-pulse. A signal porportional to the total γ-ray energy absorbed by the crystal. The pulse-height analyzer determines whether or not the gamma event corresponds to the desired energy window.

Zwitterion. An amphoteric dipolar ion possessing a positive charge at one position of its structure and a negative charge at another.

Zygote. The cell resulting from the fusion of an ovum and a spermatozoon.

Zymogen. Inactive precursor of an enzyme that, on reaction with an appropriate kinase or other chemical agent, liberates the enzyme in active form.

DATA HANDBOOK

Characteristics of the Elements

KEY TO CHART

Atomic Number →
Symbol →
1987 Atomic Weight →

50	+2	+4
Sn		
118.71		
18 18 4		

Oxidation States
Electron Configuration

New notation
Previous IUPAC form
CAS version

Group 1 IA		2 IIA		13 IIIB IIIA		14 IVB IVA		15 VB VA		16 VIB VIA		17 VIIB VIIA		18 VIIIA		Orbit
1 H 1.00794 1	+1 −1													2 He 4.002602 2	0	K
3 Li 6.941 2-1	+1	4 Be 9.012182 2-2	+2	5 B 10.811 2-3	+3	6 C 12.011 2-4		7 N 14.00674 2-5		8 O 15.9994 2-6		9 F 18.9984032 2-7	−1	10 Ne 20.1797 2-8	0	K-L
11 Na 22.989768 2-8-1	+1	12 Mg 24.3050 2-8-2	+2	13 Al 26.981539 2-8-3	+3	14 Si 28.0855 2-8-4		15 P 30.97362 2-8-5		16 S 32.066 2-8-6		17 Cl 35.4527 2-8-7		18 Ar 39.948 2-8-8	0	K-L-M

Transition metals and remaining groups 3–12:

Group 3 (IIIA/IIIB): 21 Sc 44.955910 -8-9-2 +3; 39 Y 88.90585 -18-9-2 +3; 57* La 138.9055 -18-9-2 +3; 89** Ac 227.028 -18-9-2 +3

Group 4 (IVA/IVB): 22 Ti 47.88 -8-10-2; 40 Zr 91.224 -18-10-2; 72 Hf 178.49 -32-10-2; 104 Unq (261) -32-10-2

Group 5 (VA/VB): 23 V 50.9415 -8-11-2; 41 Nb 92.90638 -18-12-1; 73 Ta 180.9479 -32-11-2; 105 Unp (262) -32-11-2

Group 6 (VIA/VIB): 24 Cr 51.9961 -8-13-1; 42 Mo 95.94 -18-13-1; 74 W 183.85 -32-12-2; 106 Unh (263) -32-12-2

Group 7 (VIIA/VIIB): 25 Mn 54.93085 -8-13-2; 43 Tc (98) -18-13-2; 75 Re 186.207 -32-13-2; 107 Uns (262) -32-13-2

Group 8 (VIII): 26 Fe 55.847 -8-14-2; 44 Ru 101.07 -18-15-1; 76 Os 190.2 -32-14-2

Group 9 (VIII): 27 Co 58.93320 -8-15-2; 45 Rh 102.90550 -18-16-1; 77 Ir 192.22 -32-15-2

Group 10 (VIII): 28 Ni 58.69 -8-16-2; 46 Pd 106.42 -18-18-0; 78 Pt 195.08 -32-16-2

Group 11 (IB): 29 Cu 63.546 -8-18-1; 47 Ag 107.8682 -18-18-1; 79 Au 196.96654 -32-18-1

Group 12 (IIB): 30 Zn 65.39 -8-18-2; 48 Cd 112.411 -18-18-2; 80 Hg 200.59 -32-18-2

Group 13 (IIIB/IIIA): 31 Ga 69.723 -8-18-3; 49 In 114.82 -18-18-3; 81 Tl 204.3833 -32-18-3

Group 14 (IVB/IVA): 32 Ge 72.61 -8-18-4; 50 Sn 118.710 -18-18-4; 82 Pb 207.2 -32-18-4

Group 15 (VB/VA): 33 As 74.92159 -8-18-5; 51 Sb 121.75 -18-18-5; 83 Bi 208.98037 -32-18-5

Group 16 (VIB/VIA): 34 Se 78.96 -8-18-6; 52 Te 127.60 -18-18-6; 84 Po (209) -32-18-6

Group 17 (VIIB/VIIA): 35 Br 79.904 -8-18-7; 53 I 126.90447 -18-18-7; 85 At (210) -32-18-7

Group 18 (VIIIA): 36 Kr 83.80 -8-18-8; 54 Xe 131.29 -18-18-8; 86 Rn (222) -32-18-8

Groups 1–2 lower rows: 19 K 39.0983 -8-8-1 +1; 37 Rb 85.4678 -18-8-1 +1; 55 Cs 132.90543 -18-8-1 +1; 87 Fr (223) -18-8-1 +1; 20 Ca 40.078 -8-8-2 +2; 38 Sr 87.62 -18-8-2 +2; 56 Ba 137.327 -18-8-2 +2; 88 Ra 226.025 -18-8-2 +2

*Lanthanides:
58 Ce 140.115 -20-8-2 +3 +4; 59 Pr 140.90765 -21-8-2 +3; 60 Nd 144.24 -22-8-2 +3; 61 Pm (145) -23-8-2 +3; 62 Sm 150.36 -24-8-2 +2 +3; 63 Eu 151.965 -25-8-2 +2 +3; 64 Gd 157.25 -25-9-2 +3; 65 Tb 158.92534 -27-8-2 +3; 66 Dy 162.50 -28-8-2 +3; 67 Ho 164.93032 -29-8-2 +3; 68 Er 167.26 -30-8-2 +3; 69 Tm 168.93421 -31-8-2 +3; 70 Yb 173.04 -32-8-2 +2 +3; 71 Lu 174.967 -32-9-2 +3

**Actinides:
90 Th 232.0381 -18-10-2 +4; 91 Pa 231.03588 -20-9-2 +4 +5; 92 U 238.0289 -21-9-2 +3 +4 +5 +6; 93 Np 237.048 -22-9-2 +3 +4 +5 +6; 94 Pu (244) -24-8-2 +3 +4 +5 +6; 95 Am (243) -25-8-2 +3 +4 +5 +6; 96 Cm (247) -25-9-2 +3; 97 Bk (247) -27-8-2 +3 +4; 98 Cf (251) -28-8-2 +3; 99 Es (252) -29-8-2 +3; 100 Fm (257) -30-8-2 +3; 101 Md (258) -31-8-2 +2 +3; 102 No (259) -32-8-2 +2 +3; 103 Lr (260) -32-9-2 +3

Orbit labels: L-M-N, M-N-O, N-O-P, O P Q, N O P

FIGURE 1. Periodic table of the elements. Numbers in parentheses are mass numbers of the most stable isotope of that element. This format numbers the groups 1 to 18. (*From Chem. Eng. News*, 63(5), 27, 1985. Copyright 1985 American Chemical Society. With permission.)

TABLE OF PROPERTIES OF THE ELEMENTS — ALPHABETIC ORDER

Name	Symbol	Atomic number (Z)	Atomic[a] weight (A)	Density[b] (g/cm^3)	K_B[c] (keV)
Actinium	Ac	89	227.028	10.07	106.759
Aluminum	Al	13	26.982	2.702	1.559
Americium	Am	95	243[d]	13.65	124.876
Antimony (Stibium)	Sb	51	121.75	6.684	30.486
Argon	Ar	18	39.948	1.784[e]	3.203
Arsenic	As	33	74.92	5.727	11.863
Astatine	At	85	210[d]	—	95.74
Barium	Ba	56	137.33	3.51	37.41
Berkelium	Bk	97	247[d]	≅14.0	131.357
Beryllium	Be	4	9.012	1.85	0.116
Bismuth	Bi	83	208.98	9.8	90.521
Boron	B	5	10.81	(2.34—2.37)	0.192
Bromine	Br	35	79.904	3.119	13.475
Cadmium	Cd	48	112.41	8.642	26.712
Calcium	Ca	20	40.08	1.54	4.038
Californium	Cf	98	251[d]	—	134.683
Carbon	C	6	12.011	(1.8—3.5)	0.283
Cerium	Ce	58	140.12	(6.66—6.76)	40.449
Cesium	Cs	55	132.905	1.879	35.959
Chlorine	Cl	17	35.453	3.214[e]	2.819
Chromium	Cr	24	51.996	7.2	5.988
Cobalt	Co	27	58.933	8.9	7.709
Copper	Cu	29	63.546	8.92	8.98
Curium	Cm	96	247[d]	13.51	128.088
Dysprosium	Dy	66	162.5	8.55	53.789
Einsteinium	Es	99	252[d]	—	138.067
Erbium	Er	68	167.26	9.006	57.483
Europium	Eu	63	151.96	5.243	48.515
Fermium	Fm	100	257[d]	—	141.51
Fluorine	F	9	18.998	1.69[e]	0.687
Francium	Fr	87	223[d]	—	101.147
Gadolinium	Gd	64	157.25	7.9	50.229
Gallium	Ga	31	69.72	(5.9—6.1)	10.368
Germanium	Ge	32	72.61	5.35	11.103
Gold	Au	79	196.966	19.3	80.713
Hafnium	Hf	72	178.49	13.31	65.313
Helium	He	2	4.003	0.179[e]	0.025
Holmium	Ho	67	164.93	8.795	55.615
Hydrogen	H	1	1.008	0.09[e]	0.014
Indium	In	49	114.82	7.3	27.928
Iodine	I	53	126.904	4.93	33.164
Iridium	Ir	77	192.22	22.421	76.097
Iron	Fe	26	55.847	7.86	7.111
Krypton	Kr	36	83.8	3.736[e]	14.323
Lanthanum	La	57	138.906	(6.14—6.17)	38.931
Lawrencium	Lr	103	260[d]	—	154.380
Lead	Pb	82	207.2	11.344	88.001
Lithium	Li	3	6.941	0.534	0.055
Lutetium	Lu	71	174.967	9.84	63.304
Magnesium	Mg	12	24.305	1.74	1.303
Manganese	Mn	25	54.938	7.20	6.537
Mendelevium	Md	101	258[d]	—	146.780
Mercury	Hg	80	200.59	13.594	83.106
Molybdenum	Mo	42	95.94	10.2	20.002

TABLE OF PROPERTIES OF THE ELEMENTS — ALPHABETIC ORDER (continued)

Name	Symbol	Atomic number (Z)	Atomic[a] weight (A)	Density[b] (g/cm³)	K$_B$[c] (keV)
Neodymium	Nd	60	144.24	(6.8—7)	43.571
Neon	Ne	10	20.179	0.9[e]	0.874
Neptunium	Np	93	237.048	(18—20.5)	118.619
Nickel	Ni	28	58.69	8.9	8.331
Niobium	Nb	41	92.906	8.57	18.987
Nitrogen	N	7	14.007	1.251[e]	0.399
Nobelium	No	102	259[d]	—	150.540
Osmium	Os	76	190.2	22.48	73.86
Oxygen	0	8	15.999	1.429[e]	0.531
Palladium	Pd	46	106.42	(11.4—12)	24.347
Phosphorus	P	15	30.974	(2.34—2.7)	2.142
Platinum	Pt	78	195.08	21.45	78.379
Plutonium	Pu	94	244[d]	(15.9—19.8)	121.72
Polonium	Po	84	209[d]	9.4	93.112
Potassium (Kalium)	K	19	39.098	0.86	3.607
Praseodymium	Pr	59	140.908	6.773	41.998
Promethium	Pm	61	145[d]	7.22	45.207
Protactinium	Pa	91	231.036	15.37	112.581
Radium	Ra	88	226.025	5	103.927
Radon	Rn	86	222[d]	9.73[e]	98.418
Rhenium	Re	75	186.207	20.53	71.662
Rhodium	Rh	45	102.906	12.4	23.224
Rubidium	Rb	37	85.468	1.532	15.201
Ruthenium	Ru	44	101.07	12.3	22.118
Samarium	Sm	62	150.36	7.52	46.846
Scandium	Sc	21	44.956	2.989	4.496
Selenium	Se	34	78.96	4.81	12.652
Silicon	Si	14	28.086	(2.32—2.34)	1.838
Silver	Ag	47	107.868	10.5	25.517
Sodium (Natrium)	Na	11	22.99	0.97	1.08
Strontium	Sr	38	87.62	2.6	16.106
Sulfur	S	16	32.06	2.07	2.47
Tantalum	Ta	73	180.948	(14.4—16.6)	67.4
Technetium	Tc	43	98[b]	11.50	21.054
Tellurium	Te	52	127.6	6.25	31.809
Terbium	Tb	65	158.925	8.229	51.998
Thallium	Tl	81	204.383	11.85	85.517
Thorium	Th	90	232.038	11.7	109.63
Thulium	Tm	69	168.934	9.321	59.335
Tin	Sn	50	118.71	(5.75—7.28)	29.19
Titanium	Ti	22	47.88	4.5	4.964
Tungsten (Wolfram)	W	74	183.85	19.35	69.508
(Unnihexium)	(Unh)	106	263[d]	—	—
(Unnilpentium)	(Unp)	105	262[d]	—	—
(Unnilquadium)	(Unq)	104	261[d]	—	—
Uranium	U	92	238.029	19.05	115.591
Vanadium	V	23	50.942	5.96	5.463
Xenon	Xe	54	131.29	5.887[e]	34.579
Ytterbium	Yb	70	173.04	6.965	61.303
Yttrium	Y	39	88.906	4.469	17.037
Zinc	Zn	30	65.38	7.14	9.66
Zirconium	Zr	40	91.22	6.49	17.998

TABLE OF PROPERTIES OF THE ELEMENTS — ATOMIC NUMBER ORDER

Atomic number (Z)	Name	Symbol	Atomic[a] weight (A)	Density[b] (g/cm^3)	K_B[c] (keV)
1	Hydrogen	H	1.008	0.09[e]	0.014
2	Helium	He	4.003	0.179[e]	0.025
3	Lithium	Li	6.941	0.534	0.055
4	Beryllium	Be	9.012	1.85	0.116
5	Boron	B	10.81	(2.34—2.37)	0.192
6	Carbon	C	12.011	(1.8—3.5)	0.283
7	Nitrogen	N	14.007	1.251[e]	0.399
8	Oxygen	O	15.999	1.429[e]	0.531
9	Fluorine	F	18.998	1.69[e]	0.687
10	Neon	Ne	20.179	0.9[e]	0.874
11	Sodium (Natrium)	Na	22.99	0.97	1.08
12	Magnesium	Mg	24.305	1.74	1.303
13	Aluminum	Al	26.982	2.702	1.559
14	Silicon	Si	28.086	(2.32—2.34)	1.838
15	Phosphorus	P	30.974	(2.34—2.7)	2.142
16	Sulfur	S	32.06	2.07	2.47
17	Chlorine	Cl	35.453	3.214[e]	2.819
18	Argon	Ar	39.948	1.784[e]	3.203
19	Potassium (Kalium)	K	39.098	0.86	3.607
20	Calcium	Ca	40.08	1.54	4.038
21	Scandium	Sc	44.956	2.989	4.496
22	Titanium	Ti	47.88	4.5	4.964
23	Vanadium	V	50.942	5.96	5.463
24	Chromium	Cr	51.996	7.2	5.988
25	Manganese	Mn	54.938	7.20	6.537
26	Iron	Fe	55.847	7.86	7.111
27	Cobalt	Co	58.933	8.9	7.709
28	Nickel	Ni	58.69	8.9	8.331
29	Copper	Cu	63.546	8.92	8.98
30	Zinc	Zn	65.38	7.14	9.66
31	Gallium	Ga	69.72	(5.9—6.1)	10.368
32	Germanium	Ge	72.61	5.35	11.103
33	Arsenic	As	74.92	5.727	11.863
34	Selenium	Se	78.96	4.81	12.652
35	Bromine	Br	79.904	3.119	13.475
36	Krypton	Kr	83.8	3.736[e]	14.323
37	Rubidium	Rb	85.468	1.532	15.201
38	Strontium	Sr	87.62	2.6	16.106
39	Yttrium	Y	88.906	4.469	17.037
40	Zirconium	Zr	91.22	6.49	17.998
41	Niobium	Nb	92.906	8.57	18.987
42	Molybdenum	Mo	95.94	10.2	20.002
43	Technetium	Tc	98[d]	11.50	21.054
44	Ruthenium	Ru	101.07	12.3	22.118
45	Rhodium	Rh	102.906	12.4	23.224
46	Palladium	Pd	106.42	(11.4—12)	24.347
47	Silver	Ag	107.868	10.5	25.517
48	Cadmium	Cd	112.41	8.642	26.712
49	Indium	In	114.82	7.3	27.928
50	Tin	Sn	118.71	(5.75—7.28)	29.19
51	Antimony (Stibium)	Sb	121.75	6.684	30.486
52	Tellurium	Te	127.6	6.25	31.809
53	Iodine	I	126.904	4.93	33.164
54	Xenon	Xe	131.29	5.887[e]	34.579

TABLE OF PROPERTIES OF THE ELEMENTS — ATOMIC NUMBER ORDER (continued)

Atomic number (Z)	Name	Symbol	Atomic[a] weight (A)	Density[b] (g/cm³)	K_B[c] (keV)
55	Cesium	Cs	132.905	1.879	35.959
56	Barium	Ba	137.33	3.51	37.41
57	Lanthanum	La	138.906	(6.14—6.17)	38.931
58	Cerium	Ce	140.12	(6.66—6.76)	40.449
59	Praseodymium	Pr	140.908	6.773	41.998
60	Neodymium	Nd	144.24	(6.8—7)	43.571
61	Promethium	Pm	145[d]	7.22	45.207
62	Samarium	Sm	150.36	7.52	46.846
63	Europium	Eu	151.96	5.243	48.515
64	Gadolinium	Gd	157.25	7.9	50.229
65	Terbium	Tb	158.925	8.229	51.998
66	Dysprosium	Dy	162.5	8.55	53.789
67	Holmium	Ho	164.93	8.795	55.615
68	Erbium	Er	167.26	9.006	57.483
69	Thulium	Tm	168.934	9.321	59.335
70	Ytterbium	Yb	173.04	6.965	61.303
71	Lutetium	Lu	174.967	9.84	63.304
72	Hafnium	Hf	178.49	13.31	65.313
73	Tantalum	Ta	180.948	(14.4—16.6)	67.4
74	Wolfram (Tungsten)	W	183.85	19.35	69.508
75	Rhenium	Re	186.207	20.53	71.662
76	Osmium	Os	190.2	22.48	73.86
77	Iridium	Ir	192.22	22.421	76.097
78	Platinum	Pt	195.08	21.45	78.379
79	Gold	Au	196.966	19.3	80.713
80	Mercury	Hg	200.59	13.594	83.106
81	Thallium	Tl	204.383	11.85	85.517
82	Lead	Pb	207.2	11.344	88.001
83	Bismuth	Bi	208.98	9.8	90.521
84	Polonium	Po	209[d]	9.4	93.112
85	Astatine	At	210[d]	—	95.74
86	Radon	Rn	222[d]	9.73[e]	98.418
87	Francium	Fr	223[d]	—	101.147
88	Radium	Ra	226.025	5	103.927
89	Actinium	Ac	227.028	10.07	106.759
90	Thorium	Th	232.038	11.7	109.63
91	Protactinium	Pa	231.036	15.37	112.581
92	Uranium	U	238.029	19.05	115.591
93	Neptunium	Np	237.048	(18—20.5)	118.619
94	Plutonium	Pu	244[d]	(15.9—19.8)	121.72
95	Americium	Am	243[d]	13.65	124.876
96	Curium	Cm	247[d]	13.51	128.088
97	Berkelium	Bk	247[d]	≅14.0	131.357
98	Californium	Cf	251[d]	—	134.683
99	Einstenium	Es	252[d]	—	138.067
100	Fermium	Fm	257[d]	—	141.51
101	Mendelevium	Md	258[d]	—	146.780
102	Nobelium	No	259[d]	—	154.380
103	Lawrencium	Lr	260[d]	—	150.540
104	(Unnilquadium)	(Unq)	261[d]	—	—
105	(Unnilpentium)	(Unp)	262[d]	—	—
106	(Unnihexium)	(Unh)	263[d]	—	—

TABLE OF PROPERTIES OF THE ELEMENTS — ATOMIC NUMBER ORDER (continued)

a Standard atomic weights 1987, based on ^{12}C scale.
b Density values in parentheses are given for elements that may exist in different crystalline forms.
c Values for k-shell binding energies (K_B) taken from *The Radiological Health Handbook*, U.S. Department of Health, Education, and Welfare, 1970, 161.
d Indicates radioactive elements whose atomic weight cannot be quoted precisely without knowledge of the origin of the elements; the value given is the atomic mass number of the isotope of that element of longest known half-life.
e Densities for gases are given in grams per liter (g/l).

Data for atomic weights and densities from Weast, Robert C., Ed., *CRC Handbook of Chemistry and Physics*, 67th ed., 1986-1987, CRC Press, Boca Raton, FL, 1986, and from *Atomic Weights of the Elements* 1987, IUPAC, 1988.

Characteristics of Practicable Radioisotopes and of Selected Radionuclides Commonly Used in Nuclear Medicine

PRACTICABLE RADIOISOTOPES

A practicable radioisotope should be

1. Simple to produce with an acceptable high specific activity
2. Of a reasonable half-life, so that it can be transported from its site of production to the user without having lost too much of its activity
3. Radiophysically and radiochemically of acceptable purity
4. Simple to detect and measure with adequate radiation counters.

ABBREVIATIONS

Half-lives		Decay mode	
y	years	α	alpha particle
d	days	β⁻	negative beta particle (negatron)
h	hours	β⁺	positive beta particle (positron)
m	minutes	γ	gamma ray
s	seconds	X	X-ray
ms	milliseconds	E.C.	electron capture
μs	microseconds	I.T.	isomeric transition

PHOTONS EMITTED

I.C. — indicates that photons of the stated energy are ~100% internally converted.

NOTE

Data from **Lederer, C. M. and Shirley, V. S., Eds.,** *Table of Isotopes*, 7th ed., John Wiley & Sons, New York, 1978; *Table of Practicable Radioisotopes*, Philips N. V. -Duphar, Petten, The Netherlands; *Chart of the Nuclides*, 3rd ed., Der Bunderminister für Wissenschaftlicheforshung, Bonn, F.D.R. 1968.

TABLE 1
Practicable Radioisotopes

Element	Radioisotope symbol	Half-life	Type of decay	Energy (Mev)
Actinium	^{227}Ac	21.6 y	β^-	0.046
			γ	0.024
			α	4.95
	^{228MsTh2}Ac	6.13 h	β^-	2.11
			γ	0.908
			γ	0.96
			γ	0.34
Aluminum	^{26}Al	7.4×10^5y	$\beta^+ + EC$	1.17
			γ	1.81
			γ	1.12
	^{28}Al	2.31 m	β^-	2.85
			γ	1.78
Americium	^{241}Am	458 y	γ	0.060
			α	5.49
Antimony	^{117}Sb	2.8 h	$\beta^+ + EC$	0.57
			γ	0.158
	^{119}Sb	38.0 h	$\gamma + EC$	0.024
	^{122}Sb	2.8 d	$\beta^- + EC$	1.97
			γ	0.56
			γ	0.69
	^{124}Sb	60 d	β^-	0.61
			β^-	2.31
			γ	0.60
			γ	1.69
			γ	0.72
	^{125}Sb	2.71 y	β^-	0.30
			β^-	0.12
			β^-	0.61
			γ	0.43
			γ	0.59
			γ	0.18
			γ	0.66
Argon	^{37}Ar	35.1 d	EC	
	^{41}Ar	1.83 h	β^-	1.20
			β^-	2.49
			γ	1.293
Arsenic	^{71}As	62 h	$\beta^+ + EC$	0.81
			γ	0.175
	^{72}As	26 h	$\beta^+ + EC$	2.5
			β^+	3.3
			γ	0.84
			γ	0.63
	^{73}As	80.3 d	$\gamma + EC$	0.054
	^{74}As	17.9 d	$\beta^+ + EC$	0.95
			β^+	1.54
			β^-	1.35
			β^-	0.72
			γ	0.60
			γ	0.64
	^{76}As	26.4 h	β^-	2.97
			β^-	2.41
			γ	0.56
			γ	0.66
			γ	1.21
	^{77}As	38.7 h	β^-	0.68
			γ	0.24

TABLE 1 (continued)
Practicable Radioisotopes

Element	Radioisotope symbol	Half-life	Type of decay	Energy (Mev)
Astatine	^{211}At	7.21 h	γ + EC	0.67
			α	5.87
Barium	^{128}Ba	58.3 h	γ + EC	0.13
			γ	0.27
	^{131}Ba	12.0 d	γ + EC	0.50
			γ	0.21
			γ	0.05
			γ	1.1
	^{133}Ba	7.2 y	γ + EC	0.36
			γ	0.08
	^{137m}Ba	2.55 m	γ + IT	0.662
	^{140}Ba	12.8 d	β$^+$	1.02
			β$^+$	0.48
			γ	0.03
			γ	0.54
Beryllium	^{7}Be	53 d	γ + EC	0.477
Bismuth	^{204}Bi	11.2 h	γ + EC	0.08
			γ	1.21
	^{205}Bi	15.3 d	γ + EC	0.70
			γ	0.26
			γ	1.91
	^{206}Bi	6.2 d	γ + EC	0.80
			γ	0.88
			γ	0.52
			γ	1.72
			γ	0.11
			γ	1.90
	^{207}Bi	30.2 y	γ + EC	0.57
			γ	1.06
			γ	1.77
Bromine	^{76}Br	16.1 h	β$^+$	3.6
			γ	0.56
			γ	3.57
	^{77}Br	57 h	β$^+$ + EC	0.34
			γ	0.24
			γ	0.52
			γ	0.58
	^{82}Br	35.3 h	β$^-$	0.44
			γ	0.78
			γ	0.55
			γ	0.62
			γ	1.48
Cadmium	^{109}Cd	1.24 y	γ + EC	0.088
	^{115m}Cd	43 d	β$^-$	1.62
			γ	0.94
			γ	1.30
			γ	0.49
	^{115}Cd	53.5 h	β$^-$	1.11
			γ	0.53
			γ	0.49
Calcium	^{45}Ca	165 d	β$^-$	0.252
	^{47}Ca	4.53 d	β$^-$	0.67
			β$^-$	1.98
			γ	1.31
			γ	0.82
			γ	0.49

TABLE 1 (continued)
Practicable Radioisotopes

Element	Radioisotope symbol	Half-life	Type of decay	Energy (Mev)
Californium	^{252}Cf	2.646 y	α	6.12
Carbon	^{11}C	20.3 m	β$^-$	0.97
	^{14}C	5730 y	β$^-$	0.156
Cerium	^{134}Ce	72 h	EC	
	^{139}Ce	140 d	γ + EC	0.165
	^{141}Ce	32.5 d	β$^-$	0.44
			β$^-$	0.58
			γ	0.145
	^{143}Ce	33.1 h	β$^-$	1.39
			γ	0.293
			γ	0.057
			γ	1.10
	^{144}Ce	284 d	β$^-$	0.31
			γ	0.134
Cesium	^{128}Cs	3.8 m	β$^+$ + EC	2.9
			γ	0.44
	^{129}Cs	32 h	γ + EC	0.37
			γ	0.42
			γ	0.55
	^{131}Cs	9.7 d	EC	
	^{132}Cs	6.6 d	β$^+$ + EC	
			β$^+$	0.40
			γ	0.67
	^{134}Cs	2.05 y	β$^-$	0.66
			γ	0.60
			γ	0.80
			γ	0.57
			γ	1.37
			γ	1.17
	^{137}Cs	30.0 y	β$^-$	0.51
			β$^-$	1.17
Chlorine	$^{34m-34}$Cl	32m—1.6 s	β$^+$ + IT	4.45
			β$^+$	2.5
			β$^+$	1.3
			γ	0.145
			γ	2.12
	^{36}Cl	3.1 × 10^5 y	β$^-$ + EC	0.714
	^{38}Cl	37.3 m	β$^-$	4.81
			β$^-$	1.11
			β$^-$	2.77
			γ	2.17
			γ	1.60
	^{39}Cl	55.5 m	β$^-$	1.91
			β$^-$	3.45
			γ	1.27
			γ	0.246
Chromium	^{48}Cr	23 h	γ + EC	0.31
			γ	0.116
	^{51}Cr	27.8 d	γ + EC	0.320
			γ	1.52
Cobalt	^{57}Co	270 d	γ + EC	0.122
			γ	0.136
	^{58}Co	71.3 d	β$^+$ + EC	0.47
			γ	0.810
	^{60}Co	5.263 y	β$^-$	0.31
			γ	1.173
			γ	1.332

TABLE 1 (continued)
Practicable Radioisotopes

Element	Radioisotope symbol	Half-life	Type of decay	Energy (Mev)
Copper	^{62}Cu	9.8 m	β^+	2.91
			γ	1.17
	^{64}Cu	12.8 h	β^- + EC	0.57
			β^+	0.66
			γ	1.34
	^{67}Cu	58.5 h	β^-	0.40
			β^-	0.48
			β^-	0.57
			γ	0.18
			γ	0.09
Curium	^{242}Cm	162.5 d	α	6.12
	^{244}Cm	17.6 y	α	5.81
Dysprosium	^{159}Dy	144 d	β^- + EC	0.058
	^{165}Dy	2.32 h	β^-	1.29
			γ	0.095
	^{166}Dy	81.5 h	β^-	0.48
			γ	0.08
Erbium	^{169}Er	9.6 d	β^-	0.34
	^{171}Er	7.52 h	β^-	1.06
			γ	0.308
			γ	0.112
			γ	0.962
Europium	$^{152m-152}$Eu	9.3 h—12.7 y	β^- + EC	1.88
			γ	0.12
			γ	1.41
	^{154}Eu	16 y	β^-	0.59
			γ	
	^{155}Eu	1.81 y	β^-	0.15
			γ	0.09
			γ	0.11
Fluorine	^{18}F	1.83 h	β^+ + EC	0.635
Gadolinium	^{148}Gd	84 y	α	318
	^{153}Gd	242 d	γ + EC	0.10
			γ	0.07
	^{159}Gd	18.0 h	β^-	0.95
			γ	0.36
			γ	0.06
Gallium	^{66}Ga	9.45 h	β^+ + EC	4.15
			β^+	0.94
			γ	1.04
			γ	2.75
			γ	0.8
			γ	4.8
	^{67}Ga	78 h	γ + EC	0.09
			γ	0.18
			γ	0.30
	^{68}Ga	68 m	β^+ + EC	1.90
			γ	1.08
	^{72}Ga	14.1 h	β^-	0.64
			β^-	0.96
			β^-	1.51
			β^-	3.15
			γ	0.83
			γ	0.63
			γ	2.20
			γ	2.50

TABLE 1 (continued)
Practicable Radioisotopes

Element	Radioisotope symbol	Half-life	Type of decay	Energy (Mev)
Germanium	^{68}Ge	275 d	EC	
	^{69}Ge	36 h	β^+ + EC	1.22
			γ	1.11
			γ	0.57
			γ	0.87
			γ	1.34
	^{71}Ge	11.4 d	EC	
Gold	^{192}Au	4.1 h	β^+ + EC	2.2
			γ	0.137
	^{193}Au	15.8 h	γ + EC	0.18
	^{194}Au	39.5 h	β^+ + EC	1.49
			γ	0.33
			γ	0.1
			γ	2.04
	^{195}Au	186 d	γ + EC	0.10
			γ	0.13
	^{196}Au	6.18 d	β^- + EC	0.259
			γ	0.356
			γ	0.333
			γ	0.426
	^{198}Au	64.7 h	β^-	0.96
			γ	0.41
	^{199}Au	75.6 h	β^-	0.30
			β^-	0.25
			β^-	0.46
			γ	0.16
			γ	0.21
			γ	0.05
Hafnium	^{172}Hf	5 y	γ + EC	0.024
			γ	0.125
			γ	0.08
	^{175}Hf	70 d	γ + EC	0.34
			γ	0.09
			γ	0.43
	^{181}Hf	42.5 d	β^-	0.41
			γ	0.48
			γ	0.13
			γ	0.34
Holmium	^{166}Ho	26.9 h	β^-	1.84
			γ	0.08
			γ	1.66
	^{166m}Ho	1200 y	β^-	0.07
			γ	0.184
			γ	0.081
			γ	1.43
Hydrogen	^{3}H	12.26 y	β^-	0.018
Indium	^{111}In	67.4 h	γ + EC	0.247
			γ	0.173
	^{113m}In	100 m	γ + IT	0.393
	$^{114-114m}$In	50 d—72 s	β^- + EC + IT	1.98
			γ	0.19
	^{115m}In	4.5 h	β^- + IT	0.83
			γ	0.34

TABLE 1 (continued)
Practicable Radioisotopes

Element	Radioisotope symbol	Half-life	Type of decay	Energy (Mev)
Iodine	^{123}I	13.3 h	γ + EC	0.159
	^{124}I	4.15 d	β⁻ + EC	0.9
			β⁻	2.14
			γ	0.60
			γ	0.73
			γ	0.64
			γ	2.26
	^{125}I	59.4 d	γ + EC	0.035
	^{126}I	12.8 d	β⁻ + EC	0.39
			β⁻	1.25
			β⁺	1.13
			γ	0.386
			γ	0.667
	^{131}I	8.05 d	β⁻	0.61
			γ	0.364
			γ	0.08
			γ	0.72
	^{132}I	2.26 h	β⁻	0.80
			β⁻	2.12
			γ	0.67
			γ	0.77
			γ	0.24
			γ	2.55
Iridium	^{189}Ir	13.3 d	γ + EC	0.245
	^{191m}Ir	4.9 s	γ + IT	0.129
	^{192}Ir	74.2 d	β⁻ + EC	0.67
			γ	0.317
			γ	0.296
			γ	0.612
	^{194}Ir	17.4 h	β⁻	2.24
			γ	0.328
			γ	0.29
			γ	2.12
Iron	^{52}Fe	8.2 h	β⁺ + EC	0.80
			γ	0.165
	^{55}Fe	2.60 y	EC	
	^{59}Fe	45.6 d	β⁻	0.47
			β⁻	0.27
			β⁻	1.57
			γ	1.095
			γ	1.292
Krypton	^{79}Kr	34.9 h	β⁺ + EC	0.60
			γ	0.398
			γ	0.606
			γ	0.261
	^{81m}Kr	13.0 s	γ + IT	0.190
	^{83m}Kr	1.86 h	γ + IT	0.009
			γ	0.032
	^{85}Kr	10.76 y	β⁻	0.67
			γ	0.514
Lanthanum	^{134}La	6.8m	β⁺ + EC	2.7
			γ	0.61
	^{135}La	19.4 h	γ + EC	0.48

TABLE 1 (continued)
Practicable Radioisotopes

Element	Radioisotope symbol	Half-life	Type of decay	Energy (Mev)
	^{140}La	40.2 h	β⁻	1.34
			β⁻	0.83
			β⁻	2.15
			γ	1.60
			γ	0.33
			γ	2.53
Lead	^{200}Pb	21.5 h	γ + EC	0.03
			γ	0.61
	^{203}Pb	52.1 h	γ + EC	0.279
	$^{210-RaO}$Pb	20.4 y	β⁻	0.015
			β⁻	0.061
			γ	0.047
Lutetium	^{173}Lu	1.37 y	γ + EC	0.272
			γ	0.079
			γ	0.637
	^{177}Lu	6.74 d	β⁻	0.50
			γ	0.21
			γ	0.11
Magnesium	^{28}Mg	21.2 h	β⁻	0.46
			γ	0.03
			γ	1.35
			γ	0.40
			γ	0.95
Manganese	^{52}Mn	5.60 d	β⁺ + EC	0.58
			γ	1.434
			γ	0.935
			γ	0.744
	^{54}Mn	303 d	γ + EC	0.835
	^{56}Mn	2.576 h	β⁻	2.85
			γ	0.847
			γ	1.81
			γ	2.11
Mercury	^{192}Hg	4.8 h	γ + EC	0.274
	^{194}Hg	1.9 y	EC	
	$^{197m-197}$Hg	24 h—65 h	γ + EC + IT	0.08
			γ	0.28
	^{203}Hg	46.9 d	β⁻	0.21
			γ	0.279
Molybdenum	^{99}Mo	66.7 h	β⁻	1.23
			β⁻	0.45
			γ	0.740
			γ	0.181
			γ	0.780
			γ	0.372
Neodymium	^{140}Nd	3.3 d	EC	
	^{147}Nd	11.1 d	β⁻	0.81
			γ	0.09
			γ	0.53
Neptunium	^{237}Np	2.14 × 10⁶ y	γ	0.086
			α	4.78
Nickel	^{56}Ni	6.10 d	γ + EC	0.16
			γ	0.81
	^{57}Ni	36 h	β⁺ + EC	0.85
			γ	1.37
			γ	0.89

TABLE 1 (continued)
Practicable Radioisotopes

Element	Radioisotope symbol	Half-life	Type of decay	Energy (Mev)
	^{63}Ni	92 y	β⁻	0.067
	^{65}Ni	2.56 h	β⁻	2.13
			γ	1.48
			γ	1.11
			γ	0.37
Niobium	^{90}Nb	14.6 h	β⁺ + EC	1.50
			γ	1.14
	^{91m}Nb	64 d	γ + EC + IT	1.21
	^{92m}Nb	10.16 d	γ + EC	0.93
	^{95}Nb	35 d	β⁻	0.16
			γ	0.76
	^{96}Nb	23.4 h	β⁻	0.75
			γ	0.78
			γ	1.09
	^{97}Nb	72 m	β⁻	1.27
			γ	0.665
Nitrogen	^{13}N	9.96 m	β⁺	1.20
Osmium	^{182}Os	21.9 h	γ + EC	0.510
	^{185}Os	93.6 d	γ + EC	0.646
			γ	0.875
	$^{191m-191}$Os	13h—15 d	β⁻ + IT	0.143
	^{193}Os	31.5 h	β⁻	0.67
			β⁻	1.13
			γ	0.460
Oxygen	^{15}O	2.05 m	β⁺	1.74
Palladium	^{100}Pd	96 h	γ + EC	0.084
	^{103}Pd	17.0 d	γ + EC	0.362
	^{109}Pd	13.47 h	β⁻	1.103
			γ	0.04
			γ	0.77
Phosphorus	^{32}P	14.2 d	β⁻	1.71
	^{33}P	24.4 d	β⁻	0.25
Platinum	^{188}Pt	10.2 d	γ + EC	0.14
			γ	0.42
	^{191}Pt	72.0 h	γ + EC	0.096
			γ	0.624
	^{193}Pt	<500 y	EC	
	^{197}Pt	18 h	β⁻	0.67
			γ	0.077
Plutonium	^{238}Pu	86.4 y	α	5.50
	^{239}Pu	2.439 × 10⁴ y	γ	0.052
			α	5.16
	^{242}Pu	3.79 × 10⁵ y	α	4.90
Polonium	^{208}Po	2.93 y	γ + EC	0.28
			γ	0.60
			α	5.11
	^{209}Po	103 y	γ + EC	0.91
			γ	0.26
			α	4.88

TABLE 1 (continued)
Practicable Radioisotopes

Element	Radioisotope symbol	Half-life	Type of decay	Energy (Mev)
Potassium	^{42}K	12.4 h	β^-	3.52
			γ	1.52
	^{43}K	22.4 h	β^-	0.82
			β^-	0.46
			β^-	1.24
			β^-	1.81
			γ	0.37
			γ	0.62
			γ	0.39
			γ	0.59
			γ	0.22
			γ	1.01
Praseodymium	^{140}Pr	3.39 m	β^+ + EC	2.32
			γ	1.60
	^{142}Pr	19.2 h	β^-	2.15
			β^-	0.64
			γ	1.57
	^{143}Pr	13.6 d	β^-	0.93
	^{144}Pr	17.3 m	β^-	2.99
			γ	0.695
Promethium	^{147}Pm	2.62 y	β^-	0.22
	^{149}Pm	53.1 h	β^-	1.07
			γ	0.286
	^{151}Pm	27.8 h	β^-	1.19
			γ	0.340
			γ	0.07
			γ	0.96
Protactinium	^{231}Pa	3.25 × 10⁴ y	γ	0.02
			γ	0.36
			α	5.01
	^{233}Pa	27.0 d	β^-	0.26
			γ	0.31
Radium	^{226}Ra	1620 y	α	4.78
			α	4.60
Radon	^{222}Rn	3.82 d	α	5.49
Rhenium	^{183}Re	71 d	γ + EC	0.046
			γ	0.292
	^{186}Re	88.9 h	β^-	1.07
			β^-	0.93
			γ	0.137
	^{188}Re	16.7 h	β^-	2.12
			β^-	1.96
			γ	0.155
Rhodium	$^{101m-101}$Rh	4.4d—3.0 y	γ + EC + IT	0.307
			γ	0.545
	^{103m}Rh	57.5 m	γ + IT	0.04
	^{105}Rh	35.9 h	β^-	0.56
			β^-	0.25
			γ	0.319
	^{106}Rh	30 s	β^-	3.54
			γ	0.512
			γ	0.612

TABLE 1 (continued)
Practicable Radioisotopes

Element	Radioisotope symbol	Half-life	Type of decay	Energy (Mev)
Rubidium	^{81}Rb	4.7 h	β^+ + EC	1.03
			γ	0.253
	^{82m}Rb	6.3 h	β^+ + EC	0.78
			γ	0.777
	^{82}Rb	1.25 m	β^+ + EC	3.15
			γ	0.777
	^{83}Rb	83 d	γ + EC	0.53
	^{84}Rb	33 d	β^+ + EC	1.66
			β^-	0.91
			γ	0.88
	^{86}Rb	18.7 d	β^-	1.78
			β^-	0.71
			γ	1.08
Ruthenium	^{97}Ru	69.1 h	γ + EC	0.215
			γ	0.324
	^{103}Ru	39.5 d	β^-	0.21
			β^-	0.69
			γ	0.497
			γ	0.610
	^{106}Ru	1.01 y	β^-	0.039
Samarium	^{145}Sm	340 d	γ + EC	0.061
	^{151}Sm	87 y	β^-	0.076
			γ	0.022
	^{153}Sm	46.8 h	β^-	0.80
			γ	0.103
			γ	0.07
Scandium	$^{44m-44}$Sc	58.6 h—3.92 h	β^+ + EC + IT	1.47
			γ	0.27
			γ	1.14
			γ	1.02
			γ	1.16
	^{44}Sc	3.92 h	β^+	1.47
			γ	1.16
	^{46}Sc	84 d	β^-	0.36
			β^-	1.48
			γ	0.89
			γ	1.12
	^{47}Sc	82.3 h	β^-	0.44
			β^-	0.60
			γ	0.16
Selenium	^{72}Se	8.4 d	γ + EC	0.046
	^{75}Se	120.4 d	γ + EC	0.27
			γ	0.14
			γ	0.28
			γ	0.07
			γ	0.40
Silicon	^{31}Si	2.62 h	β^-	1.48
			γ	1.26
	^{32}Si	650 y	β^-	0.21
Silver	^{105}Ag	40 d	γ + EC	0.34
			γ	0.28
			γ	0.44
			γ	0.06

TABLE 1 (continued)
Practicable Radioisotopes

Element	Radioisotope symbol	Half-life	Type of decay	Energy (Mev)
	^{106m}AG	8.5 d	γ + EC	0.51
			γ	0.80
			γ	0.72
			γ	0.62
	^{109m}Ag	39.2 s	γ + IT	0.088
	$^{110m-110}$Ag	225 d-24.4 s	β⁻ + IT	0.09
			β⁻	1.5
			β⁻	2.87
			β⁻	2.14
			γ	0.658
			γ	0.68
			γ	1.51
	^{111}Ag	7.5 d	β⁻	1.05
			β⁻	0.69
			β⁻	0.79
			γ	0.342
			γ	0.247
Sodium	^{22}Na	2.62 y	β⁺ + EC	0.54
			γ	1.28
	^{24}Na	15.0 h	β⁻	1.39
			γ	1.37
			γ	2.75
Strontium	^{83}Sr	32.4 h	β⁺ + EC	1.15
			γ	0.76
			γ	0.38
	^{85}Sr	64 d	γ + EC	0.514
	^{87m}Sr	2.83 h	γ + IT	0.388
	^{89}Sr	52.7 d	β⁻	1.46
	^{90}Sr	27.7 y	β⁻	0.54
Sulfur	^{35}S	87.9 d	β⁻	0.17
	^{38}S	2.87 h	β⁻	1.1
			β⁻	3.0
			γ	1.88
Tantalum	^{177}Ta	56.6 h	γ + EC	0.11
	^{178}Ta	9.35 m	β⁺ + EC	0.89
			γ	0.093
	^{179}Ta	1.64 y	EC	
	^{182}Ta	115.1 d	β⁻	0.36
			β⁻	1.71
			γ	0.03
			γ	1.6
Technetium	$^{95m-95}$Tc	61 d—20.0 h	β⁺ + EC + IT	0.68
			γ	0.204
			γ	0.504
			γ	0.78
	^{96}Tc	4.35 d	γ + EC	0.78
			γ	0.81
			γ	0.85
	^{99m}Tc	6.05 h	γ + IT	0.140
	^{99}Tc	2.12 × 10⁵ y	β⁻	0.292
Tellurium	$^{121m-121}$Te	154 d—17 d	γ + EC + IT	0.212
			γ	1.10
			γ	0.57
			γ	0.51
	^{125m}Te	58 d	γ + IT	0.035

TABLE 1 (continued)
Practicable Radioisotopes

Element	Radioisotope symbol	Half-life	Type of decay	Energy (Mev)
	$^{127m}-^{127}$Te	109 d—9.4 h	β^- + IT	0.73
			β^-	0.70
			γ	0.059
			γ	0.417
	^{132}Te	77.7 h	β^-	0.22
			γ	0.230
			γ	0.053
Terbium	^{160}TB	72.1 d	β^-	0.45
			β^-	1.74
			γ	0.88
			γ	0.09
			γ	1.31
	^{161}Tb	6.9 d	β^-	0.45
			β^-	0.58
			γ	0.02
			γ	0.13
Thallium	^{200}Tl	26.1 h	γ + EC	0.368
	^{201}Tl	73 h	γ + EC	0.135
			γ	0.167
	^{202}Tl	12.0 d	γ + EC	0.439
	^{204}Tl	3.81 y	β^- + EC	0.766
Thorium	$^{228}-^{RdTh}$Th	1.910 y	γ	0.084
			γ	5.43
	^{230}Th	8.0×10^4 y	γ	0.068
			α	4.68
	^{232}Th	1.4×10^{10} y	α	4.01
Thulium	^{167}Tm	9.6 d	γ + EC	0.208
	^{170}Tm	134 d	β^-	0.97
			β^-	0.88
			γ	0.084
	^{171}Tm	1.92 y	β^-	0.97
			γ	0.067
Tin	^{113}Sn	115 d	γ + EC	0.26
	^{117m}Sn	14 d	γ + IT	0.158
	^{121}Sn	27.5 h	β^-	0.383
Titanium	^{44}Ti	48 y	γ + EC	0.078
			γ	0.068
	^{45}Ti	3.1 h	β^+	1.04
			γ	0.72
			γ	1.41
Tungsten (Wolfram)	^{181}W	140 d	EC	
	^{185}W	75 d	β^-	0.43
	^{187}W	23.9 h	β^-	0.63
			β^-	1.31
			γ	0.69
			γ	0.48
			γ	0.04
			γ	0.87
	^{188}W	69.4 d	β^-	0.35
			γ	0.293
Uranium	^{232}U	72 y	γ	0.058
			γ	0.328
			α	5.32
	^{233}U	1.62×10^5 y	γ	0.03
			γ	0.32
			α	4.82

TABLE 1 (continued)
Practicable Radioisotopes

Element	Radioisotope symbol	Half-life	Type of decay	Energy (Mev)
	^{235}U	7.1×10^8 y	γ	0.185
			α	4.40
	^{238}U	4.5×10^9 y	α	4.20
Vanadium	^{48}V	16 d	β^+ + EC	0.70
			γ	0.98
			γ	1.31
			γ	2.24
	^{49}V	330 d	EC	
Xenon	^{127}Xe	36.41 d	γ + EC	0.203
	^{129m}Xe	8.0 d	γ + IT	0.04
			γ	0.196
	^{131m}Xe	11.8 d	γ + IT	0.164
	$^{133m—133}$Xe	2.26 d—5.2 d	β^- + IT	0.346
			γ	0.233
			γ	0.081
Ytterbium	^{166}Yb	57.5 h	γ + EC	0.082
	^{169}Yb	31.8 d	γ + EC	0.06
			γ	0.31
	^{175}Yb	4.2 d	β^-	0.466
			γ	0.40
			γ	0.28
Yttrium	$^{87m—87}$Y	14 h-80 h	β^+ + EC + IT	1.60
			β^+	0.7
			γ	0.38
			γ	0.48
	^{88}Y	108.1 d	γ + EC	1.84
			γ	0.90
	^{90}Y	64 h	β^-	2.27
	^{91}Y	58.8 d	β^-	1.55
Zinc	^{62}Zn	9.1 h	β^+ + EC	0.66
			γ	0.59
	^{65}Zn	245 d	β^+ + EC	0.33
			γ	1.11
	$^{69m—69}$Zn	13.8 h—57 m	β^- + IT	0.90
			γ	0.44
Zirconium	^{86}Zr	16.5 h	γ + EC	0.24
	^{88}Zr	85 d	γ + EC	0.394
	^{89}Zr	78 h	β^+ + EC	0.90
			γ	0.91
	^{95}Zr	65.5 d	β^-	0.40
			β^-	0.36
			β^-	0.89
			γ	0.72
			γ	0.76
	^{97}Zr	17.0 h	β^-	1.9
			γ	0.75

TABLE 2
Decay Schemes of Selected Radionuclides Used in Nuclear Medicine

Nuclide, half-life, Production method	Type of Decay	Particle energies		X or γ-Rays photons energies	
		Energy MeV	Abundance (%)	Energy MeV	Abundance (%)
Americium-241	α	5.387	1.6	0.026	2.5
(458 y)		5.442	12.5	0.033	0.1
^{241}Pu$(\alpha)^{241}$Am		5.484	85.2	0.043	0.1
		5.511	0.20	0.0595	35.9
		5.543	0.34	0.099	0.02
				0.103	0.02
				0.125	0.004
				Np X-rays	
				0.012—0.022	40.0
Antimony-124	β⁻	0.21	9	0.603	98.0
(60.2 d)		0.61	52	0.646	7.2
		0.86	4	0.709	1.4
		0.94	2	0.714	2.3
		1.57	5	0.723	11.2
		1.65	3	0.791	0.7
		2.30	23	0.968	1.9
				1.045	1.9
				1.325	1.5
				1.355	0.9
				1.368	2.5
				1.437	1.1
				1.691	50.4
				2.091	6.1
Antimony-125[a]	β⁻	0.094	13.5	0.035	4.5
(2.71 y)		0.124	5.7	0.176	6.8
		0.130	18.1	0.321	0.5
		0.241	1.5	0.381	1.5
		0.302	40.2	0.428	29.8
		0.332	0.3	0.463	10.4
		0.445	7.2	0.601	17.8
		0.621	13.5	0.607	4.9
				0.636	11.4
				0.671	1.7
				Te X-rays	
				0.027—0.031	50.0
	Daughter	^{125m}Te			
		(58d)			
		I.T.	100	0.035	7
				0.109	0.3
				Te X-rays	
				0.027—0.032	110
Arsenic-74	β⁻	0.718	15.4	0.635	15.4
(17.9 d)		1.353	18.8		
^{71}Ga$(\alpha, n)^{74}$As					
	β⁺	0.944	25.7	0.511	58.2
		1.540	3.4	0.596	59.2
	E.C.		36.7		
				Ge X-rays	
				0.010	15.0
Astatine-211	α	5.87	40.9	0.67	low
(7.21 h)	E.C.		59.1		
^{209}Bi$(\alpha, 2n)^{211}$At					
	α	7.45	99.0	0.57	0.5
				0.90	0.5

TABLE 2 (continued)
Decay Schemes of Selected Radionuclides Used in Nuclear Medicine

Nuclide, half-life, Production method	Type of decay	Particle energies		X or γ-Rays photons energies	
		Energy MeV	Abundance (%)	Energy MeV	Abundance (%)
Barium-133 (7.2 y) ^{137}Cs(β^-)^{137m}Ba	E.C.		100	0.053	2.2
				0.080	2.6
				0.081	33.9
				0.161	0.7
				0.223	0.4
				0.276	7.1
				0.303	18.4
				0.356	62.2
				0.384	8.9
				Cs X-ray 0.030—0.036	120.0
Barium-137 m (2.55 m) ^{137}Cs(β^-)^{137m}Ba	I.T.		0.032	0.662	89.8
				Ba X-rays 6.0	
				0.036	1.4
Barium-140 (12.8 d)	β^-	0.468	24.0	0.014	1.3
		0.582	10.0	0.030	14.0
		0.886	2.6	0.163	6.2
		1.005	46.0	0.305	4.5
		1.019	17.0	0.424	3.2
				0.438	2.1
				0.537	23.8
				0.602	0.6
				0.661	0.7
	Daughter ^{140}La				
Beryllium-7 (53 d)	E.C.		100	0.478	10.4
Bromine-75 (98 m) ^{78}Kr(p, α)^{75}Br	β^+ E.C.	1.740	50.8 24.5	0.511	151
				0.141	7
				0.286	92
				Se X-rays 0.11	
Bromine-77 (57 h) ^{75}As(α, 2n)^{77}Br	β^+ E.C.	0.343	0.7 99.3	0.511	1.4
				0.239	23.1
				0.250	3.0
				0.297	4.2
				0.521	22.4
				0.579	3.0
				Se X-rays	
				0.011	45.4
				0.012	7.2
Bromine-82 (35.3 h) ^{75}As(α, 2n)^{77}Br	β^-	0.263	1.7	0.221	2.3
		0.444	98.3	0.554	72.0
				0.606	1.0
				0.619	43.0
				0.698	27.0
				0.777	83.0
				0.828	24.0
				1.008	1.7
				1.044	29.0
				1.317	28.0
				1.475	17.0
				1.651	0.9

TABLE 2 (continued)
Decay Schemes of Selected Radionuclides Used in Nuclear Medicine

Nuclide, half-life, Production method	Type of decay	Particle energies		X or γ-Rays photons energies	
		Energy MeV	Abundance (%)	Energy MeV	Abundance (%)
Cadmium-109[b] (452 d)	E.C.		100	Ag X-rays 0.022—0.026	67.7
				0.088	3.8
				Ag X-rays 0.022-0.026	34.5
Calcium-45 (165 d) $^{44}Ca(n, \gamma)^{45}Ca$	β⁻	0.257	100		
Calcium-47 (4.53 d) $^{46}Ca(n, \gamma)^{47}Ca$	β⁻	0.69	82.0	0.489	6.8
		1.22	0.1	0.530	0.1
		1.99	17.9	0.767	0.2
				0.808	6.8
				1.297	75.1
	Daughter	^{47}Sc (3.48 d)			
		0.44	70	0.159	69.7
		0.60	30		
Californium-252 (2.64 y)	α	5.974	0.3	up to 9 MeV	
		6.075	15.0		
		6.118	81.6		
Carbon-11 (20.38 m) $^{10}B(d, n)^{11}C$	β⁺	0.960	99.8	0.511	199.6
Carbon-14 (5730 y) $^{14}N(n, p)^{14}C$	β⁻	0.156	100		
Cerium-139 (140 d)	E.C.		100	0.166	79.9
				La X-rays 0.033-0.039	90.0
Cerium-141 (32.5 d)	β⁻	0.436	70	0.145	48
		0.581	30	Pr X-rays 0.035—0.042	17.0
Cerium-144[c,d] (284.3 d)	β⁻	0.182	19.1	0.034	0.1
		0.216	0.2	0.040	0.4
		0.236	4.4	0.053	0.1
		0.316	76.3	0.080	1.5
				0.100	0.03
				0.134	10.8
	β⁻	1.534	0.05	0.696	0.05
	I.T		1.15	0.814	0.05
	β⁻	0.808	1.0	0.696	1.53
		2.298	1.2	1.489	0.28
		2.994	97.75	2.186	0.72
Cesium-134 (2.05 y)	β	0.09	26.0	0.475	1.5
		0.42	2.5	0.563	8.1
		0.66	71.5	0.569	14.0
				0.605	97.5
				0.796	85.4
				0.802	8.6
				1.038	1.0
				1.168	2.0
				1.365	3.3

TABLE 2 (continued)
Decay Schemes of Selected Radionuclides Used in Nuclear Medicine

Nuclide, half-life, Production method	Type of decay	Particle energies		X or γ-Rays photons energies	
		Energy MeV	Abundance (%)	Energy MeV	Abundance (%)
Cesium-137ᵉ (30 y) ²³⁵U(n, f)¹³⁷Cs	β⁻	0.512 1.174	94.6 5.4	0.662 Ba X-rays 0.032—0.038	85.1 7.0
Chlorine-36 (3.01 × 10⁵ y) ³⁵Cl(n, γ)³⁶Cl	β⁻ E.C	0.709	98.1 1.9		
Chromium-51 (27.8 d) ⁵⁰Cr(n, γ)⁵¹Cr	E.C		100	0.320 V X-rays 0.005 0.006	9.83 22
Cobalt-56 (77.3 d)	β⁺ E.C	0.4 1.5	1 18 81	0.511 0.847 0.977 1.038 1.175 1.238 1.360 1.771 2.015 2.035 2.599 3.010 3.202 3.254 3.273 3.452	from β⁺ 99.97 1.4 14.0 2.3 67.6 4.3 15.7 3.1 7.9 16.9 1.0 3.0 7.4 1.8 0.9
Cobalt-57 (270 d) ⁶⁰Ni(p, α)⁵⁷Co	E.C		100	0.014 0.122 0.136 0.570 0.692 Fe K X-rays 0.006—0.007	9.5 85.5 10.8 0.01 0.16 55
Cobalt-58 (71.3 d) ⁵⁵Mn(α, n)⁵⁸Co	β⁺ E.C.	0.475	15.0 85.0	0.511 0.811 0.864 1.675 Fe X-rays 0.006—0.007	from β⁺ 99.4 0.796 0.5 26
Cobalt-60 (5.26 y) ⁵⁹Co(n, γ)⁶⁰Co	β⁻	0.318 1.491	99.9 0.1	1.173 1.333	99.86 99.98 <0.01
Copper-62 (9.8 m) ⁵⁹Cu(p, 2n)⁶²Zn ⁶²Zn(E.C., β⁺) ⁶²Cu	β⁺ E.C.	2.917	97.6 2.2	0.511	from β⁺
Copper-64 (12.8 h)	β⁻	0.578	37.2		

TABLE 2 (continued)
Decay Schemes of Selected Radionuclides Used in Nuclear Medicine

Nuclide, half-life, Production method	Type of decay	Particle energies		X or γ-Rays photons energies	
		Energy MeV	Abundance (%)	Energy MeV	Abundance (%)
^{63}Cu(n, γ)^{64}Cu	β$^+$	0.663	17.9	0.511	35.7
	E.C		44.9	1.346	0.5
				Ni X-rays	
				0.008	16.5
Copper-67	β$^-$	0.390	57.2	0.091	7.0
(58.5 h)		0.482	21.6	0.093	16.1
^{64}Ni(α, p)^{67}Cu		0.75	20.0	0.184	48.7
				0.300	0.8
				Zn X-rays	
				0.009	6.4
Curium-244	α	5.763	23.6	0.043	0.02
(17.6 y)		5.806	76.4	0.099	0.0013
				0.152	0.0014
				Pu X-rays	8.0
				0.012—0.023	
Erbium-169	β$^-$	0.53	100	Tm X-rays	
(9.6 d)				0.1098	0.001
Europium-152	β$^-$	0.185	1.8	0.122	28.2
(12.7 y)		0.394	2.4	0.245	7.4
		0.705	13.8	0.344	26.3
		1.484	8.0	0.411	2.2
				0.444	3.1
	β$^+$		0.02	0.779	12.8
	E.C		72.3	0.867	4.1
				0.964	14.4
				1.086	10.0
				1.090	1.7
				1.112	13.6
				1.213	1.4
				1.299	1.6
				1.408	20.6
Fluorine-18	β$^+$	0.633	96.9	0.511	194
(109.7 m)					
^{20}Ne(d, α)^{18}F	E.C.		3.1		
^{16}O(^{3}H, n)^{18}F					
Gadolinium-153	E.C.		100	0.070	2.6
(242 d)				0.075	0.07
				0.083	0.23
				0.089	0.12
				0.097	30.0
				0.103	20.0
				0.173	0.04
				Eu X-rays	110.0
				0.041—0.048	
Gallium-67^f	E.C.		100	0.093	38.0
(78 h)				0.185	23.5
^{68}Zn(p, 2n)^{67}Ga				0.209	2.6
				0.300	16.7
				0.394	4.4
				0.494	0.1
				0.704	0.02
				0.795	0.06
				0.888	0.17
				Zn X-rays	

TABLE 2 (continued)
Decay Schemes of Selected Radionuclides Used in Nuclear Medicine

Nuclide, half-life, Production method	Type of decay	Particle energies		X or γ-Rays photons energies	
		Energy MeV	Abundance (%)	Energy MeV	Abundance (%)
				0.008—0.010	43
				0.093	37.6
				Zn X-rays	
				0.008—0.010	13
Gallium-68	β⁺	0.822	1.1	0.511	from β⁺
(68 m)		1.899	88.0		
⁶⁹Ga(p,2n)⁶⁸Ge	E.C.		10.9	1.077	3.3
⁶⁸Ge(E.C.)				Zn X-rays	
⁶⁸Ga			0.009	4.7	
Gold-198	β⁻	0.285	1.32	0.412	95.45
(64.7 h)		0.961	98.66	0.676	1.06
¹⁹⁷Au(n, γ)¹⁹⁸Au		1.373	0.02	1.088	0.23
Gold-199	β⁻	0.25	21	0.050	0.3
(75.6 h)		0.29	72	0.158	39.6
		0.45	7	0.208	8.8
				Hg X-rays	
				0.069—0.083	18
Hydrogen-3	β⁻	0.0186	100		
(Tritium)					
(12.26 y)					
⁶Li(n, α)³H					
Indium-111	E.C.		100	0.171	90.9
(67.4 h)				0.245	94.2
¹⁰⁹Ag(α, 2n)¹¹¹In				Cd X-rays	
				0.023—0.027	84.0
Indium-113m	I.T.	0.3917	100	0.3917	64
(100 m)					
¹¹²Sn(n, γ)¹¹³Sn					
¹¹³Sn(E.C.)¹¹³ᵐIn					
Iodine-123	E.C.		100	0.027	86.0
(13.3 h)				0.159	83.4
¹²¹Sb(α, 2n)¹²³I				0.529	1.4
Iodine-125	E.C.		100	0.035	7.0
(59.4 d)				Te X-ray	138.0
¹²⁴Xe(n, γ)¹²⁵Xe				0.027—0.032	
¹²⁵Xe(E.C.)¹²⁵I					
Iodine-129	β⁻	0.150	100	0.040	7.5
(1.57 × 10⁷ y)				Xe X-rays	69.0
				0.030—0.035	
Iodine-131ᵍʰ	β⁻	0.247	1.8	0.080	2.4
(8.05 d)		0.304	0.6	0.284	5.9
¹³⁰Te(n, γ)¹³¹Te		0.334	7.2	0.364	81.8
¹³¹Te(β⁻)¹³¹I		0.606	89.7	0.637	7.2
		0.806	0.7	0.723	1.8
	I.T		100	0.164	2
Iron-52	β⁺	0.804	56	0.511	112
(8.2 h)	E.C.		44	0.165	100
⁵⁵Mn(p, 4n)⁵²Fe					
Iron-55	E.C.		100	Mn X-rays	28.0
(2.6 y)				0.0059—0.0065	
⁵⁴Fe(n, γ)⁵⁵Fe					

TABLE 2 (continued)
Decay Schemes of Selected Radionuclides Used in Nuclear Medicine

Nuclide, half-life, Production method	Type of decay	Particle energies		X or γ-Rays photons energies	
		Energy MeV	Abundance (%)	Energy MeV	Abundance (%)
Iron-59	β⁻	0.084	0.1	0.143	0.8
(45.6 d)		0.132	1.1	0.192	2.8
^{58}Fe(n, γ)^{59}Fe		0.274	45.8	0.335	0.3
		0.467	52.7	0.383	0.02
		1.566	0.3	1.099	55.8
				1.292	43.8
				1.482	0.06
Krypton-81m	I.T.		100	0.191	66.4
(13 s)				Kr X-rays	
^{81}Rb(β⁺, E.C)^{81m}Kr				0.013	16.9
Krypton-85ⁱ	β⁻	0.158	0.43		
(10.76 y)		0.672	99.57		
				0.514	0.43
Lanthanum-140	β⁻	1.247	11	0.131	0.8
(40.2 h)		1.253	6	0.242	0.6
		1.288	1	0.266	0.7
		1.305	5	0.329	21.0
		1.357	45	0.432	3.3
		1.421	5	0.487	45.0
		1.685	18	0.752	4.4
		2.172	7	0.816	23.0
				0.868	5.5
				0.920	2.5
				0.925	6.9
				0.950	0.6
				1.597	95.6
				2.348	0.9
				2.522	3.3
Lead-203	E.C.		100	0.279	80.9
(52.1 h)				0.401	3.4
^{203}Tl(d,2n)^{203}Pb				0.680	0.7
				Tl X-rays	
				0.072	68.0
				0.083	18.9
Lead-210	α		2×10^6	0.046	4
(20.4 y)				BiL X-rays	
	β	0.015	80	0.009—0.017	21
		0.061	20		
	Daughter	^{210}Bi			
		(5.01 d)			
	α	4.67			
			1.3×10^{-4}		
	β⁻	1.161	100		
	Daughter	^{210}Po			
		(138.38 d)			
	α	5.305	100		
Manganese-52	β⁺	0.575	29.4	0.511	58.8
5.6 d	E.C.		60.6	0.744	90.0
^{52}Cr(d.2n)^{52}Mn				0.848	3.3
				0.936	94.0
				1.246	4.2
				1.334	5.1

TABLE 2 (continued)
Decay Schemes of Selected Radionuclides Used in Nuclear Medicine

Nuclide, half-life, Production method	Type of decay	Particle energies Energy MeV	Abundance (%)	X or γ-Rays photons energies Energy MeV	Abundance (%)
				1.434	100.0
				Cr X-4ay	
				0.005	15.5
Manganese-52m	β⁺	0.905	0.2	0.511	193.4
(21.1 m)		1.174	96.5		
⁵²Fe(β⁺,E.C.)⁵²Mn	E.C.		1.5	1.434	98.2
			1.8	1.728	0.2
				0.378	1.8
				Cr X-rays	
				0.005	0.4
Manganese-54	E.C.		100	0.835	100
(303 d)				Cr X-rays	
				0.0055	25
Mercury-197	E.C.	0.60	100	0.077	18
(65 h)				Au X-ray	
¹⁹⁶Hg(n,γ)¹⁹⁷Hg				0.069—0.081	72
Mercury-203	β⁻	0.212	100	0.279	81.5
(46.9 d)				Ti X-rays	
²⁰²Hg(n.γ)²⁰³Hg				0.071—0.085	12.8
Molybdenum-99ʲ	β⁻	0.454	18.3	0.041	1.2
(66.7 h)		0.866	1.4	0.141	5.4
⁹⁸Mo(n,γ)⁹⁹Mo		1.232	80.0	0.181	6.6
²³⁵U(n,f)⁹⁹Mo			0.366	1.4	
				0.412	0.02
				0.529	0.05
				0.621	0.02
				0.740	13.6
				0.778	4.7
				0.823	0.13
				0.961	0.1
				0.141	83.9
				0.143	0.03
Neptunium-237	α	4.638	6.0	0.029	12.0
(2.14 × 10⁶ y)		4.663	3.3	0.087	13.0
		4.765	8.0	0.106	0.08
		4.770	25.0	0.118	0.18
		4.787	47.0	0.131	0.09
		4.802	3.0	0.134	0.07
		4.816	2.5	0.143	0.44
		4.872	2.6	0.151	0.25
				0.155	0.10
				0.169	0.08
				0.193	0.06
				0.195	0.21
				0.202	0.05
				0.212	0.17
				0.214	0.05
				0.238	0.07
	Daughter	²³³Pa			
		(27 d)			
		0.15	27	0.075	1.3
		0.17	15	0.087	2.0
		0.23	36	0.104	0.7

TABLE 2 (continued)
Decay Schemes of Selected Radionuclides Used in Nuclear Medicine

Nuclide, half-life, Production method	Type of decay	Particle energies		X or γ-Rays photons energies	
		Energy MeV	Abundance (%)	Energy MeV	Abundance (%)
		0.26	17	0.300	6.5
		0.53	2	0.312	38.0
		0.57	3	0.340	4.3
				0.375	0.7
				0.398	1.3
				0.416	1.7
Nickel-63 (92 y)	β⁻	0.066	100		
Niobium-95 (35 d)	β⁻	0.160	>99.9	0.766	99.8
Nitrogen-13 (9.96 m) ¹²C(d,n)¹³N	β⁺	1.198	99.8	0.511	199.6
Oxygen-15 (2.05 m) ¹⁴N(d,n)¹⁵O	β⁺	1.732	99.9	0.511	199.8
Phosphorus-32 (14.3 d) ³¹P(n,γ)³²P	β⁻	1.709	100		
Plutonium-238 (86.4 y)	α	5.445	28.7	0.043	IC
		5.499	71.1	UL X-rays 0.011—0.022	13
				UK X-rays 0.094—0.115	2.1 × 10⁻⁴
Potassium-42 (12.4 h) ⁴¹K(n,γ)⁴²K	β⁻	1.683	0.3	0.312	0.3
		1.995	17.6	0.900	0.05
		3.520	82.0	1.021	0.02
				1.525	17.9
				1.921	0.04
				2.424	0.02
Potassium-43 (22.4 h) ⁴⁰Ar(α,p)⁴³K	β⁻	0.422	2.2	0.221	4.1
		0.827	92.1	0.373	87.3
		1.224	3.7	0.397	11.4
		1.444	0.8	0.593	11.0
		1.817	1.3	0.617	80.5
				1.022	1.8
Promethium-147 (2.62 y)	β⁻	0.103	low	0.121	2.85 × 10⁻³
		0.225	100		
Radium-226 (1620 y)	α	4.598	5.5	0.186	3.4
		4.781	94.5		
Rhenium-186 (88.9 h)	β⁻	0.973	21	0.1372	9
		1.077	72	0.123	0.6
				W X-ray 0.058—0.074	9
Rubidium-81 (4.7 h) ⁷⁹Br(α,2n)⁸¹Rb	β⁺ E.C.	0.601	2.0	0.511	61.5
		1.048	28.8	0.446	23.15
			69.2	0.458	3.1
				0.538	2.3
				⁸¹ᵐKr	96.0
				Kr X-rays 0.013	40.3

TABLE 2 (continued)
Decay Schemes of Selected Radionuclides Used in Nuclear Medicine

Nuclide, half-life, Production method	Type of decay	Particle energies Energy MeV	Abundance (%)	X or γ-Rays photons energies Energy MeV	Abundance (%)
Rubidium-82	β⁺	2.375	11.5	0.511	189.3
(1.25 m)		3.150	82.8	0.776	13.4
⁸⁵Rb(p,4n)⁸²Sr	E.C.		5.4	Kr X-rays	
⁸²Sr(E.C.)⁸²Rb				0.013	2.7
Rubidium-86	β⁺	0.69	8.8	1.077	8.8
(18.7 d)		1.77	91.2		
Ruthenium-97	E.C.		100	0.216	86.0
(69.1 h)				0.325	10.2
⁹⁴Mo(α,n)⁹⁷Ru					
				Tc X-rays	
				0.018	58.3
				0.021	11.5
Ruthenium-103ᵏ	β⁻	0.101	6.3	0.053	0.4
(39.5 d)		0.214	89.0	0.133	0.01
		0.456	0.3	0.242	0.01
		0.711	4.4	0.295	0.3
				0.444	0.4
				0.497	88.2
				0.557	0.8
				0.610	5.5
				Rh X-rays	
				0.020—0.023	0.9
				0.040	0.1
				Rh X-rays	
				0.020—0.023	8
Ruthenium-106ˡ	β⁻	0.039	100		
(369 d)					
	β⁻	1.98	1.7	0.512	20.6
		2.41	10.5	0.616	0.7
		3.03	8.4	0.622	9.9
		3.54	78.9	0.874	0.4
				1.050	1.5
				1.128	0.4
				1.562	0.2
Samarium-151	β⁻	0.054	1.7	0.022	0.06
(87 y)		0.076	98.3	Eu X-rays	0.2
				0.005—0.008	
Selenium-75⁽ⁿᵒᵗᵉ ᵐ⁾	E.C.		100	0.066	1.1
(120.4 d)				0.097	3.5
⁷⁴Se(n,γ)⁷⁵Se				0.121	17.3
				0.136	59.0
				0.119	1.5
				0.265	59.1
				0.280	25.2
				0.401	11.6
				As X-ray	50.0
				0.010—0.012	
				0.24	0.03
				0.280	5.4
				0.304	1.2
				As X-rays	2.6
				0.010—0.012	

TABLE 2 (continued)
Decay Schemes of Selected Radionuclides Used in Nuclear Medicine

Nuclide, half-life, Production method	Type of decay	Particle energies		X or γ-Rays photons energies	
		Energy MeV	Abundance (%)	Energy MeV	Abundance (%)
Silver-110m[n]	β^-	0.084	67.6	0.447	3.4
(255 d)		0.531	31.0	0.62	2.7
	I.T		1.4	0.658	94.2
				0.678	11.1
				0.687	6.9
				0.707	16.3
				0.744	4.5
				0.764	22.5
				0.818	7.2
				0.885	71.7
				0.937	34.4
				1.384	25.7
				1.476	4.1
				1.505	13.7
				1.562	1.2
	β^-	2.23	0.1	0.658	0.1
		1.89	1.3		
Sodium-22	β^+	0.546	90.49	0.511	from β^+
(2.62 y)	E.C.	1.820	0.05	1.275	99.95
			9.46		
Sodium-24	β^+	0.284	0.08	1.369	100.0
(15.0 h)		1.392	99.92	2.754	99.85
$^{23}Na(n,\gamma)^{24}Na$				3.861	0.08
Strontium-85[o]	E.C.		100	0.36	0.022
(64 d)				0.88	0.01
$^{84}Sr(n,\gamma)^{85}Sr$					
				Rb X-rays	
				0.013—0.015	60.0
				0.514	99.2
Strontium-87m	I.T.	99.7		0.388	82.3
(2.83 h)	E.C.	0.3		Sr X-rays	
$^{88}Sr(p.2n)^{87}Y$				0.014	8.3
$^{87}Y(E.C.)^{87m}Sr$				0.016	1.5
Strontium-89[P]	β^-	0.554	0.01		
(52.7 d)		1.463	100.0		
				0.909	0.01
Strontium-90[q]	β^-	0.546	100		
(27.7 y)					
		0.513	0.02	1.761	IC
		2.274	99.98		
Sulfur-35	β^-	0.167	100		
(87.9 d)					
Technetium-99	β^-	0.204	low	0.089	6×10^{-4}
(2.12×10^5 y)		0.293	100		
Technetium-99m	I.T.		100	0.141	88.5
(6.05 h)				0.143	0.03
$^{234}U(n,F)^{99}Mo$					
$^{98}Mo(n,\gamma)^{99}Mo$					
$^{99}Mo(\beta^-)^{99m}Tc$					
Terbium-160	β^-	0.441	4.4	0.087	13.8
(72.1 d)		0.481	10.0	0.197	5.2
		0.553	3.3	0.216	3.9
		0.575	46.4	0.299	26.9

TABLE 2 (continued)
Decay Schemes of Selected Radionuclides Used in Nuclear Medicine

Nuclide, half-life, Production method	Type of decay	Particle energies		X or γ-Rays photons energies	
		Energy MeV	Abundance (%)	Energy MeV	Abundance (%)
		0.791	6.8	0.765	2.0
		0.874	26.8	0.879	29.8
				0.962	9.9
				0.966	24.9
				1.178	15.1
				1.200	2.3
				1.272	7.6
				1.312	2.9
Thallium-201 (73 h) ^{203}Tl(p,3n)^{201}Pb ^{201}Pb(E.C.)^{201}Tl	E.C.		100	0.031	0.22
				0.032	0.22
				0.135	2.65
				0.166	0.16
				0.167	10.0
				Hg X-rays	
				0.068—0.082	95
Thallium-204 (3.85 y)	β⁻	0.763	97.4	Hg X-rays	
	E.C.		2.6	0.069—0.083	1.5
Thorium-228 (1.913 y)	α	5.140	0.03	0.085	1.6
		5.176	0.2	0.132	0.19
		5.211	0.4	0.167	0.12
		5.341	28.0	0.216	0.29
		5.424	71.0		
Thulium-170 (134 d)	β⁻	0.884	22.8	0.084	3.4
		0.968	77.0		
	E.C.		0.2		
Tin-113 (115d) ^{112}Sn(n,γ)^{113}Sn	E.C.		100	0.255	2.1
				In X-rays	
				0.024—0.028	73
	Daughter	^{113m}In	99.5	0.392	64.9
				In X-rays	
	I.T.		100.0	0.024—0.028	24.0
Tin-119m (293 d)	I.T.		100	0.024	16.3
				0.065	IC
				Sn X-rays	28.0
				0.025—0.029	
Tungsten-185 (75 d)	β⁻	0.304	low	0.125	0.005
		0.429	>99.9		
Uranium-238 (4.49 × 10⁹ y)	α	4.145	23	0.048	IC
		4.195	77		
Xenon-127 (36.41 d) ^{127}I(p,n)^{127}Xe	E.C.		100	0.058	1.3
				0.145	4.3
				0.172	25.0
				0.203	68.3
				0.374	17.2
				I X-rays	
				0.029	72
				0.032	16.4
Xenon-133 (5.27 d) ^{235}U(n,f)→^{133}Xe	β⁻	0.266	0.9	0.080	0.4
		0.346	99.1	0.081	36.6
			0.160	0.05	
				Cs X-rays	
				0.030—0.036	46.0

TABLE 2 (continued)
Decay Schemes of Selected Radionuclides Used in Nuclear Medicine

Nuclide, half-life, Production method	Type of decay	Particle energies		X or γ-Rays photons energies	
		Energy MeV	Abundance (%)	Energy MeV	Abundance (%)
Ytterbium-169 (31.8 d) ^{169}Tm(d,2n)^{169}Yb ^{168}Yb(n,γ)^{169}Yb	E.C.		100	0.063	42.0
				0.094	2.6
				0.110	17.4
			0.118	1.9	
				0.131	11.5
				0.177	22.3
				0.197	35.9
				0.261	1.7
				0.308	9.9
Yttrium-88 (108.1 d)	β$^+$ E.C.	0.763	0.2 99.8	0.511	from β$^+$
				0.898	93.2
				1.383	0.04
				1.836	99.4
				2.734	0.6
				3.219	0.009
				3.52	0.007
				Sr X-rays 0.014—0.016	60.0
Yttrium-90 (64 h) ^{89}Y(n,γ)^{90}Y	β$^-$	0.513 2.274	0.02 99.98		
Yttrium-91 (58.8 d)	β$^-$	0.340 1.545	0.3 99.7	1.205	0.3
Zinc-65 (245 d)	β$^+$ E.C.	0.325	1.46 98.54	0.345	0.003
				0.511	from β$^+$
				0.770	0.003
				1.115	50.7
				Cu X-rays 0.008—0.009	38.0
Zinc-69m (13.8 h) ^{68}Zn(n,γ)^{69m}Zn	I.T. β$^-$	0.905	100 100	0.439	94.9
				Zn X-rays 0.009	1.8
Zirconium-95^r (65.5 d)	β$^-$	0.365 0.398 0.887 1.12	54.7 44.6 0.7 low	0.724 0.757	44.5 54.6
				0.235	0.2

a   23% of ^{125}Sb decays via ^{125m}Te.
b   Cadmium-109 decays via ^{109}Ag (40 s).
c   Cerium-144 decays via ^{144m}Pr (7.2 m).
d   Cerium-144 decays via ^{144}Pr (17 m).
e   Cesium-137 decays via ^{137m}Ba (2.6 m).
f   Gallium-67 decays via ^{67m}Zn (9.2 μs).
g   1.3% of ^{131}I decays via ^{131m}Xe (12 d).
h   Percentages relate to disintegrations of ^{131m}Xe.
i   Krypton-85 decays via ^{85m}Rb (0.96 μs).
j   Molybdenum-99 decays via 6.02 h ^{99m}Tc in equilibrium.

k   Ruthenium-103 decays via ^{103m}Rh (56 m).
l   Ruthenium-106 decays via ^{100}Rh (30.4 s).
m   Selenium-75 decays via ^{75m}As (16.4 ms).
n   Silver-110m decays via ^{110}Ag (24.5 s).
o   Strontium-85 decays via ^{85m}Rb (0.096 μs).
p   Strontium-89 decays via ^{89m}Y (16 s).
q   Strontium-90 decays via ^{90}Y (64.1 h).
r   Zirconium-95 decays via ^{95m}Nb (86.6 h) in equilibrium.

Data from *Amersham Nuclear Medicine Catalogue*, Amersham International, plc., Little Chalfont, England, 1985. With permission.

Properties and Production of Radionuclides

NATURAL RADIOACTIVITY

Background radioactivity from natural sources originates from singly occurring radio-nuclides of both cosmic (Table 1) and terrestrial (Table 2) origins, and from components of the three families of heavy radioactive elements: the uranium series (starting from ^{238}U); the thorium series (starting from ^{232}U); and the actinium series (starting from ^{235}U) (Table 3). The latter chains account for much of the background radiation to which every human, animal and plant is exposed for every second of their lives.

ABBREVIATIONS

Half-lives		**Type of decay**	
y	years	α	alpha particle
d	days	β$^-$	negative beta particle (nega-tron)
h	hours	β$^+$	positive beta particle (posi-tron)
m	minutes	γ	gamma ray
s	seconds	X	X-rays
ms	milliseconds	EC	electron capture
μs	microseconds	IT	isomeric transition

Data presented in the following tables on Natural Radioactivity, Radioisotope Generators, Reactor-Produced Radionuclides, and Cyclotron-Produced Radionuclides, compiled from:

- **Gopal B. Saha**, *Fundamentals of Nuclear Pharmacy*, Springer-Verlag, New York, 1986.
- **James A. Sorensen and Michael E. Phelps**, *Physics in Nuclear Medicine*, 2nd ed., Grune & Stratton, Orlando, Florida, 1987.
- **Robert C. Weast, Ed.**, *CRC Handbook of Chemistry and Physics*, 67th ed., 1986-87, CRC Press, Boca Raton, Florida, 1986.
- *Radiological Handbook,* Department of Health, Education and Welfare, Washington, D. C., 1970.

TABLE 1
Singly Occurring Radionuclides of Cosmic Origin

Radionuclide	Half-life	Type of decay	Principal radiation Energy (MeV)	Principal radiation Abundance (%)
Beryllium (^{7}Be)	53.29 d	EC	0.862	
		γ	0.478	10.35
(^{10}Be)	1.6×10^6 y	β^-	0.555	100
Carbon (^{14}C)	5730 y	β^-	0.1565	100
Chlorine (^{36}Cl)	3×10^5 y	β^-	0.7093	98
		β^+, EC	0.115	0.002
(^{38}Cl)	37.2 m	β^-	4.91	58
		γ	1.6422	31
			2.1676	42
(^{39}Cl)	55.7 m	β^-	1.91	85
		γ	0.2503	47
			1.2672	54
			1.5174	38
Hydrogen (^{3}H)	12.26 y	β^-	0.0186	100
Phosphorus (^{32}P)	14.28 d	β^-	1.71	100
(^{33}P)	25.3 d	β^-	0.249	100
Sodium (^{22}Na)	2.6 y	β^+	0.545	90
		γ	1.2745	99.9
(^{24}Na)	14.97 h	β^-	1.389	99
		γ	1.3686	100
			2.7541	100
Sulfur (^{35}S)	87.2 d	β^-	0.1674	100
(^{38}S)	2.84 h	β^-	1.00	
		γ	1.9421	84

TABLE 2
Singly Occurring Radionuclides of Terrestrial Origin

Radionuclide	Natural abundance (%)	Half-life years	Type of decay	Principal radiation Energy (MeV)	Principal radiation Abundance (%)
Cerium (^{142}Ce)	11.08	$>5 \times 10^{16}$			
Dysprosium (^{156}Dy)	0.06	$>1 \times 10^{18}$			
Gadolinium (^{152}Gd)	0.20	1.1×10^{14}			
Hafnium (^{174}Hf)	0.16	2×10^{15}			
Indium (^{115}In)	95.8	4.4×10^{14}	β^-	0.48	100
Lanthanum (^{138}La)	0.09	1.06×10^{11}	β^-	0.26	
			Ec, γ	1.4359	66
Lutetium (^{176}Lu)	2.59	3.6×10^{10}	γ	0.2019	84
				0.306⁰	93
Neodynium (^{144}Nd)	23.80	2.1×10^{15}			
Platinum (^{190}Pt)	0.013	6.9×10^{11}			
Potassium (^{40}K)	0.017	1.25×10^9	β^-	1.312	89
			EC, γ	1.461	10.5
Rhenium (^{187}Re)	62.6	4.5×10^{10}	β^-	0.0025	
Rubidium (^{87}Rb)	27.83	4.9×10^{10}	β^-	0.273	100
Samarium (^{146}Sm)	13.82	1.03×10^8	α	2.50	
(^{147}Sm)	15.0	10.08×10^{11}	α	2.23	
(^{148}Sm)	11.3	7×10^{15}	α	1.96	
Tantalum (^{180}Ta)	0.012	$>1 \times 10^{12}$			
Tellurium (^{123}Te)	0.903	1.3×10^{13}	EC	0.052	
Vanadium (^{50}V)	0.25	$>3.9 \times 10^{17}$	EC, β^-		

TABLE 3
Chains of Naturally Occurring Radioactive Elements

Isotope	Half-life	Type of decay	Principal radiation Energy (MeV)	Abundance (%)
Uranium Series				
Uranium (^{238}U)	4.46×10^9 y	α	4.147	23
(Isotopic abundance			4.196	77
99.28%)		γ	0.0495	
Thorium (^{234}Th)	24.1 d	β^-	0.102	20
			0.198	72
		γ	0.0633	3.8
			0.0924	2.7
			0.0928	2.7
Protactinium (^{234m}Pa)	1.17 m	β^-	2.29	99.9
		IT, γ	0.7664	0.21
			1.001	0.65
Uranium (^{234}U)	2.45×10^5 y	α	4.7231	27.5
			4.776	72.5
		γ	0.0532	0.12
Thorium (^{230}Th)	7.54×10^4 y	α	4.6211	23.4
			4.6876	76.3
Radon (^{222}Rn)	3.82 d	α	5.4897	99.9
		γ	0.510	0.07
Polonium (^{218}Po)	3.11 m	α	6.002	100
Lead (^{214}Pd)	26.8 m	β^-	0.67	48
			0.73	42
		γ	0.2419	7.5
			0.295	19.2
			0.3519	37
Astatine (^{218}At)	1.6—2 s	α	6.654	6
			6.695	90
			6.748	4
Bismuth (^{214}Bi)	19.9 m	β^-	3.27	
		γ	0.6093	46.1
			1.1203	15
			1.2381	5.95
			1.7645	15.9
Polonium (^{214}Po)	163 μs	α	7.686	99.9
Thallium (^{210}Tl)	1.3 m	β^-	1.3	25
			1.9	56
		γ	0.2981	79
			0.7979	99
			1.068	12
			1.208	17
			1.315	21
Lead (^{210}Pb)	22.3 y	β^-	0.017	81
			0.061	19
Bismuth (^{210}Bi)	5.01 d	β^-	1.16	99
Polonium (^{210}Po)	138.4 d	α	5.304	100
		γ	0.8031	0.001
Thallium (^{206}Tl)	4.2 m	β^-	1.53	99.9
Lead (^{206}Pb)	Stable			
(Isotopic abundance				
24.1%)				

TABLE 3 (continued)
Chains of Naturally Occurring Radioactive Elements

Isotope	Half-life	Type of decay	Principal radiation	
			Energy (MeV)	Abundance (%)

Thorium Series

Isotope	Half-life	Type of decay	Energy (MeV)	Abundance (%)
Thorium (^{232}Th) (Isotopic abundance 100%)	1.4×10^{10} y	α	3.925	23
			4.010	77
		γ	0.059	0.19
Radium (^{228}Ra)	5.75 y	β⁻	0.045	
Actinium (^{228}Ac)	6.13 h	β⁻	1.11	32
			1.85	12
			2.18	11
		γ	0.2094	4.1
			0.3384	12.4
			0.4631	4.6
			0.7948	4.6
			0.9112	29
			0.969	17
Thorium (^{228}Th)	1.913 y	α	5.3405	26.7
			5.4233	73
Radium (^{224}Ra)	3.66 d	α	5.449	4.9
			5.685	95
		γ	0.2407	3.9
Radon (^{220}Rn)	55.6 s	α	6.2883	99.9
Polonium (^{216}Po)	0.15 s	α	6.778	99.9
Lead (^{212}Pb)	10.64 h	β⁻	0.28	83
			0.57	12
		γ	0.2386	43.6
			0.30	3.3
Bismuth (^{212}Bi)	1.009 h	β⁻	2.248	64
		α	6.051	25
			6.090	9.6
		γ	0.7272	6.6
			0.7855	1.1
			1.0787	0.53
			1.6207	1.5
Polonium (^{212}Po)	0.3μs	α	8.784	
Thallium (^{208}Tl)	3.052 m	β⁻	1.28	23
			1.52	22
			1.796	51
		γ	0.2773	6.8
			0.5106	22
			0.5830	86
			0.8603	12
			2.6145	99.8
Lead (^{208}Pb) (Isotopic abundance 52.4%)	Stable			

Actinium Series

Isotope	Half-life	Type of decay	Energy (MeV)	Abundance (%)
Uranium (^{235}U) (Isotopic abundance 0.72%)	7.04×10^8 y	α	4.2157	5.7
			4.3237	4.6
			4.3641	11
			4.37	6

TABLE 3 (continued)
Chains of Naturally Occurring Radioactive Elements

Isotope	Half-life	Type of decay	Principal radiation	
			Energy (MeV)	Abundance (%)
			4.3952	55
			4.4144	2.1
			4.5025	1.7
			4.5558	4.2
			4.5970	5.0
		γ	0.1438	10.5
			0.1634	4.7
			0.1857	53
			0.2053	4.7
Thorium (^{231}Th)	25.2 h	β$^-$	0.138	22
			0.218	20
			0.305	52
		γ	0.0256	15
			0.0842	6.6
			0.090	0.9
Protactinium (^{231}Pa)	3.27×10^4 y	α	4.7343	8.4
			4.9339	3
			4.9505	22.8
			5.0131	25.4
			5.0292	20
			5.0587	11
		γ	0.0274	9.3
			0.2837	1.6
			0.3001	2.4
			0.3301	1.3
Actinium (^{227}Ac)	21.77 y	β$^-$	0.0455	54
		α	4.938	0.52
			4.951	0.65
		γ	0.0152	0.035
			0.0997	0.03
Thorium (^{227}Th)	18.72 d	α	6.146	
		γ	0.0501	8.5
			0.2398	11.2
			0.2562	6.7
			0.2999	2.1
			0.3298	2.73
Francium (^{223}Fr)	21.8 m	β$^-$	1.17	65
		γ	0.0501	33
			0.0797	8.9
			0.0884	4.0
			0.2348	3.7
Radium (^{223}Ra)	11.43 d	α	5.433	2.3
			5.502	1.0
			5.540	9.2
			5.607	24
			5.716	52
			5.747	9
		γ	0.1442	3.3
			0.1542	5.6
			0.2694	14
			0.3239	3.9

TABLE 3 (continued)
Chains of Naturally Occurring Radioactive Elements

Isotope	Half-life	Type of decay	Principal radiation Energy (MeV)	Principal radiation Abundance (%)
Radon (^{219}Rn)	3.96 s	α	6.425	7.5
			6.553	12.2
			6.8193	81
		γ	0.2711	9.9
			0.4017	6.6
Polonium (^{215}Po)	1.78 ms	α	7.386	100
Lead (^{211}Pb)	36.1 m	β$^-$	0.57	5.0
			1.36	92
		γ	0.4049	3.8
			0.427	1.7
			0.8319	3.8
Astatine (^{215}At)	100 μs	α	8.023	99.9
		γ	0.4049	0.045
Bismuth (^{211}Bi)	2.14 m	α	6.279	16
		β$^-$	6.623	84
		γ	0.3501	12.8
Polonium (^{211}Po)	0.52 s	α	6.570	0.54
			6.892	0.55
			7.450	98.9
		γ	0.5691	0.53
			0.8972	0.52
Thallium (^{207}Tl)	4.77 m	β$^-$	1.43	99.8
		γ	0.8972	0.24
Lead (^{207}Pb) (Isotopic abundance 22.1%)	Stable			

RADIOISOTOPE GENERATORS

A radioisotope generator is based on two basic principles: (1) the decay-growth relationship between a long-lived parent radionuclide and its shorter-lived daughter radionuclide, and (2) the daughter product has distinctly different chemical properties from the parent radionuclide.

Because of these principles the daughter product may be extracted repeatedly in a carrier-free state with an adequate solvent. After elution the daughter product activity is replenished continuously by decay of the parent product in the column until an equilibrium is reached. This is evident when the daughter product appears to decay with the same half-life as that of the parent radionuclide

The great advantage of radioisotope generators is that they are compact and easily transportable sources of short-lived radionuclides to institutions distant from a reactor or a cyclotron radioisotope production center.

The tables that follow list some radioisotope generators of practical use in nuclear medicine arranged in three arbitrary categories according to the half-life of the daughter radionuclides.

TABLE 1
Characteristics of Selected Radioisotope Generators Useful in Nuclear Medicine

Ultra Short-Lived Daughter Radionuclides With a Half-Life <1 Minute

Parent-Daughter	Half-life	Principal photon		Mode of daughter decay	Method of production
		Energy (KeV)	Abundance (%)		
Thulium (^{167}Tm)	9.25 d				^{165}Ho(α,2n)
Erbium (^{167m}Er)	2.28 s	207	42	IT	
Osmium (^{191}Os)	15.4 d				^{190}Os(n,γ)
Iridium (^{191m}Ir)	4.93 s	129	26	IT	
Rhenium (^{183}Re)	70 d				^{181}Ta(α,2n)
Tungsten (^{183m}W)	5.15 s	W K X-ray 46-160	63	IT	^{184}W(p,2n)
Rubidium (^{81}Rb)	4.58 h				^{79}Br(α,2n)
Krypton (^{81m}Kr)	13.3 s	190	67	IT	
Bromine (^{77}Br)	57 h				^{75}As(α,2n)
Selenium (^{77m}Se)	17.4 s	162	52	IT	
Mercury (^{195m}Hg)	40 h				^{197}Au(p,3n)
Gold (^{195m}Au)	30.5 s	261	68	IT	
Cadmium (^{109}Cd)	462.3 d				^{108}Cd(n,γ)
Silver (^{109m}Ag)	39.8 s	88	3.6	IT	

Short-Lived Daughter Radionuclides With a Half-Life >1 Minute — <1 Day

Parent-Daughter	Half-life	Energy (KeV)	Abundance (%)	Mode of daughter decay	Method of production
Strontium (^{82}Sr)	25.6 d				^{85}Rb(p,4n)
Rubidium (^{82}Rb)	1.27 m	511	191	β^+,EC	
		766	13.6		

TABLE 1 (continued)
Characteristics of Selected Radioisotope Generators Useful in Nuclear Medicine

Ultra Short-Lived Daughter Radionuclides With a Half-Life <1 Minute

Parent-Daughter	Half-life	Principal photon Energy (KeV)	Principal photon Abundance (%)	Mode of daughter decay	Method of production
Cesium (^{137}Cs)	30.17 y				Fission
Barium (^{137m}Ba)	2.55 m	661	90	IT	
Germanium (^{68}Ge)	288 d				^{69}Ga(p,2n)
Gallium (^{68}Ga)	68.1 m	511	176	β$^+$,EC	
Tin (^{113}Sn)	115.1 d				^{112}Sn(n,γ)
Indium (^{113m}In)	1.66 h	392	64	IT	
Tellurium (^{232}Te)	78.2 h				Fission
Iodine (^{132}I)	2.3 h	670	144	β$^-$	
Yttrium (^{87}Y)	80.3 h				^{88}Sr(p,2n)
Strontium ^{87m}Sr)	2.8 h	388	82	IT	
Titanium (^{44}Ti)	47 y				^{45}Sc(p,2n)
Scandium (^{44}Sc)	3.93 h	511	188	β$^+$,EC	
		1157	100		
Molybdenum (^{99}Mo)	65.94 h				Fission
Technetium (^{99m}Tc)	6.01 h	140	89	IT	^{98}Mo(n,γ)
Tungsten (^{188}W)	69.4 d				^{187}W(n,γ)
Rhenium (^{188}Re)	16.98 h	155	15	β$^-$	

Long-Lived Daughter Radionuclides With a Half-Life >1 Day

Parent-Daughter	Half-life	Principal photon Energy (KeV)	Principal photon Abundance (%)	Mode of daughter decay	Method of production
Calcium (^{47}Ca)	4.56 d				^{46}Ca(n,γ)
Scandium (^{47}Sc)	3.42 d	159	68	β$^-$	
Barium (^{131}Ba)	11.8 d				^{130}Ba(n,γ)
Cesium (^{131}Cs)	9.69 d	Xe k X-ray	39	EC	

Note: Abbreviations:

Half-lives		Decay mode	
y	years	α	alpha particle
d	days	β$^-$	negative beta particle (negatron)
h	hours	β$^+$	positive beta particle (positron)
m	minutes	γ	gamma ray
s	seconds	X	X-rays
		EC	Electron capture
		IT	Isomeric transition

REACTOR-PRODUCED RADIONUCLIDES

A variety of practicable radionuclides are produced in nuclear reactors with the following general characteristics:

1. Because neutrons are added to the nucleus the products of neutron activation generally lie above the line of stability. Therefore, they tend to decay by β^- emission.
2. Two types of interaction with thermal neutrons are of importance in the reactor production of practicable radioisotopes: neutron capture or (n, γ) reaction, and fission of heavy elements or (n, f) reaction.
3. The most common production mode is by the (n, γ) reaction. In this reaction, the target nucleus captures one thermal neutron and emits γ rays to produce an isotope of the same element. The products of this reaction are not carrier-free because they are the same chemical element as the target material. For this same reason, chemical separation is obviously unnecessary. It is possible to produce carrier-free radioisotopes in a reactor by using (n, p) reaction, e.g., $^{14}N(n,p)^{14}C$, or by activating a short-lived intermediate product, e.g., ^{131}I from ^{131}Te by $^{130}Te(n,\gamma)^{131}Te(\beta^-) \rightarrow {}^{131}I$.
4. When a target of heavy elements, such as Uranium-235, Plutonium-239, Neptunium-237, Uranium-233, and others with atomic number greater than 92 is inserted in the nuclear reactor core, heavy elements absorb thermal neutrons and undergo fission (n,f). Some of the fission fragments produced in the fission process are radioactive. This has been one important source of Molybdenum-99, Iodine-131, and Xenon-133 for practical nuclear medicine utilization

Characteristics of some of these practicable reactor-produced radionuclides, according to mode of production and half-lives, are listed in the following tables.

TABLE 1
Characteristics of Selected, Neutron-Capture (n, γ) Reaction, Reactor-Produced Practicable Radionuclides

Short Half-Life (<1 Day)

Radionuclide	Half-life hours	Decay mode	Principal photon Energy (MeV)	Principal photon Abundance (%)
Lutetium (^{176m}Lu)	3.63	β^-	.088	8.9
Krypton (^{85m}Kr)	4.48	β^-, IT	0.15118	79
Erbium (^{171}Er)	7.52	β^-	0.1116	20
			0.29591	29
			0.30832	64
Dysprosium (^{157}Dy)	8.1	EC	0.3262	93
Xenon (^{135}Xe)	9.1	β^-	2.24975	90
Potassium (^{42}K)	12.36	β^-	1.5246	18.9
Copper (^{64}Cu)	12.8	EC, β^-, β^+	0.511	35.7
Zinc (^{69m}Zn)	13.8	IT	0.439	95
Sodium (^{24}Na)	14.97	β^-	1.3686	100
			2.7541	100
Rhenium (^{188}Re)	16.98	β^-	0.15502	15

Intermediate Half-Life (>1 Day to <1 Week)

Radionuclide	Half-life	Decay mode	Principal photon Energy (MeV)	Principal photon Abundance (%)
Barium (^{135m}Ba)	28.7 h	IT	0.2682	16

TABLE 1 (continued)
Characteristics of Selected, Neutron-Capture (n, γ) Reaction, Reactor-Produced Practicable Radionuclides

Short Half-Life (<1 Day)

Radionuclide	Half-life hours	Decay mode	Principal photon Energy (MeV)	Principal photon Abundance (%)
Bromine (^{82}Br)	35.30 h	β⁻	0.55432	71
			0.61905	43
			0.77649	83
Lanthanum (^{140}La)	40.28 h	β⁻	0.32876	20.5
			0.48701	45
			0.81577	24
			1.59617	95
Samarium ^{153}Sm)	46.7 h	β⁻	0.10318	28
Yttrium (^{90}Y)	64 h	β⁻	no γ	
Mercury (^{197}Hg)	64.1 h	EC	0.069—0.081	72
			Au X-rays	
			0.07735	18
Molybdenum (^{99}Mo)	65.94 h	β⁻	0.144048	88
			0.73947	12.6
Gold (^{198}Au)	2.69 d	β⁻	0.411794	95.5
Ruthenium (^{97}Ru)	2.89 d	EC	0.2137	10
			0.3245	86
Platinum (^{195m}Pt)	4.02 d	IT	0.0989	11
Calcium (^{47}Ca)	4.54 d	β⁻	1.2968	77
Lutetium (^{177}Lu)	6.71 d	β⁻	0.11295	6.4
			0.20836	11

Long Half-Life (>1 Week)

Radionuclide	Half-life	Decay mode	Principal photon Energy (MeV)	Principal photon Abundance (%)
Barium (^{131}Ba)	11.8 d	EC	0.49636	47
Rubidium (^{86}Rb)	18.63 d	β⁻	1.0768	8.8
Chromium (^{51}Cr)	27.7 d	EC	0.320076	10.2
Ytterbium (^{169}Yb)	32.02 d	EC	0.06306	45
			0.19795	36
Iron (^{59}Fe)	44.51 d	β⁻	1.09922	56
			1.29156	43
Mercury (^{203}Hg)	46.6 d	β⁻	0.279188	81.5
Strontium (^{85}Sr)	64.8 d	EC	0.51399	99
Tin (^{133}Sn)	115.1 d	EC	0.024—0.028	80
			In X-rays	
			0.39169	64
Selenium (^{75}Se)	118.5 d	EC	0.136	55
			0.264651	58
Cobalt (^{60}Co)	5.27 y	β⁻	1.17321	100
			1.33247	100

TABLE 2
Characteristics of Selected, Carrier-Free, Reactor-Produced Practicable Radionuclides

Radionuclide	Half-life	Mode of decay	Common production reaction	Principal photon Energy	Principal photon Abundance
Carbon (^{14}C)	5730 y	β^-	^{14}N(n,p)^{14}C	no γ	
Cesium (^{137}Cs)	30.17 y	β^-	^{235}U(n,f)^{137}Cs	0.6616	85.1
Fluorine (^{18}F)	109.7 m	β^+	^{6}Li(n,α)^{3}H ^{16}O(^{3}H,n)^{18}F	0.511	194
Hydrogen (^{3}H) (Tritium)	12.26 y	β^-	^{6}Li(n,α)^{3}H	no γ	
Iodine (^{125}I)	59.9 d	EC	^{124}Xe(n,γ)^{125}Xe ^{125}Xe(EC)^{125}I	0.0355	6.7
Iodine (^{131}I)	8.04 d	β^-	^{130}Te(n,γ)^{131}Te ^{131}Te(β^-)^{131}I	0.3644	81
Molybdenum (^{99}Mo)	65.94 h	β^-	^{235}U(n,f)^{99}Mo	0.1440 0.7394	88 12.6
Phosphorus (^{32}P)	14.28 d	β^-	^{32}S(n,p)^{32}P	no γ	
Sulfur (^{35}S)	87.2 d	β^-	^{35}Cl(n,p)^{35}S	no γ	
Xenon (^{133}Xe)	5.25 d	β^-	^{235}U(n,f)^{133}Xe	0.8099	36

CYCLOTRON-PRODUCED RADIONUCLIDES

Accelerators are devices used to accelerate electrically charged subnuclear particles (ions) to very high energies. Those used for the production of radionuclides are generally cyclotrons, which produce beams of protons (p or $^1H^+$), deuterons (d or $^2H^+$), tritons ($^3H^+$), or helions-3 ($^3He^{2+}$). These ions when directed onto a target material, cause nuclear reactions that result in the production of radionuclides.

General characteristics of cyclotron-produced radionuclides are the following:

1.   Since the bombarding particle always includes at least one proton, a positive charge is added to the nucleus. Therefore, most of the reactions form nuclides on the proton-rich side of the line of stability and tend to decay by electron capture (EC), positron (B^+) emission, or both.

2.   In all cases, because of the addition of a positive charge to the nucleus, the product is a different element which can therefore be chemically separated. This results in one general feature of cyclotron-produced radionuclides — they are carrier-free.

3.   Cyclotron products are usually more expensive than reactor products. Because of this, the former are only used when their characteristics are far superior to any other agent. The reason for this difference in price is that in a reactor there are many positions where a sample can be irradiated by thermal neutrons while the reactor is not being used exclusively for this specific purpose. Therefore, the price of radionuclides produced by reactor irradiation is cheaper, with most of the cost being related to the separation process. In the case of a cyclotron, the whole machine is utilized in the production of smaller quantities of a single radionuclide at a time, which tends to increase their cost.

4.   Recently, considerable interest has been directed to the production and clinical use of ultra-short-lived cyclotron-produced positron-emitting radionuclides. Among them are the key physiologic radionuclides such as Carbon-11 ($T^1/_2 = 20.3$ min), Nitrogen-13 ($T^1/_2 = 9.97$ min), and Oxygen-15 ($T^1/_2 = 2.03$ min) which decay by B^+ emission (annihilation radiation of 0.511 MeV). These radionuclides represent elements that are important participants of all biologic functions, and they can be used to label a wide variety of physiologically important tracers, for *in vivo* three-dimensional tomographic imaging by positron cameras (PET). Because positron-emitters have very short lifetimes, a cyclotron or a dedicated medical cyclotron must be located on-site in the nuclear medicine laboratory.

Characteristics of selected practicable cyclotron-produced radionuclides according to their mode of decay, production reaction, and half-lives are listed in the following tables.

TABLE 1
Characteristics of Selected Short-Lived Cyclotron-Produced Positron-Emitters

Radionuclide	Half-life	Decay mode (%)	Principal photon		Common production reaction
			Energy (MeV)	Abundance (%)	
Bromine (^{75}Br)	98 m	B$^+$(76)	0.511	150	^{78}Kr(p,α)
		EC(24)	0.286	92	^{74}Se(d,n)
					^{75}As(^{3}He,3n)
Carbon (^{11}C)	20.3 m	B$^+$(99.8)	0.511	199.6	^{10}B(d,n)
		EC(0.2)			^{11}B(p,n)
					^{14}N(p,α)
Cesium (^{127}Cs)	6.2 h	B$^+$(96)	0.511		^{127}P(^{3}He,3n)
		EC(4)	0.411	58	^{127}I(α,4n)
Cesium (^{128}Cs)	3.62 m	B$^+$	0.511		^{127}I(^{3}He,2n)
		EC(32)	0.443	26	
Chlorine (^{34m}Cl)	32.2 m	B$^+$	0.511		^{35}Cl(p,pn)
			0.146	42	
			2.128	42	
Chromium (^{49}Cr)	42.1 m	B$^+$,EC	0.511		^{46}Ti(α,n)
			0.091	51	^{47}Ti(α,2n)
			0.153	27	^{48}Ti(α,3n)
Cobalt (^{55}Co)	17.5 h	B$^+$,EC	0.511		^{56}Fe(p,2n)
			0.477	20	^{54}Fe(d,n)
			0.931	75	
Copper (^{60}Cu)	23.2 m	B$^+$,EC	0.511		^{60}Ni(p,n)
			1.332	88	
Fluorine (^{18}F)	109.7 m	B$^+$(96.9)	0.511	193.8	^{20}Ne(d,α)
		EC(3.1)			^{19}F(p,pn)
					^{15}O(α,pn)
Iron (^{52}Fe)	8.28 h	B$^+$(57)	0.511		^{55}Mn(p,4n)
		EC(43)	0.169	99	^{50}Cr(α,2n)
Krypton (^{77}Kr)	1.24 h	B$^+$(80)	0.511		^{79}Br(p,3n)
		EC(20)	0.13	84	^{76}Se(α,3n)
Nitrogen (^{13}N)	9.97 m	B$^+$(100)	0.511	200	^{12}C(d,n)
Oxygen (^{15}O)	122 s	B$^+$(100)	0.511	200	^{14}N(d,n)
					^{16}O(^{3}He,α)
Rubidium (^{79}Rb)	23 m	B$^+$(84)	0.511	168	^{79}Br(^{3}He,3n)
		EC(16)	0.688	24	
Selenium (^{73}Se)	7.1 h	B$^+$(65)	0.511	125	^{72}Ge(^{3}He,2n)
		EC(35)	0.067	72	^{70}Ge(α,n)
			0.361	97	^{75}As(d,4n)
Titanium (^{45}Ti)	3.078 h	B$^+$(86)	0.511		^{45}Sc(p,n)
		EC(14)			
Zinc (^{63}Zn)	38.1 m	B$^+$(93)	0.511		^{63}Cu(p,n)
		EC(7)			^{60}Ni(α,n)

TABLE 2A
Characteristics of Selected Short-Lived Cyclotron-Produced Radionuclides Decaying Primarily by Electron Capture

Half-Life <1 Day

Radionuclide	Half-life hours	Principal photon		Common production reaction
		Energy (MeV)	Abundance (%)	
Xenon (^{123}Xe)	2	0.149	49	^{127}I(p,5n)
				^{122}Te(α,3n)
Tantalum (^{178m}Ta)	2.45	0.0889	62	
		0.2134	81	
		0.3256	94	
		0.4264	97	
Antimony (^{117}Sb)	2.8	0.1586	86	^{115}In(α,2n)
Rubidium (^{81}Rb)	4.58	0.511	46	^{81}Br(^{3}He,3n)
		0.190	66	^{79}Br(α,2n)
		0.446	19	
Thallium (^{119}Tl)	7.4	0.2082	12	^{199}Hg(d,2n)
		0.4555	12	
Dysprosium (^{157}Dy)	8.1	0.3262	93	^{159}Tb(p,3n)
				^{154}Gd(α,n)
				^{155}Gd(α,2n)
Bismuth (^{204}Bi)	11.2	0.3748	81	^{206}Pb(p,3n)
		0.8992	98	^{204}Pb(d,2n)
		0.9841	58	
Iodine (^{123}I)	13.1	0.159	83	^{123}Te(p,n)
				^{122}Te(d,n)
				^{124}Te(p,2n)
				^{123}Sb(^{3}He,3n)
				^{121}Sb(α,2n)
				^{123}Xe $\rightarrow$ ^{123}I
Chromium (^{48}Cr)	21.6	0.116	95	
		0.305	100	

TABLE 2B
Characteristics of Selected Cyclotron-Produced Radionuclides of Intermediate Half-Life Decaying Primarily by Electron Capture

Half-Life >1 Day to <1 Week

| Radionuclide | Half-life hours | Principal photon | | Common production reaction |
		Energy (MeV)	Abundance (%)	
Cesium (^{129}Cs)	32.3	0.3719	31	^{127}I(α,2n)
		0.4115	23	
Lead (^{203}Pb)	52.06	0.2792	80.1	^{203}Tl(p,n)
				^{203}Tl(d,2n)
Bromine (^{77}Br)	57	0.239	23	^{75}As(α,2n)
		0.5207	22	
Arsenic (^{71}As)	62	0.511		^{70}Ge(d,n)
		0.1749	84	^{69}Ga(α,2n)
Mercury (^{197}Hg)	64.1	0.069—0.081	72	^{197}As(p,n)
		Au k X-ray		^{197}Au(d,2n)
		0.07764	18	
Indium (^{111}In)	67.34	0.1712	94	^{111}Cd(p,n)
		0.2453	90	^{109}Ag(α,2n)
Ruthenium (^{97}Ru)	69.36	0.3245	86	^{99}Tc(p,3n)
				^{94}Mo(α,n)
Thallium (^{201}Tl)	73	0.068—0.082	95	^{203}Tl(p,3n)$\rightarrow$
		Hg k X-ray		^{201}Pb $\rightarrow$ ^{201}Tl
Gallium (^{67}Ga)	78.25	0.0933	38	^{68}Zn(p,2n)
		0.1846	23	^{66}Zn(d,n)
		0.3002	19	^{64}Zn(α,p)
Yttrium (^{87}Y)	80.3	0.388	90	^{88}Sr(p,2n)
		0.487	92	^{86}Sr(d,n)
				^{85}Rb(α,2n)

TABLE 2C
Characteristics of Selected Cyclotron-Produced Radionuclides With Long Half-Life Decaying Primarily by Electron Capture

Half-Life >1 Week

Radionuclide	Half-life days	Principal photon Energy (MeV)	Principal photon Abundance (%)	Common production reaction
Thulium (^{167}Tm)	9.25	0.2077	41	^{169}Er(p,n) ^{165}Ho(α,2n)
Arsenic (^{74}As)	17.78	0.511 0.5959	60	^{71}Ga(α,n)
Strontium (^{82}Sr)	25.6	0.511 Rb X-ray		^{85}Rb(p,4n)
Xenon (^{127}Xe)	36.34	0.1721 0.2029 0.375	25 68 17	^{127}I(p,n) ^{127}I(d,2n)
Strontium (^{85}Sr)	64.8	0.514	99	^{85}Rb(p,n) ^{85}Rb(d,2n)
Cobalt (^{58}Co)	70.91	0.511 0.8108	99	^{55}Mn(α,n)
Cobalt (^{57}Co)	271	0.1221	85.6	^{60}Ni(p,α) ^{56}Fe(d,n)
Germanium (^{68}Ge)	288	0.511 Ga k X-ray	39	^{69}Ga(p,2n) ^{66}Zn(α,2n)

TABLE 3
Characteristics of Cyclotron-Produced Radionuclides With Beta (β^-) Decay

Radionuclide	Half-life hours	Principal photon Energy (MeV)	Principal photon Abundance (%)	Common production reaction
Krypton (^{85m}Kr)	4.48	0.3049 0.1512	14 79	^{84}Kr(α,p)
Potassium (^{43}K)	22.3	0.3729 0.6178	88 81	^{40}Ar(α,p)

TABLE 4
Characteristics of Selected Positron-Emitting Radioligands for *In Vivo* Receptors Studies

Receptors (Radioligand)	Synthesis radioactive precursor	Radio-chemical yield (%)	Specific radioactivity (TBq/mmol)	Ref.
Acetylcholine				
[¹¹C]-Methioididquinuclidinyl benzyl (¹¹C-MQMB)	¹¹CH₃I	8	37	36
				50
[¹¹C]-Dexetimid	C₆H₅¹¹CH₂I	8	30	19
[¹¹C]-Levetimid	C₆H₅¹¹CH₂I	8	30	19
Benzodiazepine				
[¹¹C]-Diazepam	¹¹CH₃I		50	35
[¹¹C]-Flunitrazepam	¹¹CH₃I		30	35
[¹¹C]-Fludiazepam	¹¹CH₃I		n.c.a.	1
[¹¹C]-Ro 15-1788	¹¹CH₃I		60	38
		51	>100	48
[⁷⁵Br]-7-Brombenzodiazepin	⁷⁵Br⁻	20	100	44
Dopamine				
[¹¹C]-Spiropedidol	H¹¹CN		24	27
[¹¹C]-N-Methylspiroperidol	¹¹CH₃I		10	52
				10
		21	100	17
[¹⁸F]-Haloperidol	¹⁸F⁻		n.c.a.	51
				53
				30
[¹⁸F]-Benperidol	¹⁸F⁻		n.c.a.	14
		10—20	>100	2
		10—20	>100	45
[¹⁸F]-Spiroperidol	¹⁸F⁻	10—20	>100	2
				45
[¹⁸F]-3-N-Methylspiroperidol	¹⁸F⁻	10—20	100	2
		10—20	100	45
		30	>100	29
3-N-[¹⁸F]-Fluorethylspiroperidol	¹⁸F⁻	20—50	10—100	8
		30—40	40—100	43
				12
				46
				13
3-N-[¹⁸F]-Fluoropropylspiroperidol		30—40	40—100	13
		15—20	40	12
		10—20		43
				46
[⁷⁷,⁷⁵Br]-p-Bromspiroperidol	BrBr			32
				20
				37
	⁷⁵Br⁻	20—30	>70	39
[⁷⁵Br]-Brombenperidol	⁷⁵Br⁻	30	300	40
[⁷⁵Br]-Bromperidol	⁷⁵Br⁻	35	370	41
[¹¹C]-Pimozid	¹¹COCl₂	20	10	15
[¹¹C]-Chlorpromazin	H¹¹CHO		22	4
[¹¹C]-Thioproperazin	H¹¹CHO		22	34
[¹¹C]-Raclopride	[¹¹C]₂H₅I	30—40		21
	¹¹CH₃I	40—50	5	23
SCH 23390	¹¹CH₃I	80	30	28
[¹¹C]-Dopamine	H¹¹CN		n.c.a.	24
[¹¹C]-DOPA	¹¹CO₂		c.a.	42

TABLE 4 (continued)
Characteristics of Selected Positron-Emitting Radioligands for *In Vivo* Receptors Studies

Receptors (Radioligand)	Synthesis radioactive precursor	Radio-chemical yield (%)	Specific radioactivity (TBq/mmol)	Ref.
Noradrenergic				
[^{11}C]-Epinephrine	^{11}C-Methionine		7	47
[^{11}C]-Norepinephrine	H^{11}CN		n.c.a.	25
[^{11}C]-Propanolol	(CH$_3$)$_2$^{11}CO		70	5
[^{11}C]-Prazosin	^{11}CO$_2$	30	7	22
[^{11}C]-Practolol	^{11}CO$_2$		n.c.a.	6
Opiate				
[^{11}C]-Carfentanyl	^{11}CH$_3$I	30	40	16
[^{11}C]-Morphine	^{11}CH$_3$I	70—80		49
		9	0.6	31
[^{11}C]-Heroin	^{11}CH$_3$I	4	0.6	31
[^{18}F]-3-Acetylcyclofoxy	^{18}F	35	7	11
[^{11}C]-Diprenorphin	^{11}CO$_2$	35	n.c.a.	33
[^{11}C]-Etorphine	H^{11}CHO		22	36
Serotonin				
[^{11}C]-O-Methylbufotenine	H^{11}CHO		20	3
[^{11}C]-Ketanserin	^{11}COCl$_2$	25—50	90	7
[^{11}C]-N-Methylketanserin	^{11}CH$_3$I	10	50	18
[^{18}F]-Ritanserin	^{11}F$^-$			9
[^{11}C]-Serotonin	H^{11}CN		n.c.a.	26

Note: c.a., carrier added.
n.c.a., no carrier added.

TABLE 4 REFERENCES

1. **Ariyoshi, Y., Maeda, M., Kojima, M., Suehiro, M., and Ito, M.,** Carbon-11 labeling of fludiazepam, *Radioisotopes,* 31, 431, 1982.
2. **Arnett, C. D., Shiue, C.-Y., Wolf, A. P., Fowler, J. S., Logan, J., and Watanabe, M.,** Comparison of three ^{18}F-labeled buryrophenone neuroleptic drugs in the baboon using positron emission tomography, *J. Neurochem.,* 44, 835, 1985.
3. **Berger, G., Maziere, M., Marazano, C., and Comar, D.,** Labeling of the psychoactive drug O-methyl-bufotenine and its distribution in the animal organism, *Eur. J. Nucl. Med.,* 3, 101, 1978.
4. **Berger, G., Maziere, M., Knipper, R., Prenant, C., and Comar, D.,** Synthesis of ^{11}C-labeled radi-opharmaceutical: imipramine, chlorpromazine, nicotine and methionine, *Int. J. Appl. Radiat. Isot.,* 30, 393, 1979.
5. **Berger, G., Maziere, M., Prenant, C., Sastre, J., Syrota, A., and Comar, D.,** Synthesis of ^{11}C-propranolol, *J. Radioanal. Chem.,* 74, 301, 1982.
6. **Berger, G., Prenant, C., Sastre, J., Syrota, A., and Comar, D.,** Synthesis of a B-blocker for heart visualization: (^{11}C)Proctolol, *Int. J. Appl. Radiat. Isot.,* 34, 1556, 1983.
7. **Berridge, M., Comar, D., Crouzel, C., and Baron, J. C.,** ^{11}C-labeled ketanserin: a selective serotonin S$_2$-antagonist, *J. Labeled Compd. Radiopharm.,* 20, 73, 1983.
8. **Block, D., Coenen, H. H., Laufer, P., and Stöcklim, G.,** Nca (^{18}F)-Fluoroalkylation via nucleophilic fluorination of disubstituted alkanes and application to the preparation of N-(^{18}F)-fluorethylspiperone, *J. Labelled Compd. Radiopharm.,* 23, 1042, 1986.
9. **Boullais, C., Frie, T., and Crouzel, C.,** No-carrier-added fluorine-18 labelling of neuroleptics with different ^{18}F.sources, *J. Labelled Compd. Radiopharm.,* 23, 1424, 1986.
10. **Burns, H. D., Dannals, R. F., and Langström, B., Ravert, H. T., Zemyan, S. E., Duelfer, T., Wong, D. F., Frost, J. J., Kuhar, M. J., and Wagner, H. N.,** (3-N-(^{11}C)methyl) spiperone, a ligand to dopamine receptors. Radiochemical synthesis and biodistribution studies in mice, *J. Nucl. Med.,* 25, 1222, 1984.
11. **Channing, M. A., Eckelman, W. C., Bennet, J. M., Burke, T. R., and Rice, K. C.,** Radiosynthesis of (^{18}F)3-acetylcyclofoxy: ad high affinity opiate antagonist, *Int. J. Appl. Radiat. Isot.,* 36, 429, 1985.

12. **Chi, D. Y., Kilbourne, M. R., Katzellenbogen, J. A., Brodack, J. W., and Welch, M. J.**, Synthesis of no-carrier-added N-([18F]fluoroalkyl) spiperone derivatives, *Int. J. Appl. Radiat. Isot.*, 37, 1173, 1986.

13. **Coenen, H. H., Laufer, P, Stöcklin, G., Wienhard, K., Pawlik, G., and Borcher-Schwarz, H. G.**, Heiss W-D: 3-N-(2-([18F])-Flouroethyl)-spiperone: a novel ligand for cerebral dopamine receptor studies with PET, *Life Sci.*, 40, 81, 1987.

14. **Corley, E. G., Burns, H. D., Frost, J. J., Duelfer, T., Kuhar, M. J., and Wagner, H. N.**, Synthesis of radiotracers for in vivo mapping and quantification of dopamine receptors, *J. Nucl. Med.*, 22, 12, 1981.

15. **Crouzel, C., Mestelan, G., Kraus, E., Lecomte, J. M., and Comar, D.**, Synthesis of a [11C]-labelled neuroleptic drug: pimozide, *Int. J. Appl. Radiat. Isot.*, 31, 545, 1980.

16. **Dannals, R. F., Raver, H. T., Frost, J. J., Wilson, A. A., Burns, H. D., Wagner, H. N.**, Radiosynthesis of an opiate receptor binding radio tracer: ([11C)carfentanil, *Int. J. Appl. Radiat. Isot.*, 36, 303, 1985.

17. **Dannals, R. F., Ravert, H. T., Wilson, A. A., and Wagner, H. N.**, An improved synthesis of (3-N-([11C)-methylspiperone, *Int. J. Appl. Radiat. Isot.*, 37, 433, 1986.

18. **Dannals, R. F., Frost, J. J., Ravert, H. T., Wilson, A. A., and Wagner, H. N.**, Radiosynthesis and biodistribution of a serotonin receptor radiotracer for positron emission tomography: [11C]-N-methyl-ketanserin, *J. Nucl. Med.*, 27, 983, 1986.

19. **Dannals, R. F., Langström, B., Frost, J. J., Ravert, H. T., Wilson, A. A., and Wagner, H. N.**, Synthesis of radiotracers for studying muscarinic cholinergic receptors in the living human brain using positron emission tomography: ([11C)-dexetimide and ([11C)-levetimide, *J. Labelled Compd. Radiopharm.*, 23, 1407, 1986.

20. **DeJesus, O. T., Friedman, A. M., Prasad, A., and Revenaugh, J. R.**, Preparation and purification of [77Br]-labelled p-bromspiroperidol suitable for in-vivo dopamine receptor studies, *J. Labelled Compd. Radiopharm.*, 20, 745, 1983.

21. **Ehrin, E., Farde, L., Depaulis, T., Eriksson, L., Greitz, R., Johnström, P., Litton, J. E., Nilsson, J. L. G., Sedvall, G., Stone-Elander, S. H., and Ogren S. -O.**, Preparation of [11C]-labelled raclopride, a new potent dopamine receptor antagonist: preliminary PET studies of cerebral dopamine receptors in monkey, *Int. J. Appl. Radiat. Isot.*, 36, 269, 1985.

22. **Ehrin, E., Luthra, S. K., Crouzel, C., and Pike, V. W.**, Preparation of carbon-11 labelled prazosin, apotent and selective a1-adrenoreceptor antagonist, *J. Labelled Compd. Radiopharm.*, 23, 1410, 1986.

23. **Farda, L., Ehrin, E., Eriksson, L., Greitz, T., Hall, H., Hedström, C. -G., Litton, J. -E., and Sedvall, G.**, Substituted benzamides as ligands for visualization of dopamine receptor binding in the human brain by positron emission tomography, *Proc. Natl. Acad. Sci. U.S.A.*, 82, 3863, 1985.

24. **Fowler, J. S., Ansari, A. N., Atkins, H. L., Bradley-Moore, P. R., MacGregor, R. R., and Wolf, A. P.**, Synthesis and preliminary evaluation in animals of carrier-free [11C]-dopamine hydrochloride, *J. Nucl. Med.*, 14, 867, 1973.

25. **Fowler, J. S., MacGregor, R. R., Ansari, A. N., Atkins, H. L., and Wolf, A. P.**, Radiopharmaceuticals XII. A new rapid synthesis of carbon-11 labeled norepinephrine hydrochloride, *J. Med. Chem.*, 17, 246, 1974.

26. **Fowler, J. S., Gallagher, B. M., MacGregor, R. R., and Wolf, A. P.**, [11C]-serotonin: a tracer for the pulmonary endothelial extraction of serotonin, *J. Labelled Compd. Radiopharm.*, 13, 194, 1977.

27. **Fowler, J. S., Arnett, C. D., Wolf, A. P., MacGregor, R. R., Norton, E. F., and Findley, A. M.**, [11C]-Spiroperidol: synthesis, specific activity determination, and biodistribution in mice, *J. Nucl. Med.*, 23, 437, 1982.

28. **Halldin, C., Stone-Elander, S., Farde, L., Ehrin, E., Fasth, K.-J., Langström, B., and Sedvall, G.**, Preparation of [11C]-labelled SCH 23390 for the in vivo study of domamine D-1 receptors using positron emission tomography, *Int. J. Appl., Radiat. Isot.*, 37, 1039, 1986.

29. **Hamacher, K., Coenen, H. H., and Stöcklin, G.**, Nca radiofluorination of spiperone and N-methylspiperone via aminopolyether supported direct nucleophilic substitution, *J. Labelled Compd. Radiopharm.*, 23, 1047, 1986.

30. **Kilbourn, M. R., Hood, T. J., Welch, M. J., Dence, C. S., Tewson, T. J., Saji, H., and Maeda, M.**, Carrier-added and no-carrier-added synthesis of ([18F)spiroperidol and ([18F)haloperidol, *Int. J. Appl. Radiat. Isot.*, 35, 591, 1984.

31. **Kloster, G., Röder, E., Machulla, H. -J.**, Synthesis, chromatography and tissue distribution of methyl-[11C]-morphine and methyl-[11C]-heroin, *J. Labelled Compd. Radiopharm.*, 16, 441, 1979.

32. **Kulmala, H. K., Huang, C. C., Dinerstein, R. J., and Friedman, M.**, Specific in vivo binding of [77Br]-p-bromospiroperidol in rat brain: a potential tool for gamma ray imaging, *Life Sci.*, 28, 1911, 1981.

33. **Luthra, S. K., Pike, V. W., and Brady, F.**, The preparation of Carbon-11 labelled diprenorphine: a new radioligand for the study of the opiate receptor system in vivo. *J. Chem. Soc. Chem. Commun.*, 1423, 1985.

34. **Maziere, B., Todd-Pokropek, A. E., Berger, G., and Comar, D.**, Carbon-11 labeled compounds in dynamic studies of the brain in *Medical Radionuclide Imaging*, Vol. 2, IAEA, Vienna (SM 210/155), 1977, 21.

35. **Maziere, M., Godot, J. M., Berger, G., Prenant, Ch., and Comar, D.,** High specific activity carbon-11 labeling of benzodiazepines: diazepam and flunitrazepam, *J. Radioanal. Chem.,* 56, 229, 1980.

36. **Maziere, M., Comar, D., Godot, J. M., Collard, P., Cepeda, C., and Naquet, R.,** In vivo characterization of muscarinic receptors by positron emission tomography, *Life Sci.,* 29, 2391, 1981.

37. **Maziere, B., Loc'h, C., Hantraye, P., Guillon, R., Duquesnoy, N., Soussaline, F., Naquet, R., Comar, D., and Maziere, M.,** [76]Br-Bromospiroperidol: A new tool for quantitative in vivo imaging of neuroleptic receptors, *Life Sci.,* 35, 1349, 1984.

38. **Maziere, M., Hantraye, P., Prenant, C., Sastre, J., and Comar, D.,** Synthesis of ethyl 8-fluoro-5,6-dihydro-5(^{11}C)methyl-6-oxo-4H-imidazol(1.5-a)(1.4) benzodiazepine-3-carboxylate (RO 15.1788-^{11}C): a specific radioligand for the in vivo study of central benzodiazepine receptors by positron emission tomography, *Int. J. Appl. Radiat. Isot.,* 35, 973, 1984.

39. **Moerlein, S. M., Laufer, P., Stöcklin, G., Pawlik, G., Wienhard, K., and Heiss, W.-D.,** Evaluation of [75]Br-labelled butyrophenone neuroleptics for imaging cerebral dopaminergic receptor areas using positron emission tomography, *Eur. J. Nucl. Med.,* 12, 211, 1986.

40. **Moerlein, S. M. and Stöcklin, G.,** Radiosynthesis of no-carrier-added [75,77]Br-brombenperidol, *J. Labelled Compd. Radiopharm.,* 21, 875, 1984.

41. **Moerlein, S. M., and Stöcklin, G.** Synthesis of high specific activity([75]Br)- and ([77]Br)-bromperidol and tissue distribution sudies in the rat, *J. Med. Chem.,* 28, 1319, 1985.

42. **Reiffers, S., Beerling-van der Molen, H. D., Vaalburg, W., Ten Hoeve, W., Paans, A. M. J., Korf, J., Woldring, M. G., and Wynberg, H.,** Rapid synthesis and purification of carbon-11 labelled DOPA: a potential agent for brain studies, *Int. J. Appl. Radiat. Isot.,* 18, 955, 1977.

43. **Satyamurthy, N., Bida, G. T., Luxen, A., and Barrio, J. R.,** Syntheses of 3-(2'-(^{18}F)fluoroethyl)spiperone, a dopamine receptor-binding radiopharmaceutical for positron emission tomography, *J. Labelled Compd. Radiopharm.,* 23, 1045, 1986.

44. **Scholl, H., Kloster, G., and Stöcklin, G.,** Bromine-75-labeled 1,4-benzodiazepines: potential agents for the mapping of benzodiazepine receptors in vivo: concise communication, *J. Nucl. Med.,* 24, 417, 1983.

45. **Shiue, C. Y., Fowler, J. S., Wolf, A. P., Watanabe, M., and Arnett, C. D.,** Synthesis and specific activity determinations of no-carrier-added ^{18}F-labeled butyrophenone neuroleptics — benperidol, haloperidol, spiroperidol, and pipamperone, *J. Nucl. Med.,* 26, 181, 1985.

46. **Shiue, C. Y., Bai, L.-Q., Teng, R. -R., and Wolf, A. P.,** Syntheses of no-carried-added-(^{18}F)fluoroalkylhalides and their application in the syntheses of (^{18}F)fluoroalkyl derivatives of neurotransmitter receptor compounts, *J. Labelled Compd. Radiopharm.,* 24, 55, 1987.

47. **Sisson, J., and Wieland, D. M.,** Radiolabeled metaiodobenzylguanidine: pharmacology and clinical studies, *Am. J. Physiol. Imag.,* 1, 96, 1986.

48. **Suzuki, K., Inoue, O., Hashimuto, K., Yamasaki, T., Kuchiki, M., and Tamate, K.,** Computer-controlled large scale production of high specific activity (^{11}C)RO 15-1788 for PET studies of benzodiazepine receptors, *Int. J. Appl. Radiat. Isot.,* 36, 971, 1985.

49. **Svärd, H., Nägren, K., Malmborg, P., Sohn, D., Sjöberg, S., and Langström, B.,** The synthesis of various N-(^{11}C-methyl)-pharmaceuticals using ^{11}C-methyliodide, *J. Labelled Compd. Radiopharm.,* 19, 1519, 1982.

50. **Syrota, A., Paillotin, G., Davy, J. M., and Aumont, M. C.,** Kinetics of in vivo binding of antagonist to muscarine cholinergic receptor in the human heart studies by positron emission tomography, *Life Sci.,* 35, 937, 1984.

51. **Tewson, T. J., Raichie, M. E., and Welch, M. J.,** Preliminary studies with (^{18}F)haloperidol: a radioligand for in vivo studies of the dopamine receptors, *Brain Res.,* 192, 291, 1986.

52. **Wagner, H. N., Burns, H., Dannals, R. F., Wong, D. F., Langstrom, B., Duelfer, T., Frost, J. J., Haxden, T. R., Links, J. M., Rosenbloom, S. B., and Lukas, S. F.,** Imaging dopamine receptors in the human brain by positron tomography, *Science,* 221, 1264, 1983.

53. **Welch, M. J., Kilbourn, M. R., Mathias, C. J., Mintun, M. A., and Raichle, M. E.,** Comparison in animal models of ^{18}F-spiroperidol and ^{18}F-haloperidol: potential agents for imaging the dopamine receptor, *Life Sci.,* 33, 1687, 1983.

CHARACTERISTICS OF GAMMA-RAY SOURCES AND STANDARDS FOR USE IN NUCLEAR MEDICINE

For any quality control procedure in nuclear medicine, it is necessary to have certain gamma-sources of appropriate (low, medium, high) energy in a specified form calibrated to some accuracy depending on the application. Typically, such sources will be sealed as a point source in a vial, in the form of a sheet (disk or "flood" source), line phantoms, or rigid and flexible marker sources. The following radioisotopes seem to be those most commonly used in nuclear medicine quality control:

Nuclide	Half-life	Principal gamma-radiation		Nuclide simulated
		Energy (MeV)	Abundance (%)	
Barium (^{133}Ba)	10.53 y	0.356	62	Iodine-131
				Indium-113m
Cadmium (^{109}Cd)	462.3 d	0.022—0.026 Ag K X-rays	67.7	
		0.088	3.6	
Cesium (^{137}Cs)	30.17 y	0.662	85	
Cobalt (^{57}Co)	271 d	0.122	85.6	Technetium-99m
		0.1365	10	Selenium-75
(^{60}Co)	5.272 y	1.1732	100	Iron-59
		1.3324	100	
Iodine (^{129}I)	1.6 × 10^7 y	0.030—0.035 Xe K X-rays	~69	Iodine-125
		0.0396	7.5	
Manganese (^{54}Mn)	312 d	0.834	100	
Strontium (^{85}Sr)	64.8 d	0.514	99	
Tin (^{113}Sn)	115.1 d	0.024—0.028 in K X-rays	73	
		0.3917	64	
Yttrium (^{88}Y)	106.61 d	0.487	92	
		0.898	92	
		1.836	99.3	

Adapted from *Amersham Nuclear Medicine Catalogue,* Amersham International, plc., Little Chalfont, England, 1985. With permission.

CHARACTERISTICS OF SELECTED RADIONUCLIDES COMMONLY COUNTED WITH LIQUID SCINTILLATION DETECTORS

Radionuclide	Half-life	Beta-radiation	
		Energy (MeV)	Abundance (%)
Calcium (^{45}Ca)	163.8 d	0.257	100
Carbon (^{14}C)	5730 y	0.1565	100
Chlorine (^{36}Cl)	3×10^5 y	0.7093	98
Hydrogen (^{3}H) (Tritium)	12.26 y	0.01861	100
Iodine (^{131}I)	8.04 d	0.606	98.7
Iron (^{59}Fe)	44.51 d	0.273	48
		0.475	51
Phosphorus (^{32}P)	14.28 d	1.710	100
Potassium (^{40}K)	1.25×10^9 y	1.312	89
Sodium (^{22}Na)	2.605 y	0.545	90
(^{24}Na)	14.97 h	1.389	>99
Sulfur (^{35}S)	87.2 d	0.1674	100
Zinc (^{65}Zn)	243.8 d	0.325	

Adapted from *Amersham Nuclear Medicine Catalogue,* Amersham International, plc., Little Chalfont, England, 1985. With permission.

CHARACTERISTICS OF GAMMA-RAY SOURCES COMMONLY USED FOR BONE DENSITOMETRY MEASUREMENTS

Radionuclide	Half-life	Recommended working life, years	Principal emissions	
			Energy (KeV)	Abundance (%)
Americium (^{241}Am)	432.2 y	15	59.36	35.7
Gadolinium (^{153}Gd)	241.6 d	5	41—48	61
			Eu K X-rays	
			97.43	30
			103.18	22
Iodine (^{125}I)	59.4 d	1	27—32	138
			Te K X-rays	
			35	6.7

Adapted from *Amersham Nuclear Medicine Catalogue,* Amersham International, plc., Little Chalfont, England, 1985. With permission.

NUCLEAR MAGNETIC RESONANCE (NMR) PROPERTIES OF SOME NUCLEI USED FOR MEDICAL SPECTROSCOPY AND IMAGING

Nuclide	Natural abundance	Spin (I)	Relative sensitivity	Resonance frequency (MHz)			
				0.5 T	1.0 T[a]	1.5 T	2.0 T
^1H	99.985	1/2	1.000	21.99	42.576	63.86	85.15
^2H	0.015	1	0.0096	3.268	6.536	9.804	13.07
^{13}C	1.108	1/2	0.0159	5.353	10.705	16.06	21.41
^{14}N	99.63	1	0.001	1.538	3.076	4.614	6.152
^{15}N	0.37	1/2	0.001	2.157	4.314	6.471	8.628
^{17}O	0.037	5/2	0.0291	2.886	5.772	8.658	11.54
^{19}F	100.0	1/2	0.833	20.03	40.054	60.08	80.11
^{23}Na	100.0	3/2	0.0925	5.631	11.262	16.89	22.52
^{25}Mg	10.13	5/2	0.0027	1.303	2.605	3.908	5.210
^{31}P	100.0	1/2	0.0663	8.618	17.235	25.85	34.47
^{35}Cl	75.53	3/2	0.047	2.085	4.172	6.255	8.34
^{39}K	93.10	3/2	0.0005	0.9935	1.987	2.981	3.974
^{43}Ca	0.145	7/2	0.0064	1.433	2.865	4.298	5.730

[a]   Values in this column also correspond to those of magnetogyric ratio or NMR frequency expressed as MHz/T.

Data compiled from *Magnetic Resonance Nuclei for Medical Spectroscopy and Imaging*, General Electric, (Medical Systems Group), Milwaukee, 1983, and Lee, K., and Anderson W. A., Nuclear spins, moments and magnetic resonance frequencies, in Weast, R. D., Ed., *CRC Handbook of Chemistry and Physics*, 67th ed., 1986-1987, CRC Press, Boca Raton, FL.

MASS ATTENUATION COEFFICIENTS FOR WATER, SODIUM IODIDE, AND LEAD

Photon energy (MeV)	H_2O (p = 1.0 g/cm³) u(cm²/gm)	NaI(Tl) (p = 3.67 g/cm³) u(cm²/gm)	Pb (p = 11.34 g/cm³) u(cm²/gm)
0.010	4.99	136	128
0.015	1.48	45.9	112
0.020	0.711	21.2	83.4
0.030	0.338	6.86	28.4
0.033[a]	—	5.19	—
0.033[a]	—	30.4	—
0.040	0.248	18.9	13.1
0.050	0.214	10.5	7.22
0.060	0.197	6.42	4.43
0.080	0.179	3.00	2.07
0.088[a]	—	—	1.62
0.088[a]	—	—	7.23
0.100	0.168	1.64	5.23
0.150	0.149	0.590	1.89
0.200	0.136	0.314	0.945
0.300	0.118	0.158	0.383
0.400	0.106	0.112	0.220
0.500	0.0967	0.0921	0.154
0.600	0.0895	0.0802	0.120
0.800	0.0786	0.0663	0.0856
1.000	0.0707	0.0580	0.0690
2.000	0.0494	0.0412	0.0450
4.000	0.0340	0.0350	0.0414
8.000	0.0277	0.0355	0.0459
10.000	0.0222	0.0368	0.0484

[a] K shell binding energies. L shell binding energies for lead omitted.

Values from Hubbell, J. H., Photon cross-sections, attenuation, coefficients, and energy absorption coefficients from 10 keV to 100 GeV, *National Bureau of Standards Reference Series*, National Bureau of Standards, 29, 1969, 62.

ATTENUATION DATA IN LEAD SHIELDING

This table presents the dose rate (in mSv/hour) due to gamma and X-ray radiation, at one meter from a point source containing one gigabecquerel. The effect on the dose rate of shielding by various thicknesses of lead is also shown.

These dose rates apply only to gamma and X-ray emissions. Those emissions with energies of less than 20 KeV were not taken into account. Where appropriate, beta emissions and bremsstrahlung radiation should also be considered.

The data given in this table is for guidance only, advice should be sought from local health physicists for information on potential dose rates under various conditions.

Dose Rate at 1m from 1GBq point source (mSv/hr).

Nuclide	0	1.0	2.0	5.0	7.0	10.0	20.0	50.0
Americium-241	4.2×10^{-3}	1.4×10^{-5}	6.2×10^{-8}	negligible				
Antimony-124	2.6×10^{-1}	2.5×10^{-1}	2.3×10^{-1}	1.95×10^{-1}	1.7×10^{-1}	1.45×10^{-1}	8.4×10^{-2}	1.9×10^{-2}
Antimony-125	7.6×10^{-2}	5.4×10^{-2}	4.7×10^{-2}	3.2×10^{-2}	2.5×10^{-2}	1.7×10^{-2}	4.6×10^{-3}	1.2×10^{-4}
Barium-133	7.7×10^{-2}	3.9×10^{-2}	2.9×10^{-2}	1.3×10^{-2}	7.2×10^{-3}	3.0×10^{-3}	1.7×10^{-4}	3.6×10^{-8}
Barium-140	3.0×10^{-2}	2.2×10^{-2}	1.9×10^{-2}	1.3×10^{-2}	9.6×10^{-3}	6.3×10^{-3}	1.5×10^{-3}	1.8×10^{-5}
Beryllium-7	7.5×10^{-3}	6.5×10^{-3}	5.6×10^{-3}	3.6×10^{-3}	2.6×10^{-3}	1.6×10^{-3}	3.0×10^{-4}	1.6×10^{-6}
Bromine-82	4.0×10^{-1}	3.7×10^{-1}	3.4×10^{-1}	2.8×10^{-1}	2.4×10^{-1}	2.0×10^{-1}	9.8×10^{-2}	1.4×10^{-2}
Cadmium-109	4.3×10^{-2}	6.0×10^{-8}	9.8×10^{-12}	negligible				
Calcium-47	1.5×10^{-1}	1.5×10^{-1}	1.4×10^{-1}	1.2×10^{-1}	1.11×10^{-1}	$9.7 \times ^{-2}$	6.0×10^{-2}	1.2×10^{-2}
Cerium-139	3.3×10^{-2}	3.7×10^{-3}	7.6×10^{-4}	5.6×10^{-6}	2.0×10^{-7}	1.4×10^{-9}	negligible	
Cerium-141	1.2×10^{-2}	9.9×10^{-4}	9.9×10^{-5}	9.1×10^{-8}	8.3×10^{-10}	negligible		
Cerium-144	3.9×10^{-3}	1.3×10^{-4}	8.6×10^{-6}	4.5×10^{-9}	6.3×10^{-11}	negligible		
Cesium-134	2.35×10^{-1}	2.2×10^{-1}	2.0×10^{-1}	1.6×10^{-1}	1.3×10^{-1}	1.0×10^{-1}	4.2×10^{-2}	3.1×10^{-3}
Cesium-137	8.7×10^{-2}	7.9×10^{-2}	7.2×10^{-2}	5.5×10^{-2}	4.6×10^{-2}	3.5×10^{-2}	1.3×10^{-2}	5.0×10^{-4}
Chromium-51	4.7×10^{-3}	3.5×10^{-3}	2.6×10^{-3}	9.7×10^{-4}	4.9×10^{-4}	1.7×10^{-4}	4.9×10^{-6}	9.6×10^{-11}
Cobalt-56	4.8×10^{-1}	4.6×10^{-1}	4.4×10^{-1}	3.8×10^{-1}	3.4×10^{-1}	3.0×10^{-1}	1.8×10^{-1}	4.1×10^{-2}
Cobalt-57	1.6×10^{-2}	6.6×10^{-4}	1.8×10^{-4}	1.2×10^{-4}	1.0×10^{-4}	7.8×10^{-5}	2.9×10^{-5}	1.3×10^{-5}
Cobalt-58	1.5×10^{-1}	1.4×10^{-1}	1.3×10^{-1}	1.0×10^{-1}	8.7×10^{-2}	6.9×10^{-2}	3.0×10^{-2}	2.5×10^{-3}
Cobalt-60	3.6×10^{-1}	3.5×10^{-1}	3.3×10^{-1}	2.9×10^{-1}	2.7×10^{-1}	2.3×10^{-1}	1.5×10^{-1}	2.9×10^{-2}
Europium-152	1.7×10^{-1}	1.5×10^{-1}	1.4×10^{-1}	1.1×10^{-1}	1.0×10^{-1}	8.5×10^{-2}	4.9×10^{-2}	8.7×10^{-3}

ATTENUATION DATA IN LEAD SHIELDING (continued)

Nuclide	Lead thickness (mm)							
	0	1.0	2.0	5.0	7.0	10.0	20.0	50.0
Gallium-67	2.2×10^{-2}	9.9×10^{-3}	6.5×10^{-3}	2.4×10^{-3}	1.4×10^{-3}	6.4×10^{-4}	1.1×10^{-4}	7.6×10^{-6}
Gold-198	6.10×10^{-2}	5.1×10^{-2}	4.2×10^{-2}	2.4×10^{-2}	1.6×10^{-2}	8.6×10^{-3}	1.2×10^{-3}	3.0×10^{-5}
Gold-199	1.2×10^{-2}	2.4×10^{-3}	6.6×10^{-4}	2.9×10^{-5}	4.4×10^{-6}	2.6×10^{-7}	2.0×10^{-11}	negligible
Indium-111	8.4×10^{-2}	2.4×10^{-2}	1.2×10^{-2}	1.7×10^{-3}	4.8×10^{-4}	7.0×10^{-5}	1.1×10^{-7}	negligible
Indium-113m	4.6×10^{-2}	3.1×10^{-2}	2.5×10^{-2}	1.3×10^{-2}	8.3×10^{-3}	4.0×10^{-3}	3.7×10^{-4}	2.1×10^{-7}
Indium-114	5.3×10^{-4}	3.7×10^{-4}	3.6×10^{-4}	3.1×10^{-4}	2.9×10^{-4}	2.5×10^{-4}	1.6×10^{-4}	3.3×10^{-5}
Iodine-123	4.4×10^{-2}	5.1×10^{-3}	2.3×10^{-3}	1.2×10^{-3}	9.3×10^{-4}	6.2×10^{-4}	1.6×10^{-4}	3.6×10^{-6}
Iodine-125	3.4×10^{-2}	negligible						
Iodine-129	1.7×10^{-2}	6.2×10^{-11}	negligible					
Iodine-131	5.7×10^{-2}	4.5×10^{-2}	3.7×10^{-2}	1.9×10^{-2}	1.3×10^{-2}	7.0×10^{-3}	1.5×10^{-3}	5.0×10^{-5}
Iron-59	1.7×10^{-1}	1.6×10^{-1}	1.6×10^{-1}	1.4×10^{-1}	1.3×10^{2}	1.1×10^{-1}	6.6×10^{-2}	1.2×10^{-2}
Krypton-85	3.4×10^{-4}	3.0×10^{-4}	2.6×10^{-4}	1.8×10^{-4}	1.4×10^{-4}	8.8×10^{-5}	2.0×10^{-5}	1.8×10^{-7}
Lanthanum-140	3.2×10^{-1}	3.1×10^{-1}	2.9×10^{-1}	2.5×10^{-1}	2.2×10^{-1}	1.9×10^{-1}	1.2×10^{-1}	2.9×10^{-2}
Lead-210	4.5×10^{-4}	7.9×10^{-9}	negligible					
Manganese-54	1.3×10^{-1}	1.2×10^{-1}	1.1×10^{-1}	9.1×10^{-2}	8.0×10^{-2}	6.5×10^{-2}	3.1×10^{-2}	2.7×10^{-3}
Mercury-203	3.5×10^{-2}	2.3×10^{-2}	1.5×10^{-2}	3.9×10^{-3}	1.6×10^{-3}	3.8×10^{-4}	3.5×10^{-6}	2.0×10^{-12}
Molybdenum-99[a]	4.1×10^{-2}	2.2×10^{-2}	1.9×10^{-2}	1.5×10^{-2}	1.3×10^{-2}	9.9×10^{-3}	4.2×10^{-3}	2.7×10^{-4}
Neptunium-237	4.8×10^{-3}	3.0×10^{-4}	6.5×10^{-5}	2.5×10^{-6}	4.7×10^{-7}	4.6×10^{-8}	3.5×10^{-11}	negligible
Niobium-95	1.2×10^{-1}	1.1×10^{-1}	1.0×10^{-1}	8.1×10^{-2}	7.0×10^{-2}	5.5×10^{-2}	2.4×10^{-2}	1.6×10^{-3}
Potassium-42	3.8×10^{-2}	3.7×10^{-2}	3.6×10^{-2}	3.2×10^{-2}	2.9×10^{-2}	2.6×10^{-2}	1.7×10^{-2}	4.3×10^{-2}
Radium-226[a]	2.6×10^{-1}	2.3×10^{-1}	2.2×10^{-1}	1.7×10^{-1}	1.5×10^{-1}	1.3×10^{-1}	7.4×10^{-2}	1.6×10^{-2}
Rubidium-86	1.4×10^{-2}	1.3×10^{-2}	1.3×10^{-2}	1.1×10^{-2}	10.0×10^{-3}	8.6×10^{-3}	4.9×10^{-3}	8.0×10^{-4}
Ruthenium-103	7.1×10^{-2}	6.3×10^{-2}	5.5×10^{-2}	3.7×10^{-2}	2.8×10^{-2}	1.8×10^{-2}	3.9×10^{-3}	4.0×10^{-5}
Scandium-46	3.0×10^{-1}	2.8×10^{-1}	2.7×10^{-1}	2.3×10^{-1}	2.1×10^{-1}	1.8×10^{-1}	9.7×10^{-2}	1.4×10^{-2}
Selenium-75	5.6×10^{-2}	2.9×10^{-2}	1.9×10^{-2}	5.9×10^{-3}	2.9×10^{-3}	1.1×10^{-3}	8.5×10^{-3}	6.5×10^{-8}
Silver-110m	4.1×10^{-1}	3.8×10^{-1}	3.6×10^{-1}	3.2×10^{-1}	2.6×10^{-1}	1.2×10^{-1}	1.1×10^{-1}	1.5×10^{-2}
Sodium-22	2.2×10^{-1}	3.0×10^{-1}	2.8×10^{-1}	2.2×10^{-1}	1.9×10^{-1}	1.6×10^{-1}	8.3×10^{-2}	1.5×10^{-2}
Sodium-24	5.0×10^{-1}	4.9×10^{-1}	4.7×10^{-1}	4.1×10^{-1}	3.9×10^{-1}	3.5×10^{-1}	2.4×10^{-1}	7.1×10^{-2}
Strontium-85	7.7×10^{-2}	6.8×10^{-2}	6.8×10^{-2}	4.0×10^{-2}	3.1×10^{-2}	2.0×10^{-2}	4.5×10^{-3}	4.2×10^{-5}
Technetium-99m	1.7×10^{-2}	1.5×10^{-3}	1.2×10^{-4}	6.6×10^{-8}	4.3×10^{-10}	negligible		
Terbium-160	1.7×10^{-1}	1.5×10^{-1}	1.4×10^{-1}	1.2×10^{-1}	1.0×10^{-1}	8.7×10^{-2}	4.8×10^{-2}	7.2×10^{-3}
Thallium-201	1.2×10^{-2}	9.5×10^{-4}	1.3×10^{-4}	8.8×10^{-7}	3.4×10^{-8}	2.6×10^{-10}	negligible	

Thorium-228[a]	1.8×10^{-1}	1.6×10^{-1}	1.5×10^{-1}	1.3×10^{-1}	1.1×10^{-1}	9.8×10^{-2}	6.3×10^{-2}	1.9×10^{-2}
Thullium-170	8.0×10^{-4}	4.3×10^{-5}	5.3×10^{-6}	1.1×10^{-8}	1.7×10^{-10}	negligible	8.7×10^{-9}	negligible
Tin-113	2.6×10^{-2}	2.2×10^{-4}	2.5×10^{-4}	4.8×10^{-5}	1.6×10^{-5}	2.8×10^{-6}	6.3×10^{-5}	2.0×10^{-8}
Xenon-127	5.8×10^{-2}	1.7×10^{-2}	9.7×10^{-3}	3.3×10^{-3}	1.9×10^{-3}	8.7×10^{-4}		
Xenon-133	1.2×10^{-2}	3.7×10^{-4}	3.7×10^{-5}	3.8×10^{-8}	4.1×10^{-10}	negligible		
Yttrium-88	3.7×10^{-1}	3.5×10^{-1}	3.4×10^{-1}	3.0×10^{-1}	2.7×10^{-1}	2.4×10^{-1}	1.5×10^{-1}	3.8×10^{-2}
Yttrium-91	5.2×10^{-4}	5.0×10^{-4}	4.8×10^{-4}	4.2×10^{-4}	3.9×10^{-4}	3.4×10^{-4}	2.1×10^{-4}	3.9×10^{-5}
Ytterbium-169	4.8×10^{-2}	8.9×10^{-3}	4.5×10^{-3}	1.4×10^{-4}	4.4×10^{-4}	2.4×10^{-11}	2.9×10^{-6}	2.4×10^{-11}
Zinc-65	8.5×10^{-2}	8.1×10^{-2}	7.7×10^{-2}	6.7×10^{-2}	6.1×10^{-2}	5.2×10^{-2}	3.0×10^{-2}	5.2×10^{-3}
Zirconium-95	1.1×10^{-1}	1.0×10^{-1}	9.6×10^{-2}	7.7×10^{-2}	6.5×10^{-2}	5.1×10^{-2}	2.2×10^{-2}	1.3×10^{-3}

[a] Isotope in equilibrium with daughter nuclides.

From *Amersham Nuclear Medicine Catalogue*, Amersham International, plc., Little Chalfont, England, 1985. With permission.

Radioactive Decay

INTRODUCTION

Radionuclides are unstable and decay by particle emission, electron capture, or γ-ray emission. The decay of radionuclides is a spontaneous, random process, that is, there is no way to predict with certainty the exact moment at which an unstable nucleus will undergo its active transformation into another, more stable nucleus. Therefore, one can only talk about the average number of radionuclides disintegrating per unit time.

The number of disintegrations per unit time (disintegration rate or D), $\Delta N/\Delta t$, of a radionuclide at any time is proportional to the total number of radionuclides present at that time.

THE DECAY CONSTANT FACTOR

$$\Delta N/\Delta t = -\lambda N$$

where N is the number of radionuclides (radioactive atoms of a certain radionuclide), and λ is the "decay constant" which is defined as the probability of disintegration per unit time for a single radionuclide (the decay constant has a characteristic value for each radionuclide). The units of λ are (time) $^{-1}$, while the disintegration rate (D) is negative; that is, N is decreasing with time. Furthermore, the disintegration rate $\Delta N/\Delta T$, expressed as disintegrations per second (dps) or disintegrations per minute (dpm), is basically a measure of the (radio) "activity" (A) of the sample.

$$D = \lambda N$$
$$A = \lambda N$$

The SI unit of activity is the becquerel (Bq), which is equal to s^{-1}, or one nuclear transformation (disintegration) per second (dps). The traditional, non SI unit of activity is the curie (Ci), which is equal to 3.7×10^{10} dps. Thus, 1 Bq = 0.27×10^{-10} Ci, and 1 Ci = 3.7×10^{10} Bq.

As the number of radioactive atoms (N) disintegrate with time (t), the activity (A) of a sample also decreases continuously. An exact mathematical expression for N(t) can be derived using methods of calculus. The result is

$$N(t) = N(0)e^{-\lambda t}$$

Thus N(t), the number of radioactive atoms remaining after a period of time t is equal to N(0), the number of atoms at time t = 0, multiplied by the factor $e^{-\lambda t}$. This factor $e^{-\lambda t}$, the fraction of radioactive atoms after time t, is called the "decay factor" (DF). The DF is a number equal to e, the base of natural logarithms (2.718), raised to the power $-\lambda t$, and is an "exponential function" of a time t. Since activity (A) is proportional to the number of radioactive atoms (N), the DF also applies to activity, therefore:

$$A(t) = A(0)e^{-\lambda t}$$

HALF-LIFE

$T_{1/2}$ is the unique characteristic of a radionuclide, defined by the time during which an initial activity (of the sample) is reduced to $^{1}/_{2}$. The $T_{1/2}$ is related to the decay constant λ, in that:

$$T_{1/2} = 0.693*/\lambda$$
$$= 0.693/T_{1/2}$$
[* natural logarithm of 2 (ln 2)]

AVERAGE LIFE

Average life is the reciprocal of the disintegration constant and is equal to 1.443 times the half life ($T_{1/2}$).

$$\tau = 1.443\ T_{1/2}$$

RADIOACTIVE DECAY DETERMINATION

Graphics — Exponential decay is characterized by the disappearance of a constant fraction of activity or number of atoms present per unit time interval. On linear graph paper, this is expressed as a curve that gradually approaches zero; on semilogarithmic graph paper, it is a straight line. From this line can be calculated the half-lives elapsed of any radionuclide or activity remaining after a known period of time.

Tables — Decay factors and for various elapsed times have been tabulated for specific radionuclides. Decay factors also can be determined by the use of tables of exponential functions found in many scientific reference books. However, the following Universal Decay Table can be used to measure the fraction of activity remaining of any radionuclide, from 0.001 to 1.00 $T_{1/2}$.

UNIVERSAL DECAY TABLE

To use this table follow these steps.

1. Divide the elapsed time (t) by the known physical half-life ($T_{1/2}$) of the radionuclide in question, where $t/T_{1/2}$ must be expressed in the same time unit, i.e. seconds, hours, days, etc.
2. Use the answer (to three significant figures) in locating the fraction of the original activity remaining. The first two significant figures are listed in the vertical column at the left of the table; the third significant figure is listed horizontally, across the top of the table.
3. Multiply the original activity by this decimal fraction to the obtain amount remaining. Example: What is the remaining activity of 800 mBq (21.6 mCi) of ^{99m}Tc after 4 hours? (^{99m}Tc half-life = 6 h)

1. $t/T_{1/2}$ = 4/6 = 0.666
2. Fraction remaining from decay table = 0.63025
3. 800 MBq × 0.63025 = 504.2 MBq
    (21.6 mCi × 0.63025 = 13.6 mCi)

If the $t/T_{1/2}$ is greater than the unit, multiple the decay factor of the excess by the decay factor of the unit.

Example: What is the remaining activity of 800 MBq of ^{99m}Tc after 8 hours?

1. $t/T_{1/2}$ = 8/6 = $1^{1}/_{3}$ = 1.33
2. The decay factor for 1 = 0.5
3. The decay factor for the excess of the unit, 0.333 = 0.79388
4. 0.79388 × 0.5 = 0.39694
5. 800 MBq × 0.39694 = 317.552 MBq

UNIVERSAL DECAY TABLE

Activity Remaining for $t/T_{1/2}$ from 0 to 1.00

	.000	.001	.002	.003	.004	.005	.006	.007	.008	.009
	1.00000	.99931	.99861	.99792	.99723	.99654	.99585	.99516	.99447	.99378
.01	.99309	.99240	.99172	.99103	.99034	.98966	.98897	.98829	.98760	.98692
.02	.98263	.98555	.98487	.98418	.98350	.98282	.98214	.98146	.98078	.98010
.03	.97942	.97874	.97806	.97739	.97671	.97603	.97536	.97468	.97400	.97333
.04	.97265	.97198	.97131	.97063	.96996	.96929	.96862	.96795	.96728	.96661
.05	.96594	.96527	.96460	.96393	.96326	.96259	.96193	.96126	.96059	.95993
.06	.95926	.95860	.95794	.95727	.95661	.95595	.95528	.95462	.95396	.95330
.07	.95264	.95198	.95132	.95066	.95000	.94934	.94868	.94803	.94737	.94671
.08	.94606	.94540	.94475	.94409	.94344	.94278	.94213	.94148	.94083	.94017
.09	.93952	.93887	.93822	.93757	.93692	.93627	.93562	.93498	.93433	.93368
.10	.93303	.93239	.93174	.93109	.93045	.92980	.92916	.92852	.92787	.92723
.11	.92659	.92595	.92530	.92466	.92402	.92338	.92274	.92210	.92146	.92083
.12	.92019	.91955	.91891	.91828	.91764	.91700	.91637	.91573	.91510	.91447
.13	.91383	.91320	.91257	.91193	.91130	.91067	.91004	.90941	.90878	.90815
.14	.90752	.90689	.90626	.90563	.90501	.90438	.90375	.90313	.90250	.90188
.15	.90125	.90063	.90000	.89938	.89876	.89813	.89751	.89689	.89627	.89565
.16	.89503	.89440	.89379	.89317	.89255	.89193	.89131	.89069	.89008	.88946
.17	.88884	.88823	.88761	.88700	.88638	.88577	.88515	.88454	.88393	.88332
.18	.88270	.88209	.88148	.88087	.88026	.87065	.87904	.87843	.87782	.87721
.19	.87661	.87600	.87539	.87478	.87418	.87357	.87297	.87236	.87176	.87115
.20	.87055	.86995	.86934	.86874	.86814	.86754	.86694	.86634	.86574	.86514
.21	.86454	.86394	.86334	.86274	.86214	.86155	.86095	.86035	.85976	.85916
.22	.85857	.85797	.85738	.85678	.85619	.85559	.85500	.85441	.85382	.85323
.23	.85263	.85204	.85145	.85086	.85027	.84968	.84910	.84851	.84792	.84733
.24	.84675	.84616	.84557	.84499	.84440	.84382	.84323	.84265	.84206	.84148
.25	.84090	.84031	.83973	.83915	.83857	.83799	.83741	.83683	.83265	.83567
.26	.83509	.83451	.83393	.83335	.83278	.83220	.83162	.83105	.83047	.82989
.27	.82932	.82874	.82817	.82760	.82702	.82645	.82588	.82531	.82473	.82416
.28	.82359	.82302	.82245	.82188	.82131	.82074	.82017	.81960	.81904	.81847
.29	.81790	.81734	.81677	.81620	.81564	.81507	.81451	.81394	.81338	.81282
.30	.81225	.81169	.81113	.81057	.81000	.80944	.80888	.80832	.80776	.80720
.31	.80664	.80608	.80552	.80497	.80441	.80385	.80329	.80274	.80218	.80163
.32	.80107	.80051	.79996	.79941	.79885	.79830	.79775	.79719	.79664	.79609
.33	.79554	.79499	.79443	.79388	.79333	.79278	.79223	.79169	.79114	.79059
.34	.79004	.78949	.78895	.78840	.78785	.78731	.78676	.78622	.78567	.78513
.35	.78548	.78404	.78350	.78295	.78241	.78187	.78133	.78079	.78025	.79970
.36	.77916	.77862	.77809	.77755	.77701	.77647	.77593	.77539	.77486	.77432
.37	.77378	.77325	.77271	.77218	.77164	.77111	.77057	.77004	.76950	.76897
.38	.76844	.76791	.76737	.76684	.76631	.76578	.76525	.76472	.76419	.76366
.39	.76313	.76260	.76207	.76154	.76102	.76049	.75996	.75944	.75891	.75838
.40	.75786	.75733	.75681	.75628	.75576	.75524	.75471	.75419	.75367	.75315
.41	.75262	.75210	.75158	.75106	.75054	.75002	.74950	.74898	.74846	.74794
.42	.74742	.74691	.74639	.74587	.74536	.74484	.74432	.74381	.74329	.74278
.43	.74226	.74175	.74123	.74072	.74021	.73969	.73918	.73867	.73816	.73765
.44	.73713	.73662	.73611	.73560	.73509	.73458	.73408	.73357	.73306	.73255
.45	.73204	.73154	.73103	.73052	.73002	.72951	.72900	.72850	.72799	.72749
.46	.72699	.72648	.72598	.72548	.72497	.72447	.72397	.72347	.72297	.72247
.47	.72196	.72146	.72096	.72047	.71997	.71947	.71897	.71847	.71797	.71747
.48	.71698	.71648	.71598	.71549	.71499	.71450	.71400	.71351	.71301	.71252
.49	.71203	.71153	.71104	.71055	.71005	.70956	.70907	.70858	.70809	.70760
.50	.70711	.70662	.70613	.70564	.70515	.70466	.70417	.70368	.70320	.70271
.51	.70222	.70174	.70125	.70076	.70028	.69979	.69931	.69882	.69834	.69786
.52	.69737	.69689	.69641	.69592	.69544	.69496	.69448	.69400	.69352	.69304
.53	.69255	.69208	.69160	.69112	.69064	.69016	.68968	.68920	.68873	.68825
.54	.68777	.68729	.68682	.68634	.68587	.68539	.68492	.68444	.68397	.68349

UNIVERSAL DECAY TABLE (continued)

Activity Remaining for $t/T_{1/2}$ from 0 to 1.00

	.000	.001	.002	.003	.004	.005	.006	.007	.008	.009
.55	.68302	.68255	.68207	.68160	.68113	.68066	.68019	.67971	.67924	.67877
.56	.67830	.67783	.67736	.67689	.76742	.67596	.67549	.67502	.67455	.67408
.57	.67362	.67315	.67268	.67222	.67175	.67129	.67082	.67036	.66989	.66843
.58	.66896	.66850	.66804	.66757	.66711	.66665	.66619	.66573	.66526	.66480
.59	.66434	.66388	.66342	.66296	.66250	.66204	.66159	.66113	.66067	.66021
.50	.65975	.65930	.65884	.65838	.65793	.65747	.65702	.65656	.65611	.65565
.61	.65520	.65474	.65429	.65384	.65338	.65293	.65248	.65203	.65157	.65112
.62	.65067	.65022	.64977	.64932	.64887	.64842	.64797	.64752	.64707	.64662
.63	.64618	.64573	.64528	.64483	.64439	.64394	.64349	.64305	.64260	.64216
.64	.64171	.64127	.64082	.64038	.63994	.63949	.63905	.63861	.63816	.63772
.65	.63728	.63684	.63640	.63596	.63552	.63508	.63464	.63420	.63376	.63332
.66	.63288	.63244	.63200	.63156	.63113	.63069	.63025	.62982	.62938	.62894
.67	.62851	.62807	.62764	.62720	.62677	.62633	.62590	.62546	.62503	.62460
.68	.62417	.62373	.62330	.62287	.62244	.62201	.62157	.62114	.62071	.62028
.69	.61985	.61942	.61900	.61857	.61814	.61771	.61728	.61685	.61643	.61600
.70	.61557	.61515	.61472	.61429	.61387	.61344	.61302	.61259	.61217	.61174
.71	.61132	.61090	.61047	.61005	.60963	.60921	.60878	.60836	.60794	.60752
.72	.60710	.60668	.60626	.60584	.60542	.60500	.60458	.60416	.60374	.60332
.73	.60290	.60249	.60207	.60165	.60123	.60082	.60040	.59999	.59957	.59915
.74	.59874	.59832	.59791	.59750	.59708	.59667	.59625	.59584	.59543	.59502
.75	.59460	.59419	.59378	.59337	.59296	.59255	.59214	.59173	.59132	.59091
.76	.59050	.59009	.58968	.58927	.58886	.58845	.58805	.58764	.58723	.58682
.77	.58642	.58601	.58561	.58520	.58479	.58439	.58398	.58358	.58317	.58277
.78	.58237	.58196	.58156	.58116	.58075	.58035	.57995	.57955	.57915	.57875
.79	.57834	.57794	.57754	.57714	.57674	.57634	.57594	.57554	.57515	.57475
.80	.57435	.57395	.57355	.57316	.57276	.57236	.57197	.57157	.57117	.57078
.81	.57038	.56999	.56959	.56920	.56880	.56841	.56801	.56762	.56723	.56683
.82	.56644	.56605	.56566	.56527	.56487	.56448	.56409	.56370	.56331	.56292
.83	.56253	.56214	.56175	.56136	.56097	.56058	.56019	.55981	.55942	.55903
.84	.55864	.55826	.55787	.55748	.55710	.55671	.55632	.55594	.55555	.55517
.85	.55478	.55440	.55402	.55363	.55325	.55287	.55248	.55210	.55172	.55133
.86	.55095	.55057	.55019	.54981	.54943	.54905	.54867	.54829	.54791	.54753
.87	.54715	.54677	.54639	.54601	.54563	.54525	.54488	.54450	.54112	.54374
.88	.54337	.54299	.54261	.54224	.54186	.54149	.54111	.54074	.54036	.53999
.89	.53961	.53924	.53887	.53849	.53812	.53775	.53737	.53700	.53633	.53626
.90	.53589	.53552	.53514	.53477	.53440	.53403	.53366	.53329	.53292	.53255
.91	.53218	.53182	.53145	.53108	.53071	.53034	.52998	.52961	.52924	.52888
.92	.52851	.52814	.52778	.52741	.52705	.52668	.52632	.52595	.52559	.52522
.93	.52486	.52449	.52413	.52377	.52340	.52304	.52268	.52232	.52196	.52159
.94	.52123	.52087	.52051	.52015	.51979	.51943	.51907	.51871	.51835	.51799
.95	.51763	.51727	.51692	.51656	.51620	.51584	.51548	.51513	.51477	.51441
.96	.51406	.51370	.51334	.51299	.51263	.51228	.51192	.51157	.51121	.51086
.97	.51051	.51015	.50980	.50945	.50909	.50874	.50839	.50803	.50768	.50733
.98	.50698	.60663	.50628	.50593	.50558	.50523	.50488	.50453	.50418	.50383
.99	.50348	.50313	.50278	.50243	.50208	.50174	.50139	.50104	.50069	.50035
100	.50000									

From Harbert, J. and Goncalves da Rocha, A. F., *Textbook of Nuclear Medicine,* Vol. 1, Basic Science, 2nd ed., Lea & Febiger, Philadelphia, 1984. With permission.

EXPONENTIAL RADIOACTIVITY DECAY TABLE

x	e^{-x}	x	e^{-x}	x	e^{-x}
0.00	1.000	0.40	0.670	1.0	0.368
0.01	0.990	0.41	0.664	1.1	0.333
0.02	0.980	0.42	0.657	1.2	0.301
0.03	0.970	0.43	0.651	1.3	0.273
0.04	0.961	0.44	0.644	1.4	0.247
0.05	0.951	0.45	0.638	1.5	0.223
0.06	0.942	0.46	0.631	1.6	0.202
0.07	0.932	0.47	0.625	1.7	0.183
0.08	0.923	0.48	0.619	1.8	0.165
0.09	0.914	0.49	0.613	1.9	0.150
0.10	0.905	0.50	0.607	2.0	0.135
0.11	0.896	0.52	0.595	2.1	0.122
0.12	0.887	0.54	0.583	2.2	0.111
0.13	0.878	0.56	0.571	2.3	0.100
0.14	0.869	0.58	0.560	2.4	0.0907
0.15	0.861			2.5	0.0821
0.16	0.852	0.60	0.549	2.6	0.0743
0.17	0.844	0.62	0.538	2.7	0.0672
0.18	0.835	0.64	0.527	2.8	0.0608
0.19	0.827	0.66	0.517	2.9	0.0550
		0.68	0.507		
0.20	0.819			3.0	0.0498
0.21	0.811	0.70	0.497	3.2	0.0408
0.22	0.803	0.72	0.487	3.4	0.0334
0.23	0.795	0.74	0.477	3.6	0.0273
0.24	0.787	0.76	0.468	3.8	0.0224
0.25	0.779	0.78	0.458		
0.26	0.771			4.0	0.0183
0.27	0.763	0.80	0.449	4.2	0.0150
0.28	0.756	0.82	0.440	4.4	0.0123
0.29	0.748	0.84	0.432	4.6	0.0101
		0.86	0.423		
0.30	0.741				
0.31	0.733			5.0	0.0067
0.32	0.726	0.90	0.407	5.5	0.0041
0.33	0.719	0.92	0.399	6.0	0.0025
0.34	0.712	0.94	0.391	6.5	0.0015
0.35	0.705	0.96	0.383	7.0	0.0009
0.36	0.698	0.98	0.375	7.5	0.0006
0.37	0.691			8.0	0.0003
0.38	0.684			8.5	0.0002
0.39	0.677			9.0	0.0001

Note: To determine the fraction of radioactivity remaining (A) at time t, the equation $A = A_o e^{t}$ can be used where A_o = original activity and = $0.693/T1/2$. The exponential table can be used by allowing t = x, then locating the corresponding e^{-t} value. The value obtained is employed as the decay factor.

Data compiled from Radioactive decay, in *The Radiochemical Manual*, 2nd ed., Amersham, England, 1966, 308, and Weast, Robert C., Ed., *CRC Handbook of Chemistry and Physics*, 67th ed., 1986—1987, CRC Press, Boca Raton, FL.

Radiopharmaceuticals

CHARACTERISTICS OF RADIOPHARMACEUTICALS COMMONLY USED IN NUCLEAR MEDICINE

BROMINE-82

Decay of bromine-82 (half-life = 35.3 h)

Time (h)	Factor (%)	Time (h)	Factor (%)
−30	180	15	74
−20	148	20	67
−10	121	25	61
−5	110	30	55
0	100	35	50
5	90	50	37
10	82	70	25

Note: Hours before (−) or hours after the reference date.

Principal γ-energies — 554 (72%), 777 (83%) keV

Sodium bromide (^{82}Br)

- **Chemical form** — Sodium bromide (^{82}Br) in sterile NaCl solution, for injection or oral administration.
- **pH** — 4 to 7.
- **Use** — Determination of extracellular liquids. Measurement of partition ratio of orally administered bromide between CSF and blood to determine the permeability of the blood brain barrier, specially in the diagnosis of tuberculous meningitis.
- **Dosage and procedure** — The adult dose is 1.85 MBq (50 μCi) administered orally in 50 ml of water. Forty eight hours later CSF is drawn by lumbar puncture and equal volumes of CSF and blood serum are counted in a well scintillation counter. The serum/CSF ^{82}Bromide ratio in TB meningitis patients is usually below 1.6.

CALCIUM-47

Decay of Calcium-47 (Half-life = 4.53 d)

Time (h)	Factor (%)	Time (h)	Factor (%)	Time (h)	Factor (%)	Time (h)	Factor (%)
−48	136	−12	108	24	86	72	64
−42	130	−6	104	30	83	84	58
−36	126	0	100	36	79	96	54
−30	121	6	96	42	76	120	46
−24	116	12	93	48	74	144	40
−18	112	18	89	60	68	168	34

Note: Hours before (−) or hours after the reference date.

Principal γ-energy — 1297 (75%) keV

Calcium (^{47}Ca) chloride injection

- **Chemical form** — Calcium chloride in a sterile solution, made isotonic with sodium chloride.
- **pH** — 4 to 8.

- **Use** — Calcium (^{47}Ca) chloride is used to investigate the gastro-intestinal absorption and metabolism of calcium, in particular the exchangeable calcium pool-size can be estimated using intravenously injected calcium-47. Increased calcium absorption has been found in primary hyperparathyroidism, idiopathic hypercalciuria, sarcoidosis, Paget's disease and invasive bone disease. Decreased absorption has been found in Cushing's disease and various renal diseases.
- **Dosage and procedure** — Reference should be made to the literature for information on techniques for different types of metabolic studies. The normal adult dose is 185 to 740 kBq, (5 to 20 μCi), but this can be varied according to the type of study being carried out.

CHROMIUM-51

Decay of chromium-51 (Half-life = 27.8 d)

Time (d)	Factor (%)	Time (d)	Factor (%)	Time (d)	Factor (%)	Time (d)	Factor (%)
−28	202	−10	128	8	82	26	52
−26	192	−8	122	10	78	28	50
−24	182	−6	116	12	74	30	47
−22	173	−4	110	14	70	35	42
−20	165	−2	105	16	67	40	37
−18	157	0	100	18	64	45	32
−16	149	2	95	20	61	50	29
−14	142	4	90	22	58	55	25
−12	135	6	86	24	55	60	22

Note: Days before (−) or days after the reference date.

Principal γ-energy — 320 (9.8%) keV

Chromic (^{51}Cr) chloride injection

- **Chemical form** — Sterile solution of chromic chloride in isotonic saline
- **pH** — 2 to 4.
- **Use** — For the determination of loss of serum protein into the gastrointestinal tract by direct intravenous injection. The chromium-51 becomes nonspecifically attached to plasma proteins *in vivo*. If there is any leakage from the gastrointestinal tract, chromium-51 will be detected in the stool in 5 d. As a clinical test the chromic (^{51}Cr) chloride method is robust and reliable, and can provide a clear diagnosis in patients with an unexplained low serum albumin level.
- **Dosage and procedure** — Adult doses of 1.11 to 3.7 MBq (30 to 100 μCi) are recommended. In infants the dose should be reduced to 0.185 to 0.370 MBq, (5 to 10 μCi). The material is given intravenously and stools are saved (free of urine) for 5 d. The whole stool sample must be counted preferably in a large-sample scintillation counter. Excretion of more than 2% of the administered activity in 5 d is indicative of significant protein loss.

Chromium (^{51}Cr) Ethylenediaminetetraacetic acid (EDTA) injection

- **Chemical form** — Sterile aqueous solution of chromium EDTA containing 1% benzyl alcohol and the disodium salt of EDTA.
- **pH** — 3.0 to 4.5

- **Use** — Chromium (^{51}Cr) EDTA injection is widely used for the determination of GFR (glomerular filtration rate), particularly when simplicity of procedure is important, or complete urine collection is difficult or impossible. Chromium (^{51}Cr) EDTA offers significant advantages over inulin and creatinine clearance measurements of GFR since it is less time-consuming for the physician and less disturbing and hazardous for the patient.
- **Dosage and administration** — The recommended dose using a single intravenous injection or continuous infusion is 1.3 to 3 MBq (35 to 80 µCi.) Half the adult dose is adequate for children. The single shot injection technique has proved to be very accurate for most routine clinical work, and results correlate well with those from continuous infusion procedures.
- **Procedure — glomerular filtration rate**
  Equipment — Sample counting (well scintillation counter).
  Technique — Timed 10 ml venous blood samples at 2, 3 and 4 h.
  Quantitative analysis — Centrifuge and measure radioactivity of plasma samples and standard of ^{51}Cr EDTA. Plot counts/time on semi log paper, calculate $T_{1/2}$ and estimate intercept at Time = 0.
  Calculate:

$$\text{Volume of Distribution VD in liters } = \frac{S \times D \times V}{A \times 1000}$$

  where S = count rate of standard, D = dilution factor of stand, V = volume injected, and A = estimated count rate at Time = 0.

$$\text{GFR} = \frac{VD \times 1000 \times 0.693 \times 0.8}{T_{1/2}} \text{ml m}^{-1}$$

  Comment — Great care must be taken to inject exact measured volume and to time the blood samples accurately.

Sodium chromate (^{51}Cr) solution

- **Chemical form** — Sterile solution of sodium chromate in isotonic saline, suitable for injection.
- **pH** — 6.0 to 8.5.
- **Use** — *In vitro* labeling of red blood cells for the determination of red cell volume or mass, and for the study of red cell survival time. Also used to study the amount and site of blood loss via the gastrointestinal tract and for the preparation of labeled damaged red blood cells for spleen scintigraphy.
- **Dosage and administration** — The usual dosage for the determination of red blood cell volume or mass is 0.555 to 0.740 MBq, (15 to 20 µCi), and for the study of red cell survival time up to 1.85 MBq (50 µCi). The method recommended of labeling for determination of red cell survival time is described in the report on Recommended Methods for Radioisotope Red Cell Survival Studies, published by the International Committee for Standardisation in Haematology, in the *British Journal of Haematology*, 21, 378, 1971.
- **Procedure — red cell mass determination**
  Equipment — Well scintillation counter
  Technique — Preinjection 10 ml heparinized blood sample then samples at 30, 60, 90 minutes. Whole blood and plasma samples are counted.
  Quantitative analysis:

Red blood cell volume = volume injected × whole blood std CPM/1 ml × dilution − plasma std CPM/1 ml × std plasmacrit WB CPM/1 ml − $\dfrac{\text{plasma CPM/1 ml} \times \text{plasmacrit}}{\text{hematocrit}}$

> Comment — Normal red cell volume
> males 25 to 35 ml kg^{-1}
> females 20 to 30 ml kg^{-1}
>   — Total blood volume
> males: 55 to 80 ml kg^{-1}
> females: 50 to 75 ml kg^{-1}

- **Procedure — Red cell survival determination**
  Equipment — Well scintillation counter, collimated scintillation detector.
  Technique — Blood sample taken at 24 h and then 3 times each week for 3 weeks. Counts are recorded over the precordium, spleen and liver at the same times as blood samples.
  Quantitative analysis — Plot blood sample count rates on semi log paper and estimate $T_{1/2}$. Sequestration results expressed as ratio of precordial to spleen and spleen to liver ratio.
  Comment — Normal value 25 to 35 d.

COBALT-57

Decay of cobalt-57 (Half-life = 270 d)

Time (d)	Factor (%)	Time (d)	Factor (%)	Time (d)	Factor (%)	Time (d)	Factor (%)
−28	107	−4	101	18	95	40	91
−24	106	0	100	22	95	45	89
−20	105	2	99	24	94	50	88
−16	104	6	98	28	93	55	87
−12	103	10	97	35	92	60	86
−8	102	14	96				

Note: Days before (−) or days after the reference date.

Principal γ-energy — 122 (85.5%) keV

Cyanocobalamin (^{57}Co) oral solution
- **Chemical form** — Aqueous solution of cyanocobalamin containing 0.9% benzyl alcohol.
- **pH** — 4 to 6.
- **Use** — Measurement of vitamin B$_{12}$ absorption in the diagnosis of pernicious anemia and other malabsorption syndromes.
- **Dosage and procedure** — The Schilling test is the most commonly used procedure and involves the administration of cobalt-57 (or cobalt-58) labeled cyanocobalamin followed by a flushing dose of inactive cyanocobalamin. Quantification of subsequent urinary B$_{12}$ excretion is then carried out.

  If absorption is abnormally low the test is repeated with the addition of intrinsic factor to correct the intrinsic factor deficiency that characterizes pernicious anemia. The normal dose of Cyanocobalamin (^{57}Co) Solution is 18.5 to 37 kBq (0.5 to 1 μCi) taken orally.

Cyanocobalamin (^{57}Co) capsules

*   **Chemical form** — Gelatin capsules each containing 1 µg cyanocobalamin.
*   **Use** — The capsules are for use in the measurement of vitamin B$_{12}$ absorption in the diagnosis of pernicious anemia and other malabsorption syndromes. Capsules offer an advantage over Cyanocobalamin (^{57}Co) solution by allowing a precalculated quantity of labeled cyanocobalamin to be administered, thus improving the convenience of the test for both the patient and the hospital staff.
*   **Dosage and Administration** — 1 capsule should be used per stage in the Schilling test. The procedure and dosimetry are exactly the same as stated under Cyanocobalamin (^{57}Co) Solution.
*   **Procedure** — **Vitamin B$_{12}$ absorption**
    Equipment — Well scintillation counter.
    Technique — Administer ^{57}Co B$_{12}$. Inject 1 mg stable B$_{12}$ 2 h later. Collect urine for 24 h twice. Prepare a ^{57}Co B$_{12}$ standard.
    Quantitative analysis — Measure radioactivity of a 5 ml aliquot of urine and standard.

$$\% \text{ in 24 hours} = \frac{\text{CPM in 5ml of urine} \times \text{urine vol}/5}{\text{CPM in 5ml of std} \times \text{dilution factor} \times 100}$$

Comment — Normal value 9% in 1st 24 h, <1% in 2nd 24 h. If less than 6% excreted repeat with intrinsic factor. The two tests can be combined with two different radioactive cobalt labels.

COBALT-58

Decay of cobalt-58 (Half-life = 71.3 d)

Time (d)	Factor (%)	Time (d)	Factor (%)	Time (d)	Factor (%)	Time (d)	Factor (%)
− 14	115	2	98	16	86	30	75
− 12	112	4	96	18	84	35	71
− 10	110	6	94	20	82	40	68
− 8	108	8	92	22	81	45	64
− 6	106	10	91	24	79	50	61
− 4	104	12	89	26	77	55	58
− 2	102	14	87	28	76	60	56
0	100						

Note: Days before (−) or days after the reference date.

Principal γ-energies — 511 (from β$^+$), 811 (99.4%) keV.

Cyanocobalamin (^{58}Co) Oral Solution

*   **Chemical form** — Aqueous solution of cyanocobalamin 0.9% benzyl alcohol.
*   **Use** — Measurement of vitamin B$_{12}$ absorption in the diagnosis of pernicious anemia and other malabsorption syndromes. Cyanocobalamin (^{58}Co) solution has also been used to determine the cause of postirradiation chronic diarrhea.
*   **Dosage and procedure** — The recommended dose for adults is 18.5 to 37 kBq (0.5 to 1 µCi) taken orally. The procedure for carrying out the Schilling test for the diagnosis of vitamin B$_{12}$ malabsorption is described in more detail under the section on Cyanocobalamin (^{57}Co) Solution.

Cyanocobalamin (^{58}Co) and Cyanocobalamin (^{57}Co) + Intrinsic Factor

*   **Basis of the dual cobalt test** — The test uses two cobalt isotopes to achieve differential diagnosis of vitamin B_{12} malabsorption. Free cyanocobalamin is labeled with cobalt-58. Absorption of this, and hence the appearance of cobalt-58 in urine, will be impaired if the patient has intrinsic factor deficiency.

    Cyanocobalamin, which is bound to intrinsic factor (human gastric juice), is labeled with cobalt-57. Absorption of this, and the subsequent level of cobalt-57 in urine, is independent of the patient's ability to secrete intrinsic factor, but dependent on his ability to absorb the vitamin in the ileum. The patient is given an oral tracer dose of both the free vitamin Cobalt-58 and the bound vitamin Cobalt-57. Absorbed isotope-labeled vitamin is flushed from the bloodstream by simultaneous intramuscular administration of a relatively large amount of nonradioactive cyanocobalamin, as in the classical Schilling test.

    Urine is collected over the next 24 h and cobalt-57 and cobalt-58 are measured in an aliquot. The two isotopes are easily measured in the presence of each other and the percentage of each tracer dose excreted in 24 h is readily calculated.

    Diagnosis of pernicious anemia is usually evident from the ratio of cobalt-57% to cobalt-58%. The overall picture of the patient's ability to absorb cyanocobalamin can be assessed from the figures for percentages excreted.

*   **Uses** — The dual cobalt isotope test is used to assess vitamin B_{12} malabsorption and to determine whether it is due to defective secretion of intrinsic factor by the stomach or to defective intestinal absorption.

GALLIUM-67

Decay of gallium-67 (Half-life = 78 h)

Time (d)	Factor (%)	Time (d)	Factor (%)	Time (d)	Factor (%)
−5	290	0	100	5	34
−4	234	1	81	6	28
−3	189	2	65	7	23
−2	153	3	53	8	18
−1	124	4	43	9	15

Note: Days before (−) or days after the reference date.

Principal γ-energies — 93 (38%), 185 (23.5%), 300 (16.7%), 394 (4.4%) keV

Gallium (^{67}Ga) citrate injection

*   **Chemical form** — Sterile aqueous solution of gallium citrate containing 2.6% w/v sodium citrate dihydrate and 0.1% w/v sodium chloride.
*   **pH** — 5 to 8.
*   **Use** — Gallium (^{67}Ga) Citrate Injection is a widely nonspecific tumor localizing agent. It is used in a variety of neoplastic conditions of soft tissue, including Hodgkin's disease, non-Hodgkin's lymphoma, testicular tumors, carcinoma of the bronchus, and liver tumors. Gallium-67 is concentrated in most sites of active infection, including abscesses, and also in various noninfective, inflammatory conditions, including sarcoidosis, interstitial pulmonary fibrosis, and many others.
*   **Dosage and administration** — The recommended adult dose for scintiscanning is 74 to 148 MBq (2 to 4 mCi). In all instances the dosage should, of course, be the minimum to provide a clear scintigram.

Because of the initially high levels of activity in the blood, scanning is not normally attempted earlier than 24 h after injection; optimum tumor visualization is likely to be obtained if scanning is performed 48 to 72 h postinjection.

- **Procedure — Gallium-67 whole body imaging**   Equipment — LFOV Gamma camera with 1, 2, or 3 pulse height analyzers and high energy collimator.

  Technique — 300 K count images. Views to cover whole body or local areas as clinically appropriate. Repeat at 72 h.

  Quantitative analysis — Possibly use subtraction technique with colloid liver scan for liver lesions.

GOLD-195m

Decay of mercury-195m generator (Half-life 40 h)

Time (h)	Factor (%)	Time (h)	Factor (%)
−24	149	24	67
−12	122	36	55
−8	114	48	45
0	100	60	37
8	88	72	30
12	82	84	24

Note: Hours before (−) or hours after a given reference point. The rate of regeneration of Gold-195m is fast; within 3 min more than 98% of the theoretical maximum amount has been formed.

Decay of Gold (^{195m}Au) (Half-life = 30.5 s)

Principal γ-energy — 261 (68%) keV

- **Chemical form** — Sterile, pyrogen-free sodium thiosulphate/sodiumnitrate solution. ^{195m}Au is present in the eluate as gold (^{195m}Au) thiosulphate complex.
- **pH** — 5 to 8.
- **Use** — After intravenous injection of the eluate of the ^{195m}Hg/^{195m}Au generator, gold-195m remains in the vascular bed, at least during the first passage from the right to the left cardiac cavities. In nuclear cardiology this allows multiple first-pass studies at 3-min intervals and visualization of the individual cardiac chambers from different angles without any overlap of activity from neighboring structures. Studies can be repeated after exercise or pharmacologic interventions without interference of background activity due to the short half-life of ^{195m}Au. Organ perfusion studies can also be made by intravenous or intra-arterial bolus injection.
- **Dosage and administration** — Cardiac performance studies by first-pass technique can be performed by repeated intravenous injection of 370 to 1110 MBq (10 to 30 mCi).

GOLD-198

Decay of gold-198 (Half-life = 64.7 h)

Time (h)	Factor (%)	Time (h)	Factor (%)	Time (h)	Factor (%)	Time (h)	Factor (%)
−72	216	−8	109	56	55	112	30
−64	198	0	100	64	50	120	28
−56	182	8	92	72	46	128	25
−48	167	16	84	80	42	136	23
−40	154	24	77	88	39	144	21
−32	141	32	71	96	36	168	16
−24	129	40	65	104	33	192	13
−16	119	48	60				

Note: Hours before (−) or hours after the reference date.

Principal γ-energy — 412 (95.4%) keV.
Principal β-energy — 961 (99%) keV.

Gold (^{198}Au) injection

- **Chemical form** — Sterile colloidal suspension of metallic gold stabilized with gelatin (22 mg/ml) and glucose (220 mg/ml).
- **pH** — 4 to 8.
- **Use** — Intracavity therapy — The growth of metastatic disease in the intraperitoneal and intrapleural cavities can be limited by the instillation of radioactive gold colloid.

  Treatment of synovial effusions — Intraarticular treatment with colloidal gold is reported to be therapeutically effective in relieving persistent synovial effusion in knee joints, as it achieves partial synovectomy due to irradiation.

  Gold (^{198}Au) colloid has been used in the past for liver scintigraphy and general studies of the reticuloendothelial system; however, the radiation dose to the liver is considerable and its use has been entirely superseded by technetium-99m colloid where the radiation dose is significantly less.

- **Dosage and procedure** — Therapeutic use — Up to 5.5 GBq (250 mCi) have been used for intracavity injection, but the more usual range is 1.29 to 2.77 GBq (37 - 75 mCi).

  Treatment of synovial effusions — Doses vary from 22.2 MBq (0.6 mCi) for treatment of interphalangeal joints, to 370 MBq (10 mCi) for knees.

HYDROGEN-3 (TRITIUM)

Decay of hydrogen-3 (Half-life = 12.26 years)

Time (years)	Factor (%)	Time (years)	Factor (%)
−6	140	4	80
−4	125	5	76
−2	112	6	71
−1	106	8	64
0	100	10	57
1	95	12	51
2	89	14	46
3	84		

Note: Years before (−) or years after reference date

Principal β-energy — 18.6 (100%) keV

Tritiated (³H) water injection
- **Chemical form** — Tritiated water sterile injectable solution.
- **Use** — Measurement of whole body water.
- **Dosage and procedure** — The normal adult dose is 3.7 MBq (100 μCi) administered intravenously.

INDIUM-111

Decay of indium-111 (Half-life = 67.4 h)

Time (d)	Factor (%)	Time (d)	Factor (%)	Time (d)	Factor (%)	Time (d)	Factor (%)
−4	268	−1	128	2	61	5	29
−3	209	0	100	3	47	6	23
−2	164	1	78	4	37	7	17

Note: Days before (−) or days after the reference date.

Principal γ-energies — 171 (91%), 245, (94%) keV.

Indium (¹¹¹In) bleomycin injection
- **Chemical form** — Sterile solution of indium bleomycin complex in isotonic saline containing 0.66 mg bleomycin per ml.
- **pH** — 4 to 7.
- **Use** — The indium-111 bleomycin complex shows a useful degree of tumor uptake and is of potential value in scintigraphic studies involving the thorax, abdomen and pelvis.

    Visualization of primary and secondary carcinomas of the breast, bronchus, cervix, colon, ovary, prostate and rectum have been reported. Uptake has been observed by adenocarcinomas, lymphomas, (including Hodgkin's disease), malignant melanomas and various sarcomas.
- **Dosage and procedure** — The adult dose administered for diagnostic scintigraphy is 74 MBq (2 mCi). The dose is given by intravenous injection. Scanning is performed 48 h or 72 h after injection.

Indium (¹¹¹In) Chloride
- **Chemical form** — Sterile solution of indium chloride in 0.04M HCl.
- **Use** — For use as an ingredient in injectable preparations, such as indium-111 labeled proteins and cells. Indium (¹¹¹In) chloride is particularly recommended for use in labeling monoclonal antibodies for immunoscintigraphy.
- **Dosage and procedure** — The quantities of isotope required for labeling depends primarily on the material being labeled and its intended use. There are many published protocols for labeling particular types of cells and monoclonal antibodies which may give guidelines, but each type of labeling requires careful evaluation by the operator to ensure that the optimum conditions exist for the particular type of work being carried out.

Indium (¹¹¹In) Diethylenetriamine-penta acetate (DTPA) injection
- **Chemical form** — Sterile, isotonic, pyrogen-free solution, of indium (¹¹¹In), calcium DTPA, containing 0.72 mg/ml sodium bicarbonate complex and sodium chloride to render the solution isotonic.

- **pH** — 7.0 to 7.6.
- **Use** — Diagnostic scintigraphy in cerebrospinal fluid (CSF) studies, cisternography and ventriculography. Indications include CSF rhinorrhea, otorrhea, extra-axial cysts, porencephalic cysts, subdural effusions, ventricular obstructing lesions, meningocele, hydrocephalus, and the testing of ventriculosomatic shunt patency.
- **Dosage and administration** — The adult dose administered for diagnostic scintigraphy is 18.5 to 37 mBq (0.5 to 1.0 mCi). As the radioactive half-life is 2.8 d, the larger dose may be required if serial scanning over more than 48 h is envisaged. The route of administration may be lumbar, intracisternal, intraventricular, or by injection into neurosurgical shunts, depending on the condition under investigation.

  In cisternography, serial scanning can usefully be commenced 1 to 2 h after lumbar administration, or within 1 h after cisternal administration. The early scan serves to confirm that the injection was subarachnoid. Further scans are usually performed at 3 to 6 h, 24 h, and 48 h after administration to monitor CSF movement. Later scans may be useful where clearance is slow.
- **Procedure — Cisternogram**

  Equipment — Standard field of view gamma camera with high energy collimator.

  Technique — 5 min images of cisterns (A, P, RL, LL) views at 2 h, 6 h, 24 h, and 48 h.

  Comment — Nasal or ear packs may be used to detect and measure CSF leakage.

Indium (^{111}In) oxine solution

- **Chemical form** — Sterile, isotonic, aqueous solution of indium oxine complex containing 100 μg/ml polysorbate 80, 6 mg/ml buffer, and 0.75% (w/v) sodium chloride to render the solution isotonic.
- **pH** — 6.5 to 7.5.
- **Use** — Indium (^{111}In) oxine is an effective labeling agent for a variety of blood cells, including granulocytes, platelets, and lymphocytes. Indium-111 labeled leukocyte imaging is used clinically to detect sites of abscess and inflammation. Indium-111 labeled platelets provide a measure of platelet survival and distribution, and have been used to visualize venous and arterial accumulation of platelets in aneurysms, venous thrombi, and thrombophlebitis.

  Indium-111 labeled platelets have also been used to provide an early indication of renal transplant rejection and to assess the thrombogenicity of arterial grafts.

  The distribution and circulation of Indium-111 labeled autologous lymphocytes can also be visualized and measured.
- **Dosage** — The normal adult dose of indium-111 labeled leukocytes for location of sites of infection is 18.5 to 37 MBq, (500 to 1000 μCi). A dose of 3.7 MBq (100 μCi) has been proposed for studies of granulocyte kinetics.

  A dose of 5.55 to 11.1 MBq (150 to 300 μCi) is appropriate for visualization studies using indium-111 labeled lymphocytes. The dose should not exceed 740 kBq (20 μCi) per 10^8 cells to avoid impaired recirculation.

  The normal adult dose of indium-111 labeled platelets is 1.85 to 3.7 MBq (50 to 100 μCi) for platelet survival and distribution studies, and 3.7 to 9.25 MBq (100 to 250 μCi) for scintigraphic detection of platelet accumulation. In all instances the dose should, of course, be the minimum needed to provide a clear scintigram.
- **Procedure — Focal sepsis white cells localization**

  Equipment — LFOV gamma camera preferably with dual PHA, with high energy collimator.

  Technique — Anterior and posterior views of chest and abdomen collecting 250,000 counts per view at 3 h; other views as clinically indicated. Repeat at 24 h.

INDIUM-133m

Decay of indium-133m (Half-life = 100 min)

Time (min)	Factor (%)	Time (min)	Factor (%)	Time (min)	Factor (%)	Time (min)	Factor (%)
− 300	808	− 120	231	60	66	240	19
− 270	656	− 90	187	90	53	270	15
− 240	532	− 60	152	120	43	300	12
− 210	432	− 30	123	150	35		
− 180	350	0	100	180	28		
− 150	284	30	81	210	23		

Note: Minutes before (−) or minutes after a given reference point.

Principal γ-energy — 392 (65%) keV

Indium (^{113m}In) sterile generator eluate

- **pH** — pH of eluate is 1.4 ± 0.1.
- **Use** — Indium-113m can be used in a number of diagnostic scanning procedures. The ionic species eluted from the generator is used for labeling injectable preparations for brain and liver scanning.

   The short half-life of indium-113m and its simple decay scheme involving only isometric transition and monoenergetic emission at 392 keV combine to produce excellent scanning characteristics with very little patient radiation dose. In addition, the long half-life (115 d) of the tin-113 parent gives the generator a useful life of several months.

- **Dosage and administration — Liver and spleen scanning**

   A variety of indium-113m labeled colloidal preparations have been described as liver scanning agents as such materials are removed from the circulation by the hepatic reticuloendothelial cells. Normal administered doses are about 37 to 74 MBq (1 to 2 mCi) for liver scanning, and up to 195 MBq (5 mCi) for bone marrow visualization. Scanning can be commenced immediately after injection.

   Lung scanning — Indium-113m can be incorporated into particulate preparations in the size range 30 to 60 μm, which are removed from the circulation by trapping in the pulmonary capillary bed. Areas of poor vascularity are detected as photopenic areas on the lung scan.

   Normal administered doses are about 74 MBq (2 mCi), and scanning is commenced within a few minutes of injection.

   Brain scanning and kidney scanning — Indium-133m chelate complexes have been widely used to delineate brain tumors in which increased target/nontarget activity ratios are observed because of a breakdown of the blood/brain barrier. Such complexes are rapidly cleared from the circulation by urinary excretion, and consequently can be used to evaluate renal function. The combination of short physical half-life of the isotope and the rapid excretion rate permits the safe administration of larger doses, that is up to 370 MBq (10 mCi).

IODINE-123

Decay of Iodine-123 (Half-life = 13.3 h)

Time (h)	Factor (%)	Time (h)	Factor (%)	Time (h)	Factor (%)	Time (h)	Factor (%)
−3	117	2	90	7	69	23	30
−2	111	3	85	8	66	24	28
−1	105	4	81	21	33	25	27
0	100	5	77	22	32	26	26
1	95	6	73				

Note: Hours before (−) or hours after the reference date.

Principal γ-energy — 159 (83%) keV

Sodium iodide (^{123}I) injection
- **Chemical form** — Sterile isotonic solution of carrier free sodium iodide (^{123}I) containing sodium thiosulphate in phosphate buffer.

Sodium iodide (^{123}I) capsules
- **Chemical form** — Gelatin capsules containing carrier free sodium iodide (^{123}I) solution absorbed onto partly dehydrated disodium hydrogen phosphate as an inert carrier.
- **Use** — Investigation of thyroid function.
- **Dosage and procedure** — The usual adult dose is 5.5 MBq (150 μCi) given orally as a capsule, solution, or intravenous injection.

Sodium orthoiodohippurate (^{123}I) injection
- **Chemical form** — Sterile isotonic solution of o-iodohippuric acid (^{123}I) containing 0.1% hydroxy benzoic acid ester.
- **Use** — Scintigraphic investigation of kidney function.
- **Dosage and procedure** — The usual adult dose for renal functional studies is 18.5 to 37 MBq (0.5 to 1 mCi). The procedure is the same as described for Iodine-131 Hippuran.

Iodine (^{123}I) iofetamine HCI (IMP) injection
- **Chemical form** — Sterile, pyrogen-free solution of N-isopropyl-p-(^{123}I) iodoamphetamine hydrochloride.
- **Use** — Amphetamine HCl Iodine (^{123}I) by intravenous injection is used for regional cerebral blood flow scintigraphy. Indications for this study are described in detail in ^{99m}Tc-HM PAO, another lipophilic agent also used for cerebral blood flow studies.
- **Dosage and administration** — The normal adult dose is 185 MBq (5 mCi) by bolus intravenous injection. Twenty minutes later, emission tomography can be started with a rotating tomographic gamma camera. Ni-isopropyl-p-(^{123}I) iodoamphetamine (I-123 IMP) has a number of attributes that make it an attractive choice for cerebral perfusion imaging. It is lipophilic, and after i.v. injection it passes efficiently into the cerebral parenchyma. Once there, it is either bound to nonspecific receptor sites or is converted to a nonlipophilic metabolite. Washout from the brain is slow, permitting substantial time for static imaging of cerebral perfusion. Its initial distribution is proportional to cerebral blood flow over a wide range of flows. The percent injected dose reaching the brain is between 7% and 8% in man, enough to permit high-resolution tomographic and planar imaging.

IODINE-125

Decay of iodine-125 (Half-life = 59.4 d)

Time (d)	Factor (%)	Time (d)	Factor (%)	Time (d)	Factor (%)	Time (d)	Factor (%)
−25	134	−2	102	5	94	40	63
−20	126	−1	101	10	89	45	60
−15	119	0	100	15	84	50	56
−10	112	1	99	20	79	55	53
−5	106	2	98	25	75	60	50
−4	105	3	97	30	71		
−3	104	4	96	35	67		

Note: Days before (−) or days after the reference date.

Principal γ-energies — 27 to 32 (138%, Te X-rays), 35 (7%) keV

Sodium iothalamate (^{125}I) injection
- **Chemical form** — Sterile aqueous solution of sodium iothalamate containing 1% alcohol and citrate-EDTA buffer.
- **pH** — 5 to 8.
- **Use** — Sodium iothalamate (^{125}I) is used in the determination of glomerular filtration rate (GFR), to determine the extent and severity of renal impairment.
- **Dosage and administration** — A normal adult dose of 0.185 to 1.85 MBq (5 to 50 μCi) is recommended for the determination of GFR.

  The clearance of radiolabeled iothalamate (^{125}I) can be measured using the constant intravenous infusion technique (traditional method) or by subcutaneous injection. The latter method can be performed over a shorter time period in a greater number of patients. Either method will produce a good estimate of the GFR.

Iodinated (^{125}I) human serum albumin injection
- **Chemical form** — Sterile solution of iodinated human albumin containing 0.9% benzyl alcohol and made isotonic with sodium chloride.
- **pH** — 6.5 to 8.5.
- **Use** — Iodinated (^{125}I) human albumin injection BP is used for the determination of plasma volume. It is most frequently used in situations where hematocrit measurements or hemoglobin levels do not correspond to the true plasma volume, for example, after the loss of blood by hemorrhage or the loss of plasma and red cells at varying rates in patients injured by burning.
- **Dosage and administration** — The normal adult dose for blood volume determinations is 185 kBq (5 μCi). The material is injected intravenously and blood samples are taken at regular time intervals. The plasma volume is then estimated by dividing the total activity injected intravenously by the activity per milliliter of plasma at zero time (extrapolated from samples taken during the first few minutes of the study).
- **Procedure** — Plasma volume determination

  Equipment — Well scintillation counter.

  Technique — 10 ml heparinized blood sample before injection. Administration of ^{125}I HSA. 10 ml heparinized blood samples at 10, 20, 30 minutes. Count 1 ml plasma samples and standard from opposite veins to injections.

Quantitative analysis. Plasma volume

$$= \frac{\text{vol injected (10)} \times \text{CPM standard} \times \text{dilution of standard}}{\text{extrapolated CPM/1 ml plasma at time 0}}$$

Comment — Normal range 30 - 40 ml kg^{-1} body weight. Whole blood volume can be calculated by:

$$\text{Blood volume} = \frac{\text{plasma volume}}{1.00 - \text{Hematocrit} \times 0.90}$$

Iodinated (^{125}I) human fibrinogen injection

*   **Chemical form** — Freeze-dried preparation of iodinated human fibrinogen containing albumin together with sodium citrate, which when reconstituted will yield an isotonic solution.
*   **Use** — Iodinated (^{125}I) human fibrinogen is indicated for the detection of deep vein thrombosis of the legs.

    Iodine-125 labeled fibrinogen is incorporated into a thrombus, whose existence can then be detected by external radioactivity monitoring. The early detection of DVT is important for the prevention of pulmonary embolism.
*   **Dosage and procedure** — 3.7 MBq (100 µCi) of iodinated (^{125}I) human fibrinogen injected intravenously.

    Radioactive measurements are best performed with a collimated scintillation counter fitted with a thin sodium iodide crystal. The measurements are made on the legs, elevated to 10° above the horizontal, on the medial surface starting at the mid-inguinal point and proceeding down the limb at constant intervals (usually 7 to 10 cm, depending upon the dimensions of the collimator), so that radiation from all parts of the principal veins of the leg is detected.

    At least 1,000 counts should be recorded at each site, and the count rate is expressed as a percentage of the count rate over the heart (fourth left intercostal space over the left sternal edge) measured on the same occasion. This factor is known as the "percentage uptake".

    The presence of a thrombus is indicated when the "percentage uptake" is 20 or more greater than that observed on the previous day, although a definitive diagnosis of whether deep vein thrombosis is present or not can usually be made within 12 h of injection of iodine-125 labeled fibrinogen. Subsequent monitoring shows whether the thrombus is extending, remaining stationary, or undergoing lysis.

Iodinated (^{125}I) polyvinylpyrrolidone (PVP) injection

*   **Chemical form** — Sterile aqueous solution of iodinated polyvinylpyrrolidone (Povidone) containing 1% benzyl alcohol and sodium succinate buffer.
*   **Use** — Iodinated (^{125}I) PVP is used to study protein losing enteropathy. Such disorders may be secondary to disorders of gastrointestinal lymphatic channels, ulceration of the gastrointestinal mucosa, or mechanisms as yet undefined. When serum proteins are lost via the gastrointestinal tract they are catabolized quickly into their respective amino acid subunits, which are then reabsorbed. Hypoproteinemia can develop if the rate of protein loss and catabolism exceeds the body protein synthetic capacity. By administering labeled macromolecules such as PVP the amount of activity excreted in the feces gives an estimate of the level of serum protein which is lost into the gastrointestinal tract.

    Iodinated (^{125}I) PVP is also used for permeability studies in investigations of the glomerular filtration barrier.
*   **Dosage and administration** — The iodinated (^{125}I) PVP is administered intravenously and the percentage of administered activity excreted over the following few days is monitored. Normal subjects excrete 0 to 1.5% and patients with gastrointestinal protein loss may excrete up to 35% of the administered dose.

    The recommended adult dose for protein-losing enteropathy studies is 185 to 925 kBq (5 to 25 µCi).

IODINE-131

Decay of Iodine-131 (Half-life = 8.05 d)

Time (d)	Factor (%)	Time (d)	Factor (%)	Time (d)	Factor (%)	Time (d)	Factor (%)
−6	168	0	100	6	60	12	36
−5	154	1	92	7	55	13	33
−4	141	2	84	8	50	14	30
−3	130	3	77	9	46		
−2	119	4	71	10	42		
−1	109	5	65	11	39		

Note: Days before (−) or days after the reference date.

Principal γ-energy — 364 (82%) keV
Principal β-energy — 606 (90%) keV

Sodium orthoiodohippurate (^{131}I) injection

• **Chemical form** — Sterile aqueous solution of sodium iodohippurate containing 1% benzyl alcohol and phosphate buffer.
• **pH** — 7.0 to 8.5
• **Use** — Sodium iodohippurate (^{131}I) is used in renal investigations to study the uptake and tubular secretory function of the kidneys. By using external radiation detectors a serial record of the counting rate over each kidney can be produced and used to construct a renogram.
• **Dosage and administration** — Doses of 0.37 to 3.7 MBq (10 — 100 μCi) administered intravenously are recommended for renography studies.

Sodium iodide (^{131}I) solution

• **Chemical form** — Sodium iodide solution for oral administration containing sodium thiosulphate, phosphate buffer and sodium chloride.
• **pH** — 7 to 8.
• **Use** — Sodium iodide (^{131}I) is indicated in the diagnosis of various thyroid disorders by gamma camera imaging or counting.

Disorders of the thyroid, including toxic nodules, multinodular goiter, solitary hypofunctioning nodule, and carcinoma of the thyroid can all be identified by performing a simple thyroid scan and radioiodine uptake.

• **Dosage and administration — Thyrotoxicosis**

In order to obtain an estimate of thyroid size and iodide uptake, a diagnostic dose of approximately 0.185 MBq (5 μCi) is recommended. For diagnostic thyroid imaging a dose of 1.85 MBq (50 μCi) is commonly used. Therapeutic doses for hyperthyroidism vary from 185 to 555 MBq (5 to 15 mCi). Ablation doses of thyroid remnants following thyroidectomy are in the region of 1.85 to 7.4 GBq (50 to 200 mCi).

Sodium iodide (^{131}I) solution is normally administered by instructing the patient to drink the liquid through a straw.

• **Procedure — Whole body radioiodine imaging for thyroid cancer**

Equipment — LVOF gamma camera with high energy collimator or whole body imaging device.

Technique — 5 min images to cover whole body.

Comment — Simultaneous serum. Thyroglobulin levels will improve accuracy.

Sodium iodide (^{131}I) injection
- **Chemical form** — Sterile solution of sodium iodide containing sodium thiosulfate and phosphate buffer, made isotonic with sodium chloride.
- **pH** — 7 to 8.
- **Use** — Same indications as for the oral (^{131}I) solution.
- **Dosage and administration** — Same dosage as for the oral (^{131}I) solution, given i.v.

Sodium iodide (^{131}I) diagnostic capsules
- **Formulation** — Gelatin capsules containing sodium iodide solution absorbed onto partly dehydrated disodium hydrogen phosphate as an inert carrier.
- **Use** — Same indications as for the oral (^{131}I) solution. It has been confirmed that thyroid uptake of sodium iodide (^{131}I) is the same whether the isotope is administered in solution or capsule form. The capsules provide a convenient way of administering diagnostic doses by eliminating the need for dispensing and thus reducing the risk of contamination.
- **Dosage and administration** — Same dosage as for the oral (^{131}I) solution. The patient is normally instructed to swallow the capsules with a small volume of liquid.

Sodium iodide (^{131}I) therapy capsules
- **Formulation** — Gelatin capsules containing sodium iodide (^{131}I) solution absorbed on to partly dehydrated disodium hydrogen phosphate as an inert carrier.
- **Use** — Sodium iodide (^{131}I) therapy capsules can be used in place of sodium iodide (^{131}I) solution for radioiodine therapy. This includes treatment of hyperthyroidism in cases where surgery is contraindicated, and the elimination of residual thyroid activity after thyroidectomy in cases of thyroid carcinoma.
- **Dosage and administration — Thyrotoxicosis**

  In order to obtain an estimate of thyroid size and iodide uptake, a diagnostic dose of approximately 0.185 MBq (5 μCi) is recommended. This is followed by the appropriate therapeutic dose, usually in the range 185 to 555 MBq (5 to 15 mCi).

  Ablation of normal thyroid function — 0.925 to 1.85 GBq (25 to 50 mCi).

  Thyroid carcinoma — For total thyroid ablation following thyroidectomy, 2.22 to 7.4 GBq (60 to 200 mCi) repeated after an interval if necessary. The recommended therapy doses are for guidance only, the activity per administration is a matter for clinical judgment, and caution is advised on all treatments of nonmalignant disease, especially in young patients.

  The use of capsules obviates the need for medical staff to come in contact with them, thus minimizing radiation exposure.

Meta-Iodobenzylguanidine (^{131}I) (MIBG)
- **Chemical form** — The sterile aqueous solution contains 9mg/ml of sodium chloride and 10mg/ml of benzyl alcohol.
- **pH** — 4.0 to 7.0.
- **Use** — MIBG (^{131}I) is indicated for adrenal medulla scintigraphy in the investigations of pheochromocytoma, neuroblastoma, and for the assessment of adrenal medullary hyperplasia. Therapeutically, MIBG (^{131}I) is a useful radiopharmaceutical in the treatment of malignant pheochromocytoma and neuroblastoma.
- **Dosage and administration** — The normal adult diagnostic dose is between 18.5 to 37 MBq (0.5 to 1 mCi). A proportionally lower dose is required for infants.

  Imaging is normally performed 24 to 48 h after administration. Most tumours are obvious after 24 h but the decline of background (especially in the liver) may permit optimal imaging at 48 or 72 h.

  The therapeutic dose needs to be decided by the physician, according to plasma and urine catecholamine measurements and determinations of tumor volumes. However, the dose is normally between 3.7 and 7.4 GBq (100 and 200 mCi).

The number of therapy doses administered can vary between 1 and 5 doses at 3 to 6 month intervals, and hence the cummulative dose can vary between 3.7 and 37 GBq (100 and 1000 mCi).

It is recommended that the therapeutic dose be diluted in 50 ml physiological saline immediately after if has been thawed, and then administered within 2 h.

Therapy doses are generally delivered over a 1.5 to 2 h infusion process.

6-Iodomethylnorcholesterol (^{131}I)

- **Chemical form** — Sterile solution of [6-iodomethy-19-norcholest-5 (10)-ene-3-ol] labeled with Iodine-131.
- **Use** — Adrenal cortex imaging.
- **Dosage and administration** — 18.5 to 37 MBq (0.3 to 1 mCi) by intravenous injection. Adrenal images are optimally obtained within 7 d after administration.

Human fibrinogen (^{131}I)

- **Chemical form** — Human fibrinogen (^{131}I) in lyophilized sterile preparation which when reconstituted will yield an isotonic solution.
- **pH** — 7 to 8.
- **Use** — Localization of deep vein thrombosis and tumors.
- **Dosage and administration** 18.5 to 37 MBq (0.5 to 1 mCi) by intravenous injection. Images are best obtained 24 to 48 h post injection.

Rose bengal (^{131}I)

- **Chemical form** — In sterile injection of tetraiodotetrachlorofluorescein sodium salt.
- **pH** — 7 to 8.5.
- **Use** — Investigation of hepatobiliary function specially in evaluating infants for obstructive jaundice.
- **Dosage and administration** — The pattern of rose bengal excretion can be used as a test of biliary patency. Following the i.v. injection of 37 to 185 kBq (1 to 5 μCi) of (^{131}I) rose bengal, the patient's feces and urine are collected, and relative amounts of radioactivity in each are measured. In cases of biliary tract obstruction fecal excretion is impaired and the kidneys become the major route of exit from the body.

Human Serum albumin (^{131}I)

- **Chemical form** — In sterile injectable solution, radioiodinated serum albumin (RISA).
- **pH** — 7 to 8.5.
- **Use** — Determination of plasma volume.
- **Dosage and administration** — The usual dosage for the determination of plasma volume is 185 to 555 kBq (5 to 15 μCi).

IRON-59

Decay of iron-59 (Half-life = 45.6 d)

Time (d)	Factor (%)	Time (d)	Factor (%)	Time (d)	Factor (%)	Time (d)	Factor (%)
−28	154	−12	120	4	94	20	73
−26	150	−10	117	6	91	22	71
−24	145	− 8	113	8	88	24	69
−22	141	− 6	110	10	86	26	67
−20	136	− 4	106	12	83	28	65
−18	132	− 2	103	14	80	30	63
−16	128	0	100	16	78	35	58
−14	124	2	97	18	76	40	54

Note: Days before (−) or days after the reference date.

Principal γ-energies — 1099 (56%), 1292, (44%) keV.

Ferric (⁵⁹Fe) citrate injection

- **Chemical form** — Sterile solution of ferric containing 1% w/v sodium citrate dihydrate and made isotonic with sodium chloride.
- **pH** — 6 to 8.
- **Use** — Ferric (⁵⁹Fe) citrate is used for the investigation of ferrokinetics, which provides insight into the mechanism of anemia and helps in the diagnosis of various hematological disorders.

    There are several indices which can be calculated in ferrokinetic studies, including plasma iron clearance, plasma iron turnover rate, maximum red blood cell utilization of iron-59, and occasionally, a whole-body iron scan.

- **Dosage and administration** — A normal adult dose for ferrokinetic studies is 111 to 370 kBq (3 to 10 μCi), either directly administered intravenously or after incubation with 20 to 30 ml autologous plasma. Blood samples are taken at various time intervals after injection and the hematocrit is determined on all samples. The data obtained from the blood counting can be used to calculate the plasma disappearance time. In addition, external surface counts can be taken by placing a probe over the liver, spleen, heart, and sacral bone marrow.

    A reduced rate of disappearance (normal rate is $T^{1}/_{2}$ 80 to 120 min) of iron from the blood indicates that iron is not being taken up by the bone marrow and is not being utilized in hemoglobin synthesis. An increased rate is due to accelerated iron utilization.

- **Procedure — Ferrokinetics study**

    Equipment — Well scintillation counter.

    Technique — Draw 6 ml sample heparinized blood at 10, 30, 60, and 90 min after injection from another vein, and then at 24 h and alternate days for 3 weeks.

    Quantitative analysis — Plot on semi-log paper determine $T_{1/2}$.

$$\% \text{ RBC incorporation of } ^{59}\text{Fe per day} = \frac{\text{CPM 5 ml blood} \times \text{RBC mass}/5 \times 100}{\text{CPM} \times 20 \times \text{decimal hematocrit}}$$

Comment — Normal $T^{1}_{/2}$ = 6 to 120 min. Red cell incorporation = 60 to 80% of dose in 7 to 10 d. Red cell mass and survival and sequestration can be measured simultaneously.

KRYPTON-81m

Rubidium-81/krypton-81m generator

Decay of Rubidium-81 (Half life = 4.58 h)

Time (h)	Factor (%)	Time (h)	Factor (%)	Time (h)	Factor (%)
−12	620	−2	136	4	55
−10	460	0	100	6	41
−8	340	1	80	8	30
−6	250	2	75	10	22
−4	184	3	64	12	16

Note: Hours before (−) or after the reference date.

Decay of krypton (⁸¹ᵐKr) (Half-life = 13.3 s)

Principal γ-energy — 190 (67%) keV.

- **Chemical form** — Krypton-81m in the liquid phase is obtained through elution of the Rubidium-81/Krypton-81m generator at a predetermined rate with a 5% dextrose solution, while the gas is obtained by passing a continuous air stream through the generator. The air must be adequately humidified before it passes across the ion-exchange resin column containing the Rubidium-81.

• **Use** — Ultra short-lived radiotracers such as Krypton-81m can be inhaled or continuously infused into the circulatory system to obtain dynamic images representing regional organ ventilation or perfusion after radioactive equilibrium has been reached. Two additional advantages of Krypton-81m are that a study can be repeated numerous times at one sitting (in different positions or following interventions), and that the radiation dose is relatively low.

• **Dosage and administration** — The optimum Rubidium-81 activity to be used with the standard generator is 1.5 to 2.2 GBq (40 to 60 mCi). The presence of sodium as NaBr precludes the use of higher ^{81}Rb activities, since the sodium competes with ^{81}Rb for binding sites on the cation exchange resin. (NaBr is the target bombarded with α particles in a cycloton for the production of rubidium-81 — ^{79}Br[^{4}He, 2n]^{81}Rb.) The removal of sodium ions before loading of the column increases the amount of ^{81}Rb which can be used and thus leads to a higher krypton-81m yield. Alternatively, a smaller-volume generator with less resin can be used, resulting in the same yield of ^{81m}Kr with less ^{81}Rb.

   Krypton-81m is ideal for the measurement of regional pulmonary ventilatory rate. High quality images are obtained during steady-state tidal inhalation through a mouth-piece of this radiogas. Multiple views can be obtained with minimal patient cooperation. Perfusion images with ^{99m}Tc-HAM can also be acquired immediately before the ventilation images without having to move the patient. This greatly facilitates ventilation/perfusion imaging for the diagnosis of pulmonary embolism.

   To measure regional perfusion, the ^{81}Rb generator is perfused with sterile 5% dextrose and ^{81m}Kr eluted in solution for intravenous or intra-arterial infusion. In addition, imaging can be repeated within minutes before and after pharmacologic or physiologic interventions.

• **Procedure — Lung ventilation imaging**

   Equipment — LVOF Gamma camera with GAP collimator or high energy collimator.

   Technique — Views obtained with camera peaked to ^{81m}Kr.

   Comment — This examination is usually done with a perfusion lung scan. The combination of these tests increases the sensitivity and specificity of the findings.

MERCURY 197

Decay of Mercury-197 (Half-life = 65 h)

Time (d)	Factor (%)	Time (d)	Factor (%)
−48	167	30	73
−36	147	36	68
−24	129	42	64
−12	114	48	60
0	100	60	53
6	94	72	46
12	88	72	46
24	77	84	40

Note: Day before (−) or after date of reference.

Principal γ-energy — 77 (18%) keV.

Mercury (^{197}Hg) chlormerodrin

- **Chemical form** — Mercuric (^{197}Hg) chlormerodrin in sterile injectable isotonic saline solution.
- **pH** — 2 to 3.
- **Use** — Mercurial diuretics such as chlormerodrine are removed from the blood by the cells of the proximal renal tubules. Part of this radiopharmaceutical is cleared rapidly from the kidneys in the urine, but a significant fraction remains bound in the renal cortex for prolonged periods of time, therefore allowing for diagnostic imaging of the kidneys.
- **Dosage and procedure** — The normal adult dose is 7.4 MBq (200 μCi) given intravenously. Imaging can start 1 h later.

PHOSPHORUS-32

Decay of phosphorus-32 (Half-life = 14.3 d)

Time (d)	Factor (%)	Time (d)	Factor (%)	Time (d)	Factor (%)	Time (d)	Factor (%)
−15	207	−3	116	5	78	25	30
−10	162	−2	110	6	75	30	23
−9	155	−1	105	7	71	35	18
−8	147	0	100	8	68	40	14
−7	140	1	95	9	65	45	11
−6	134	2	91	10	62	50	9
−5	127	3	86	15	48	55	7
−4	121	4	82	20	38	60	6

Note: Days before (−) or days after the reference date.

Principal β-energy — 1709 (100%) keV.

Sodium phosphate (^{32}P) injection

- **Chemical form** — Sterile solution of sodium phosphate made isotonic with phosphate buffer.
- **pH** — 6 to 8.
- **Use** — Sodium Phosphate (^{32}P) is indicated in the treatment of polycythemia vera, a condition in which there is an abnormal increase in the number of red blood cells in the circulation. A further indication is the diagnosis of superficial tumors.

    Following intravenous injection, phosphorus-32 is incorporated into the phosphorus metabolic pathway. The quantity of phosphorus-32 taken up by individual tissues will depend on the rate of proliferation of the tissue cells. Those cells with active proliferation, such as bone marrow, or those cells where mitotic activity is abnormally accelerated, such as malignant cells, will exhibit high uptake.

    The effectiveness of phosphorus-32 therapy is the result of this selective uptake of phosphorus-32 by the hemopoietic tissues, thus providing a continuous field of radiation in the region of the sensitive dividing cells, of sufficient strength to interfere significantly with their viability.

- **Dosage and administration** — For the treatment of polycythemia vera a normal initial dose of 185 MBq (5 mCi) is administered intravenously. Further doses may be given if necessary. However, the life-span of erythrocytes can be up to 4 months, so no further administration of sodium phosphate (^{32}P) should be attempted until the true effect to the first dose has been assessed.

POTASSIUM 42

Decay of potassium-42 (Half-life = 12.4 h)

Time (d)	Factor (%)	Time (d)	Factor (%)
−24	384	2	89
−20	307	6	71
−16	245	10	57
−10	175	16	40
−6	140	20	32
−2	111	24	26
0	100		

Note: Hours before (−) or hours after the reference date.

Principal γ-energy — 1525 (18%) keV.

Potassium (^{42}K) chloride injection

- **Chemical form** — Potassium chloride (^{42}K) in sterile injectable isotonic saline solution.
- **pH** — 6 to 8.
- **Use** — Measurement of exchangeable potassium and coronary blood flow.
- **Dosage and procedure** — Normal adult dose 3.7 MBq (100 μCi) injected intravenously.

SELENIUM-75

Decay of Selenium-75 (Half-life = 120.4 d)

Time (d)	Factor (%)	Time (d)	Factor (%)	Time (d)	Factor (%)	Time (d)	Factor (%)
−30	119	−5	103	1	99	15	92
−20	112	−3	102	3	98	20	89
−15	109	−1	101	5	97	30	84
−10	106	0	100	10	94		

Note: Days before (−) or days after the reference date.

Principal γ-energies — 136 (59%), 265 (59%), 280 (25%) keV.

Selenomethyl (^{75}Se) Norcholesterol

- **Chemical form** — Sterile solution of 6-methyl selenomethyl-19-norcholest-5(10)-en-3 β ol. Containing 8 mg ascorbic acid, 16 mg Polysorbate 80, 80 μl ethanol and isotonic saline.
- **pH** — 2.5 to 3.5.
- **Use** — When administered intravenously, Selenomethyl (^{75}Se) norcholesterol provides a means of imaging the adrenal cortex by gamma-scintigraphy. The diagnostic information gained from the technique is probably of most value in distinguishing unilateral adrenocortical dysfunction from bilateral dysfunction in Cushing's disease, and for the lateral location of other steroid secreting tumors.
- **Dosage and administration** — The normal adult dose is 7.4 MBq (200 μCi) by intravenous injection. For children the dose should be limited to 111 Bq/kg (3 μCi/kg) body mass. Patients suffering from bilateral adrenal hyperplasia have the greatest and most rapid uptake, while those showing symptoms of adrenal insufficiency have

the smallest and slowest uptake. Visualization may be made 2 to 4 d postinjection, and if necessary, repeated at 6 to 10 d postinjection. Prior renal scintigraphy may assist in the localization of the adrenals. Longer term studies are also possible since selenium-75 has a sufficiently long half-life.

- **Procedure — Adrenal cortex scintigraphy**

    Equipment — LFOV gamma camera medium energy high sensitivity collimator. Computer may be used.

    Technique — At 7 d a 300 K count image is obtained centered over the upper poles of kidneys.

    Quantitative analysis — The percentage uptake in each gland may be measured by previously measuring the syringe containing [75]Secholesterol and depth correction.

    Comment — [75]Secholesterol scan may be made after 7 d of suppression with dexamethasone for detection of aldosterone secreting tumor.

L-Selenomethionine (^{75}Se) injection

- **Chemical form** — Sterile aqueous solution of L-selenomethionine.
- **pH** — 5 to 8.
- **Use** — L-Selenomethionine (^{75}Se) injection is indicated for pancreatic scanning when gross impairment of the exocrine function of the gland is suspected. It is also used to detect hyperactive, enlarged parathyroid glands in cases of confirmed hyperparathyroidism.
- **Dosage and administration** — For pancreatic scanning an intravenous injection of approximately 9.25 MBq (250 μCi) is normally administered, followed by scintigraphic examination of the appropriate area; a second scan may be performed 1 to 2 h later.

    L-Selenomethionine (^{75}Se) has also been used to detect hyperactive parathyroid glands with a normal dose of 7.4 to 9.25 MBq (200 to 250 μCi) administered intravenously.

Selenium (^{75}Se) taurocholic acid

- **Chemical form** — <0.1 mg tauroselcholic acid absorbed on inert carrier, disodium hydrogen phosphate dihydrate.
- **Use** — Selenium (^{75}Se) taurocholic acid provides a means for measuring the rate of bile acid loss from the endogenous pool. This can be achieved by determining either the excretion of activity in feces, or the retention of activity in the body over a period of days. The results may be expressed as a rate of loss if several measurements are taken, or, more simply, as a retained percentage after a fixed period.

    Since Selenium (^{75}Se) taurocholic acid is specifically absorbed by the ileum, the extent of loss of ileal bile acid absorptive function in cases of suspected Crohn's disease can be determined.

    A major sympton of bile acid malabsorption is chronic diarrhea (cholegenic diarrhea) due to the inhibitory effect of bile acids on colonic absorption. This may be treated by oral administration of cholestyramine and insoluble bile acid binding resin. Chronic diarrhea can also arise from other causes, for example, ulcerative colitis or infections of the small intestine. Selenium (^{75}Se) taurocholic acid can therefore be used in assisting the classification of patients presenting with chronic diarrhea.

- **Dosage and administration** — The adult dose is one capsule of either 37 kBq (1 μCi) or 370 kBq (10 μCi) administered orally for a single diagnostic procedure.

    The amount of activity retained can be measured using a whole body counter or a counter with a field of view encompassing the abdomen. Measurements are usually made 3 h after administration of the capsule and again after 7 d.

    The alternative method of estimating bile acid loss is by γ scintillation counting of total feacal samples collected over a period of time. Selenium (^{75}Se) has also been used in scintigraphic studies of the enterohepatic circulation.

SODIUM-24

Decay of sodium-24 (Half-life = 14.97 h)

Time (h)	Factor (%)	Time (h)	Factor (%)	Time (h)	Factor (%)
−4	120	3	87	10	63
−3	115	4	83	11	60
−2	110	5	79	12	58
−1	105	6	76	24	33
0	100	7	72	48	11
1	96	8	69	72	4
2	91	9	66	96	1

Note: Hours before (−) or hours after the reference date.

Principal γ-energies — 1369 (100%), 2754 (99.8%) keV.

Sodium (^{24}Na) chloride injection
* **Chemical form** — Sterile isotonic solution of sodium chloride.
* **pH** — 5 to 8.
* **Use** — Determination of exchangeable sodium and sodium space.
* **Dosage and procedure** — The normal adult dose is 185 KBq to 3.7 MBq (5 to 100 μCi) administered orally or intravenously.

STRONTIUM-85

Decay of strontium-85 (Half-life = 64 d)

Time (d)	Factor (%)	Time (d)	Factor (%)	Time (d)	Factor (%)	Time (d)	Factor (%)
−25	131	−5	106	15	85	100	34
−20	124	0	100	20	81	150	20
−15	117	5	95	25	76	200	12
−19	111	10	90	50	59		

Note: Days before (−) or days after the reference date.

Principal γ-energy — 514 (99%) keV.

Strontium (^{85}Sr) Chloride injection
* **Chemical form** — Sterile aqueous solution of strontium chloride.
* **pH** — 4 to 8.
* **Use** — Strontium (^{85}Sr) chloride can be used for bone scintigraphy studies. It is of particular value in assessing the affinity of bone tumors for strontium in cases where the use of strontium-89 is indicated.
* **Dosage and administration** — The normal adult dose for bone scintigraphy is 0.74 to 3.7 MBq (20 to 100 μCi) administered intravenously.

STRONTIUM-89

Decay of strontium-89 (Half-life = 52.7 d)

Time (d)	Factor (%)	Time (d)	Factor (%)	Time (d)	Factor (%)	Time (d)	Factor (%)
−28	147	−14	121	0	100	14	82
−26	143	−12	118	2	97	16	80
−24	139	−10	115	4	95	18	78
−22	135	−8	112	6	92	20	76
−20	132	−6	109	8	90	22	74
−18	128	−4	106	10	87	24	72
−16	125	−2	103	12	85	26	70

Note: Days before (−) or days after the reference date.

Principal β-energy — 1463 (100%) keV.

Strontium (^{89}Sr) Chloride injection
- **Chemical form** — Sterile aqueous solution of strontium chloride.
- **pH** — 4 to 7.5.
- **Use** — Strontium (^{89}Sr) chloride injection is indicated for the palliation of pain in patients suffering from bone metastases.
- **Dosage and administration** — The normal dose is 1.48 MBq (40 μCi) per kilogram of body weight or 111-148 MBq (3 to 4 mCi) per injection.

SULFUR-35

Decay of sulfur-35 (Half-life = 87.9 d)

Time (d)	Factor (%)	Time (d)	Factor (%)	Time (d)	Factor (%)	Time (d)	Factor (%)
−25	122	−5	104	15	89	100	45
−20	117	0	100	20	85	150	30
−15	113	5	96	25	82	200	20
−10	108	10	92	50	67		

Note: Days before (−) or days after the reference date.

Principal β-energy — 167 (100%) keV.

Sodium sulfate (^{35}S) injection
- **Chemical form** — Sterile solution of sodium sulfate in isotonic saline.
- **pH** — 5 to 9.
- **Use** — Sodium sulfate (^{35}S) injection is used for the measurement of extracellular fluid volume.
- **Dosage and administration** — The normal adult dose is 3.7 MBq (100 μCi) administered intravenously.

Following injection the labeled sulfate mixes with the naturally occuring sulfate in the extra-cellular fluid; equilibrium is reached in about 2 h. Provided that the patient does not drink fluids during the mixing stage and does not void, it is not necessary to make a correction for excretion. A single measurement of the specific activity of the plasma or serum enables a calculation of the extracellular fluid volume to be performed.

$$\text{extra-cellular fluid volume} = \frac{\text{activity administered}}{\text{plasma (or serum specific activity)}}$$

TECHNETIUM-99m

Molybdenum-99 decay factors at various times from generator reference time (Molybdenum-99 half-life 66.7 h)

Hours	\multicolumn{9}{c}{Days from generator reference time}
	−2	−1	0	+1	+2	+3	+4	+5	+6
0200	1.8354	1.4276	1.1104	0.8637	0.6717	0.5225	0.4064	0.3161	0.2458
0400	1.7974	1.3980	1.0874	0.8458	0.6578	0.5117	0.3980	0.3095	0.2408
0600	1.7602	1.3690	1.0648	0.8282	0.6442	0.5010	0.3897	0.3031	0.2358
0800	1.7237	1.3407	1.0428	0.8111	0.6308	0.4907	0.3816	0.2968	0.2309
1000	1.6880	1.3129	1.0212	0.7943	0.6178	0.4805	0.3737	0.2907	0.2261
1200	1.6530	1.2857	1.0000	0.7778	0.6050	0.4705	0.3660	0.2847	0.2214
1400	1.6187	1.2590	0.9793	0.7617	0.5924	0.4608	0.3584	0.2788	0.2168
1600	1.5852	1.2330	0.9590	0.7459	0.5802	0.4512	0.3510	0.2730	0.2123
1800	1.5523	1.2074	0.9391	0.7304	0.5681	0.4419	0.3437	0.2673	0.2079
2000	1.5202	1.1824	0.9196	0.7153	0.5564	0.4327	0.3366	0.2618	0.2036
2200	1.4887	1.1579	0.9006	0.7005	0.5448	0.4238	0.3296	0.2564	0.1994
2400	1.4578	1.1339	0.8819	0.6860	0.5335	0.4150	0.3228	0.2510	0.1953

Decay of Technetium-99m (Half life = 6.05 h)

Time (min)	Factor (%)	Time (min)	Factor (%)	Time (min)	Factor (%)	Time (min)	Factor (%)
−330	178	−120	126	60	89	240	63
−270	168	−90	119	90	84	270	60
−240	158	−60	112	120	79	300	56
−210	150	−30	106	150	75		
−180	141	0	100	180	71		
−150	133	30	94	210	67		

Note: Minutes before (−) or days after a given reference point.

Principal γ-energy — 140 (88%) keV.

Factors allowing for growth of technetium-99m at various times following the previous elution

Time (h)	Factor (%)	Time (h)	Factor (%)	Time (h)	Factor (%)	Time (h)	Factor (%)
1	9	11	65	20	83	32	92
2	18	12	68	21	84	34	92
3	26	13	70	22	85	36	93
4	33	14	73	23	86	38	93
5	39	15	75	24	87	40	94
6	44	16	77	25	88	42	94
7	49	17	79	26	89	44	94
8	54	18	80	28	90	46	94
9	58	19	82	30	91	48	94
10	62						

Technetium (^{99m}Tc) sodium pertechnetate

- **Chemical form** — Sterile, pyrogen-free isotomic solution of technetium (^{99m}Tc) per-technetate.

- **Use** — Sodium pertechnetate (^{99m}Tc) is used for scintigraphy, particularly of the brain and thyroid. It can also be used to prepare various technetium-99m labeled radiopharmaceuticals for selective organ imaging, especially of the liver, lung, bone, kidney, and brain.
- **Dosage and administration** — Technetium-99m is normally administered by intravenous injection with doses which vary widely according to the clinical information required and the equipment employed. The table below shows the recommended maximum adult activity per test, although for clinical reasons other amounts may be necessary.

Brain imaging (static pertechnetate)	740 MBq (20 mCi)
Thyroid imaging (pertechnetate)	37 MBq (1 mCi)
Hepatobiliary preparations	148 MBq (4 mCi)
Liver preparations	74 MBq (2 mCi)
Lung preparations	74 MBq (2 mCi)
Bone preparations	740 MBq (20 mCi)
Kidney preparations for static imaging	74 MBq (2 mCi)
Kidney preparations for dynamic studies	185 MBq (5 mCi)

- **Procedures — 1. Thyroid scintigraphy**

  Equipment — Standard gamma camera with pinhole collimator, computer if measuring uptake simultaneously.

  Technique — Wash esophagus with glass of water; anterior view with maximum magnification 200 K counts of 15 min. LAO and RAO if indicated. Repeat with ^{57}Co marker on nodule or suprasternal notch if indicated.

  Quantitative analysis — Measure uptake using ROI around thyroid and also a background ROI and express as percentage of a standard or the syringe measured in a thyroid phantom at a set distance from the gamma camera.

  Comment — Scan must be combined with manual examination of the gland.

- **Procedures — 2. Salivary gland scintigraphy**

  Equipment — Standard field of view gamma camera with GAP or high resolution collimator and computer.

  Technique — 2 min images of anterior neck to include all 4 glands for 30 min. Continuous data collection. If obstruction is suspected a stimulant (acid drop or lemon) is given and recording continued for 15 min. If mass lesion is suspected magnified images of the gland or glands using pinhole or converging collimator with oblique views and 300 K counts are obtained.

  Quantitative analysis — Using ROI over glands, measure rate of accumulated activity and rate of discharge with stimulant.

- **Procedures — 3. Meckel's diverticulum imaging**

  Equipment — LFOV gamma camera.

  Technique — Anterior abdominal images every 5 min up to 30 min. Lateral and posterior images as indicated.

  Comment — Pentagastrin with or without nasogastric suction may also be used to enhance ectopic uptake while removing intragastric activity.

- **Procedures — 4. Testicular and scrotal imaging**

  Equipment — LFOV gamma camera with GAP collimator.

  Technique — Anterior blood flow 1 s frames. Static images 5, 10 and 15 min postinjection acquiring 300 K images.

  Comment — Penis should be positioned cephalad and taped to the abdominal wall. Scrotum can be raised with cotton wool padding, or plastic foam sponge.

- **Procedures — 5. First pass angiocardiography**

  Equipment — Standard field of view gamma camera with high resolution collimator. Computer, R wave trigger.

Technique — Rapid sequence imaging during first pass with data acquisition in list, frame, or histogram mode. View depends on clinical problem, RAO or A. If using autologous red blood cells proceed to routine gated blood pool study.

Quantitative analysis — Measure ejection fraction and L — R shunting.

Technetium (^{99m}Tc) Mercapto-acetyltriglycine (MAG 3)

- **Chemical form** — Sterile and nonpyrogenic vial containing benzoylmercaptoacetyltriglicine, disodium tartrate, and stannous chloride, which, when reconstituted with ^{99m}Tc-sodium pertechnetate, produces a ^{99m}Tc-MAG 3 complex suitable for diagnostic renal function studies.
- **pH** — 5 to 6.
- **Uses** — After intravenous injection ^{99m}Tc-labeled MAG 3 is rapidly cleared from the blood by the kidneys in a manner similar to that of hippuran. Recording of individual renal activity enables the measurement of blood flow, tubular transit time, and excretion.
- **Dosage and administration** — The suggested dose for intravenous administration to a normal adult for the study of nephrological and urological disorders 74 to 185 MBq (2 to 5 mCi).

Colloidal (^{99m}Tc) Antimony or Rhenium Sulfide

- **Chemical form** — Sterile, pyrogen-free solution of antimony or rhenium sulfide, gelatin, ascorbic acid, and water for injection, which when reconstituted with sodium pyrophaste, stannous chloride, and technetium-99m pertechnetate, renders a colloidal ^{99m}Tc Antimony or Rhenium sulfide solution ready for scintigraphy of the lymphatic system.
- **pH** — 5 to 7.
- **Use** — Colloidal (^{99m}Tc) antimony or rhenium sulfide is used in the evaluation of and diagnosis of peripheral edema, lymphoadenoid investigation of the limbs, extension evaluation of visceral and breast cancers, investigation of thoracic ganglia for localization of radiotherapy fields, extension and evaluation of malignant hematolymphopaties, and drainage of cutaneous malignant melanoma.
- **Dosage and administration** — The doses administered are 74 to 185 MBq (2 to 5 mCi) in a volume of 0.2 to 0.5 ml per injection site. For studying the lymphatic draining system of limbs: superficial subcutaneous injection in the first interdigital space of the hand or of the foot. For studying the thoracic ganglia: deep intramuscular abdominal injection in the sheath of rectus below the subcostal margin on the side explored.
- **Procedure — Lymphoscintigraphy**

  Equipment — LFOV gamma camera with GAP or high sensitivity collimator.

  Technique — Image regional lymph nodes, covering the injection site with lead if in field of view.

  Comment — Obtain delayed images up to 6 hrs post injection.

Hexakis (isonitrile) technetium (^{99m}Tc) complexes

- **Chemical form** — Hexakis (alkylisonitrile) agents, such as carbomethoxyisopropyl isonitrile (CPI) or 2-Methoxyisobutyl isonitrile (MIBI) are prepared in sterile, pyrogen-free vials which when reconstituted with ^{99m}Tc Pertechnetate form ^{99m}Tc-CPI, MIBI complexes.
- **pH** — 7.4.
- **Use** — Hexakis (alkyloisonitrile) complexes of Technetium-99m are used to study myocardial blood flow for the scintigraphic assessment of coronary artery disease and

myocardial infarction. Scintigraphy with these agents provides an elegant method to assess the efficacy of revascularization.

- **Dosage and administration** — Myocardial perfusion studies with ^{99m}Tc-CPI, MIBI can be performed during exercise stress or at rest. Following an intravenous injection of 185 to 370 MBq (5 to 10 mCi) of the complex imaging can be started ten minutes later with a planar or SPECT rotating gamma camera. Exercise protocols and data processing programs are similar to those used with thallium-201 myocardial perfusion studies. The rapid myocardial clearance of ^{99m}Tc-CPI, MIBI permits reinjection of the tracer 3 to 4 hours after the first injection and completion of the stress and rest studies within the same day.

It appears that ^{99m}Tc-isonitrile complexes distribute proportionally to myocardial blood flow, but because of the slow lung clearance, they redistribute into zones of transient hyperemia with time. It is possible that the mechanism of ^{99m}Tc-isonitriles is less dependent on an active process than ^{201}Tl.

Technetium (^{99m}Tc) human albumin microspheres (HAM)

- **Chemical form** — Sterile pyrogen free vial containing freeze-dried human serum albumin microspheres (23 to 45 μm), stannous chloride and sodium chloride, which when reconstituted with ^{99m}Tc pertechnetate provides a suspension of human albumin microsphere labeled with technetium-99m.
- **pH** — 7 to 9.
- **Use** — Technetium (^{99m}Tc) human albumin microsphere are used for the quantitative scintigraphic assessment of organs tissues perfusion.
- **Dosage and administration** — The dose of intravenous or intra-arterial administration to an adult patient is 37 to 111 MBq (1 to 3 mCi). When injected intra-arterially, the microspheres are stopped completely at the level of the first microcirculatory network present downstream to the injection point. Assuming that they have totally mixed with the inflowing blood stream, the distribution of the microsphere will reflect the blood flow within the organ. When injected intravenously, the microspheres mix uniformly with the blood before they reach the main pulmonary artery; they are then extracted completely from the circulation as the blood makes its first passage through the lung capillaries, allowing quantitative lung imaging to be performed.

The normal applications of lung scintigraphy are for diagnosis of pulmonary embolism, chronic obstructive airways disease, space occupying lesions such as carcinoma and abscess, and other pulmonary diseases, such as pneumonia and tuberculosis.

The ^{99m}Tc-HAM can also be used in radionuclide venography.

- **Procedure — 1. Lung perfusion imaging**

  Equipment — LFOV Gamma camera with GAP or HIGH resolution collimator.

  Technique — 500 K count images of A, P, RL, LL, RPO, LPO.

  Quantitative analysis — Useful in determining relative pulmonary arterial perfusion in patients with compromised lung function in order to predict post-operative lung function prior to pneumonectomy.

  Comment — This is usually done with ventilation scan. When combined with a perfusion lung scan, increases the sensitivity and specificity of the findings.

- **Procedure — 2. Radionuclide venogram**

  Equipment — Large field of view gamma camera with GAP collimator.

  Technique — With tourniquets on obtain sequential 10 to 20 K count images of calves, knees, thighs, and abdomen. Repeat with tourniquets off, and again after lung scan or after leg raising.

  Comment — Performed in conjunction with lung scan.

Technetium (⁹⁹ᵐTc) human serum albumin (HSA)

- **Chemical form** — Sterile pyrogen-free vial containing freeze-dried human serum albumin and stannous chloride, which, when reconstituted with ^{99m}Tc-pertechnetate, provides a suspension complex of Technetium-99m human serum albumin.
- **pH** — 6.5 to 8.5
- **Use** — Technetium (^{99m}Tc) human serum albumin is used as a blood pool imaging agent, i.e., cardiac blood pool scintigraphy and measurement of blood volume.
- **Dosage and administration** — The dose for intravenous administration to an adult patient is 185 to 740 MBq (5 to 20 mCi). Following intravenous injection ^{99m}Tc-HSA remains in the blood stream long enough for usual blood pool procedures to be carried out. About 16% of the complex is cleared from the plasma in the first hour, and about 50% in 6 h.

Technetium (⁹⁹ᵐTc) human fibrinogen

- **Chemical form** — Sterile and pyrogen-free vial containing freeze-dried human fibrinogen, stannous chloride, glycine buffer, and sodium chloride, which, when reconstituted with ^{99m}Tc-pertechnetate, forms a Technetium 99m-Fibrinogen complex.
- **pH** — 9 to 10.5.
- **Use** — Technetium (^{99m}Tc) human fibrinogen is indicated for the detection of deep venous thrombosis, detection of tumors, as well as for differentiation of malignancies from inflammatory processes.
- **Dosage and administration** — The dose for intravenous administration to an adult patient is 370 to 740 MBq (10 to 20 mCi).

  At 6 h post injection 35 % of the injected dose is still circulating in the blood and an amount greater than 60% of this activity is still clottable. Apart from the circulating activity ^{99m}Tc-Fibrinogen is observed in the liver where it is metabolized. Excretion occurs through the kidneys. This radiopharmaceutical behaves like endogenous fibrinogen, transforming into fibrin under thrombin reaction. Images of thrombi or tumors are usually obtained 3 to 6 h post-injection.

Technetium (⁹⁹ᵐTc) iminodiacetic acid (IDA)

- **Chemical form** — Sterile and nonpyrogenic vial containing freeze-dried N-(2.6 dimethylphenylcarboylmethyl) iminodiacetic acid (IDA) or derivatives and stannous chloride (as Sn $Cl_2 \cdot 2H_2O$), for use by addition of sodium pertechnetate (^{99m}Tc). Other derivatives of IDA are carbamolmethyl iminodiacetic acid (HIDA), para-isopropyl iminodiacetic acid (PIPIDA), diethyl iminodiacetic acid (DIDA), diisopropyl iminodiacetic acid (DISIDA), or paraisopropyl iminodiacetic acid (BIDA).
- **pH** — 5.5 to 6.5.
- **Use** — The injection of this radiopharmaceutical is indicated for the investigation of hepatic function and for the scintigraphic imaging of the hepatobiliary system. Patients with liver cell disease or partial biliary blockage exhibit delayed hepatic transport of the tracer with an increase in urinary excretion and accompanying kidney visualization. Differential diagnosis of hepatocellular and obstructive jaundice is possible by obtaining delayed images. Extrahepatic bile duct disease may cause visualization of dilated bile ducts. Hepatobiliary imaging with technetium (^{99m}Tc) IDA has been demonstrated to be of value in neonatal jaundice.

  The functioning gall bladder is imaged during technetium (^{99m}Tc) IDA scintigraphy. It has been reported that in fasting patients the absence of accumulated activity in the gall bladder is diagnostic of common bile duct obstruction or cholecystitis.

  Technetium (^{99m}Tc) IDA may also be used for postsurgical detection of duodeno-gastric or jejuno-gastric reflux.

- **Dosage and administration** — The normal adult dose is 74 to 150 MBq (2 to 4 mCi). Imaging should commence immediately following injection. Sequential images can be obtained of the liver, gall bladder, and bile ducts for the detection of abnormalities in these structures.
- **Procedure — Hepatobiliary imaging**

    Equipment — LFOV gamma camera with GAP collimator.

    Technique — 300 K count image of liver anteriorly at 2 min. Right lateral views as indicated. Repeat for the same time every 5 min to 45 min. If gallbladder and duodenum are not visualized, continue intermittently up to 4 h.

    Comment — Gallbladder response to cholecystokinin or fatty meal may be measured after gallbladder filling.

Technetium (^{99m}Tc) glucoheptonate

- **Chemical form** — Sterile and nonpyrogenic vial containing freeze-dried calcium gluconate and stannous chloride, which when reconstituted with sodium pertechnetate (^{99m}Tc) produces a labeled complex suitable for kidney/brain imaging.
- **pH** — 6.0 to 7.0.
- **Use** — Scintigraphy with this agent provides information on the shape, size, and anatomical position of the kidneys. Perfusion defects arising from lesions or vascular diseases are visualized and sequential imaging provides information on the patency of the ureters and ureteral reflux. The tracer can also be used for the evaluation of renal transplants.

    Technetium (^{99m}) glucoheptonate may be used for imaging of brain tumors, particularly those located in regions of high vascularity, such as the posterior fossa, orbits, and base of the skull. It is also useful in localizing other brain lesions in which the blood-brain-barrier has been impaired.

- **Dosage and administration** — For kidney studies the normal adult dose is 74 to 200 MBq (2 to 5 mCi). Serial imaging to obtain data on the vascular phase of renal clearance should begin immediately after injection. Delayed images at 1 to 2 h post-injection provide optimum static, morphological visualization.

    For brain studies the normal adult dose is 370 to 740 MBq (10 to 20 mCi). Static images are obtained 1 to 2 h postinjection.

Technetium (^{99m}TC) Stannous, Pyrophosphate (PYP)

- **Chemical form** — Sterile and nonpyrogenic vial containing lyophilized sodium pyrophosphate (PYP) and stannous chloride for reconstitution with isotonic saline providing a solution for *in vivo* or semi *in vitro* loading of erythrocytes with stannous ions, preparatory to ^{99m}Tc labeling.
- **pH** — 5.5 to 7.5.
- **Uses** — The agent enables blood pool scintigraphic studies to be performed. Visualization of the cardiac chambers allows evaluation of cardiac ventricular function.

    The stannous (PYP) agent may be used in evaluating the patency of the peripheral vascular system and to detect gastrointestinal bleeding.

    While the "cold" nonradioactive PYP is used for loading of erythrocytes with stannous ions, the radioactively labeled Technetium (^{99m}) pyrophosphate is also used for bone scintigraphy, and myocardial scintigraphy as the agent is suited for the recognition of acute (24 h to 7 d) myocardial infarctions.

- **Dosage and administration** — The recommended dose of the reconstituted nonradioactive injection is 0.03 ml/kg body weight. The normal adult dose of pertechnetate (^{99m}Tc) is 370 to 740 MBq (10 to 20 mCi). Imaging is normally commenced a few minutes after injection of either pertechnetate (^{99m}Tc) or technetium-99m labeled red cells (depending on the labeling method chosen).

- **Procedure — 1. Multiple gated blood pool imaging**

    Equipment — Standard field of view gamma camera, high resolution or slant hole collimator and computer with R wave trigger.

    Technique — Image to attain a count density of greater than 250 counts/pixel over the left ventrile in each frame. Views are RAO, A, LAO, possible LPO. Repeat during stress (isometric hand grip, cold stimulation, exercise) or drug intervention.

    Quantitative analysis — Measure ejection fraction routinely. There are many other parameters which may be used.

- **Procedure — 2. Myocardial infarct scintigraphy**

    Equipment — Standard field of view gamma camera with high resolution collimator. Technique — 500 K count images in A, LAO 35° and 70°, LL views.

    Comment — Single photon emission tomography is helpful.

- **Procedure — 3. Localization of lower GI bleeding**

    Equipment — LFOV gamma camera with GAP collimator.

    Technique — Anterior abdomen images every 5 min for 30 min. Then as indicated up to 24 h; lateral views as necessary.

Technetium (^{99m}Tc) dimercaptosuccinic acid (DMSA)

- **Chemical form** — Sterile and nonpyrogenic vial containing freeze-dried dimercaptosuccinic acid, stannous chloride, ascorbic acid, sodium chloride, and inositol, which when recontituted with ^{99m}Tc sodium pertechnetate produces a ^{99m}Tc-DMSA complex suitable for diagnostic renal functional studies.
- **pH** — 2.3 to 3.3.
- **Uses** — The injection is used for visualization of the kidneys and may also be used in the determination of individual renal function.
- **Dosage and administration** — Kidney imaging — The usual adult dose is 37 to 74 MBq (1 to 2 mCi) by intravenous injection. Optimal kidney imaging is obtained between 1 and 3 h following injection.

    Assessment of kidney function — The usual adult dose is 74 MBq (2 mCi) by intravenous injection. Quantitative measurements should be carried out between 6 and 24 h following administration.

- **Procedure — Static renal scintigraphy**

    Equipment — LFOV Gamma Camera with high resolution collimator.

    Technique — 500 K count images posterior view oblique and lateral views as indicated. Quantitative analysis — Analysis of differential uptake with background subtracted.

    Comment — Using large doses blood flow image may be obtained.

Technetium (^{99m}Tc) diethylenetriamine-penta acetate (DTPA)

- **Chemical form** — Sterile and nonpyrogenic vial containing freeze-dried calcium trisodium diethylenetriamine-penta acetate, stannous chloride and sodium para-aminobenzoate, which, when recontituted with ^{99m}Tc sodium pertechnetate, produces a solution containing a ^{99m}Tc-DTPA complex suitable for diagnostic kidney/brain scintigraphy
- **pH** — 4.0 to 5.0.
- **Uses** — The agent is indicated for renal studies providing both anatomical and functional information.

    Measurement of individual kidney function is of particular interest in the management of unilateral and bilateral uropathy, staging of disease, assessment of unilateral compensatory hypertrophy, and cases where X-ray examinations (i.v. pyelography, etc.) are contraindicated.

Technetium (^{99m}Tc) DTPA is also suitable for conventional cerebral scintigraphy studies and is indicated for the detection of vascular and neoplastic brain lesions.

- **Dosage and administration** — The suggested dose for intravenous administration to a normal adult is as follows: for kidney imaging and GFR determination, up to 200 MBq (5.4 mCi); for brain imaging 740 MBq (20 mCi).
- **Procedure — 1. Dynamic renal imaging**

    Equipment — LFOV gamma camera, GAP collimator, computer.

    Technique — Posterior views (anterior for transplant) at 0 to 30 s, images for at least 20 min.

    Quantitative analysis — Analysis of relative blood flow, divided GFR, parenchymal transit time.

    Comment — Fluids + + and empty bladder frequently after study to reduce bladder dose.
- **Procedure — 2. Dynamic renal imaging with furosemide**

    Equipment — As per dynamic renal scan with ^{99m}Tc DTPA.

    Technique — Image kidneys for at least 5 min after administration of Furosemide.
    Quantitative analysis — Measure percentage and rate of washout from renal pelvis.

    Comment — Warn patient of diuretic effect of furosemide.
- **Procedure — 3. Vesico ureteric reflux imaging**

    Equipment — LFOV gamma camera with GAP collimator. Large storage data logging device.

    Technique — Record data before, during and for 2 min post micturition.

    Quantitative analysis — Measure change in activity in kidneys and ureters before, during and after micturition.

    Comment — Female technicians for females and vice versa for males. Only suitable for children 3 years and older.
- **Procedure — 4. Brain scintigraphy**

    Equipment — Standard field of view gamma camera with GAP collimator and computer.

    Technique — One second images usually in the anterior view during the first pass with continuous data acquisition. Anterior view (or full 5 view) blood equilibrium image immediately after dynamic scan each for 500 K counts. At 90 min 500 K count images in A, P, LL, PL and vertex positions.

    Quantitative analysis — Time activity curves plotted from ROI over the two hemispheres.

    Comment — Delayed views may be helpful in equivocal cases when using technetium-99m pertechnetate.

Technetium (^{99m}Tc) hexamethyl propyleneamineoxime (HM0-PAO)

- **Chemical form** — Sterile and nonpyrogenic vial containing a freeze-dried mixture of hexamethyl propyleneamineoxime (HM-PAO) stannous chloride and sodium chloride, sealed under an inert nitrogen atmosphere, which, when reconstituted with ^{99m}Tc-sodium pertechnetate, produces a lipophilic, low molecular weight solution containing a ^{99m}T-HM-PAO complex suitable for cerebral blood flow scintigraphy by single photon emission computerized tomography techniques.
- **pH** — 9 to 9.8.
- **Uses** — Technetium (^{99m}Tc) HM-PAO intravenous injection is used for regional cerebral blood flow scintigraphy. In stroke, reduced cerebral blood flow appears as photopenic areas on scintigrams. Technetium (^{99m}Tc) HM-PAO scintigraphy may also be useful in investigations of transient ischaemic attack, migraine and tumors of the brain.

In epilepsy, areas of both ictally increased and interictally decreased perfusion have been demonstrated. Characteristic areas of reduced perfusion have been demonstrated in Alzheimer's disease, which may provide the basis for differential diagnosis of dementia.

- **Dosage and administration** — The normal adult (70 kg) dose is 350 to 500 MBq (9.5 to 13.5 mCi) by intravenous injection. Although gross abnormalities of regional cerebral blood flow may be visualized by planar imaging, it is strongly recommended that SPECT imaging be carried out to maximize the value of the study.

Technetium (⁹⁹ᵐTc) macroaggregate albumin (MAA)

- **Chemical form** — Sterile and non pyrogenic vial containing a freeze-dried mixture of human albumin macroaggregates, hydrated stannous oxide, and poloxamer, which, when reconstituted with ⁹⁹Tc-sodium pertechnetate, provides a suspension of macroaggregated albumin labeled with technetium-99m suitable for intravenous or arterial diagnostic use. Particle size, 10 to 60 μm diameter.
- **pH** — 5.0 to 7.0.
- **Use** — Technetium (⁹⁹ᵐTc) MAA is indicated for the scintigraphic detection lung perfusion patterns.

    Lung scintigraphy is important in the diagnosis of pulmonary embolism and in the management of patients with carcinoma of the bronchus, emphysema, pleural effusions, and congestive heart failure.
- **Dosage and administration** — The dose for intravenous administration to an adult patient is 37 to 74 MBq (1 to 2 mCi). Imaging should commence promptly after injection.

    The suggested number of MAA particles per adult injection is 0.5×10^6. For general guidance the nominal particle number present in 74 MBq (2 mCi) dose at various times after preparation can be estimated from the table given below.

Number of particles ($\times 10^6$) per 74 MBq (2 mCi) dose at various times after preparation

Technetium-99m added to vial		Time after preparation (h)				
GBq	mCi	0	2	4	6	8
0.74	20	0.60	0.76	0.95	1.20	1.51
1.11	30	0.40	0.50	0.63	0.81	1.01
1.48	40	0.30	0.40	0.48	0.60	0.75
1.85	50	0.24	0.30	0.38	0.48	0.60
2.22	60	0.20	0.25	0.32	0.40	0.50
2.59	70	0.17	0.22	0.27	0.34	0.43
2.96	80	0.15	0.19	0.24	0.30	0.38
3.33	90	0.13	0.17	0.21	0.27	0.33
3.70	100	0.12	0.15	0.19	0.24	0.30
4.07	110	0.11	0.14	0.17	0.22	0.27
4.44	120	0.10	0.13	0.16	0.20	0.25
4.81	130	0.09	0.12	0.15	0.18	0.23
5.18	140	0.09	0.11	0.14	0.17	0.22
5.55	150	0.08	0.10	0.13	0.16	0.20

Technetium (⁹⁹ᵐTc) colloid agent

- **Chemical form** — Sterile and nonpyrogenic vial containing a freeze-dried mixture of stannous fluoride (chloride), sodium fluoride, and poloxamer, which, when reconstituted with ^{99m}Tc sodium pertechnetate, produces a suspension of technetium-^{99m} labeled colloid, of a size range 0.05 to 0.6 μm, for diagnostic use.

- **pH** — 4.0 to 6.0.
- **Use** — The agent is indicated for scintigraphic studies of the liver and spleen reticuloendothelial system (RES).

   Both benign and malignant tumors, as well as abscesses and cysts, are observed as regions of reduced uptake of radioactivity on the liver scintigram. Nonhomogenous colloidal uptake may be observed in other hepatocellular disease states. Increased splenic, lung, or bone marrow uptake may be diagnostic of diffuse liver disease such as cirrhosis, hepatitis, and fatty infiltration. The anatomical position, size, and shape of the liver and spleen may also be assessed from the scintigram.

- **Dosage and administration** — The normal adult dose is up to 80 MBq (2.2 mCi) by intravenous injection. Imaging should commence 10 min after injection.
- **Procedure — 1. Liver-spleen scintigraphy**

   Equipment — LFOV gamma camera with GAP collimator.

   Technique — Standard 4 views (A, P, RL, LL). 500 K counts each with extra anterior view with costal margin marker.

   Comment — May be combined with ''first pass'' blood flow study.
- **Procedure — 2. Bone marrow scintigraphy**

   Equipment — LFOV gamma camera with GAP collimator or whole body imaging device.

   Technique — 5 minute images of posterior thoracic and lumbar spine, posterior pelvis, both shoulders, both upper femora (distal limbs if indicated).

   Comment — Do routine liver/spleen scan.

Technetium (^{99m}Tc) methylene diphosphonic acid (MDP)

- **Chemical form** — Sterile and non-pyrogenic vial containing freeze-dried methylene diphosphonic acid (as sodium salt), stannous chloride and preservative, which when reconstituted with ^{99m}Tc sodium pertechnetate produces a solution of technetium-99m MDP complex suitable for bone imaging.
- **pH** — 5.5 to 7.5.
- **Uses** — The injection is indicated for skeletal scintigraphy, especially for the detection of pathological osteogenesis. Scintigraphy has proved valuable in the detection of primary and metastatic bone disease. Additionally it has been found useful in the detection and delineation of lesions of inflammatory, infectious, degenerative and metabolic bone and joints disease.
- **Dosage and administration** — The normal adult dose is 370-740 MBq (10 to 20 mCi) by intravenous injection. Scanning should commence at least 2 h after injection.
- **Procedure — 1. Skeletal scintigraphy**

   Equipment — LFOV gamma camera, high resolution collimator or coverging collimator/pinhole for hips or whole body imaging device.

   Technique — 500 K count images of anterior chest for fixed time to cover the body anteriorly and posteriorly depending on size of patient and field of view or equivalent count density for whole body imaging device.

   Quantitative analysis — Sacroiliac activity quantitation if indicated.

   Comment — Advise patient to drink and empty bladder frequently to reduce bladder dose.
- **Procedure — 2. Three phase bone imaging**

   Equipment — LFOV or standard field camera, depending on size of area to be examined. High resolution or converging collimator.

Technique — Begin immediately 1 s sequential images for "flow" study. Static images commenced within 1 min for "blood pool" phase, then 3 h delay for static bone scan images. 500 K count delayed images of involved side. Comparison contralateral side for same time.

Comment — May be done in association with whole body images for additional assessment of particular symptomatic site.

THALLIUM-201

Decay of thallium-201 (Half-life = 73 h)

Time (d)	Factor (%)	Time (d)	Factor (%)	Time (d)	Factor (%)	Time (d)	Factor (%)
−6	392	−3	198	0	100	3	50
−5	312	−2	158	1	80		
−4	248	−1	126	2	63		

Note: Days before (−) or days after the reference date.

Principal γ-energy — 68 to 82 (95% Hg X-rays) keV.

Thallous (^{201}Tl) chloride injection

- Chemical form — Sterile isotonic aqueous solution of thallous (^{201}Tl) chloride containing 0.9% (v/v) benzyl alcohol as preservative and 0.75% (w/v) sodium chloride to achieve isotonicity.
- pH — 4.5 to 7.0.
- Use — Thallous (^{201}Tl) chloride injection is indicated for myocardial perfusion scintigraphy in the investigation of coronary artery disease, acute myocardial infarction, and postsurgical assessment of coronary artery bypass graft patency.

  Resting thallium-201 images have intrinsically poor myocardial to background ratios. There are, however, a number of ways in which exercise testing and dypiridamole can be used in order to optimize the diagnostic information by improving the ratios of uptake between myocardium and background, and between damaged and healthy regions of myocardial tissue, and comparison with resting reperfusion images.

- **Dosage and administration** — Thallous (^{201}Tl) chloride injection is supplied ready for intravenous injection. The normal adult dose is 55.5 MBq (1.5 mCi). The rapid clearance of intravenously administered thallium-201 from the blood (half-time less than 1 min) ensures minimal interference with myocardial imaging.

  The intracellular distribution will show higher accumulation of activity in viable myocardium than in surrounding tissues. Reduced uptake is indicative of poorly perfused myocardium.

- **Procedure — Myocardial perfusion scintigraphy**

  Equipment — Standard field of view gamma camera, GAP collimator, computer, SPECT.

  Technique — 600 K count images screening the extracardiac structures with lead sheet. Views are A, LAO (45 and 55°), LL delayed views at 4 h, as indicated.

  Quantitative analysis — Varies from background subtraction to various filters and count density measurements.

  Comment — Pharmacological stress with dipyridamole may be substituted for exercise.

Thallium (^{201}Tl) Diethyldithiocarbamate (DDC)

- Chemical form — Sodium diethyldithiocarbamate is in sterile solution made isotonic with sodium chloride, and stabilized with dithiothreitol. When mixed with Thallous (^{201}Tl) chloride it forms a lipophylic complex for studies of brain blood flow.
- pH — 7.4 to 9.
- Use — The ^{201}Tl-DDC complex has lipophylic properties which make it suitable for regional cerebral blood flow studies with single photon emission tomography (SPECT). This agent is easy to prepare with chemicals of analytical grade, low priced and available 24 h.
- **Dosage and procedure** — After intravenous injection of the adult dose of 111 MBq (3 mCi) of ^{201}Tl-DDC imaging can be started immediately with a SPECT rotating gamma camera.

XENON-127

Decay of Xenon-127 (Half life = 36.4 d)

Time (d)	Factor (%)	Time (d)	Factor (%)	Time (d)	Factor (%)
−60	310	−6	112	8	87
−50	258	−4	108	10	84
−40	212	−2	104	20	69
−30	178	0	100	30	57
−20	146	2	98	40	48
−10	122	4	94	50	40
−8	117	6	90	60	33

Note: Days before (−) or days after the reference date.

Principal γ-energies 172 (22%), 203, (65%), 375 (20%) keV.

Xenon (^{127}Xe) gas

- **Uses** — Xenon (^{127}Xe) gas is used for evaluation of pulmonary ventilation and measurement of regional cerebral blood flow. Inhaled xenon passes into the pulmonary venous circulation. It exchanges freely between blood and tissues, locating preferentially in body fat rather than blood, plasma, water or protein solutions. The major portion of xenon-127 entering the circulation from a single breath is released through the lungs by an alveolo-capillary diffusion mechanism after a single pass through the peripheral circulation.
- **Dosage and administration** — In practice a wide range of doses can be used, the final choice depending on the investigation, apparatus available, and sensitivity of detecting equipment. The recommended maximum administered dose is 37 MBq (1 mCi) per liter rebreathed for 2 min. Xenon-127 should be superior to Xenon-133 because of its higher photon yield per becquerel of activity, better photon energy for imaging with gamma-camera systems, lower radiation dose to the patient per useful photon detected, and longer shelf-life.

XENON-133

Decay of xenon-133 (Half life = 5.27 d)

Time (d)	Factor (%)	Time (d)	Factor (%)	Time (d)	Factor (%)	Time (d)	Factor (%)
−4	170	1	88	6	45	11	23
−3	149	2	77	7	40	12	20
−2	130	3	67	8	35	13	18
−1	114	4	59	9	30	14	16
0	100	5	52	10	27		

Note: Days before (−) or days after the reference date.

Principal γ-energy — 81 (37%) keV.

Xenon (^{133}Xe) gas

- **Uses** — Xenon (^{133}Xe) gas is used for evaluation of pulmonary ventilation.

    Inhaled xenon passes into the pulmonary circulation. It exchanges freely between blood and tissue, locating preferentially in body fat rather than blood, plasma, water or protein solutions. The major portion of xenon-133 entering the circulation from a single breath is released through the lungs by an alveolo-capillary diffusion mechanism after a single pass through the peripheral circulation.

- **Dosage and administration** — In practice a wide range of doses can be used, the final choice depending on the investigation, apparatus available and sensitivity of detecting equipment. The recommended maximum administered dose is 37 MBq (1 mCi) per liter rebreathed for 2 min. A knowledge of the exact amount of xenon-133 administered is not important as this does not normally enter into subsequent calculations. The two essential measurements are the distribution of activity over a particular body area and its rate of elimination.

    Xenon-133 gas is administered by inhalation of a mixture of xenon-133 and a nonradioactive gas, usually air or oxygen.

Xenon (^{133}Xe) injection

- **Chemical form** — Sterile and non-pyrogenic vial containing xenon-133 gas dissolved in sterile isotonic saline.

- **Use** — Xenon-133 in saline is used as an indicator for the measurement of local blood flow in brain, muscle, skin, and other organs.

    Xenon is soluble in water and body fluids, such as blood. It is also freely diffusible in most tissues and readily passes through the alveolar membrane of the lung. A large proportion of xenon-133 will transfer from a liquid solution into any gas phase coming into contact with it. The clearance of xenon-133 from the body is therefore extremely rapid, 95% of the blood activity being cleared in a single passge through the lung.

- **Dosage and administration** — In practice a wide range of dosages can be used; the final choice depending on the investigation, apparatus available, and sensitivity of detecting equipment. The maximum recommended dose is 185 MBq (5 mCi).

    A knowledge of the exact amount of xenon-133 administered is not important as this does not normally enter into calculations. The two essential measurements are the distribution of activity over a particular body area and its rate of elimination.

    After administration of xenon-133 to a particular organ, either by direct injection or in blood entering it, the flow of blood through the organ can be assessed by measuring the wash out of xenon-133.

    Because of the rapid excretion of radioactivity via the lungs, the background activity in blood recirculating to the organ is minimal and calculations are simplified.

YTTERBIUM-169

Decay of Ytterbium-169 (Half-life = 31.8 d)

Time (d)	Factor (%)	Time (d)	Factor (%)	Time (d)	Factor (%)
−60	366	−6	115	8	84
−50	295	−4	110	10	80
−40	240	−2	105	20	65
−30	191	0	100	30	52
−20	155	2	96	40	42
−10	125	4	92	50	34
−8	120	6	88	60	27

Note: Days before (−) or days after the reference date.

Principal γ-energies — 63 (45%), 177 (22%), 197 (36%), 307 (11%) keV.

Ytterbium (^{169}Yb) diethylenetriamine-penta acetate (DTPA)
- **Chemical form** — Sterile, isotonic, pyrogen-free solution of Ytterbium (^{169}Yb) DTPA and sodium chloride to render the solution isotonic.
- **Use** — Diagnostic scintigraphy in cerebrospinal fluid (CSF) studies, cisternography and ventriculography.
- **Dosage and procedure** — The adult dose administered for diagnostic scintigraphy is 18.5 to 37 MBq (0.5 to 1 mCi). The route of administration may be lumbar, intra-cisternal, intraventricular, or by injection into neurosurgical shunts, depending on the condition under investigation.

YTTRIUM-90
Decay of yttrium-90 (Half-life = 64 d)

Time (h)	Factor (%)	Time (h)	Factor (%)	Time (h)	Factor (%)	Time (h)	Factor (%)
−48	168	−16	119	16	84	60	52
−44	161	−12	114	20	81	72	46
−40	154	−8	109	24	77	96	35
−36	148	−4	104	28	74	120	27
−32	141	0	100	32	71	144	21
−28	135	4	96	36	68	168	16
−24	130	8	92	48	60	192	12
−20	124	12	88				

Note: Hours before (−) or days after the reference date.

Principal β-energy — 2274 (99.9%) keV.

Yttrium (^{90}Y) silicate injection
- **Chemical form** — Sterile suspension of colloidal yttrium silicate in aqueous solution containing 204 mg sodium silicate per ml.
- **pH** — 10 to 11.5.
- **Use** — Yttrium (^{90}Y) silicate injection is indicated in the treatment of patients with chronic synovitis and effusions of joints and viscera. It is of particular value in the treatment of conditions of the knee, such as rheumatoid arthritis, chronic pyrophosphate arthropathy, osteoarthritis, psoriatic arthritis, and ankylosing spondylitis. Treatment is thought to be effective because it achieves partial synovectomy due to irradiation, and is significantly less traumatic to the patient than surgical synovectomy.

Yttrium-90 colloids are also indicated in the treatment of neoplastic visceral effusions by intrapleural or intraperitoneal injection in those patients who have failed to respond to conventional radiotherapy or chemotherapy.

The local therapeutic action of radioisotopes, such as Yttrium-90, is based on the principle that the emitted beta rays transfer their energy to tissue over a short distance. This transfer of energy is largely in the form of production of ion pairs and the breaking of chemical bonds within the cells. As the energy transfer is biodestructive, it leads to impairment of cellular reproductive potential and/or to cell death. This is the ideal desired effect of a radiotherapeutic agent, provided it is the target tissue cells which are so affected.

* **Dosage and administration** — For the treatment of synovial effusion conditions of the knee, a standard dose of 185 MBq (5 mCi) is recommended. A repeat dose may be administered after 6 months if the initial injection does not cause any significant improvement in the condition. The knee should be immobilized in a light splint following injection. Doses between 2.6 to 3.7 GBq (70 to 100 mCi) are used for intrapleural or intraperitoneal injection. These recommended doses are for guidance only; the activity per administration is a matter for clinical judgment; caution is advised on all treatments for nonmalignant disease, especially in young patients.

REFERENCES

Adapted from *Amersham Nuclear Medicine Catalogue*, Amersham International, plc., Little Chalfont, England, 1986. With permission.

Other references obtained from package inserts of radiopharmaceutical products from:

* Atomic Energy Corporation of South Africa, Isotope Production Centre, Pelindaba, South Africa.
* Byk Mallinckrodt CIL B.V., Petten, Holland.
  International CIS, Gif-Sur-Yvette, France.
* NEN Medical Products — Du Pont, Billerica, MA.

Radiation Dosimetry

RADIATION DOSIMETRY

INTRODUCTION

Absorption of energy from ionizing radiation, produced by the primary radiation or by secondary electrons, may cause damage to living tissues. Such ionization occurring within a living cell may lead to changes in the nucleus resulting in abnormal reproduction or its death. Cellular destruction by radiation is used to advantage in radionuclide therapy, but becomes a limiting factor for diagnostic applications because of the potential hazard for the patient. For this reason, it is of primary importance to determine as exactly as possible the absorbed radiation dose to different organs from internally administered radiopharmaceuticals in order to balance the expected value of diagnostic information to be gained from nuclear medicine procedures against the potential radiation effects on a patient.

No specific dose limit has been established for patients undergoing diagnostic nuclear medicine procedures since the risks involved must be weighed against the potential benefits to the patient. However, as a general principle, the dose must be kept as low as reasonably achievably (the ALARA principle) consistent with the need to obtain reliable results that will benefit the patient's medical care. Special attention should be taken with women of reproductive age, avoiding in particular nonurgent studies in pregnancy and lactation which might involve a significant and unnecessary dose to the fetus or infant, respectively.

RADIATION DOSIMETRY UNITS

Exposure — The quantity of *exposure* is a measure of the intensity of X or gamma radiation and the time for which it has been acting. This is measured by the amount of ionization that is produced in air. The SI unit of exposure is the coulomb per kilogram (C/kg), while the traditional unit, the *roentgen* (R), is equal to one electrostatic unit of charge per cm^3. The relationship between the two units is:

$$1 \text{ Ckg} = 3876 \text{ R}$$

The intensity of an X or gamma ray beam is measured by its *exposure rate* in $C \text{ kg}^{-1}s^{-1}$ (or $R \text{ s}^{-1}$).

Absorbed dose — However, the biological effect of radiation depends not just on its intensity, but more on how much of its energy is absorbed by tissue. Therefore, the quantity *absorbed dose* is defined as the energy absorbed per unit mass of material. The SI unit of absorbed dose is the *gray* (Gy), which is equal to one joule per kilogram, although the traditional unit is the rad (from roentgen-absorbed dose), equal to 100 erg/g. The conversion between traditional and SI units is therefore:

$$1 \text{ Gy} = 100 \text{ rad}$$

Dose Equivalent — The biological effect of radiation on tissue depends primarily on the absorbed dose, but also on other factors such as how quickly this dose was delivered, how uniformly it was distributed, and the type of radiation involved. To take account of this a third quantity, the dose equivalent, is used. This is defined by:

$$\text{Dose equivalent} = \text{Absorbed dose} \times \text{Modifying quality factors} \qquad (1)$$

The SI unit of dose equivalent is the sievert (Sv), and the traditional unit is the rem (from roentgen equivalent in man):

$$1 \text{ Sv} = 100 \text{ rem}$$

Quality Factor — The most important modifying factor in equation (1) is the *quality factor* which allows for the different densities of ionization produced by different types of radiation. All X-rays and gamma rays and most beta particles are assigned a quality factor of 1, but alpha particles, which produce very dense ionization, have a quality factor of 20 (IRCP, 1977).

Effective Dose Equivalent — If the dose distribution is nonuniform — as it is usually in nuclear medicine — the different susceptibilities of each organ must be allowed for taking a weighed sum over all irradiated organs. This sum defines the *effective dose equivalent* — the uniformly distributed dose which would involve the same overall risk.

The *effective dose equivalent* = (sum, all tissues) Weighting factor × Dose equivalent.

(2)

METHOD OF CALCULATING ABSORBED DOSE

From the foregoing definition of absorbed dose it follows that

Absorbed dose = Total energy absorbed / Mass of absorbing organ   (3)

Therefore, the process of calculating the absorbed dose for a particular organ is really one of calculating the total energy absorbed by that organ.

The absorbed radiation fraction dosimetry allows the calculation of the dose delivered to a *target organ* from radioactivity contained in one or more *source organs* in the body. The source and target may be the same organ. In fact, the largest contribution is very often from activity within the target organ itself. Organs other than the target organ are considered to be source organs if they contain concentrations of radioactivity greater than the average concentration in the body.

The absorbed dose to a given target organ due to radiation from a particular source organ depends on factors such as:

1. The energy of the radiation
2. The type of radiation — in particular, the numbers of gamma rays, beta particles, and X-rays emitted on average from each disintegration of the radionuclide
3. Source and target organ shapes, source-to-target distance, and the nature of the intervening tissues
4. Target organ mass, which is needed in the denominator of equation (3)
5. Administered dose of radiopharmaceutical
6. Physical half-life of decay of the radionuclide
7. Physiological handling of the radiopharmaceutical, i.e., the uptake by the source organ and its biological half-life

The first four factors together determine a quantity, S, called the absorbed dose per unit cumulated activity. This would be measured in units of μGy/MBq.s (or rad/μCi h). Since it depends only on physical and anatomical data, for a given target organ and source organ, S will only depend on the radionuclide used and the size of the patient.

The quantity S, can be calculated from purely physical and anatomical data. This has been done by Snyder et al. and published in a report by the Medical Internal Radiation Dose Committee (MIRD) of the Society of Nuclear Medicine (Snyder et al., 1975). They have tabulated S for 20 different source organs and 20 target organs of a standard adult human phantom for a range of radionuclides likely to be encountered in nuclear medicine. One of the limitations of their method is that it only gives the average dose to an organ, and, in cases where the activity is not distributed uniformly throughout the organ, this will underestimate the local dose.

The last three factors determine a quantity, $\widetilde{A}$, called the cumulated activity, measured in units such as MBq.s (or μCi h). Since this depends largely on physiological data which may not be accurately known, it is the major source of uncertainty in the calculation of absorbed dose.

Finally, the absorbed dose can be calculated from the following equations:

Absorbed dose to target organ = (Sum over all source organs) S.A   (4)

$\widetilde{A}$ is equal to the activity in the source organ multiplied by the time that it remains there, or, if the activity is varying continuously with time.

$$\widetilde{A} = \int_0^\infty A(t)dt$$

(5)

where A(t) is the activity in the source organ at any time t.

RADIATION DOSIMETRY: TABLE 1

Estimated Absorbed Radiation Doses to Adults From Selected Radioactive Agents Commonly Used in Nuclear Medicine Procedures (Technetium-99m Radiopharmaceuticals Listed Separately)

Radionuclide Physical half-life Agents	Clinical application	Route of administration	Administered activity kBq (uCi)	Organ	Radiation absorbed dose for administered activity	
					mGy	rads
Calcium (^{47}Ca) 4.53 d Chloride	Calcium absorption and metabolism	I.v.	370 (10)	Bone surfaces	5.1	0.51
				Red marrow	1.9	0.19
				Whole body	0.4	0.04
Chromium (^{51}Cr) 27.8 d Sodium chromate	Determination of red blood cell mass and survival time	I.v.	740 (20)	Red cell survival (740 kBq)		
			1 850 (50)	Blood	0.155	0.0155
				Ovaries	0.145	0.0145
				Testes	0.115	0.115
				Red marrow	0.155	0.0155
				Spleen	7.0	0.70
				Whole body	0.155	0.0155
Chromic chloride	Detection of gastrointestinal protein loss	I.v.	3 700 (100)	Whole body	0.07	0.007
EDTA	Glomerular filtration rate (GFR)	I.v.	1 300 (35)	Kidney, normal	0.05	0.005
				Kidney, severe insufficiency	0.25	0.025
Cobalt (^{57}Co) 270 d Cyanocobalamin	Vitamin B12 absorption	Oral	37 (1)	Liver	1.10	0.110
				Stomach wall	0.17	0.017
				Spleen	0.10	0.010
				Kidneys	0.25	0.025
				Total bone	0.03	0.003
				Ovaries	0.06	0.006
				Testes	0.61	0.061
				Red marrow	0.04	0.004
				Whole body	0.06	0.006
Cobalt (^{58}Co) 71.3 d Cyanocobalamin	Vitamin B12 absorption	Oral	37 (1)	Testes	0.03	0.003
				Ovaries	0.08	0.008
				Liver	2.10	0.210
				Whole body	0.15	0.015

Radionuclide	Chemical form	Application	Route	Activity	Organ		
Fluorine (18F) 109.7 m	Fluoro-deoxy glucose (2FDG)	Determination of the regional cerebral metabolic rate for glucose	I.v.	260 MBq (7 mCi)	Kidneys	5.95	0.595
					Lungs	5.46	0.546
					Liver	5.25	0.525
					Spleen	11.06	1.106
					Red marrow	3.57	0.357
					Ovaries	3.71	0.371
					Testes	4.76	0.476
					Bladder	30.45	3.045
					Brain	5.6	0.56
					Lens of eye	2.87	0.287
					Heart	11.13	1.113
					Whole body	2.73	0.273
Gallium (67Ga) 78 h	Citrate	Tumor and inflammation scintigraphy	I.v.	148 MBq (4 mCi)	Red marrow	24.0	2.40
					Bone surfaces	144.0	14.40
					Liver	30.0	3.00
					Spleen	28.0	2.80
					Stomach	8.8	0.88
					Small intestine	14.4	1.44
					Large intestine	58.4	5.84
					Whole body	10.0	1.00
Gold (195mAu) 30.5 s	Thiosulphate solution	Angiocardiography	I.v.	925 MBq (25 mCi)	Heart wall	0.25	0.025
					Lungs	0.33	0.033
					Kidneys	3.33	0.333
					Liver	0.33	0.033
					Spleen	0.42	0.042
					Gonads	0.25	0.025
					Whole body	0.16	0.016
Gold (198Au) 64.7 h	Colloid	Treatment of metastasis and synovial effusions / Liver scintigraphy	Intracavitary / Intra-articular / I.v.	5.5 GBq (150 mCi) / 370 MBq (10 mCi) / 3 700 (100)	Liver scintigraphy		
					Liver	39.0	3.90
					Ovaries	0.14	0.014
					Testes	0.03	0.003
					Red marrow	2.70	0.270
					Spleen	12.00	1.2
					Whole body	1.40	0.14
Hydrogen (3H) 12.26 y	Tritiated water	Total body water determination	I.v.	3 700 (100)	Gonads	0.20	0.02
					Whole body	0.13	0.013

RADIATION DOSIMETRY: TABLE 1 (continued)

Estimated Absorbed Radiation Doses to Adults From Selected Radioactive Agents Commonly Used in Nuclear Medicine Procedures (Technetium-99m Radiopharmaceuticals Listed Separately)

Radionuclide Physical half-life Agents	Clinical application	Route of administration	Administered activity kBq (uCi)	Organ	Radiation absorbed dose for administered activity	
					mGy	rads
Indium (^{111}In) 67.4 h Bleomycin	Localization of tumors	I.v.	74 MBq(2 mCi)	Liver	20.6	2.06
				Spleen	19.6	1.96
				Kidney	18.4	1.84
				Bladder	16.0	1.60
				Red marrow	18.8	1.88
				Whole body	5.2	0.52
DTPA	Study of cerebrospinal fluid (CSF) circulation	Intrathecal	37 MBq(1 mCi)	Spinalcord/brain surfaces, normal	120.0	12.0
				spinalcord/brain hydrocephalus surfaces,	200.0	20.0
				Gonads	0.6	0.06
				Whole body	1.0	0.10
Oxine	Blood cells labeling	I.v.	7 400 (200)	Labeled leukocytes		
				Spleen	23.0	2.3
				Liver	9.8	0.98
				Whole body	0.8	0.08
				Labeled platelets		
				Spleen	52.0	5.2
				Liver	7.2	0.72
				Whole body	1.4	0.14
Chloride	Labeling agent for protein, cells, monoclonal antibodies	I.v.	37 MBq (1 mCi)	Labeled protein		
				Liver	45.0	4.5
				Spleen	4.1	0.41
				Red marrow	28.0	2.8
				Ovaries	5.2	0.52
				Testes	2.1	0.21
				Whole body	6.0	0.6
Indium (^{113m}In) 100 m DTPA	Brain scintigraphy	I.v.	370 MBq (10 mCi)	Kidneys	190	19.0
				Whole body	3	0.3

Compound	Application	Route	Activity	Organ		
Colloid	Liver scintigraphy	I.v.	37 MBq (1 mCi)	Liver	10.0	1.0
				Red marrow	0.6	0.06
				Ovaries	0.2	0.02
				Testes	0.1	0.01
				Whole body	0.4	0.04
Macroaggregated albumin	Lung scintigraphy	I.v.	74 MBq (2 mCi)	Lungs	16.0	1.6
				Liver	0.6	0.06
				Ovaries	0.4	0.04
				Testes	0.2	0.02
				Whole body	0.4	0.04
Iodine (^{123}I) 13.3 h Sodium iodide	Thyroid function studies	Oral	3 700 (100)	Liver	0.028	0.0028
				Red marrow	0.03	0.003
				Ovaries	0.034	0.0034
				Testes	0.012	0.0012
				Stomach wall	0.23	0.023
				Thyroid	7.5	0.75
				Whole body	0.027	0.0027
Orthoiodohippurate	Renal (tubular) function (renography)	I.v.	74 (2)	Kidney	0.51	0.051
				Red marrow	0.2	0.02
				Ovaries	0.61	0.061
				Testes	0.38	0.038
				Bladder wall	17.0	1.7
				Whole body	0.2	0.02
Sodium rose bengal	Hepatobiliary function	I.v.	37 (1)	Gall bladder	2.5	0.25
				Small intestine	6.0	0.60
				Large intestine	25.0	2.5
				Liver	1.9	0.19
				Ovaries	2.8	0.28
				Testes	0.14	0.014
				Red marrow	0.80	0.08
Iofetamine	Cerebral blood flow imaging	I.v.	222 (6)	At time of reference		
				Brain	5.8	0.585
				Retina	44.0	4.4
				Lens	7.6	0.76
				Lungs	14.0	1.4
				Liver	13.0	1.3

RADIATION DOSIMETRY: TABLE 1 (continued)

Estimated Absorbed Radiation Doses to Adults From Selected Radioactive Agents Commonly Used in Nuclear Medicine Procedures (Technetium-99m Radiopharmaceuticals Listed Separately)

Radionuclide Physical half-life Agents	Clinical application	Route of administration	Administered activity kBq (uCi)	Radiation absorbed dose for administered activity		
				Organ	mGy	rads
				Kidneys	4.2	0.42
				Bladder	22.0	2.2
				Thyroid	2.0	0.2
				Red marrow	5.2	0.52
				Ovaries	4.7	0.47
				Testes	3.8	0.38
				Whole body	4.6	0.46
Murine monoclonal antibody, antigranulocyte (Mab gc) (Example of Mab dosimetry)	Localization of inflammatory processes	I.v.	185 (5)	Spleen	15.72	1.572
				Liver	10.91	1.091
				Red marrow	14.43	1.443
				Thyroid	1.48	0.148
				Ovaries	2.59	0.259
				Whole body	2.78	0.278
Iodine (^{125}I) 59.4 d Human serum albumin	Measurement of plasma volume	I.v.	185 (5)	Bladder wall	0.06	0.006
				Red marrow	0.05	0.005
				Gonads	0.03	0.003
				Blood	0.16	0.016
				Whole body	0.03	0.003
Human fibrinogen	Detection of deep venous thrombosis	I.v.	3700 (100)	Blood	0.81	0.081
				Bladder	0.32	0.032
				Kidneys	0.05	0.005
				Whole body	0.17	0.017
Polyvinylpyrrolidone (PVP)	Detection of gastrointestinal protein loss	I.v.	370 (10)	Liver	4.1	0.41
				Ovaries	0.01	0.001
				Testes	0.003	0.0003
				Whole body	0.2	0.02

Compound	Application	Route	Activity MBq (µCi)	Organ		
Oleic acid	Fat absorption	Oral	900 (25)			
Sodium iodide	Thyroid function	Oral	900 (25)	Whole body	0.01	0.001
				Liver	0.06	0.006
				Ovaries	0.01	0.001
				Testes	0.005	0.0005
				Red marrow	0.02	0.0002
				Stomach wall	0.06	0.006
				Thyroid	112.5	11.25
Iodine (^{131}I) 8.05 days	Thyroid function studies and treatment	Oral	370 (10)	Whole body	0.07	0.007
Sodium iodide				Liver	0.04	0.004
				Gonads	0.01	0.001
				Red marrow	0.02	0.002
				Stomach wall	0.16	0.016
				Thyroid	80.0	8.0
Orthoiodohippurate	Renal function (renography)	I.v.	3700 (100)	Whole body	4.7	0.47
				Bladder wall	13.0	1.3
				Kidneys	0.4	0.04
				Ovaries	0.07	0.007
				Testes	0.05	0.005
				Red marrow	0.02	0.002
				Whole body	0.03	0.003
Iodomethylnorcholesterol	Adrenal cortex imaging	I.v.	18.5 MBq (500)	Ovaries	40	4.0
				Testes	11.5	1.15
				Adrenals	125	12.5
Metaiodobenzylguanidine (MIBG)	Adrenal medullary scintigraphy and therapy	I.v.	18.5 MBq (500)	Whole body	6	0.6
				Ovaries	2.18	0.218
				Testes	2.0	0.2
				Thyroid	105.26	10.526
				Lungs	3.26	0.326
				Skeleton	2.02	0.202
				Red marrow	2.22	0.222
				Adrenal medulla	345.39	34.539
				Liver	2.8	0.281
				Kidneys	2.53	0.253
				Spleen	2.39	0.239
				Pancreas	2.35	0.235
				Stomach wall	2.18	0.218
				Whole body	2.07	0.207

RADIATION DOSIMETRY: TABLE 1 (continued)

Estimated Absorbed Radiation Doses to Adults From Selected Radioactive Agents Commonly Used in Nuclear Medicine Procedures (Technetium-99m Radiopharmaceuticals Listed Separately)

Radionuclide Physical half-life Agents	Clinical application	Route of administration	Administered activity kBq (uCi)	Organ	Radiation absorbed dose for administered activity	
					mGy	rads
Human fibrinogen	Localization of deep venous thrombosis and tumors	I.v.	18.5 MBq (500)	Gonads	9.5	0.95
				Thyroid	175.0	17.50
				Whole body	8.5	0.85
Rose bengal	Hepatobiliary function	I.v.	370 (10)	Gall bladder	0.11	0.011
				Large intestine	4.9	0.49
				Small intestine	0.35	0.035
				Liver	0.08	0.008
				Ovaries	0.16	0.016
				Testes	0.014	0.0014
				Red marrow	0.032	0.0032
				Whole body	0.06	0.006
Human serum albumin	Determination of plasma volume	I.v.	370 (10)	Thyroid	3.5	0.350
				Blood	1.2	0.120
				Liver	0.12	0.012
				Spleen	0.13	0.013
				Ovaries	0.9	0.090
				Testes	0.9	0.090
				Whole body	0.2	0.020
Macroaggregate albumin	Lung perfusion imaging	I.v.	11.1 MBq (300)	Ovaries	3.9	0.39
				Testes	0.9	0.09
				Lung	11.2	1.12
				Kidneys	18.0	1.8
				Liver	0.9	0.09
				Spleen	9.0	0.9
				Thyroid	300.0	30.0
				Whole body	0.9	0.09
Triolein	Fats absorption	Oral	925 (25)	Gonads	0.05	0.005
				Whole body	0.04	0.004
Iron (^{52}Fe) 82 h Citrate	Ferrokinetics, bone marrow scintigraphy	I.v.	3700 (100)	Red marrow	21.42	2.142
				Liver	4.0	0.4
				Whole body	1.0	0.1

Radionuclide / Agent	Use	Route	Activity MBq (mCi)	Organ		
Iron (^{59}Fe) 45.6 d, Citrate	Ferrokinetics, bone marrow scintigraphy		370 (10)	Gonads	2.2	0.22
				Red marrow	1.3	0.13
				Liver	10.0	1.0
				Spleen	14.0	1.4
				Blood	9.0	0.9
				Whole body	2.0	0.2
Krypton (^{81m}Kr) 13.3 s, Gas	Lung ventilation imaging	Inhalation and rebreathing	650 MBq (18 mCi)/m	Per minute of rebreathing		
				Lungs	0.45	0.045
				Liver	2.16	0.216
				Red marrow	0.02	0.002
				Spleen	0.03	0.003
				Whole body	0.05	0.005
Mercury (^{197}Hg) 65 h, Chlormerodrin	Renal scintigraphy	I.v.	7400 (200)	Kidneys	30.0	3.0
				Gonads	0.16	0.016
				Whole body	0.20	0.02
Phosphorus (^{32}P) 14.3 d, Sodium phosphate	Treatment of polycythemia vera	I.v.	185 MBq (5 mCi)	Liver	315	31.5
				Spleen	3150	315.0
				Skeleton	2800	280.0
				Gonads	150	15.0
				Red marrow	2850	285.0
				Whole body	405	40.5
Potassium (^{42}K) 12.4 h, Chloride	Measurement of exchangeable potassium	I.v.	3700 (100)	Liver	0.7	0.07
				Muscle	1.3	0.13
				Heart	1.0	0.1
				Gonads	1.0	0.1
				Whole body	1.0	0.1
Selenium (^{75}Se) 120.4 d, Cholesterol	Adrenal cortex imaging	I.v.	7400 (200)	Liver	23	2.3
				Ovaries	19	1.9
				Adrenals (normal)	40	4.0
				Adrenals (hyperplasia)	200	20.0
				Whole body	17	1.7
Methionine	Pancreatic imaging	I.v.	9250 (250)	Blood	22.5	2.25
				Kidney	57.5	5.75
				Liver	62.5	6.25
				Ovaries	12.5	1.25
				Testes	30.0	3.0
				Spleen	40.0	4.0
				Pancreas	30.0	3.0
				Whole body	2.5	0.25

RADIATION DOSIMETRY: TABLE 1 (continued)

Estimated Absorbed Radiation Doses to Adults From Selected Radioactive Agents Commonly Used in Nuclear Medicine Procedures (Technetium-99m Radiopharmaceuticals Listed Separately)

Radionuclide Physical half-life Agents	Clinical application	Route of administration	Administered activity kBq (uCi)	Radiation absorbed dose for administered activity		
				Organ	mGy	rads
Taurocholic acid	Biliary acids metabolism	Oral	37 (1)	Normal health		
				Liver	0.01	0.001
				Gall bladder	0.12	0.012
				Small intestine	0.11	0.011
				Large intestine	0.16	0.016
				Ovaries	0.04	0.004
				Whole body	0.01	0.001
				Severe jaundice		
				Liver	2.04	0.204
				Gall bladder	0.42	0.042
				Small intestine	0.22	0.022
				Large intestine	0.40	0.040
				Ovaries	0.14	0.014
				Whole body	0.21	0.021
Sodium (^{24}Na) Chloride 14.97 h	Exchangeable sodium	I.v., oral	370 (10)	Gonads	0.20	0.020
				Whole body	0.17	0.017
Strontium (^{85}Sr) Chloride 64 d	Bone scintigraphy	I.v.	7400 (200)	Bone	100	10
				Whole body	40	4
Strontium (^{89}Sr) Chloride 52.7 d	Palliation of bone pain in malignancy	I.v.	74 MBq (2 mCi)	Bone	1186	118.6
				Red marrow	792	79.2
				Bladder	4	0.4
				Whole body	60	6.0
Sulfur (^{35}S) Sodium sulfate 87.9 d	Extracellular fluid volume	I.v.	3700 (100)	Cartilage	1.9	0.19
				Bone marrow	0.5	0.05
				Whole body	0.03	0.003
Thallium (^{201}Tl) Chloride 73 h	Myocardial perfusion parathyroid scintigraphy	I.v.	55.5 MBq (1.5 mCi)	Liver	4.0	0.4
				Kidneys	14.5	1.45
				Bladder	4.4	0.44

Radionuclide	Administration	Activity	Application	Organ		
Xenon (^{127}Xe) 36.4 d Gas	Inhalation	37 MBq (1 mCi)	Lung ventilation imaging	Small intestine	5.5	0.55
				Large intestine	41.0	4.1
				Thyroid	11.6	1.16
				Ovaries	3.7	0.37
				Testes	1.8	0.18
				Heart	3.6	0.36
				Red marrow	3.75	0.375
				Whole body	2.4	0.24
				Lungs	0.04	0.004
				Red marrow	0.02	0.002
				Gonads	0.01	0.001
				Whole body	0.02	0.002
Xenon (^{133}Xe) 5.27 d Gas	Inhalation	185 MBq (5 mCi)/5L spirometer	Lung ventilation imaging	Rebreath and washout		
				Bronchial mucosa	6.42	0.642
				Lung	0.39	0.039
				Blood	0.037	0.0037
				Fat	0.247	0.0247
				Gonads	0.037	0.0037
				Single breath		
				Bronchial mucosa	2.61	0.261
				Lung	0.30	0.030
				Blood	0.013	0.0013
				Fat	0.083	0.0083
				Gonads	0.013	0.0013
Saline solution	I.v., i.a.	37 MBq (1 mCi)	Lung perfusion/ventilation and tissues perfusion	Bronchial mucosa	2.57	0.257
				Lung	0.4	0.040
				Blood	0.824	0.0824
				Fat	0.104	0.104
				Gonads	0.013	0.0013
				Whole body	0.03	0.003
Ytterbium (^{169}Yb) 31.8 d DTPA	Intrathecal	37 MBq (1 mCi)	Cerebrospinal fluid (CSF) circulation imaging	Spinal cord	120 — 140	12 — 14
				Brain	11.0	1.1
				Blood	10.0	1.0
Yttrium (^{90}Y) 64 d Silicate	Intra-articular	185 MBq (5 mCi)	Treatment of synovitis	Whole body	0.2 — 0.7	0.2 — 0.07
				Knee	4×10^6	4×10^5
				Regional lymph nodes	4.5×10^4	4.5×10^3
				Liver	25	2.5
				Whole body	65	6.5

RADIATION DOSIMETRY: TABLE 2

Estimated Absorbed Radiation Doses to Adults From Selected Technetium-99m Tc Radiopharmaceuticals Commonly Used in Nuclear Medicine Procedures (Physical Half-Life of ^{99m}Tc = 6.05 Hours)

Technetium (^{99m}Tc) Radiopharmaceutical	Clinical application	Route of administration	Administered activity MBq (mCi)	Organ	Radiation absorbed dose for administered activity	
					mGy	rads
					(mGy/MBq)	(rads/mCi)
Sodium pertechnetate	Brain, thyroid, and tissues perfusion	I.v.	Different doses according to study	Bladder wall	0.014	0.053
				Stomach wall	0.068	0.250
				Large intestine	0.34	0.129
				Ovaries	0.006	0.022
				Testes	0.002	0.009
				Thyroid	0.035	0.130
				Red marrow	0.005	0.019
				Whole body	0.004	0.014
Hexamethylpropylene amine oxime (HM-PAO)	Cerebral blood flow imaging	I.v.	740 (20)	Brain	7.62	0.762
				Bone	3.48	0.348
				Red marrow	3.99	0.399
				Ovaries	3.09	0.309
				Testes	2.21	0.221
				Whole body	2.78	0.278
Glucoheptonate	Brain, kidney imaging	I.v.	Kidney 370 (10) Brain 740 (20)	Kidney (370 MBq)	17.0	1.7
				Bladder wall	28.0	2.8
				Red marrow	1.2	0.12
				Ovaries	1.6	0.16
				Testes	1.0	0.1
				Whole body	0.73	0.073
Diethylenetriamine-penta acetate (DTPA)	Brain, kidney imaging (glomerular filtration)	I.v.	Kidney 185 (5) Brain 740 (20)	Kidney (185 MBq)	2.0	0.20
				Bladder wall	22.5	2.25
				Red marrow	0.47	0.047
				Ovaries	1.35	0.135
				Testes	1.0	0.100
				Whole body	0.8	0.08

Substance	Use	Route	MBq (mCi)	Organ		
Mercapto-acetyltriglycine (MAG-3)	Renal (tubular) function	I.v.	185 (5)	Bladder wall		
				2 h void	10.5	1.05
				5 h void	23.5	2.35
				Gall bladder	8.0	0.8
				Kidneys	3.1	0.31
				Liver	0.85	0.085
				Ovaries		
				Bladder void 2 h	0.6	0.06
				Bladder void 5 h	1.2	0.12
				Testes		
				Bladder void 2 h	0.35	0.035
				Bladder void 5 h	0.75	0.075
				Whole body	0.25	0.025
Dimercaptosuccinic acid (DMSA)	Renal imaging	I.v.	370 (10)	Kidney	75.0	7.5
				Bladder wall	28.0	2.8
				Red marrow	3.5	0.35
				Ovaries	2.3	0.23
				Testes	1.4	0.14
				Whole body	1.6	0.16
Iminodiacetates (IDA)	Hepatobiliary function imaging	I.v.	148 (4)	Gall bladder	76.0	7.6
				Liver	5.2	0.52
				Small intestine	4.0	0.40
				Upper large intestine	7.6	0.76
				Lower large intestine	4.8	0.48
				Red marrow	0.96	0.096
				Ovaries	1.52	0.152
				Testes	0.12	0.012
				Kidney	0.8	0.08
				Bladder wall	2.9	0.29
				Whole body	0.64	0.064
Stannous or sulfur colloid	Reticuloendothelial system, RES (liver, spleen, bone marrow) imaging	I.v.	111 (3)	Liver	10.2	1.02
				Spleen	6.3	0.63
				Red marrow	0.81	0.081
				Ovaries	0.168	0.168
				Testes	0.033	0.0033
				Whole body	0.057	0.0057

RADIATION DOSIMETRY: TABLE 2 (continued)

Estimated Absorbed Radiation Doses to Adults From Selected Technetium-99m Tc Radiopharmaceuticals Commonly Used in Nuclear Medicine Procedures (Physical Half-Life of ^{99m}Tc = 6.05 Hours)

Technetium (^{99m}Tc) Radiopharmaceutical	Clinical application	Route of administration	Administered activity MBq (mCi)	Organ	Radiation absorbed dose for administered activity	
					mGy	rads
Antimony or rhenium sulfide colloid	Lymphatic system imaging	Subcutaneous injection	148 (4)	Lymph nodes	11.2	1.2
				Liver	0.2	0.02
				Gonads	0.04	0.004
				Whole body	0.04	0.004
Human fibrinogen	Detection of deep venous thrombosis	I.v.	370 (10)	Liver	8	0.8
				Kidneys	60	6.0
				Bladder wall	22	2.2
				Stomach wall	4	0.4
				Small intestine	5	0.5
				Large intestine	8	0.8
				Red marrow	3	0.3
				Ovaries	3	0.3
				Testes	1	0.1
				Whole body	2	0.2
Human serum albumin (HSA)	Blood pool imaging	I.v.	370 (10)	Brain	0.47	0.047
				Kidneys	0.63	0.063
				Bladder wall	1.66	0.166
				Red marrow	0.76	0.076
				Ovaries	0.82	0.082
				Testes	0.79	0.079
				Whole body	0.73	0.073
Red blood cells (PYP + ^{99m}Tc O$_4$ labeling)	Blood pool imaging	I.v.	740 (20)	Heart	0.6	0.06
				Blood	11.6	1.16
				Liver	3.8	0.38
				Spleen	3.8	0.38
				Red marrow	0.46	0.046
				Ovaries	4.0	0.4
				Testes	2.4	0.24
				Whole body	3.4	0.34

Hexakis methody isobutyl isonitrile (HEXAMIBI)

Myocardial perfusion

I.v.

740 (20)

Exercise		
Bladder wall	16.8	1.68
Small intestine	4.2	0.42
Upper large intestinal wall	6.0	0.6
Lower large intestinal wall	4.8	0.48
Gall bladder	8.1	0.81
Heart wall	8.1	0.81
Kidneys	12.9	1.29
Liver	3.0	0.3
Lungs	5.7	0.57
Spleen	6.3	0.63
Thyroid	17.1	1.71
Ovaries	3.0	0.3
Testes	1.5	0.15
Red marrow	2.8	0.28
Whole body	2.0	0.2
Rest		
Bladder wall	23.7	2.37
Small intestine	7.2	0.72
Upper large intestine	11.1	1.11
Lower large intestine	8.4	0.84
Gall bladder	16.2	1.62
Heart wall	8.1	0.81
Kidneys	24.9	2.49
Liver	4.2	0.42
Lungs	5.7	0.57
Spleen	7.8	0.78
Thyroid	28.5	2.85
Ovaries	4.2	0.42
Testes	1.5	0.15
Red marrow	3.0	0.30
Whole body	2.1	0.21

RADIATION DOSIMETRY: TABLE 2 (continued)

Estimated Absorbed Radiation Doses to Adults From Selected Technetium-99m Tc Radiopharmaceuticals Commonly Used in Nuclear Medicine Procedures (Physical Half-Life of ^{99m}Tc = 6.05 Hours)

Technetium (^{99m}Tc) Radiopharmaceutical	Clinical application	Route of administration	Administered activity MBq (mCi)	Organ	Radiation absorbed dose for administered activity	
					mGy	rads
Human albumin micros-pheres (HAM) Macroaggregate albumin (MAA)	Lungs and tissue perfusion	I.v., i.a.	111 (3)	Lungs	6.9	0.69
				Kidneys	4.2	0.42
				Stomach	2.16	0.216
				Thyroid	2.16	0.216
				Bladder wall	12.0	1.2
				Red marrow	0.6	0.06
				Ovaries	0.39	0.039
				Testes	0.15	0.015
				Whole body	0.26	0.026
Methylenediphosphonic acid (MDP)	Skeletal scintigraphy	I.v.	740 (20)	Bone	7.6	0.760
				Kidneys	6.2	0.620
				Bladder wall	88.0	8.8
				Red marrow	5.0	0.5
				Ovaries	3.4	0.34
				Testes	2.4	0.24
				Whole body	1.4	0.140
Stannous pyrophosphate (PYP)	Skeletal, myocardial infarction imaging	I.v.	740 (20)	Bone	8.0	0.8
				Kidney	20.0	2.0
				Bladder wall	28.0	2.8
				Red marrow	5.58	0.558
				Ovaries	2.0	0.2
				Testes	2.0	0.2
				Whole body	1.8	0.180

REFERENCES (TABLES 1 AND 2)

Note: Estimated Absorbed Radiation Doses (Tables 1 and 2) were compiled from the following reference sources:

- *Amersham Nuclear Medicine Catalogue,* Amersham International, plc., Little Chalfont, England, 1986.
- **Maisey, M. N., Britton, K. E., and Gilday, D. L., Eds.,** *Clinical Nuclear Medicine,* Chapman and Hall, London, 1983.
- *CRC Handbook Series in Clinical Laboratory Science. Section A: Nuclear Medicine,* Vol. II, Selingson, David, Editor-in-Chief; Spencer, Richard P., Section Editor, CRC Press, Boca Raton, FL, 1982.
- **Fitzgerald, M., Ed.,** *Dosimetry in Diagnostic Radiology,* The Hospital Physicists' Association, London, 1982.
- **Freeman, Leonard M., Ed.,** *Freeman and Johnson's Clinical Radionuclide Imaging,* 3rd ed., Grune & Stratton, Orlando, Florida, 1984.
- **Saha, Gopal B.,** *Fundamentals of Nuclear Pharmacy,* 2nd ed., Springer-Verlag, New York, 1984.
- **J. R. Greening, Ed.,** *Fundamentals of Radiation Dosimetry,* 2nd ed., Adam Hilger Ltd., Bristol and Boston, in collaboration with the Hospital Physicists' Association, 1981.
- **Attix, Frank Herbert,** *Introduction to Radiological Physics and Radiation Dosimetry,* John Wiley & Sons, New York, 1986.
- **Pizzarello, Donald J. and Witcofski, Richard L.,** *Medical Radiation Biology,* 2nd ed., Lea & Febiger, Philadelphia, 1982.
- **Sorensen, James A. and Phelps, Michael E.,** *Physics in Nuclear Medicine,* 2nd ed., Grune & Stratton, Harcourt Brace Jovanovich, Publishers, Orlando, Florida, 1987.

RADIATION DOSIMETRY: TABLE 3

Weighting Factors Recommended for Calculating Effective Dose Equivalent[a]

Tissue	Weighting factor
Whole body (uniform)	1.00
Gonads	0.25
Breast	0.15
Red bone marrow	0.12
Lung	0.12
Thyroid	0.03
Bone surfaces	0.03
Any other organ (up to 5 organs)	0.06

[a]   ICRP 1977 Recommendations of the International Commission on Radiological Protection.

Adapted from Fitzgerald, M., Ed., *Dosimetry in Diagnostic Radiology,* The Hospital Physicists Association, CR-Series 40, London, 1984.

RADIATION DOSIMETRY: TABLE 4

Estimated Absorbed Radiation Dose to Adults From Selected Radiological Examinations

Type of examination	Mean skin dose per film mGy (rads)	Mean red marrow[a] dose per film mGy (rads)	Mean gonadal dose per exam M mGy (rads)	F mGy (rads)
Skull	3.0 (0.3)	0.8 (0.08)	—	—
Cervical spine	2.5 (0.25)	0.5 (0.05)	—	—
Thoracic spine	13 (1.3)	2.4 (0.24)	—	—
Lumbar spine	25 (2.5)	4.5 (0.45)	2.2 (0.22)	7.2 (0.72)
Pelvis	5.0 (0.5)	0.9 (0.09)	3.6 (0.36)	2.1 (0.21)
Hip joints	10 (1.0)	0.7 (0.07)	6.0 (0.6)	1.2 (0.12)
Upper extremity	1.3 (0.13)	—	—	—
Lower extremity	1.1 (0.11)	0.2 (0.02)	—	—
Brain CT scan	50 (5.0)	3.0 (0.3)	—	—
Chest	0.5 (0.05)	0.1 (0.01)	—	—
Mammography	13 (1.3)	—	—	—
Upper GI series	8.0 (0.8)	5.4 (0.54)	—	3 (0.3)
Barium enema	6.3 (0.63)	8.8 (0.88)	3.0 (0.3)	17 (1.7)
Cholecystography/ Cholangiogram	7.7 (0.77)	1.7 (0.17)	—	0.8 (0.08)
IV pyelogram	5.0 (0.05)	4.2 (0.42)	2.1 (0.21)	5.9 (0.59)
Abdomen, kidneys, urinary bladder	7.7 (0.77)	1.5 (0.15)	1.0 (0.1)	2.2 (0.22)

[a]   "Mean Red Marrow Dose" is the average over the whole mass of red marrow to compensate for regional organ irradiation.

Adapted from Pizzarello, Donald J. and Witcofski, Richard L., *Medical Radiation Biology,* 2nd ed., Lea & Febiger, Philadelphia, 1982.

RADIATION DOSIMETRY: TABLE 5

Maximum Permissible Dose Limits Recommended by the NCRP

Maximum permissible dose equivalent for occupation
exposure

Whole body	50 mSv	(5 rem) in any one year after age 18
Skin	150 mSv	(15 rem) in any one year
Hands	750 mSv	(75 rem) in any one year (not more than 250 mSv per quarter)
Forearms	300 mSv	(30 rem) in any one year (not more than 100 mSv per quarter)
Other organs	150 mSv	(15 rem) in any one year
Pregnant woman (with respect to the fetus)	5 mSv	(0.5 rem) during gestation period

Dose Limits for the general public or occasionally exposed persons[a]

Whole body	5 mSv	(0.5 rem) in any one year

[a] Nonoccupational exposures.

From NCRP Report No. 39, *Basic Radiation Protection Criteria,* National Council on Radiation Protection and Measurements, Bethesda, MD, 1971, 106.

RADIATION DOSIMETRY: TABLE 6

U.S. General Population Exposure Estimates

Source	Average individual dose	
	(μSv/year)	(mrem/year)
Natural background (Cosmic, terrestrial, internal)	820	82
Medical[a]	930	93
X-rays-790 μSv/yr		
Radiopharmaceuticals-140 μSv/yr		
Fallout (Weapons testing)	40—50	4—5
Consumer products	30—40	3—4
Nuclear industry	<10	<1
Airline	6.1	0.61
Travel-6 μSv/yr		
Radiopharmaceutical		
Transportation—0.1 μSv/yr		
Total	1850	185

[a] Note that the dose from medical exposure is 50 % of the total.

Adapted from National Research Council, Advisory Committee on the Biological Effects of Ionizing Radiations (BEIR III), The effects on population of exposure to low levels of Ionizing Radiation, National Academy of Sciences, Washington, D.C., 1980.

RADIATION DOSIMETRY: TABLE 7

Typical Ranges for Electromagnetic Radiation

Type of radiation	Wavelength[a] (m)	Frequency range (Hz)	Energy range (eV)
Electricity	∞—3×10^5	0—10^3	0—4.1×10^{-1}
Radio, TV, radar	3×10^4—3×10^{-4}	10^4—10^{12}	4.1×10^{-11}—4.1×10^{-7}
NMR	6×10^2—0.43	0.5×10^6—7×10^8	2.0×10^{-4}—29×10^{-7}
Electron spin resonance	0.3—0.003	10^9—10^{11}	4.1×10^{-6}—4.1×10^{-4}
Infrared	3×10^{-3}—7.6×10^{-7}	10^{11}—10^{14}	4.1×10^{-4}—1.6
Visible light	7.6×10^{-7}—3.8×10^{-7}	4×10^{14}—7.9×10^{14}	1.6—3.3
Ultraviolet	3.8×10^{-7}—3×10^{-9}	7.9×10^{14}—10^{17}	3.3—410
X-rays	1.2×10^{-7}—4.1×10^{-17}	2.5×10^{15}—7.3×10^{24}	10—3×10^7
Gamma rays	1.5×10^{-17}—1.2×10^{-11}	2×10^{18}—2.5×10^{21}	8×10^3—10^7
Cosmic rays	1.2×10^{-7}— . . .	2.5×10^{15}— . . .	10— . . .

[a]   Ranges are approximate.

Note: The energy E of a photon of frequency v is calculated by Planck's equation: $E = h v$ where h is Planck's constant.

Adapted from Sorenson, James A. and Phelps, Michael E., Eds., *Wavelength of Electromagnetic Radiation in Physics in Nuclear Medicine,* 2nd ed., Grune & Stratton, Orlando, FL, 1987, and Chart of various types of electromagnetic radiations showing relative energies and frequencies, in Rollo, David F., Ed., *Nuclear Medicine Physics Instrumentation and Agents,* C. V. Mosby, St. Louis, 1977.

RADIATION DOSIMETRY: TABLE 8

Linear Energy Transfer (LET) Values of Ionizing Particles

Particle	Charge	Energy (MeV)	LET (keV/μm)
Electron	-1	0.001	12.3
		0.01	2.3
		0.1	0.42
		1	0.25
		200 keV X-rays[a]	0.4—36
		Cobalt 60[a] gamma rays	0.2—2
Proton	$+1$	Small	92
		2	16
		5	8
		10	4
Alpha	$+2$	Small	260
		3.4	140
		5	95
Neutron[b]		2.5	15—80 (peak at 20)
		14.1	3—30 (peak at 7)

[a]   This applies to the LET of secondary electrons ejected by photons.
[b]   Neutrons produce no ionization directly in passing through tissue. These values are for the protons ejected in collisions.

From Pizarello, Donald J. and Witcofski, Richard L., *Medical Radiation Biology,* 2nd ed., Lea & Febiger, Philadelphia, 1982. With permission.

RADIATION DOSIMETRY: TABLE 9

Types of Ionizing Radiation

Type	Mass	Charge	Description	Produced by
Alpha	4	+2	Doubly ionized helium atom	Radioactive decay primarily of heavy atoms
Beta (negatron)	0.00055	−1	Negative electron	Radioactive decay and betatrons
Beta (positron)	0.00055	+1	Positive electron	Radioactive decay and pair production
Gamma rays	0	0	Electromagnetic radiation	Radioactive decay
Heavy nuclei	Have a range of masses	Have a range of charges	Any atom stripped of one or more electrons and accelerated will be an ionizing particle. Deuterons and carbon atoms are examples	Accelerators
Negative mesons	0.15	−1	Negatively charged particle with a mass 273 times an electron	Accelerators
Neutrons	1	0	Neutral	Atomic reactors, cyclotrons
Protons	1	+1	Hydrogen nuclei	Van de Graaff generators and cyclotrons
X-rays	0	0	Electromagnetic radiation	X-ray machines and from the rearrangement of orbital electrons

From Pizarello, Donald J. and Witcofski, Richard L., *Medical Radiation Biology*, 2nd ed., Lea & Febiger, Philadelphia. With permission.

Characteristics of the Adult Reference Man

CHARACTERISTICS OF THE ADULT REFERENCE MAN

Note: These tables are excerpted, and printed with permission from ICRP Report No. 23, *Report of the Task Group on Reference Man,* Pergamon Press, Ltd. 1975, and *Radiological Health Handbook,* U.S. Department of Health, Education, and Welfare, Division of Radiological Health, Washington, D.C., 1970.

	Male	Female
Mass	70 kg	58 kg
Length	1.7 m	1.6 m
Surface area	1.8 m²	1.6 m²

ANATOMICAL AND PHYSIOLOGICAL DATA: TABLE 1

MASS OF ORGANS AND TISSUES

Organs—tissues	Mass (g)	% of total body
Adipose tissue	15,000	21
Subcutaneous	7,500	11
Other separable	5,000	7.1
Yellow Marrow (included with skeleton)	1,500	2.1
Interstitial	1,000	1.4
Adrenal glands (2)	14	0.02
Aorta	100	0.14
Contents (blood)	190	0.27
	(180 ml)	
Blood—total	5,500	7.8
	(5,200 ml)	
Plasma	3,100	4.4
	(3,000 ml)	
Erythrocytes	2,400	3.4
	(2,200 ml)	
Blood vessels (Excluding aorta and pulmonary artery)	200	0.29
Contents (blood)	3000	4.3
	(2900 ml)	
Cartilage (included with skeletal)	1100	1.6
Connective tissue	3400	4.8
Tendons and fascia	1400	2.0
Periarticular tissue	1500	2.1
Separable connective tissue	1600	2.3
Central Nervous System	1430	2.04
Brain	1400	2.0
Spinal cord	30	0.04
Contents—cerebrospinal fluid	120	0.17
	(120 ml)	
Eyes (2)	15	0.02
Lenses (2)	0.4	
Gallbladder	10	0.01
Contents (bile)	62	0.09
	(60 ml)	

ANATOMICAL AND PHYSIOLOGICAL DATA: TABLE 1
(continued)

MASS OF ORGANS AND TISSUES

Organs—tissues	Mass (g)	% of total body
GI tract	1200	1.7
Esophagus	40	0.06
Stomach	150	0.21
Intestine	1000	1.4
Small	640	0.91
Upper large	210	0.30
Lower large	160	0.23
Hair	20	0.03
Heart	330	0.47
Contents (blood)	500	0.71
	(470 ml)	
Kidneys (2)	310	0.44
Larynx	28	0.04
Liver	1800	2.6
Lung (2)	1000	1.4
Parenchyma (includes bronchial tree, capillary blood, and associated lymph nodes)	570	0.81
Pulmonary blood	430	0.61
	(400 ml)	
Lymphocytes	1500	2.1
Lymphatic tissue	700	1.0
Lymph nodes (dissectible)	250	0.36
Muscles (skeletal)	28000	40.0
Nails	3	0.004
Pancreas	100	0.14
Parathyroid (4)	0.12	
Pineal	0.18	
Pituitary	0.6	
Prostate	16	0.023
Salivary glands (6)	85	0.12
Skeleton	10000	14
Bone	5000	7.2
Cortical	4000	5.7
Trabecular	1000	1.4
Red marrow	1500	2.1
Yellow marrow	1500	2.1
Cartilage	1100	1.6
Periarticular tissue (skeletal)	900	1.3
Skin	2600	3.7
Epidermis	100	0.14
Dermis	2500	3.6
Spleen	180	0.26
Teeth	46	0.066
Testes (2)	35	0.05
Thymus	20	0.029
Thyroid	20	0.029
Tongue	70	0.10
Tonsils (2)	4	0.006
Trachea	10	0.014
Ureters (2)	16	0.023
Urethra	10	0.014
Urinary bladder	45	0.064
Contents (urine)	102	0.15
	(100 ml)	
Whole body	70000	100

ANATOMICAL AND PHYSIOLOGICAL DATA: TABLE 1
(continued)

MASS OF ORGANS AND TISSUES

Organs—tissues	Mass (g)	% of total body

Mass of Organs and Tissues of an Adult Female

Organs—tissues	Mass (g)	% of total body
Breasts (2)	360	0.62
Fallopian tubes (2)	2	0.0034
Ovaries (2)	11	0.019
Placenta (at term)	510	0.87
Uterus	80	0.14

ANATOMICAL AND PHYSIOLOGICAL DATA: TABLE 2

Dimensions of Organs

Spleen

	Length (cm)	Width (cm)	Thickness (cm)
Newborn	4.6	2.7	1.3
Adult	10—14	6—10	3—4

Heart

	Length (cm)		Transverse diameter (cm)		Anteroposterior diameter (cm)	
	M	F	M	F	M	F
Newborn	2.9—3.1	2.5—2.9	3.3—4.0	2.6—3.9	1.9	1.7
Adult	9.7—14	8.7—9.3	7.5—10.7	9.6—9.9	5—8	

Esophagus

Age (y)	Length (cm)
Newborn	8—10
1	12
5	16
10	18
15	19
Adult M	25
Adult F	23

Stomach (Fully distended)

	Cranial to caudal diameter (cm)	Transverse diameter (cm)
Newborn	3	5
Adult	37	15

Intestines

	Anatomical length (cm)	
Age (y)	Small intestine	Large intestine
Newborn	339	66
1	460	89

ANATOMICAL AND PHYSIOLOGICAL DATA: TABLE 2
(continued)

Dimensions of Organs

| Age (y) | Anatomical length (cm) | |
	Small intestine	Large intestine
5	470	100
10	579	116
Adult	654	160

Liver

	Transverse diameter or length (cm)	Vertical diameter or height (cm)	Anteroposterior diameter or width (cm)
Newborn	11	8	7.5
Adult	20—30	7—15	10—21

Pancreas

	Transverse diameter or length (cm)	Vertical diameter or thickness (cm)	Anteroposterior diameter or width (cm)
Newborn	4—6	1—2	
Adult	14—18	2—3	3—9

Trachea

| Age (y) | Length (cm) | Diameter of lumen (mm) | |
		Transverse	Anteroposterior
Newborn	4.0	5.0	3.6
1	4.5	7.6	6.5
5	5.4	9.2	8.0
10	6.3	10.5	9.4
15	7.2	14.0	12.7
Adult	9—15	12—18	13—23

Lungs

		Sagittal diameter or length (cm)	Transverse diameter at the base (cm)	Anteroposterior diameter (cm)
Adult male	R	27	14	20
	L	30	13	18
Adult female	R	22	12	18
	L	23	11	16

Lungs

Age (y)	Lung volume (ml)	Alveolar air volume (ml)	Capillary volume (ml)	No. of alveoli ($\times 10^6$)	No. of Respiratory Airways ($\times 10^6$)	Generations of airways
Newborn	200	81	2	24	1.5	21
1	550	303	11	129	4.5	22
5	990	582	13	257	7.9	
Adult	5,500	2,945	35	297	14	23

ANATOMICAL AND PHYSIOLOGICAL DATA: TABLE 2
(continued)

Dimensions of Organs

Main Bronchi

| | Length (mm) | | Diameter (mm) | | | |
| | | | Right | | Left | |
Age (y)	Right	Left	Sagittal	Transverse	Sagittal	Transverse
Newborn	9	21	4.6	5.0	3.9	4.1
1	11	19	5.9	6.2	4.4	5.1
5	13.5	34	8.5	9.1	6.3	7.0
10	14	35	8.6	9.2	7.3	8.4
Adult Male	23	54	17		15	
Adult Female	21	50	15		12	

Kidney

| | Length (cm) | Transverse diameter (cm) | Anteroposterior diameter (cm) | Width (cm) | |
				Cortex	Medulla
Newborn	4—6	2—2.5	1.2—1.5	0.8—1.5	0.8
Adult	10—12	5—6	3—4	0.8—1.5	1.6—1.9

Urinary System

Age (y)	Length of urethra (cm)	Weight of ureters (cm)	Capacity of the urinary bladder (ml)
Male			
Newborn	6	6—7	80
1	6.7	9—10	100
Adult	15—17	27—30	200—400
Female			
Newborn	2.2	6—7	80
1	2.3	9—10	100
5	2.6	15—17	200
Adult	3.8	27—30	200—400

Urinary Bladder

	Length (cm)	Transverse diameter (cm)	Anteroposterior diameter (cm)
Contracted bladder			
0—1 year	2.5—3	2	0.5—1.5
Adult	5—6	4—5	2—2.5
Distended bladder			
0—1 year	5—5.5	3—5	3—4
Adult	12—14	8—10	8—10

Testes

	Vertical diameter (cm)	Transverse diameter (cm)	Anteroposterior diameter (cm)
Newborn	1	0.4	0.5
Adult	4—5	2—2.7	2.5—3.5

ANATOMICAL AND PHYSIOLOGICAL DATA: TABLE 2
(continued)

Dimensions of Organs

Prostate

	Vertical diameter (cm)	Transverse diameter (cm)	Anteroposterior diameter (cm)
Adult (range)	2.1—3.7	1.7—4.7	1.1—6
(mean)	3.18	3.8	2.7

Ovaries

	Length or vertical axis (cm)	Diameter (cm)	
		transverse	anteroposterior
Newborn	1.5—3	0.3	0.4—0.8
Adult	2.2—5.5	1.5—2	1.5—3

Fallopian Tubes

	Length (cm)	Diameter of lumen (mm)
Newborn	3.46	
Adult	10.67	2—4

Uterus

	Length or long axis (cm)	Transverse diameter (cm)		Anteroposterior thickness (cm)	
		At the fundus	At the isthmus	At the fundus	At the isthmus
Newborn	2.5—5	1		0.25	
Adult nulliparous	6—7.5	4—5.5	1.5—3	2.2—3	1.5—2.5
Adult multiparous	7—8.5	5—6.5	2.5—4	3.2—4	2.5—3.5

Breast

	Diameter (cm)		Protrusion from chest wall (cm)
	Transverse	Cephalocaudal	
Newborn	0.8—1		
Adult male	1.5—2.5	0.3—0.5	
Adult female before lactation	12—13	10—11	5—6

Vagina

	Length (cm)
Newborn	3.2
Adult	
Anterior wall	5.5—7.5
Posterior wall	7—9

Thyroid gland

	Transverse diameter (cm)	Vertical diameter (cm)	Anteroposterior diameter (cm)
Newborn	1—1.5	2—3	0.18—1.2
Adult (each lobe)	2—4	5—8	1—2.5
Adult (isthmus)	2	2	0.2—0.6

ANATOMICAL AND PHYSIOLOGICAL DATA: TABLE 2
(continued)

Dimensions of Organs

Parathyroid Gland

	Transverse diameter (mm)	Vertical diameter (mm)	Anteroposterior diameter (mm)
Newborn	2.18	2.95	1.35
Adult	3—4	4—15	1.5—2

Adrenal Gland

	Transverse diameter (cm)	Vertical diameter (cm)	Anteroposterior diameter (cm)
Newborn	3.3—3.5	2.3—2.8	1.2—1.3
Adult	3—7	2—3.5	0.3—0.8

Pineal Gland (Epiphysis)

	Transverse diameter (mm)	Vertical diameter (mm)	Anteroposterior diameter (mm)
Newborn	2.5	2	3
Adult	2—4	3—6	5—9

Pituitary Gland

	Transverse diameter (mm)	Vertical diameter (mm)	Sagittal diameter (mm)
Newborn	7.9—8.5	4—4.9	5.7—7.5
Adult	10.5—17	5—9.7	5—15

Brain

	Transverse diameter (cm)	Vertical diameter (cm)	Anteroposterior diameter (cm)
Adult male	14	13	16.5
Adult female	13	12.5	15.5

Spinal Cord (Adult)

Segment	Length (cm)	Transverse diameter (mm)	Anteroposterior diameter (mm)	Circumference (mm)
Total	44.8—46.8			
Cervical	11.5	12—14	9	38
Thoracic	27.5	10	8	27
Lumbar	7.0	11—13	9	33

ANATOMICAL AND PHYSIOLOGICAL DATA: TABLE 2
(continued)

Dimensions of Organs

Eyes

Age (y)	Diameters of the eyeball (mm)		
	Transverse	**Vertical**	**Sagittal**
Newborn	17.1	16.5	17.7
1	20.5	20.2	20.2
5	21.8	21.3	21.8
10	21.9	21.5	21.2
Adult male	24.2	23.6	24.5
Adult female	23.4	23.0	23.9

ANATOMICAL AND PHYSIOLOGICAL DATA: TABLE 3

Other Anatomical Data

Alveoli (surface area)	75 m²
Blood (distribution in total body)	
Arterial system	1,000 ml
Venous system	3,200 ml
Pulmonary system	500 ml
Heart cavity	500 ml
Blood volume (total)	5,200 ml
Volume of red blood cells	2,200 ml
Volume of plasma	3,000 ml
Body (length)	170 cm
Body water (total)	600 ml/kg
Extracellular water	260 ml/kg
Intracellular water	340 ml/kg
Bronchial tree (mean wall thickness)	75 μm
Bronchial tree, surface area	3,950 cm²
Cerebrospinal fluid, volume	120 ml
Hypodermis (thickness)	3,750 μm
Lens (depth and size)	
Anterior aspect of lens to anterior pole of cornea	3—4 mm
Anterior aspect of lens to anterior aspect of closed lid	8 mm
Equator of lens to anterior of corneal border	3 mm
Equatorial diameter of lens	9 mm
Axial thickness of lens	4 mm
Nose specifications	
Surface area of both vestibules	21 cm²
Surface area of turbinates and nasal passages	160 cm²
Thickness of mucus	0.5 mm
Thickness of epithelium	0.1 mm
Thickness of entire mucosa	2 mm
Skin (total thickness)	1,300 μm
Epidermis	50 μm
Dermis	1,250 μm
Specific gravity of total body	1.07
Surface area of body	1.8 m²
Urinary bladder capacity	
Capacity (distress)	500 ml
Physiological capacity	200 ml

ANATOMICAL AND PHYSIOLOGICAL DATA: TABLE 4

Mass of Organs in Children

Age	Body length (cm)	Heart (g)	Lungs (2) (g)	Spleen (g)	Liver (g)	Kidneys (2) (g)	Brain (g)
Birth—3 d	49	17	39	8	78	27	335
3—5 weeks	52	20	58	12	127	32	413
3 months	56	23	65	14	140	39	516
6 months	62	31	81	17	200	51	660
12 months	73	44	121	26	288	71	925
18 months	78	52	137	30	345	83	1042
24 months	84	56	164	33	394	93	1060
6 years	109	94	243	58	642	135	1200
10 years	130	116	343	85	852	187	1290
12 years	139	124	391	93	936	191	1350

ANATOMICAL AND PHYSIOLOGICAL DATA: TABLE 5

Applied Physiological Data

Carbon dioxide exhaled	1,000 g/day
Dietary intake (nutrients)	
Protein	95 g/day
Carbohydrates	390 g/day
Fat	120 g/day
Dietary intake (major elements)	
Carbon	300 g/day
Hydrogen	350 g/day
Nitrogen	16 g/day
Oxygen	2,600 g/day
Sulfur	1 g/day
Energy expenditure	3,000 kcal/day
Feces, weight of	135 g/day
Feces, components of	
Water	105 g/day
Solids	30 g/day
Ash	17 g/day
Fats	5 g/day
Nitrogen	1.5 g/day
Other substances	6.5 g/day
Feces, major elements in	
Carbon	7 g/day
Hydrogen	13 g/day
Nitrogen	1.5 g/day
Oxygen	100 g/day
Intake of milk	300 ml/day
Lung capacities	
Total capacity	6.0 l
Functional residual capacity	2.4 l
Vital capacity	4.8 l
Dead space	160 ml
Lung volume and respiration	
Minute volume, resting	7.5 l/min
Minute volume, light activity	20 l/min
Air breathed, 8 h light work activity	9,600 l
Air breathed, 8 h nonoccupational activity	9,600 l
Air breathed, 8 h resting	3,600 l

ANATOMICAL AND PHYSIOLOGICAL DATA:
TABLE 5 (continued)

Applied Physiological Data

Metabolic rate	17 cal/min/kg W
Nasal secretion, composition of (major elements)	
Water	95—97 g/100 ml
Calcium	11 g/100 ml
Chlorine	495 g/100 ml
Potassium	69 g/100 ml
Sodium	295 g/100 ml
Oxygen inhaled	
Urine valves	920 g/day
Volume	1,400 ml/day
Specific gravity	1.02
pH	6.2
Solids	60 g/day
Urea	22 g/day
"Sugars"	1 g/day
Bicarbonates	0.14 g/day
Urinary loss of major elements	
Nitrogen	15 g/day
Hydrogen	160 g/day
Oxygen	1,300 g/day
Carbon	5 g/day
Water balance (gains)	
Total fluid intake	1,950 ml/day
Milk	300 ml/day
Tap water	150 ml/day
Other	1,500 ml/day
In food	700 ml/day
By oxidation of food	350 ml/day
Total	3,000 ml/day
Water balance (losses)	
In urine	1,400 ml/day
In feces	100 ml/day
Insensible loss	850 ml/day
In sweat	650 ml/day
Total	3,000 ml/day

ANATOMICAL AND PHYSIOLOGICAL DATA: TABLE 6

Surface Area of the Total Body and Subdivisions of the Total Body as a Function of Age

Age (y)	SA of total body (cm²)	Percentage SA of			
		Head	Trunk	Extremities	
				Upper	Lower
Birth	2,115	20.8	31.9	16.8	30.5
2	5,275	15.2	33.6	18.5	32.7
3	6,250	14.4	33.6	18.8	33.2
4	6,950	13.7	33.1	19.4	33.8
5	7,510	13.1	33.0	19.6	34.3
7	8,275	12.4	33.5	19.3	34.7
9	9,100	11.5	33.5	19.2	35.7
11	10,165	10.4	33.4	19.5	36.6
13	11,425	9.6	33.0	19.7	37.6
15	13,325	8.8	31.9	21.4	37.9
17	15,200	8.2	31.7	21.2	38.8
19	16,435	7.7	33.5	20.5	38.3
21	17,050	7.5	34.3	19.9	38.3
Adult	17,535	7.5	34.6	19.4	38.5

ANATOMICAL AND PHYSIOLOGICAL DATA: TABLE 7

Elemental Distribution of Body Components

Component	Carbon (%)	Hydrogen (%)	Nitrogen (%)	Oxygen (%)
Water		11		89
Fat	77	12		11
Protein	52	7	16	23
Carbohydrate	42	6		52
Bone ash				40

ANATOMICAL AND PHYSIOLOGICAL DATA: TABLE 8

Water and Fat Content of the Adult Body

Organ	% Water	% Fat
Skin	62	19
Hair	4—13	2.3
Nails	0.07—13	—
Skeleton	28—40	18—25
Cartilage	78	1.3
Bone marrow		
Red	40	40
Yellow	15	35—80
Lymphocytes	80	—
Spleen	72—79	0.85—3
Thymus	82	2.8
Skeletal muscle	79	2.2—3
Heart	63—83	2.7—17
Tongue	60—72	15—24
Esophagus	76	—
Stomach	60—78	—
Intestine	77—82	1—9
Liver	63—74	1—12
Gallbladder	6	—
Pancreas	66—73	3—20
Larynx	68	—
Trachea	60	—
Lung	72—84	1—1.5
Kidneys	71—81	2—7
Bladder	65	—
Filled with urine	90	—
Testes	81	3
Prostate	83	1.2
Ovaries	78	1—2
Uterus	79	1—2.2
Breast		
Male	50	3
Female	39	40
Thyroid	72—78	—
Adrenals	64	6—26
Brain		
Total	76—79	9—17
Gray matter	84—86	5.3
White matter	68—77	18
Spinal cord	63—75	2—19
Cerebrospinal fluid	99	
Cornea stroma	78	
Aqueous humor	98	—
Vitreous humor	99	—
Lens	68	1—3
Placenta	84	0.11

ANATOMICAL AND PHYSIOLOGICAL DATA: TABLE 9

Body Water Content

Total body water (TBW)

Fetus mass (g)	% Water
10	92—94
100	90
200	88
1000	82—84
3500	70—72

Post natal male:

$$TBW(l) = \frac{Mass\ (kg)\ [79.45 - 0.24\ Mass\ (kg) - 0.15\ age\ (yr)]}{100}$$

Post natal female:

$$TBW(l) = \frac{Mass\ (kg)\ [69.81 - 0.26\ Mass\ (kg) - 0.12\ age\ (yr)]}{100}$$

Average adult: 600 ml/kg

Extracellular water (ECW)

Age		% Water
Prenatal		70—95
Infant		ECW = 0.239 Mass (kg) + 0.325 kg
Child	(M)	ECW = 0.277 Mass (kg) + 0.916 kg
	(F)	ECW = 0.211 Mass (kg) + 0.989 kg
Adult	(M)	ECW = 7.35 + 0.135 Mass (kg)
	(F)	ECW = 5.27 + 0.135 Mass (kg)
Average adult:		260 ml/kg

Intracellular water (ICW = TBW − ECW)

Age		% Water
Prenatal		17—38
Child	(M)	ICW = 0.3236 Mass (kg) + 1.773
	(F)	ICW = 0.3288 Mass (kg) + 0.930
Adult	(M)	ICW = TBW [55.3 − 0.07 (yr)]/100
Adult	(F)	ICW = TBW [62.3 − 0.16 (yr)]/100
Average adult:		340 ml/kg

ANATOMICAL AND PHYSIOLOGICAL DATA: TABLE 10

Changes in Body Fat With Age

Male: age	% Fat	Female: age	% Fat
20	11	20	29
—	—	35	29
47	21	45	35
51	26	56	41
70	31	65	45

ANATOMICAL AND PHYSIOLOGICAL DATA: TABLE 11

Chemical Composition of the Body (70 kg)

Element	Amount (g)	% of total body mass	Element	Amount (g)	% of total body weight
Oxygen	43500	61	Lead	0.12	0.00017
Carbon	16000	23	Copper	0.072	0.00010
Hydrogen	7000	10	Aluminum	0.061	0.00009
Nitrogen	1800	2.6	Cadmium	0.050	0.00007
Calcium	1000	1.4	Boron	<0.048	0.00007
Phosphorus	780	1.1	Barium	0.022	0.00003
Sulfur	140	0.20	Tin	<0.017	0.00002
Potassium	140	0.20	Manganese	0.012	0.00002
Sodium	100	0.14	Iodine	0.013	0.00002
Chlorine	95	0.12	Nickel	0.010	0.00001
Magnesium	19	0.027	Gold	<0.010	0.00001
Silicon	18	0.026	Molybdenum	<0.0093	0.00001
Iron	4.2	0.006	Chromium	<0.0018	0.000003
Fluorine	2.6	0.0037	Cesium	0.0015	0.000002
Zinc	2.3	0.0033	Cobalt	0.0015	0.000002
Rubidium	0.32	0.00046	Uranium	0.00009	0.0000001
Strontium	0.32	0.00046	Beryllium	0.000036	
Bromine	0.20	0.00029	Radium	3.1×10^{-11}	

ANATOMICAL AND PHYSIOLOGICAL DATA: TABLE 12

Average Normal Blood Pressure (mm Hg)

Age	Systolic	Diastolic	Pulse pressure
10 years	103	70	33
15 years	113	75	38
20 years	120	80	40
25 years	122	81	41
30 years	123	82	41
35 years	124	83	41
40 years	126	84	42
45 years	128	85	43
50 years	130	86	44
55 years	132	87	45
60 years	135	89	46

Temperature of the Body

The average normal temperature of adults is 36.8°C (98.6°F). The daily variation is from 0.2° — 0.3°, the maximum temperature being reached between 5 and 7 p.m.

ANATOMICAL AND PHYSIOLOGICAL DATA: TABLE 13

The Pulse, Average Frequency at Different Ages in Health

Age	Beats per minute	
In the fetus in utero	between	140—150
Newborn infants	between	130—150
During the first year	from	108—130
During second year	from	90—108
During third year	from	80—90
From 7th to 14th year	from	72—80
From 14th to 21st year	from	80—85
From 21st to 60th year	average	72
In old age	average	67

Note: The pulse rate is faster in females, by 10—14 beats per minute; during and after exertion, unless long continued; during digestion or mental excitement; and generally more frequent in the morning.

ANATOMICAL AND PHYSIOLOGICAL DATA: TABLE 14

Physiological Changes During Maturation

Parameter	Neonate	Infant	Child	Adult
Hemoglobin (gram/l)	170—200	105—125	120—140	140—160
Heart rate (beats/min)	130—150	90—110	72—80	70—80
Blood pressure (average: mm Hg)	80/45	85/50	100/70	120/80
Breathing rate (breaths/min)	30—50	20—30	16—20	14—16
Urine volume (ml/24 h)	100—300	400—500	600—1,000	1,000—1,500
Urine specific gravity	1.002—1.008	1.002—1.008	1.015—1.025	1.015—1.025

Note: (Neonate, period that extends from birth until the end of the 4th week of life; infant, the period extending from 4 weeks until 2 years of age; child, the period extending from 2 years until 12 years of age.)

ANATOMICAL AND PHYSIOLOGICAL DATA: TABLE 15A

Normal Blood Volume Values in Milliliters for Men

	Height in meters (parentheses indicate height in inches)									
Wt(kg)	1.52 (60)	1.57 (62)	1.63 (64)	1.68 (66)	1.73 (68)	1.78 (70)	1.83 (72)	1.88 (74)	1.93 (76)	Wt(lb)
40.8	3,150	3,250	3,350	3,450	3,550	3,650	3,750	3,850	3,950	90
43.1	3,250	3,350	3,450	3,550	3,650	3,750	3,850	4,000	4,100	95
45.4	3,350	3,450	3,550	3,650	3,800	3,900	4,000	4,100	4,200	100
47.6	3,450	3,550	3,650	3,750	3,900	4,000	4,100	4,200	4,300	105
49.9	3,500	3,650	3,750	3,850	4,000	4,100	4,200	4,300	4,400	110
52.2	3,600	3,750	3,850	3,950	4,100	4,200	4,300	4,400	4,500	115
54.4	3,700	3,850	3,950	4,050	4,200	4,300	4,400	4,500	4,650	120
56.7	3,800	3,900	4,050	4,150	4,250	4,400	4,500	4,600	4,750	125
59.9	3,900	4,000	4,150	4,250	4,350	4,500	4,600	4,700	4,850	130
61.2	3,950	4,100	4,200	4,350	4,450	4,600	4,700	4,800	4,950	135
63.5	4,050	4,150	4,300	4,400	4,550	4,650	4,800	4,900	4,050	140
65.8	4,100	4,250	4,400	4,500	4,650	4,750	4,900	5,000	5,150	145
68.0	4,200	4,350	4,450	4,600	4,700	4,850	4,950	5,100	5,200	150
70.3	4,300	4,440	4,550	4,650	4,800	4,950	5,050	5,200	5,300	155
72.6	4,350	4,500	4,600	4,750	4,900	5,000	5,150	5,250	5,400	160
74.8	4,450	4,550	4,700	4,850	4,950	5,100	5,220	5,350	5,500	165
77.1	4,550	4,650	4,750	4,900	5,050	5,150	5,300	5,450	5,550	170
79.4	4,550	4,700	4,850	5,000	5,100	5,250	5,400	5,500	5,650	175
81.6	4,650	4,800	4,900	5,050	5,200	5,350	5,450	5,600	5,750	180
83.9	4,700	4,850	5,000	5,150	5,250	5,400	5,550	5,700	5,800	185
86.2	4,800	4,900	5,050	5,200	5,350	5,500	5,600	5,750	5,900	190
88.5	4,850	5,000	5,150	5,300	5,400	5,500	5,700	5,850	6,000	195
90.7	4,900	5,050	5,200	5,350	5,550	5,650	5,750	5,900	6,050	200
93.0	4,950	5,100	5,250	5,400	5,550	5,700	5,850	6,000	6,150	205
95.3	5,050	5,200	5,350	5,500	5,650	5,800	5,900	6,050	6,200	210
97.5	5,100	5,250	5,400	5,550	5,700	5,850	6,000	6,150	6,300	215
99.8	5,150	5,300	5,450	5,600	5,750	5,900	6,050	6,200	6,350	220
102.1	5,200	5,400	5,550	5,700	5,850	6,000	6,150	6,300	6,450	225
104.3	5,300	5,450	5,600	5,750	5,900	6,050	6,200	6,350	6,500	230
106.6	5,350	5,550	5,650	5,800	5,950	6,100	6,250	6,400	6,550	235
108.9	5,400	5,550	5,700	5,900	6,050	6,200	6,350	6,500	6,650	240
111.1	5,450	5,600	5,800	5,950	6,100	6,250	6,400	6,550	6,700	245
113.4	5,500	5,700	5,850	6,000	6,150	6,300	6,450	6,650	6,800	250
115.7	5,600	5,750	5,900	6,050	6,200	6,400	6,550	6,700	6,850	255
117.9	5,650	5,800	5,950	6,100	6,300	6,450	6,600	6,750	6,900	260
120.2	5,700	5,850	6,000	6,200	6,350	6,500	6,650	6,800	7,000	265
122.5	5,750	5,900	6,100	6,250	6,400	6,550	6,750	6,900	7,050	270
124.7	5,800	5,950	6,150	6,300	6,450	6,650	6,800	6,950	7,100	275
127.0	5,850	6,000	6,200	6,350	6,500	6,700	6,850	7,000	7,150	280
129.3	5,900	6,100	6,250	6,400	6,600	6,750	6,900	7,100	7,250	285
131.5	5,950	6,150	6,300	6,450	6,650	6,800	6,950	7,150	7,300	290
133.8	6,000	6,200	6,350	6,550	6,700	6,850	7,050	7,200	7,350	295
136.1	6,050	6,250	6,400	6,600	6,750	6,900	7,100	7,250	7,450	300
138.3	6,100	6,300	6,450	6,650	6,811	7,000	7,150	7,300	7,500	305
140.6	6,150	6,350	6,500	6,700	6,850	7,050	7,200	7,400	7,550	310
142.9	6,200	6,400	6,550	6,750	6,900	7,100	7,250	7,450	7,600	315

From Hidalgo, J. U., Nadler, S. B., and Bloch, T., *J. Nucl. Med.*, 3, 94, 1962. With permission.

ANATOMICAL AND PHYSIOLOGICAL DATA: TABLE 15B

Normal Blood Volume Values in Milliliters for Women

Wt(kg)	1.47 (58)	1.52 (60)	1.57 (62)	1.63 (64)	1.68 (66)	1.73 (68)	1.78 (70)	1.83 (72)	1.88 (74)	Wt(lb)
36.3	2,300	2,400	2,500	2,600	2,750	2,850	2,950	3,050	3,150	80
38.6	2,400	2,550	2,650	2,750	2,850	2,950	3,050	3,150	3,250	85
40.8	2,550	2,650	2,750	2,850	2,950	3,050	3,200	3,300	3,400	90
43.1	2,650	2,750	2,860	2,950	3,100	3,200	3,300	3,400	3,500	95
45.4	2,750	2,850	2,950	3,100	3,200	3,300	3,400	3,500	3,650	100
47.6	2,850	2,950	3,050	3,200	3,300	3,400	3,500	3,650	3,750	105
49.9	2,950	3,050	3,150	3,300	3,400	3,500	3,650	3,750	3,850	110
52.2	3,000	3,150	3,250	3,350	3,500	3,650	3,750	3,850	4,000	115
54.4	3,100	3,250	3,350	3,500	3,600	3,750	3,850	3,950	4,100	120
56.7	3,200	3,350	3,450	3,600	3,700	3,850	3,950	4,050	4,200	125
59.0	3,300	3,400	3,550	3,650	3,800	3,950	4,050	4,200	4,300	130
61.2	3,350	3,500	3,650	3,750	3,900	4,000	4,150	4,250	4,400	135
63.5	3,450	3,600	3,700	3,850	4,000	4,100	4,250	4,350	4,500	140
65.8	3,550	3,650	3,800	3,950	4,050	4,200	4,350	4,450	4,600	145
68.0	3,600	3,750	3,900	4,050	4,150	4,300	4,450	4,550	4,700	150
70.3	3,700	3,850	3,950	4,100	4,250	4,400	4,500	4,650	4,800	155
72.5	3,750	3,900	4,050	4,200	4,350	4,450	4,600	4,750	4,900	160
74.8	3,850	4,000	4,150	4,250	4,400	4,550	4,700	4,850	4,950	165
77.1	3,900	4,050	4,200	4,350	4,500	4,650	4,800	4,900	5,050	170
79.4	4,000	4,150	4,300	4,450	4,600	4,700	4,850	5,000	5,150	175
81.6	4,050	4,200	4,350	4,500	4,650	4,800	4,950	5,100	5,250	180
83.9	4,150	4,300	4,450	4,600	4,750	4,900	5,000	5,150	5,300	185
86.2	4,200	4,350	4,500	4,650	4,800	5,000	5,100	5,250	5,400	190
88.5	4,250	4,450	4,600	4,750	4,900	5,050	5,200	5,350	5,450	195
90.7	4,350	4,500	4,650	4,800	4,950	5,100	5,250	5,400	5,500	200
93.0	4,400	4,550	4,700	4,900	5,000	5,200	5,350	5,500	5,560	205
95.3	4,450	4,650	4,800	4,950	5,100	5,250	5,400	5,550	5,700	210
97.5	4,550	4,700	4,850	5,000	5,150	5,350	5,500	5,650	5,800	215
99.8	4,600	4,750	4,900	5,100	5,250	5,400	5,550	5,700	5,850	220
102.1	4,650	4,850	5,000	5,150	5,300	5,450	5,650	5,800	5,950	225
104.3	4,700	4,900	5,050	5,200	5,400	5,550	5,700	5,850	6,000	230
106.6	4,800	4,950	5,100	5,300	5,450	5,600	5,750	5,950	6,100	235
108.9	4,850	5,000	5,200	5,350	5,500	5,700	5,850	6,000	6,150	240
111.1	4,900	5,100	5,250	5,400	5,600	5,750	5,900	6,050	6,250	245
114.1	4,950	5,150	5,300	5,550	5,650	5,800	6,000	6,150	6,300	250
115.7	5,000	5,200	5,350	5,550	5,700	5,900	6,050	6,200	6,350	255
117.9	5,100	5,250	5,450	5,600	5,750	5,950	6,100	6,300	6,450	260
120.2	5,150	5,300	5,500	5,650	5,850	6,000	6,150	6,350	6,500	265
122.5	5,200	5,350	5,550	5,700	5,900	6,050	6,250	6,400	6,600	270
124.7	5,250	5,450	5,600	5,800	5,950	6,150	6,300	7,450	6,650	275
127.0	5,300	5,500	5,650	5,850	6,000	6,200	6,350	6,500	6,700	280
129.3	5,350	5,550	5,700	5,900	6,100	6,250	6,450	6,600	6,750	285
131.5	5,400	5,600	5,800	5,950	6,150	6,300	6,500	6,650	6,850	290
133.8	5,450	5,650	5,850	6,000	6,200	6,400	6,550	6,750	6,900	295
136.1	5,500	5,700	5,900	6,100	6,250	6,450	6,600	6,800	6,950	300
138.3	5,600	5,750	5,950	6,150	6,300	6,500	6,650	6,850	7,050	305
140.6	5,650	5,800	6,000	6,200	6,350	6,550	6,750	6,900	7,100	310
142.9	5,700	5,850	6,050	6,250	6,450	6,600	6,800	6,950	7,150	315

Height in meters (parentheses indicate height in inches)

From Hidalgo, J. U., Nadler, S. B., and Bloch, T., *J. Nucl. Med.*, 3, 94, 1962. With permission.

ANATOMICAL AND PHYSIOLOGICAL DATA: TABLE 16

Desirable Body Mass in Kilograms

	Height in cm	Small bones	Medium bones	Heavy bones
Male (in typical indoor clothing; shoes with 2.5 cm heels)	157.5	50.9—54.5	53.4—58.6	57.3—64.1
	160.0	52.3—55.9	55.0—60.5	58.6—65.5
	162.5	53.6—57.3	56.4—61.8	60.0—67.3
	165.0	55.0—58.6	57.7—63.2	61.4—69.1
	167.5	56.4—60.5	59.1—65.0	62.7—70.9
	170.0	58.2—62.3	60.9—66.8	64.5—73.2
	172.5	60.0—64.1	62.7—69.1	66.8—75.5
	175.0	61.8—65.9	64.5—70.9	68.6—77.3
	177.5	63.5—68.2	66.4—72.7	70.5—79.1
	180.0	65.4—70.0	68.2—75.0	72.3—81.4
	182.5	67.3—71.8	70.0—77.3	74.5—83.6
	185.0	69.1—73.6	71.8—79.5	76.4—85.9
	187.5	70.9—75.9	73.6—81.8	78.6—88.2
	190.0	72.7—77.7	75.9—84.1	80.9—90.5
	192.5	74.5—79.5	78.2—86.2	82.7—92.7
Female (in typical indoor clothing in shoes with 5 cm heels)	147.5	41.8—44.5	43.6—48.6	47.3—54.1
	150.0	42.7—45.9	44.5—50.0	48.2—55.5
	152.5	43.6—47.3	45.9—51.4	49.5—56.8
	155.0	45.0—48.6	47.3—52.7	50.9—58.2
	157.5	46.4—50.0	48.6—54.1	52.3—59.5
	160.0	47.7—51.4	50.0—55.5	53.6—60.9
	162.5	49.1—52.7	51.4—57.3	55.0—62.7
	165.0	50.5—54.1	52.7—59.1	56.8—64.5
	167.5	51.8—55.9	54.5—61.4	58.6—66.4
	170.0	53.6—57.7	56.4—63.2	60.5—68.2
	172.5	55.5—59.5	58.2—65.0	62.3—70.0
	175.0	57.3—61.4	60.0—66.8	64.1—71.8
	177.5	59.1—63.6	61.8—68.6	65.9—74.1
	180.0	60.9—65.5	63.6—70.5	67.7—76.4
	182.5	62.7—67.3	65.5—72.3	69.5—78.6

From the Department of Physiology, University of Pretoria, Pretoria.

COMMONLY PERFORMED LABORATORY TESTS

THE FORMAT OF LABORATORY REPORTS

System Codes

B	Blood
P	Plasma
S	Serum
U	Urine
F	Feces
Sf	Spinal fluid
E	Erythrocyte
Lkc	Leukocyte
Pt	Patient
fPt	fasting patient
a	arterial
c	capillary
v	venous
d	day (24 h)

(a,c,v,d are prefixes to other codes)

For example:

1. A glucose estimation on plasma from a fasting patient is reported as (fPt)P-Glucose 4.0 mmol/l
2. The same test done on whole blood obtained by a fingerprick would appear as (fPt)-cB-Glucose 4.0 mmol/l
3. A 24 h urinary creatinine excretion would be reported as dU-Creatinine 10 mmol
4. S (serum) is named where either serum or plasma (P) may be used.

The symbols $-$, $+$, $++$, etc., have been replaced by the following:

1. Where a result distinguishes only between the presence or absence of a reaction it is reported as 0 or 1. For example, if antibodies are detected by the direct Coombs test the report will read:

   S — Incomplete antibody (0—1) 1
   (Indirect Coombs)

2. Alternatively, if a qualitative test has a known lower limit of sensitivity it can be reported as such. A urine that fails to react to a test for glucose could be reported as:

   U-Glucose <12 mmol/l

3. Where a graded response is possible, for example Benedict's test on urine, it may be reported as:

   U-Reducing substances (0—4) 3

Note that the possible responses (0—1) or (0—4) are incorporated as part of the test description.

4. Titers are reported as follows:

   E-Incomplete antibody (titer) 64
   (Direct Coombs)

From the Institute for Pathology, University of Pretoria, Pretoria.

COMMONLY PERFORMED LABORATORY TESTS:
TABLE 1

Blood Chemistry

Component	Units	Reference values		
		Male		Female
S-Albumin	g/l		35—50	
aB-Base excess	mmol/l		0—3	
S-Bilibrubin (total)	μmol/l		3.4—17.1	
S-Bilirubin (conjugated)	μmol/l		0—3.4	
S-CO$_2$ (total)	mmol/l		23—29	
aB-pC$_{O2}$	kPa		4.8—6.3	
S-Ceruloplasmin	g/l		1.8—4.5	
S-Calcium (total)	mmol/l		2.10—2.55	
S-Calcium (ionized)	mmol/l		1.2—1.23	
S-B-Carotene	μmol/l		1.12—3.72	
S-Chloride	mmol/l		98—108	
S-Cholesterol	mmol/l		3.6—6.4	
P-Cortisol	nmol/l		170—700 (08:00 h)	
S-Creatinine	μmol/l	62—115		53—106
(fPt)P-Glucose	mmol/l		3.89—5.83	
S-Globulin	g/l		22-40	
alpha[1]	g/l		1—3	
alpha[2]	g/l		6—10	
beta	g/l		7—11	
gamma	g/l		8—16	
S-Iron	μmol/l	8.95—28.64		7.16—26.85
S-Iron-binding capacity	μmol/l		44.75—71.60	
S-Magnesium	mmol/l		0.65—1.05	
S-Osmolality	mmol/kg		275—295	
aB-p$_{O2}$	kPa		11.4—14.36	
S-Phospholipids	g/l		1.5—2.5	
S-Phosphorus (inorganic)	mmol/l	0.74—1.20		0.90—1.32
S-Potassium	mmol/l		3.6—5.1	
S-Protein (total)	g/l		64—83	
S-Sodium	mmol/l		136—146	
S-Thyroxine	nmol/l	65—129		71—135
S-Triglyceride	mmol/l	0.45—1.81		0.40—1.53
S-Urate	mmol/l	0.21—0.42		0.15—0.35
S-Urea	mmol/l		2.5—6.4	
S-Vitamin A	μmol/l		1.05—2.27	

COMMONLY PERFORMED LABORATORY TESTS: TABLE 2

Urine

Component	Units	Reference values Male	Reference values Female
dU-Calcium	mmol	2.5—7.5	
dU-Coproporphyrins I and III	μmol	150—450	
dU-Cortisol	nmol	27.6—48.3	
dU-Creatine	mmol	0—0.3	0—0.61
dU-Creatinine	mmol	7.1—17.7	5.3—15.9
dU-5-Hydroxyindolyl acetate (5-HIAA)	μmol	10.4—31.4	
dU-4-Hyrodxy 3-methoxy mandelate (HMMA)	μmol	10.1—35.4	
dU-Ketones	mmol	0.1—0.3	
dU-Phosphorus (inorganic)	mmol	12.9—42	
dU-17-Oxosteroids (as DHEA)	μmol	20—70	16—52
dU-Total-17-oxogenic steroids (as DHEA)	μmol	14-54	12—41
dU-Urate	mmol	<2.48	
dU-Urea	mmol	430—700	
Glomerular filtration rate (GFR)	ml/min/1.73 m^2	106—154	97—144
Maximum urine concentration	mOsmol/kg	>800	
Minimal urine pH		<5.3	

COMMONLY PERFORMED LABORATORY TESTS: TABLE 3

Cerebrospinal fluid

Component	Units	Reference values
Sf-Chloride	mmol/l	118—132
Sf-Glucose	mmol/l	2.22—3.89
Sf-Protein (lumbar)	mg/l	150—450
Cells		
Polymorphs	no./l	0
Lymphocytes	no./l	0—5 × 10^6
Erythrocytes	no./l	0—5 × 10^6

COMMONLY PERFORMED LABORATORY TESTS: TABLE 4A

Blood Counts — Adults at Sea Level

		Reference values	Units
B-Erythrocytes (RBC)	Male	4.5—5.9	$\times 10^{12}$/l
	Female	4.0—5.2	$\times 10^{12}$/l
B-Hemoglobin (Hb)	Male	13.5—17.5	g/dl
	Female	12—16	g/dl
B-Hematocrit	Male	0.41—0.53	—
	Female	0.36—0.46	—
B-ESR (Westergren 1 h at 17-23°C)	Male	0—15	mm
	Female	0—20	mm
(B)E-Mean corpuscular volume (MCV)		77—93	fl
(B)E-Mean corpuscular hemoglobin (MCH)		27—32	pg
(B)E-Mean corpuscular hemoglobin concentration (MCHC)		31—35	g/dl
(B)E-Reticulocytes (0.5-2.0%)		25—100	$\times 10^9$/l
B-Leucocytes	Male	3.9—10.6	$\times 10^9$/l
	Female	3.5—11	$\times 10^9$/l
Differential leucocyte count:			
B-Neutrophils (40-75%)		2.0—7.5	$\times 10^9$/l
B-Lymphocytes (20-45%)		1.5—4.0	$\times 10^9$/l
B-Monocytes (2-10%)		0.18—0.8	$\times 10^9$/l
B-Eosinophils (1-6%)		0.04—0.45	$\times 10^9$/l
B-Basophils (<1%)		<0.1	$\times 10^9$/l
B-Platelets		150—400	$\times 10^9$/l

COMMONLY PERFORMED LABORATORY TESTS: TABLE 4B

Hematology

Component	Units	Reference values Male	Female
E-Folate	μg/l	150—450	
S-Folate	μg/l	1.8—9	
S-Haptoglobin	g/l	0.83—2.67	
S-Lysozyme	mg/l	4—13	
S-Vitamin B$_{12}$	ng/l	100—700	
S-Ferritin	μg/l	15—200	12—150
S:Transferrin	μmol/l	31—52	33—63
dU-Schilling test		>10% of dose excreted	
Immunoglobulins			
IgG	g/l	6—15	
IgM	g/l	0.43—3.23	0.66—3.52
IgA	g/l	1—4.5	
Total blood volume	ml/kg	52—83	50—75
Red cell volume	ml/kg	20—36	19—31
Plasma volume	ml/kg	25—43	28—45
Red blood cell T$_{1/2}$	d	25—33	
Plasma iron clearance T$_{1/2}$	min	80—120	
Red cell iron utilization		>80% in 10 d	
pH		arterial 7.35—7.45	
		mixed venous 7.34—7.42	

COMMONLY PERFORMED LABORATORY TESTS: TABLE 5

Hemostasis

Component	Units	Reference values
Pt-Capillary bleeding time	min	1—7
P-Fibrinogen	g/l	2—4
S-Fibrinogen degradation products	mg/l	<10
P-Prothrombin time	s	10—14
B-Clotting time	min	<10
P-Thrombin time	s	10—12

COMMONLY PERFORMED LABORATORY TESTS: TABLE 6

Enzymes

Enzyme	(Abbreviation)	Reference values		Units
		Male	Female	
Acid phosphatase	(ACP)	2.5—11.7	0.3—9.2	U/l
Alanine transaminase	(ALT)		8—20	U/l
Alkaline phosphatase	(ALP)		32—92	U/l
Aspartate transaminase	(AST)		10—30	U/l
Cholinesterase	(CHS)		8—18	kU/l
Creatine kinase	(CK)	38—174	96—140	U/l
γ-Glutamyltransferase	(GGT)	5—38	5—29	U/l
Glucose-6-phosphate dehydrogenase	(GPD)		1.16—2.72	kU/l RBC
Glutamate dehydrogenase	(GMD)		0—0.9	U/l
Isocitrate dehydrogenase	(ICD)		3—8.5	U/l
Lactate dehydrogenase	(LD)		210—420	U/l
5'-Nucleotidase	(NTP)		2—17	U/l
Pyruvate kinase	(PK)		4.42—5.78	kU/l RBC

Note: There is no international agreement on enzyme units. These are the recommended names and abbreviations for the common enzymes estimations.

COMMONLY PERFORMED LABORATORY TESTS: TABLE 7

Hormones

Hormone	Unit	Reference values Male	Female	Comments
P-Adrenocorticotrophin (ACTH)	ng/l	25—100		08:00 Adult
		<50		18:00 Adult
P-Aldosterone	nmol/l	0.17—0.61	0.14—0.83	Adult
S-Androstenedione	nmol/l	2.86—4.60	3.94—6.60	Adult
				In females, specimen to be collected 1 week before or after menstruation
aP-Angiotensin II	pmol/l	12—36		Adult
P-Antidiuretic hormone (ADH)	pmol/l	0.9—4.6		Adult
P-Calcitonin	pmol/l	<27		Adult
dU-Chorionic Gonadotropin (CG)	1U/l	13,000—20,000		Pregnancy from 6th wk to term (mean).
S-Cortisol	μmol/l	0.14—0.64		08:00 h
				16:00h
				20:00 h
dU-Cortisol-free	nmol	27.6—276		Adult
S-Estradiol, total	pmol/l	29—132		Adult
			0—1100	Puberty
			37—330	Follicular
			367—1835	Midcycle
			184—881	Luteal
			37—110	Postmenopausal
dU-Estrogens	μg	2.5—652		Puberty
		5—25		Adult
			5—25	Preovulation
			28—100	Ovulation
			22—80	Luteal
			<10	Post menopausal
			up to 45,000	Pregnant, term
S-Follicle stimulating hormone (FSH)	IU/l	4—25		Adult
			4—30	Premenopause
			10—90	Midcycle peak
			40—250	Post menopause
P-Gastrin	pmol/l	<27		Adult
P-Glucagon	pmol/l	15—44		Adult
S-Growth hormone (GH)	μg/l	<2 <1—10	<10	Adult
fP-Insulin	mIU/l	6—24		Adult
S-Luteinizing hormone (LH)	IU/l	6—23		Adult
P-Parathyroid hormone	pmol/l	16—62		N-terminal assay
		16—125		C-terminal assay
S-Placental lactogen	mg/l		<0.5	Non-pregnant
				Pregnant wk
			1—3.8	22
			1.5—4.5	26
			2.8—5.8	30
			3.6—82	38

COMMONLY PERFORMED LABORATORY TESTS: TABLE 7
(continued)

Hormones

Hormone	Unit	Reference values		Comments
		Male	**Female**	
			3—8	42
S-Progesterone	nmol/l	0.35—0.83		Puberty
		0.38—0.95		Adult
			0—1.91	Puberty
			0.06—2.86	Follicular phase
			19.08—95.4	Luteal phase
			254—636	Pregnancy term
			0.09—0.95	Post menopausal
S-Prolactin	µg/l	<20		Adult
			<23	Follicular phase
			5—40	Luteal phase
			<400	Pregnancy term
S-Thyroxine (T4)	nmol/l	65—129	71—135	Adult
S-Thyroxine, free	pmol/l	10.3—3.31		Adult
S-Thyroxine binding globulin (TBG)	mg/l	15—34		Adult
S-Thyroid stimulating hormone (TSH)	mIU/l	2—7.3	2—16.8	Adult
S-Testosterone, total	nmol/l	15.17—24.53	0.93—1.63	Adult
S-Tri-iodothyronine (T3)				
Free	pmol/l	3.54—10.16		Adult
Total	nmol/l	1.77—2.93		Adult
P-Vaso-active intestinal polypeptide (VIP)	pmol/l	8—17		

COMMONLY PERFORMED LABORATORY TESTS: TABLE 8

Cardiac Function Normal Values

Pressures (mm Hg)

Systemic arterial	
Peak systolic	100—140
End diastolic	60—90
Left ventricle	
Peak systolic	100—140
End diastolic	3—12
Systolic mean	80—130
Diastolic mean	1—10
Left atrium (pulmonary capillary wedge)	
Mean	2—10
Diastolic mean	1—10
Pulmonary artery	
Peak systolic	15—30
End diastolic	4—12
Systolic mean	10—20
Right ventricle	
Peak systolic	15—30
End diastolic	2—8
Systolic mean	10—20
Diastolic mean	0—4
Right atrium	
Mean	2—8
Cardiac output	Varies with individual's size and heart rate
Cardiac index	2.6—4.2 $l/m/m^2$
Stroke index	30—65 $ml/min/m^2$
End-diastolic volume	53—83 ml/m^2
End-systolic volume	17—33 ml/m^2
Left ventricular ejection fraction (LVEF)	56—74%
Right ventricular ejection fraction (RVEF)	48—68%
Mean pulmonary transit time	5.5—7.7 s

COMMONLY PERFORMED LABORATORY TESTS: TABLE 9

Blood Flow, Fractional Cardiac Output, and Oxygen Utilization of Major Organs

Organ	Blood flow during rest				Oxygen usage during rest			
	Weight (kg)	ml/min	mil/min/ 100 g	% Total cardiac output	A-V O$_2$ Difference (ml/100 ml Blood)	ml/min	ml/min/ 100 g	% Total O$_2$ usage
Brain	1.4	750(1,500)ᵃ	55	14	6	45	3	18
Heart	0.3	250(1,200)	80	5	10	25	8	10
Liver	1.8	1,300(5,000)	85	23	6	75	2	30
GI tract	1.2	1,000(4,000)	40					
Kidneys	0.3	1,200(1,800)	400	22	1.3	15	5	6
Muscle	35	1,000(20,000)	3	18	5	50	0.15	20
Skin	2	200(3,000)	10	4	2.5	5	0.2	2
Remainder (skeleton, bone marrow, fat connective tissue, etc.)	27	800(4,000)	3	14	5	35	0.15	
Total	70 kg	5,500 ml/min		100		250		100

Note: The values in the table are rounded figures and roughly describe the situation in an average man.

ᵃ Figures in parentheses give in very approximate terms organ blood flows as maximal vasodilation of the respective circuits.

From Folkow, B. and Neil, E., *Circulation*, London, Oxford University Press, 1971, 12. With permission.

COMMONLY PERFORMED LABORATORY TESTS: TABLE 10

Typical Values for Pulmonary Function Tests: Mechanics of Breathing

Measurement and units	Mean value/range
Maximum voluntary ventilation BTPS, l/min	170
Forced expiratory volume%1 s	83
%3 s	97
Maximal expiratory flow rate (for 1 liter (AIPS), l/min	>400
Maximal inspiratory flow rate (for 1 liter) (AIPS), l/min	>300
Compliance of lungs and thoracic cage, l/H_2O	0.1
Compliance of lungs, L/H_2O	0.2
Airway resistance, H_2O/l/s	1.6
Pulmonary resistance, H_2O/l/s	1.9
Work of quiet breathing, kg·m/min	0.5
Maximal work of breathing, kg·m/b	10
Maximal inspiratory and expiratory pressures, mmHg	60—100 (7.99—13.33 kPa)

Ventilation (BTPS)

Tidal volume, ml	500
Frequency respirations, /min	12
Minute volume, ml/min	6,000
Respiratory dead space, ml	150
Alveolar ventilation, ml/min	4,200

Distribution of Inspired Gas

Single-breath test (% increase N_2 for 500 ml, expired alveolar gas, % N_2)	<1.5
Pulmonary nitrogen emptying rate, (7 min. test), % N_2	<2.5
Helium closed circuit % (mixing efficiency related to perfect mixing)	76

Pulmonary Circulation

Pulmonary capillary blood flow, ml/min	5,400
Pulmonary artery pressure, mmHg	25/8 (3.33—3.73 kPa)
Pulmonary capillary blood volume, ml	90
Pulmonary "capillary" blood pressure, (wedge), mmHg	8 (1.06 kPa)

Alveolar Gas

Oxygen partial pressure, mmHg	104 (13.86 kPa)
Co_2 partial pressure, mmHg	40 (5.33 kPa)

Diffusion and Gas Exchange

O_2 consumption (STPD), ml/min	240
Co_2 output (STPD), ml/min	192
Respiratory exchange ratio, R (CO_2 output/O_2 uptake)	0.8
Diffusing capacity, O_2 (STPD), resting, ml O_2/min/mmHg	>15
Diffusing capacity, O_2 (steady-state) (STPD), resting, ml O_2/min/mmHg	17
Diffusing capacity CO (single-breath) (STPD), resting, ml CO/min/mmHg	25
Diffusing capacity, CO (rebreathing), (STPD), resting, ml CO/min/mmHg	25
Fractional CO uptake, resting, %	53
Maximal diffusing capacity, O_2 (exercise) (STPD), ml O_2/min/mmHg	60

COMMONLY PERFORMED LABORATORY TESTS: TABLE 10
(continued)

Typical Values for Pulmonary Function Tests: Mechanics of Breathing

Arterial Blood

O_2 saturation (percent saturation of Hb with O_2), %	97.1
O_2 tension, mmHg	95
	(12.66 kPa)
CO_2 tension, mmHg	40
	(5.33 kPa)
Alveolar-arterial PO_2 difference, mmHg	9
	(1.2 kPa)
Alveolar-arterial PO_2 difference, (12—14% O_2), mmHg	10
	(1.33 kPa)
Alveolar-arterial PO_2 difference, (100% O_2), mmHg	35
	(4.66 kPa)
O_2 saturation, (100% O_2), % (+1.9 ml dissolved O_2/100 ml blood)	100
O_2 tension, (100% O_2), mmHg	640
	(7.99 kPa)
pH	7.4

Alveolar Ventilation/Pulmonary Capillary Blood Flow

Alveolar ventilation, (l/min)/blood flow (l/min)	0.8
Physiologic shunt/cardiac output $\times$ 100%	<7
Physiologic dead space/tidal volume $\times$ 100%	<30

Note: These are values for a healthy, resting, recumbent young male (1.7 square meters of surface area), breathing air at sea level, unless other conditions are specified. They are presented merely to give approximate figures. These values may change with position, age, size, sex and altitude; variability occurs among members of the homogeneous group under standard conditions. Reference Departments of Physiology and Internal Medicine (Division of Pulmonology), University of Pretoria, Pretoria.

COMMONLY PERFORMED LABORATORY TESTS: TABLE 11

Symbols and Abbreviations Used by Pulmonary Physiologists: American College of Chest Physicians/American Thoracic Society (ACCP/ATS)

A	Alveolar
a	Arterial
an	Anatomic
ATPD	Ambient temperature and pressure, dry
ATPS	Ambient temperature and pressure, saturated with water vapor at these conditions
B	Barometric
BTPS	Body conditions: Body temperature, ambient pressure, and saturated with water vapor at these conditions
C	A general symbol for compliance, volume change per unit of applied pressure
c	Capillary
C/V_L	Specific compliance
CD	Cumulative inhalation dose. The total dose of an agent inhaled during bronchial challenge testing; it is the sum of the products of concentration multiplied by the number of breaths at that concentration
c_{dyn}	Dynamic compliance, compliance measured at point of zero gas flow at the mouth during active breathing. The respiratory frequency should be designated, e.g., $C_{dyn}40$
C_{st}	Stactic compliance, compliance determined from measurements made during conditions of prolonged interruption of air flow
D	Dead space or wasted ventilation
D/V_A	Diffusion per unit of alveolar volume
D_k	Diffusion coefficient or permeability constant
Dm	Diffusing capacity of the alveolar capillary membrane (STPD)
D_x	Diffusing capacity of the lung expressed as volume (STPD) of gas (x) uptake per unit alveolar-capillary pressure difference for the gas used. Unless otherwise stated, carbon monoxide is assumed to be the test gas, i.e., D is D_{CO}.
E	Expired
ERV	Expiratory reserve volume; the maximal volume of air exhaled from the end-expiratory level
est	Estimated
f	Respiratory frequency per minute
F	Fractional concentration of a gas
FEFmax	The maximal forced expiratory flow achieved during an FVC
$FEF_{25-75\%}$	Mean forced expiratory flow during the middle half of the FVC
$FEF_{75\%}$	Instantaneous forced expiratory flow after 75% of the FVC has been exhaled
$FEF_{200-1200}$	Mean forced expiratory flow between 200 ml and 1200 ml of the FVC
FEF_x	Forced expiratory flow, related to some portion of the FVC curve. Modifiers refer to the amount of the FVC already exhaled when the measurement is made
FET_x	The forced expiratory time for a specified portion of the FVC
$FEV_t/FVC\%$	Forced expiratory volume (timed) to forced vital capacity ratio, expressed as a percentage
FIF_x	Forced inspiratory flow. As in the case of the FEF, the appropriate modifiers must be used to designate the volume at which flow is being measured
Q_c	Capillary blood volume (usually expressed as V_c in the literature, a symbol inconsistent with those recommended for blood volumes)
R	A general symbol for resistance, pressure per unit flow
R_{aw}	Airway resistance
rb	Rebreathing
RQ	Respiratory quotient
R_{us}	Resistance of the airways on the alveolar side (upstream) of the point in the airways where intraluminal pressure equals Ppl, measured under conditions of maximal expiratory flow
RV	Residual volume: that volume of air remaining in the lungs after maximal exhalation. The method of measurement should be indicated in the text or, when necessary, by appropriate qualifying symbols
SBN	Single breath nitrogen test; a test in which plots of expired N_2 concentration vs. expired volume after inspiration of 100% O_2 are recorded
STPD	Standard conditions: temperature 0°C, pressure 760 mmHg, and dry (0 water vapor)
t	Time

COMMONLY PERFORMED LABORATORY TESTS: TABLE 11
(continued)

Symbols and Abbreviations Used by Pulmonary Physiologists: American College of Chest Physicians/American Thoracic Society (ACCP/ATS)

T	Tidal
TGV	Thoracic gas volume; the volume of gas within the thoracic cage as measured by body plethysmography
TLC	Total lung capacity; the sum of all volume compartments or the volume of air in the lungs after maximal inspiration
V	Gas volume. The particular gas as well as its pressure, water vapor conditions, and other special conditions must be specified in text or indicated by appropriate qualifying symbols
v	Venous
$\bar{v}$	Mixed venous
$\dot{V}_A$	Alveolar ventilation per minute (BIPS)
$\dot{V}_{CO2}$	Carbon dioxide production per minute (STPD)
$\dot{V}_D$	Ventilation per minute of the physiologic dead space
V_D	The physiologic dead-space volume defined as V_D/f
$V_D$an	Volume of the anatomic dead space (BTPS)
$\dot{V}_E$	Expired volume per minute (BTPS)
$\dot{V}_I$	Inspired volume per minute (BTPS)
Viso$\dot{V}$	Volume of isoflow; the volume when the expiratory flow rates become identical when flow-volume loops performed after breathing room air and helium-oxygen mixtures are compared
$\dot{V}_{O2}$	Oxygen consumption per minute (STPD)
$\dot{V}_{max}X$	Forced expiratory flow, related to the total lung capacity or the actual volume of the lung at which the measurement is made
V_T	Tidal volume; TV is also commonly used
X_A or Xa	A small capital letter or lower case letter on the same line following a primary symbol is a qualifier to further define the primary symbol. When small capital letters are not available on typewriters or printers, large capital letters may be used as subscripts, e.g., X_A = XA

Blood-gas Measurements
Abbreviations for these values are composed by combining the general recommended symbols:

$PaCO_2$	Arterial carbon dioxide tension
$C(a-v)O_2$	Arteriovenous oxygen content difference
CcO_2	Oxygen content of pulmonary end-capillary blood
F_ECO	Fractional concentration of CO in expired gas
$P(A-a)O_2$	Alveolar-arterial oxygen pressure difference; the previously used symbol, $A-aD_2$ is not recommended
SaO_2	Arterial oxygen saturation of hemoglobin
Q_{sp}	Physiologic shunt flow (total venous admixture) defined by the following equation when gas and blood data are collected during ambient air breathing

$$Qsp = \frac{CcO_2 - CaO_2}{CcO_2 - CvO_2} \cdot Q$$

$P_{ET}O_2$	PO2 of end tidal expired gas
$TCPO_2$	Transcutaneous PO2

International System (SI) Units for the Measurement of
Radioactivity and Ionizing Radiation

INTERNATIONAL SYSTEM (SI) UNITS FOR THE MEASUREMENT OF RADIOACTIVITY AND IONIZING RADIATION

INTRODUCTION

The General Conference on Weights and Measures in 1960 approved a comprehensive set of units — for use in all branches of science, trade, industry and government — called the Système International d'Unites (SI Units). Essentially, these units are an extension of the metric system and are derived by the mathematical relationship between appropriate physical quantities. Under the SI, a set of seven base and two supplementary units have been defined. From these, all other components of the system are derived. For convenience, the mathematicals expressions so derived are given special names. Perhaps the most important advantage obtained from the use of the SI Units has been promoting the standardization of units between the different branches of science and technology in most countries in the world. In 1974, the International Commission on Radiological Units (ICRU) recommended to the General Conference on Weights and Measures the adoption of special names for SI Units used for the measurement of radioactivity and radiation protection. These were approved in 1975, and the definitions of these new quantities and units were published in the ICRU Reports.

SI BASE AND SUPPLEMENTARY QUANTITIES

The International System of Units (SI) is based on seven basic and two supplementary physical quantities together with their units. These are defined as follows:

SI Base Units

1. **Mass:** The kilogram (symbol kg), is equal to the mass of the international prototype of the kilogram.
2. **Time:** The second (symbol s) is the duration of 9 192 631 770 periods of the radiation corresponding to the transition between the 2 hyperfine levels of the ground state of the cesium-133 atom.
3. **Length:** The meter (symbol m) is the length of the path traveled by light in vacuum during a time interval of 1/299 792 458 of a second.
4. **Electric Current:** The ampere (symbol A) is that constant current which, if maintained in two straight parallel conductors of infinite length of negligible circular cross section, and placed one meter apart in vacuum, would produce between these conductors a force equal to 2×10^{-7} newton per meter of length.
5. **Thermodynamic Temperature:** The kelvin (symbol K) is the fraction 1/273.16 of the thermodynamic temperature of the triple point of water.
5. **Amount of Substance:** The mole (symbol mol) is the amount of substance of a system which contains as many elementary entities as there are atoms in 0.012 kilogram of carbon-12. When the mole is used, the elementary entities must be specified, and may be atoms, molecules, ions, electrons, other particles, or specified groups of such particles.
7. **Luminous Intensity:** The candela (symbol cd) is the luminous intensity, in a given direction, of a source that emits monochromatic radiation of frequency 540×10^{12} hertz and that has a radiant intensity in that direction of (1/683) watt per steradian.

SI Supplementary Units

1. **Plane Angle:** The radian (symbol rad) is the plane angle between two radii of a circle which cut off on the circumference an arc equal in length to the radius.

TABLE 1
Summary of SI Base and Supplementary
Units

Quantity	Name	Symbol
SI base units		
Mass	Kilogram	kg
Time	Second	s
Length	Meter	m
Electric current	Ampere	A
Thermodynamic temperature	Kelvin	K
Amount of substance	Mole	mol
Luminous intensity	Candela	cd
SI Supplementary Units		
Plane angle	Radian	rad
Solid angle	Steradian	sr

From Radiation Quantities and Units, International Commission on Radiological Units and Measurements Report No. 33, Washington, D.C., ICRU, 1980.

2. **Solid Angle:** The steradian (symbol sr) is the solid angle which, having its vertex in the center of a sphere, cuts off an area of the surface of the sphere equal to that of a square with sides of length equal to the radius of the sphere.

SI UNITS FOR THE MEASUREMENT OF RADIOACTIVITY AND IONIZING RADIATION

SI units for the measurement of radiation and ionizing radiation are regarded as derived from the seven basic units. Many of these have special names:

1. **Activity:** The becquerel (symbol Bq) is equal to s^{-1}, or one nuclear transformation (disintegration) per second (dps). This replaces the non-SI unit, the curie.
2. **Absorbed Dose:** The gray (symbol Gy) is equal to the joule per kilogram (J/kg). The gray may also be used for other physical quantities, such as kerma and specific energy imparted, expressed in joules per kilogram, provided these quantities are used in connection with ionizing radiation. This replaces the non-SI unit, the rad.
3. **Dose Equivalent:** The sievert (symbol Sv) is defined as the radiation dose equivalent to the joule per kilogram (J/kg). This replaces the non-SI unit, the rem.
4. **Exposure:** The coulomb per kilogram (symbol C/kg) is the unit of exposure. It replaces the roentgen (R). The roentgen may still be used as the unit of exposure.

SI UNITS FOR RADIATION SOURCES

The quantity exposure rate is replaced by the quantity air kerma rate. The preferred SI units for air kerma rate are submultiples of gray per second, but brachytherapy sources will be specified in submultiples of gray per hour and teletherapy sources will be specified in submultiples of gray per minute. This maintains consistency with the units of time which have been used previously in these applications.

The quantity equivalent activity has hitherto been used as a convenient way of specifying exposure rate by the use of the appropriate exposure rate constant. This quantity will also be replaced by air kerma rate. The SI unit of activity, the becquerel, will be used to specify the content activity of a source.

Sources previously specified in terms of equivalent activity may be converted to the new quantity and units by first converting to exposure rate using the appropriate rate constant.

The new SI Unit and quantity for the specification of output by radiation sources are the gray per second (Gy/s), and the "air kerma rate", respectively. These replace the old unit of roentgen per hour (R/h) and the old quantity of exposure rate or equivalent activity exposure rate constant. The following should be noted:

1. Brachytherapy sources will be specified in submultiples of gray per hour.
2. Teletherapy sources will be specified in submultiples of gray per minute.
3. Outputs will be specified at a distance from the center of the source, unless otherwise stated.
4. The specified output will refer to an axial direction for disk source and a radial direction for all other sources, unless otherwise stated.

For most radiation sources, a constant factor may be used to convert from exposure rate to air kerma rate. Quite simply, an exposure of 1 roentgen per hour (1R/h) becomes 2.425 microgray per second (μGy/s), or for brachytherapy sources, 8.73 milligray per hour (mGy/h). Radiation sources are specified in terms of the exposure rate of air kerma rate at a distance of 1 meter from the source, and at this distance the strength of most sources is such that exposure rate will be in units for mR/h and air kerma rate will be in units of μGy/h. A conversion factor of 8.73 should therefore be used to convert from mR/h to μGy/h. It must be noted that the above mentioned conversion factors and equivalences only hold good providing that charged particle equilibrium is maintained and also that bremsstrahlung production is negligible.

Conversion for Industrial Sources

Multiply value by 2.425 to convert from R/h to μGy/s. Multiply value by 412.4 to convert from μG/s to mR/h.

Conversion for Brachytherapy Sources

Multiple value by 8.73 to convert from R/h to mGy/h. Multiply value by 114.5 to convert from mGy/h to mR/h.

Conversion for Teletherapy Sources

Multiply value by 8.73 to convert from R/min to mGy/min. Multiply value by 114.5 to convert from mGy/min to mR/min.

OTHER DERIVED SI UNITS FOR THE MEASUREMENT OF IONIZING RADIATION AND RADIATION PROTECTION

1. **Absorbed Dose Rate:** The gray per second (Gy/s) is the unit of absorbed dose rate. It replaces the rad per second (rad s^{-1}).
2. **Exposure Rate:** The coulomb per kilogram second (C/kg·s) is the unit of exposure rate. It replaces the roentgen per second (R s^{-1}).
3. **Transport Index:** The radiation dose rate in μSv/h at 1 meter from package surface, divided by ten is the transport index.
4. **Electronvolt** (eV): A non-SI unit of energy, the electronvolt, with its multiples, is still used extensively. In the absence of international moves to abandon it in favor of the joule(J) and its submultiples, the electronvolt will be retained.

$$1 \text{ eV} = 1.6022 \times 10^{-19} \text{ J: } 1\text{J} = 6.24 \times 10^{18} \text{ eV}$$

TABLE 2
Relationship Between SI and Non-SI Units in Ionizing Radiation and Radiation Protection

Physical quantity	SI unit	Non-SI unit		Relationship
Activity	Becquerel (Bq) (1 Becquerel = s^{-1})	Curie (Ci)	1 Ci	= 3.7 × 10^{10} Bq = 37 GBq
			1 Bq	= 2.7 × 10^{-11} Ci = 27 pCi
Absorbed dose, kerma, Specific energy Imparted, etc.	Gray (Gy) (1 Gy = 1 J/kg)	Rad (rad)	1 rad	= 0.01 Gy
			1 Gy	= 100 rad
Dose equivalent	Sievert (Sv) (1 Sv = J/kg)	Rem	1 rem	= 0.01 Sv
			1 Sv	= 100 rem
Exposure	Coulomb per Kilogram (C/kg)	Roentgen (R)	1 R	= 2.58 × 10^{-4} C/kg = 0.258 mC/kg
			1 C/kg	= 3876 R
Absorbed dose rate	Gray per second (Gy/s)	Rad per second (rad/s)	1 rad/s	= 0.01 Gy/s
		Rad per minute (rad/min)	1 rad/min	= 1.67 × 10^{-4} Gy/s
		Rad per hour (rad/h)	1 rad/h	= 2.78 × 10^{-6} Gy/s
			1 Gy/s	= 100 rad/s, 6000 rad/min = 3.6 × 10^5 rad/h
Exposure rate	Coulomb per kilogram second (C/kg·s)	Roentgen per second (R/s)	1 R/s	= 2.58 × 10^{-4} C/kg·s = 0.258 mC/kg·s
		Roentgen per min (R/min)	1 R/min	= 4.30 × 10^{-6} C/kg·s = 4.30 uC/kg·s
		Roentgen per hour (R/h)	1 R/h	= 7.17 × 10^{-8} C/kg·s = 71.7 nC/kg·s
			1 C/kg·s	= 3876 R/s = 233 × 10^3 R/min = 233 kR/min = 1.40 × 10^7 R/h = 14.0 MR/h

From *Amersham Nuclear Medicine Catalogue,* Amersham International, plc., Little Chalfont, England, 1985.

TABLE 3A
Radiation Quantities and Units

Quantity	Symbol	Unit symbols SI	Special[a]
Particle number	N	1	
Radiant energy	R	J	
(Particle) fluence	Φ	m^{-2}	
Energy fluence	ψ	$J\ m^{-2}$	
(Particle) fluence rate	ϕ	$m^{-2}\ s^{-1}$	
Energy fluence rate	ψ	$W\ m^{-2}$	
Cross section	σ	m^2	b
Mass attenuation coefficient	U/ρ	$m^2\ kg^{-1}$	
Mass energy transfer coefficient	U_{tr}/ρ	$m^2\ kg^{-1}$	
Mass energy absorption coefficient	U_{en}/ρ	$m^2\ kg^{-1}$	
Total mass stopping power	S/ρ	$J\ m^2\ kg^{-1}$	$eV\ m^2\ kg^{-1}$

TABLE 3B
Radiation Quantities and Units

Quantity	Symbol	Unit symbols SI	SI restricted name	Special[a]
Linear energy transfer	L_Δ	Jm^{-1}		eVm^{-1} $keV\mu m^{-1}$
Radiation chemical yield	G(x)	$molJ^{-1}$		
Mean energy expended per ion pair	W	J		
Energy imparted	ϵ	J		
Specific energy (imparted)	z	Jkg^{-1}	Gy	rad
Absorbed dose	D	Jkg^{-1}	Gy	rad
Absorbed dose rate	D	$Jkg^{-1}s^{-1}$	Gys^{-1}	$rad\ s^{-1}$
Kerma	K	Jkg^{-1}	Gy	rad
Kerma rate	K	$Jkg^{-1}s^{-1}$	Gys^{-1}	$rad\ s^{-1}$
Exposure	X	Ckg^{-1}		R
Exposure rate	X	$Ckg^{-1}s^{-1}$		Rs^{-1}
Activity	A	s^{-1}	Bq	Ci
Air kerma-rate constant	Γ_σ	m^2Jkg^{-1}	$m^2GyBq^{-1}s^{-1}$	$m^2radCi^{-1}s^{-1}$

Note: Day (d), hour (h), and minute (min) may be used instead of seconds (s).

[a] One should not infer that the size of a unit given in this column is equal to the size of a unit on the same line in other columns. The symbol for the special name of the SI Unit restricted to specified quantities.

From Radiation Quantities and Units, International Commission on Radiological Units and Measurements Report No. 33, Washington, D.C., ICRU 1980.

TABLE 4
Quantities and Units for Radiation Protection

| | | Unit symbols | | |
| | | | | |
Quantity	Symbol	SI	SI restricted name	Special[a]
Dose equivalent	H	Jkg^{-1}	Sv	rem
Dose equivalent rate	H	$Jkg^{-1}s^{-1}$	Svs^{-1}	$rems^{-1}$
Absorbed dose index	D_1	Jkg^{-1}	Gy	rad
Aosorbed dose index rate	D_1	$Jkg^{-1}s^{-1}$	Gys^{-1}	$rads^{-1}$
Dose equivalent index	H_1	Jkg^{-1}	Sv	rem
Dose equivalent rate	H_1	$Jkg^{-1}s^{-1}$	Svs^{-1}	$rems^{-1}$
Shallow dose equivalent index	$H_{1,s}$	Jkg^{-1}	Sv	rem
Deep dose equivalent index	$H_{1,d}$	Jkg^{-1}	Sv	rem
Ambient dose equivalent	H (d)	Jkg^{-1}	Sv	rem
Directional dose equivalent	H'(d)	Jkg^{-1}	Sv	rem
Individual dose equivalent, penetrating	$H_p(d)$	Jkg^{-1}	Sv	rem
Individual dose equivalent, superficial	$H_s(d)$	Jkg^{-1}	Sv	rem

Note: Day (d), hour (h), and minute (min) may be used instead of seconds (s).

[a]   One should not infer that the size of a unit given in this column is equal to the size of a unit on the same line in other columns. The symbol for the special name of the SI Unit restricted to specified quantities.

From Radiation Quantities and Units, International Commission on Radiological Units and Measurements Report No. 33, Washington, D.C., ICRU, 1980.

RADIOACTIVITY CONVERSION TABLES:
SI Units to Conventional Units and Conventional Units to SI Units

Becquerels (Bq) to curies (Ci) and curies to becquerels.
1 Bq = 1 disintegration per second = 2.7×10^{-11} curie (Ci)
1 Ci = 3.7×10^{10} becquerel = 37 GBq

Megacuries (MCi) are converted to petabecquerels (PBq)
Kilocuries (kCi) are converted to terabecquerels (TBq)
Curies (Ci) are converted to gigabecquerels (GBq)
Millicuries (mCi) are converted to to megabecquerels (MBq)
Microcuries (μCi) are converted to kilobecquerels (kBq)
Nanocuries (nCi) are converted to becquerels (Bq)
Picocuries (pCi) are converted to millibecquerels (mBq)
Femtocuries (fCi) are converted to microbecquerels (μBq)

Note: The prefix associated with the becquerel unit is 10^9 greater than the corresponding prefix associated with the curie unit.

TABLE 5
Conversion Table to Convert Curie
(Ci) Activities to Becquerels (Bq)

μCi mCi Ci	kBq MBq GBq	μCi mCi Ci	MBq GBq TBq
0.1	3.7	30	1.11
0.2	7.4	40	1.48
0.25	9.25	50	1.85
0.3	11.1	60	2.22
0.4	14.8	70	2.59
0.5	18.5	80	2.96
1	37	90	3.33
2	74	100	3.7
2.5	92.5	125	4.625
3	111	150	5.55
4	148	200	7.4
5	185	250	9.25
6	222	300	11.1
7	259	400	14.8
8	296	500	18.5
9	333	600	22.2
10	370	700	25.9
12	444	750	27.75
15	555	800	29.6
20	740	900	33.3
25	925	1000	37

From *Amersham Nuclear Medicine Catalogue*, Amersham International, plc., Little Chalfont, England, 1985. With permission.

TABLE 6
Conversion Table to Convert Becquerel (Bq) Activities to Curie (Ci)

0.1 MBq = 2.7 μCi	500.0 MBq = 13.5 mCi
0.2 MBq = 5.4 μCi	525.0 MBq = 14.9 mCi
0.3 MBq = 8.1 μCi	550.0 MBq = 14.9 mCi
0.4 MBq = 10.8 μCi	575.0 MBq = 15.5 mCi
0.5 MBq = 13.5 μCi	600.0 MBq = 16.2 mCi
0.6 MBq = 16.2 μCi	625.0 MBq = 16.9 mCi
0.7 MBq = 18.9 μCi	650.0 MBq = 17.6 mCi
0.8 MBq = 21.6 μCi	675.0 MBq = 18.2 mCi
0.9 MBq = 24.3 μCi	700.0 MBq = 18.9 mCi
1.0 MBq = 27.0 μCi	725.0 MBq = 19.6 mCi
2.0 MBq = 54.1 μCi	750.0 MBq = 20.3 mCi
3.0 MBq = 81.1 μCi	775.0 MBq = 20.9 mCi
4.0 MBq = 108 μCi	800.0 MBq = 21.6 mCi
5.0 MBq = 135 μCi	825.0 MBq = 22.3 mCi
6.0 MBq = 162 μCi	850.0 MBq = 23.0 mCi
7.0 MBq = 189 μCi	875.0 MBq = 23.7 mCi
8.0 MBq = 216 μCi	900.0 MBq = 24.3 mCi
9.0 MBq = 243 μCi	925.0 MBq = 25.0 mCi
10.0 MBq = 270 μCi	950.0 MBq = 25.7 mCi
15.0 MBq = 405 μCi	975.0 MBq = 26.4 mCi
20.0 MBq = 541 μCi	1.0 GBq = 27.0 mCi
25.0 MBq = 676 μCi	1.1 GBq = 29.7 mCi
30.0 MBq = 811 μCi	1.2 GBq = 32.4 mCi
35.0 MBq = 946 μCi	1.3 GBq = 35.1 mCi
40.0 MBq = 1.08 mCi	1.4 GBq = 37.8 mCi
45.0 MBq = 1.22 mCi	1.5 GBq = 40.5 mCi
50.0 MBq = 1.35 mCi	1.6 GBq = 43.2 mCi
60.0 MBq = 1.62 mCi	1.7 GBq = 46.0 mCi
70.0 MBq = 1.89 mCi	1.8 GBq = 48.7 mCi
80.0 MBq = 2.16 mCi	1.9 GBq = 51.3 mCi
90.0 MBq = 2.43 mCi	2.0 GBq = 54.1 mCi
100.0 MBq = 2.70 mCi	2.2 GBq = 59.5 mCi
125.0 MBq = 3.38 mCi	2.4 GBq = 64.9 mCi
150.0 MBq = 4.05 mCi	2.6 GBq = 70.3 mCi
175.0 MBq = 4.73 mCi	2.8 GBq = 75.5 mCi
200.0 MBq = 5.41 mCi	3.0 GBq = 81.1 mCi
225.0 MBq = 6.08 mCi	3.2 GBq = 86.5 mCi
250.0 MBq = 6.76 mCi	3.4 GBq = 91.9 mCi
275.0 MBq = 7.43 mCi	3.6 GBq = 97.3 mCi
300.0 MBq = 8.11 mCi	3.8 GBq = 103 mCi
325.0 MBq = 8.78 mCi	4.0 GBq = 108 mCi
350.0 MBq = 9.46 mCi	5.0 GBq = 135 mCi
375.0 MBq = 10.1 mCi	6.0 GBq = 162 mCi
400.0 MBq = 10.8 mCi	7.0 GBq = 189 mCi
425.0 MBq = 11.5 mCi	8.0 GBq = 216 mCi
450.0 MBq = 12.2 mCi	9.0 GBq = 243 mCi
475.0 MBq = 12.8 mCi	10.0 GBq = 270 mCi

From *Amersham Nuclear Medicine Catalogue*, Amersham International, plc., Little Chalfont, England, 1985. With permission.

TABLE 7
Examples of Typical Activities of Radionuclide Applications

Radionuclide	Application	Typical activities
Iodine-125	*In vitro* test for radioimmunoassay	50 nCi = 1850 Bq; approx. 2 kBq
Iodine-131	Thyroid uptake	5 μCi = 185 kBq; approx. 200 kBq
Iodine-131	Treatment of thyrotoxicosis	20 mCi = 740 MBq
Iodine-131	Thyroid cancer ablation	100 mCi = 3700 MBq; approx. 4 GBq
Cobalt-60	Source for teletherapy	3 kCi = 111 TBq

From *Amersham Nuclear Medicine Catalogue,* Amersham International, plc., Little Chalfont, England, 1985. With permission.

TABLE 8
Conversion of Absorbed Dose Units

SI Units	Non-SI units
100 Gy (10^2Gy)	= 10,000 rad (10^4 rad)
10 Gy (10^1Gy)	= 1,000 rad (10^3 rad)
1 Gy(10^0 Gy)	= 100 rad (10^2 rad)
100 mGy (10^{-1} Gy)	= 10 rad (10^1 rad)
10 mGy (10^{-2} Gy)	= 1 rad (10^0 rad)
1 mGy (10^{-3} Gy)	= 100 mrad (10^{-1} rad)
100 μGy (10^{-4} Gy)	= 10 mrad(10^{-2} rad)
10μGy (10^{-5} Gy)	= 1 mrad (10^{-3} rad)
1 μGy (10^{-6} Gy)	= 100 μrad (10^{-4} rad)
100 nGy (10^{-7} Gy)	= 10 μrad (10^{-5} rad)
10 nGy (10^{-8} Gy)	= 1 μrad (10^{-6} rad)
1 nGy (10^{-9} Gy)	= 100 nrad (10^{-7} rad)

From *Amersham Nuclear Medicine Catalogue,* Amersham International, plc., Little Chalfont, England, 1985. With permission.

TABLE 9
Conversion of Dose Equivalent Units

SI units	Non-SI units
100 Sv (10^2 Sv)	= 10,000 rem (10^4 rem)
10 Sv (10^1 Sv)	= 1,000 rem (10^3 rem)
1 Sv (10^0 Sv)	= 100 rem (10^2 rem)
100 mSv (10^{-1} Sv)	= 10 rem (10^1 rem)
10 mSv (10^{-2} Sv)	= 1 rem (10^0 rem)
1 mSv (10^{-3} Sv)	= 100 mrem (10^{-1} rem)
100 μSv (10^{-4} Sv)	= 10 mrem (10^{-2} rem)
10 μSv (10^{-5} Sv)	= 1 mrem (10^{-3} rem)
1 μSv (10^{-6} Sv)	= 100 μrem (10^{-4} rem)
100 nSv (10^{-7} Sv)	= 10 μrem (10^{-5} rem)
10 nSv (10^{-8} Sv)	= 1 μrem (10^{-6} rem)
1 nSv (10^{-9} Sv)	= 100 nrem (10^{-7} rem)

From *Amersham Nuclear Medicine Catalogue,* Amersham International, plc., Little Chalfont, England, 1985. With permission.

TABLE 10
SI Derived Units With Special Names

Quantity	Name	Symbol	Definition
Activity	Becquerel	Bq	s^{-1}
Absorbed dose	Gray	Gy	Jkg^{-1}
Capacitance	Farad	F	$m^{-2} \cdot kg^{-1} \cdot s^4 \cdot A^2$
Temperature, Celsius[a]	Degree, Celsius	°C	K
Conductance	Siemens	S	$m^{-2} \cdot kg^{-1} \cdot s^3 \cdot A^2$
Dose equivalent	Sievert	Sv	Jkg^{-1}
Electric resistance	Ohm	Ω	$m^2 \cdot kg \cdot s^{-3} \cdot A^{-2}$
Flux density	Tesla	T	$kg \cdot s^{-2} \cdot A^{-1}$
Force	Newton	N	$m \cdot kg \cdot s^{-2}$
Frequency	Hertz	Hz	s^{-1}
Illuminance	Lux	lx	$m^{-2} \cdot cd \cdot sr$
Inductance	Henry	H	$m^2 \cdot kg \cdot s^{-2} A^{-2}$
Luminous flux	Lumen	lm	cd·sr
Magnetic flux	Weber	Wb	$m^2 \cdot kg \cdot s^{-2} \cdot A^{-1}$
Potential difference	Volt	V	$m^2 \cdot kg \cdot s^{-3} \cdot A^{-1}$
Power	Watt	W	$m^2 \cdot kg \cdot s^{-3}$
Pressure	Pascal	Pa	$m^{-1} \cdot kg \cdot s^{-2}$
Quantity of electricity	Coulomb	C	s·A
Work, energy	Joule	J	$m^2 \cdot kg \cdot s^{-2}$

[a]   The unit "degree Celsius" is equal to the unit "kelvin". A temperature interval or a Celsius temperature difference can be expressed in degrees Celsius as well as in kelvins. The term "degree centigrade" is obsolete and no longer acceptable.

Adapted from Radiation Quantities and Units, Radiological Commission on Radiological Units and Measurements Report No. 33, Washington, D.C., ICRU, 1980.

TABLE 11
Multiples and Submultiples of SI Units Having Special Names

Quantity	Name of unit	Symbol	Definition of unit
Area	Barn	b	10^{-28} m²
Energy	Erg	erg	10^{-7} J
Force	Dyne	dyn	10^{-5} N
Length	Angstrom	Å	10^{-10} m
Length	Micron[a]	μ	10^{-6} m
Mass	Ton	t	10^3 kg
Pressure	Bar	bar	10^5 Pa
Volume	Liter	L(ℓ)	dm³

[a]   The names millimicron (mμ) for nonometer (nm), and micron (μ) for micrometer (μm) should no longer be used. (Resolution 7 of the 13th General Conference on Weights and Measures, 1967.)

TABLE 12
Units Continuing in Use With the International System

Defined in Terms of SI Units

Quantity	Name	Symbol	Definition or equivalent
Angle	Degree	°	$1° = (\pi/180)$ rad
Angle	Minute	'	$1' = (1/60)°$
			$= (\pi/10800)$ rad
Mass	Metric ton	t	$1\ t = 10^3$ kg
Time	Minute	min	1 min = 60 s
Time	Hour	h	1 h = 60 min = 3 600 s
Time	Day	d	1 d = 24 h = 86 400 s
Volume	Liter	L(l)	$1L(\ell) = dm^3 = 10^{-3}\ m^3$

Defined Empirically

Energy	Electronvolt	eV	1.602×10^{-19} J
Length	Astronomical unit	AU	$149\ 600 \times 10^6$ m
Mass	Atomic mass unit	μ(amu)	1.660531×10^{-27} kg

TABLE 13
Relationship Between CGS and SI Units

Quantity	Unit	Symbol	Equivalent in SI units
Length	Centimeter	cm	0.01 meter
Mass	Gram	g	0.001 kilogram
Time	Second	s	1 second
Length	Angstrom unit	Å	1 nanometer
Work, energy	Erg	erg	10^{-7} joule
Energy	Calorie(lT)	cal(lT)	4.1868 joule
Force	Dyne	dyn	10^{-5} newton
Force	Gram-force	gf	9.807×10^{-5} newton

TABLE 14
Other Quantities of SI Derived Units

Quantity	Name of unit	Definition or equivalent
Absorbed dose rate	Gray per second	$Jkg^{-1}s^{-1}$
Acceleration	Meter per square second	ms^{-2}
Angular velocity	Radian per second	$rads^{-1}$
Area	Square meter, hectare	m^2
		$10^4 \ m^2$
Concentration	Mole per cubic meter, liter	$mol \ m^{-3}$
		$mol \ \ell^{-1}$
Density	Kilogram per cubic meter	kgm^{-3}
Dose equivalent rate	Sievert per second	$Jkg^{-1}s^{-1}$
Electric charge density	Coulomb per cubic meter	Asm^{-3}
Electric displacement, Electric flux density	Coulomb per square meter	Asm^{-2}
Energy density	Joule per cubic meter	$kgs^{-2}m^{-1}$
Exposure	Coulomb per kilogram	$Askg^{-1}$
Exposure rate	Coulomb per kilogram second	$Ckg^{-1}s^{-1}$
		Akg^{-1}
Fluence	1 per meter squared	m^{-2}
Fluence rate	1 per meter squared second	$m^{-2}s^{-1}$
Heat capacity, entropy	Joule per kelvin	m^2kgKs^{-2}
Heat flux density, irradiance	Watt per square meter	kgs^{-3}
Kerma rate	Gray per second	$Jkg^{-1}s^{-1}$
Linear energy	Joule per meter	$mkgs^{-2}$
Luminance	Candela per square meter	cdm^{-2}
Mass attenuation coefficient	Meter squared per kilogram	m^2kg^{-1}
Mass energy transfer coefficient		
Mass energy absorption coefficient		
Mass stopping power	Joule meter squared per kilogram	Jm^2kg^{-1}
Molality	Mole per kilogram	$mol \ kg^{-1}$
Molar energy	Joule per mole	$m^2kgs^{-2}mol^{-1}$
Molar heat capacity	Joule per mole kelvin	$m^2kgs^{-2}mol^{-1}K^{-1}$
Permittivity	Farad per meter	$m^{-3}kg^{-1}s^4A^2$
Specific heat capacity	Joule per kilogram kelvin	$Jkg^{-1}K^{-1}$
Surface tension	Newton per meter	kgs^{-2}
Thermal conductivity	Watt per meter kelvin	$mkgs^{-3}K^{-1}$
Velocity	Meter per second	ms^{-1}
Viscosity (dynamic)	Pascal second	$m^{-1} \ kgs^{-1}$
Viscosity (kinematic)	Meter squared per second	m^2s^{-1}
Wave number	1 per meter	m^{-1}

Adapted from Weast, R. C., *CRC Handbook of Chemistry and Physics,* 67th ed., 1986-1987, CRC Press, Boca Raton, FL, 1986.

TABLE 15
Electromagnetic Quantities

Quantity	Unit symbol	Name of SI (and other common) unit
Capacitance	C	Farad
Charge	Q	Coulomb
Current	I	Ampere
Current density	J	Ampere/meter^2
Electric field	$\overline{E}$	Volt/meter
Electric potential or electromotive force (emf)	V	Volt
Inductance	L	Henry
Magnetic dipole moment	$\overline{m}$	Ampere/meter^2
Magnetic field	$\overline{H}$	Ampere/meter
Magnetic field gradient	$\theta B_z/\theta_z$	Tesla/meter (.01 tesla/meter = 1 gauss/cm)
Magnetic flux	ϕ	Volt-second
Magnetic induction or flux density	$\overline{B}$	Tesla
Magnetic susceptibility	χ	Dimensionless
Magnetization	$\overline{M}$	Ampere/meter
Permeability	μ	Henry/meter
Permeability of free space	μ_o	Henry/meter
Relative permeability		Dimensionless
Resistance	R	Ohm

Adapted from Vigoreux, P., *Units and Standards for Electromagnetism,* Wykeham, London, 1971.

TABLE 16
Acoustics Quantities

Quantity	Unit symbol	Unit
Attenuation	dB	Decibles
Attenuation coefficient	dB/m	Decibels/meter
Beam area	m^2	Meters^2
Pulse duration	s	Seconds
Pulse repetition frequency	Hz	Hertz
Pulse repetition period	s	Seconds
Cosine	—	Unitless
Depth of penetration	m	Meters
Displacement	m	Meters
Doppler shift	Hz	Hertz
Duty factor	—	Unitless
Fractional volume change	—	Unitless
Frequency	Hz	Hertz
Gain	dB	Decibles
Impedance	—	Rayls
Intensity	W/m^2	Watts/meter^2
Intensity reflection coefficient	—	Unitless
Intensity transmission coefficient	—	Unitless
Pressure	N/m^2	Newtons/meter^2
Propagation speed	m/s	Meters/second
Sine	—	Unitless
Spatial pulse length	m	Meters
Speed	m/s	Meters/second
Stiffness	N/m^2	Newtons/meter^2
Voltage	V	Volts
Volume	m^3	Meters^3
Wavelength	m	Meters

Adapted from Sarti, D. A. and Sample, W. F., Eds., *Diagnostic Ultrasound,* Martinus Nijhoff, The Hague, Netherlands, 1985.

TABLE 17
Prefixes for SI Units

Factor	Prefix	Symbol	Origin
		Multiples	
10^{18}	exa	E	Greek "six" (10^3 to sixth power is 10^{18})
10^{15}	peta	P	Greek "five" (10^3 to fifth power is 10^{15})
10^{12}	tera	T	Greek "monster"
10^9	giga	G	Greek "giant"
10^6	mega	M	Greek "large"
10^3	kilo	k	Greek "thousand"
10^2	hecto	h	Greek "hundred"
10^1	deca	da	Greek "ten"
		Sub multiples	
10^{-1}	deci	d	Latin "tenth"
10^{-2}	centi	c	Latin "hundredth"
10^{-3}	milli	m	Latin "thousandth"
10^{-6}	micro	μ	Greek "little"
10^{-9}	nano	n	Latin "dwarf"
10^{-12}	pico	p	Latin "pike, spear"
10^{-15}	femto	f	Danish, Norwegian "fifteen"
10^{-18}	atto	a	Danish, Norwegian "eighteen"

TABLE 18
Abbreviations of the System, Tissue or Excretory Product Preceding or Following a Unit Expression

B	Blood
P	Plasma
S	Serum
U	Urine
F	Feces
Sf	Cerebrospinal fluid
Lkc	Leukocyte (leucocyte)
E (or Erc)	Erythrocyte
Pt	Patient
fPt	Fasting patient

As prefixes to other codes

c	capillary
v	venous
a	arterial
d	day (24 h)

From Institute for Pathology, University of Pretoria, Pretoria.

TABLE 19
Other International Accepted Abbreviations and Symbols

	Abbreviation	Symbol	Unit
Amount of substance	ams.	n	mol
Mass concentration	massc.	p	g/ℓ
			kg/ℓ
Substance concentration	substc.	c	mol/ℓ
Number concentration	numberc.	C	1^{-1}
Number fraction	numberfr.	δ	dimensionless
Volume fraction	volfr.	φ	ℓ/ℓ
Arbitrary (e.g., unit)	arb.		
Difference	diff.		
Relative	rel.		

From Institute for Pathology, University of Pretoria, Pretoria.

GUIDANCE ON THE USE OF SI UNITS

1. Units, prefixes and their symbols are printed in roman (upright) type, and with a few exceptions, in the lower case, when a unit begins a sentence. Symbols derived from proper names begin with capital letters, but the name itself does not (i.e. Bq, but becquerel). Another exception is the symbol for the liter "l" which should be clearly different from the numeral "1". Accordingly, the symbol "L" may be used for clarity when required.

2. Prefixes appear directly before the unit, without a space, thus forming a new unit or symbol. For example: millisievert "mSv" not m Sv.

3. Only one prefix may be used at a time with each unit. However, more than one prefix may be used in expressions containing several units; for example, a radionuclide concentration may be expressed in megabecquerels per milliliter, MBqml^{-1}.

4. Prefixes should be used to express convenient numerical values in relation to common usage, e.g., the megabecquerel, starting from 0.1 to 999 MBq could cover most situations in nuclear medicine practice. However, when dealing with a higher activity source such as a ^{99}Mo/^{99m}Tc generator, the use of the prefix giga is more appropriate: 17.5 GBq, instead of 17 500 MBq.

5. As symbols are not abbreviations, they are not followed by a full stop except at the end of a sentence. Similarly, they do not change in the plural.

6. The expression "per", e.g., coulomb per kilogram, may be written C/kg; or Ckg^{-1}. Only one solidus (/) may be used.

7. The product of two or more symbols is best indicated by a point on or above the line: N . m, or N · m.

8. A single space is left between the numerical value and the unit symbol: 20 mg/l, not 20mg/l.

9. The decimal sign is a point on the line. For a value less than 1 a zero (0) should precede the decimal sign (0.7 not .7). Numbers with more than 3 digits are written with spaces separating groups of 3, starting from the decimal sign. No point or comma is used for separation, e.g., 299 792 458.32.

10. The symbols > and < are usually unambiguous when typed or printed. In written reports it may be safer to express "less than" or "greater than" to avoid misinterpretations. The symbols + and − are not recommended.

11. Because of the everyday language meaning of the words quantity and unit, care must be taken to avoid any possible confusion. The common meaning of "quantity" is that of amount, while in the field of metrology (the science of art and measurement), the

word quantity means "to characterize a physical phenomenon in terms that are suitable for numerical specification", such as time and length. On the other hand, a unit is a selected reference sample of a quantity. The second and the meter are units of time and length, respectively. However, a defined quantity can have many units, i.e., seconds, minutes, and hours are all units of time.

12. Because it is common practice to use the single word "dose" rather than the proper terms "absorbed dose" or "dose equivalent", possible ambiguity may be alleviated if the special names of the units for these two quantities are used, thus the "absorbed dose in Gy," and "dose equivalent in Sv."

13. A large volume of evidence in the scientific literature points to the fact that the use of dual (non-SI Units) serves no educational purpose and can actually delay a familiarity and competence in the use of the new SI units. However, in areas where safety is involved, dual units could be acceptable for a reasonable period of time. Related values should all be changed together.

BIBLIOGRAPHY

1. British Standards Institution Conversion Factors, BS350, British Standards Institution, London, 1974.
2. **Goldman, D. T. and Bell, R. J., Eds.,** SI: The International System of Units, 4th ed., HMSO, London (Translation of BIPM's Le Systeme International d'Unites), 1982.
3. **Kaye, G. W. C. and Laby, T. H.,** *Tables of Physical and Chemical Constants,* 15th ed., Longman, London, 1986.
4. **Royal Society,** *Quantities, Units and Symbols: A Report,* 2nd ed., Royal Society, London, 1975.
5. **Vigoureux, P.,** *Units and Standards for Electromagnetism,* Wykeham, London, 1971.
6. **Attix, F. H., Roesch, W. C., and Tochilin, E., Eds.,** *Radiation Dosimetry,* 2nd ed., Academic Press, New York, 1968—1969.
7. International Commission on Radiation Units and Measurements, Radiation Quantities and Units, ICRU Report 33, International Commission on Radiation Units and Measurements, Washington, D.C., 1980.
8. International Commission on Radiation Units and Measurements, Determination of Dose Equivalent Resulting from External Radiation Sources, ICRU Report 39, International Commission on Radiation Units and Measurements. Washington, D.C., 1985.
9. National Physical Laboratory, SI: *The International System of Units,* 4th ed., HMSO, London, 1982.
10. **Greening, J. R.,** *Fundamentals of Radiation Dosimetry,* 2nd ed., Hilger, Bristol, 1985.
11. International Commission on Radiation Units and Measurements, Neutron Fluence, Neutron Spectra and Kerma, ICRU Report No. 13, ICRU, Washington, D.C., 1969.
12. International Commission on Radiation Units and Measurements, Radiation Dosimetry, X-Rays and Gamma Rays with Maximum Photon Energies between 0.6 and 50 MeV, ICRU Report No. 14, ICRU, Washington, D.C., 1969.
13. International Commission on Radiation Units and Measurements, Quantitative Concepts and Dosimetry in Radiobiology, ICRU Report No. 30, ICRU, Washington, D.C., 1979.
14. International Commission on Radiation Units and Measurements, Determination of Dose Equivalents Resulting from External Radiation Sources, ICRU Report No. 39, ICRU, Washington, D.C., 1985.
15. **Jennings, W. A., Smith, D., and Axton, E. J.,** The development of international measurement standards, *J. Soc. Radiol. Protection,* 4(3), 166, 1984.
16. International Commission on Radiological Protection, *Recommendations of the International Commission on Radiological Protection,* ICRP Publication 26, Annals of the ICRP, 1,(3), Pergamon Press, New York, 1977.
17. International Commission on Radiological Protection, Statement from the 1978 Stockholm Meeting of the ICRP, in *Annals of the ICRP,* 2,(1), Pergamon Press, New York, 1978.
18. International Commission on Radiological Protection, Statement and Recommendation of the 1980 Brighton Meeting of the ICRP, in *Annals of the ICRP,* 4(3/4), Pergamon Press, New York, 1980.
19. International Commission on Radiation Units and Measurements, Radiation Quantities and Units, ICRU Report 33, International Commission on Radiation Units and Measurements, Bethesda, Maryland, 1980.
20. Le Bureau International Des Poids et Mesures, The International Bureau of Weights and Measures, Translation of the BIPM Centennial Volume, NBS Special Publication 420, Page, D. H. and Vigoureux, P., Eds. National Bureau of Standards, Washington, D.C., 1975.

21. Comite Consultatif pour les Etalons de Mesure des Rayonnements Ionisants (CCEMRI), Section I, Rayons X and gamma, electrons, 5ᵉ Reunion, OFFILIB, Paris, 1979.
22. Comite Consultatif pour les Etalons de Mesure des Rayonnements Ionisants (CCEMRI), Section I., Rayons X and y, electrons, 6ᵉ Reunion, OFFILIB, Paris, 1981.
23. **Danloux-Dumesnils, M.,** *The Metric System,* translated by Garrett and Rowlinson, Athlone Press, London, 1969.
24. EEC, Council Directive of 20 December 1979, Official Journal of the European Communities, L, 39/40, 15 February 1980.
25. International Commission on Radiation Units and Measurements, Radiation Quantities and Units, ICRU Report 19, International Commission on Radiation Units and Measurements, Bethesda, Maryland, 1971.
26. International Commission on Radiation Units and Measurements, Methods of Assessment of Absorbed Dose in Clinical Use of Radionuclides, ICRU Report 32, International Commission on Radiation Units and Measurements, Bethesda, Maryland, 1979.
27. International Union of Pure and Applied Chemistry (IUPAC), *Manual of Symbols and Terminology for Physico-Chemical Quantities and Units,* Pergamon Press, Oxford, 1979.
28. International Union of Pure and Applied Physics (IUPAP), Symbols, Units, and Nomenclature in Physics, Document U.I.P. 20, International Union of Pure and Applied Physics, Quebec, Canada, 1978.
29. Metric Commission Canada, The SI Manual in Health Care, 2nd edition, Publication Services Section, Ontario Government Bookstore, Toronto, 1982.
30. National Bureau of Standards, The International System of Units (SI), translation approved by the International Bureau of Weights and Measures (BIPM) of its publication "Le Systeme International d'Unites", NBS Special Publication 330, National Bureau of Standards, Gaithersburg, Maryland, 1981.
31. **Roedler, H. D., Kaul, A., and Hine, G. J.,** Internal Radiation Dose in Diagnostic Nuclear Medicine, Verlag H. Hoffmann, Berlin, 1978.
32. *Amersham Nuclear Medicine Catalogue,* Amersham International, plc., Little Chalfont, England, 1985.
33. **Weast, R. C., Ed.,** *CRC Handbook of Chemistry and Physics,* 67th ed., CRC Press, Boca Raton, FL, 1986.

Physical Constants and Conversion Factors

PHYSICAL CONSTANTS AND CONVERSION FACTORS: TABLE 1
Fundamental Physical Constants

Physical Constant	Symbol	Value in SI units
Acceleration due to gravity	g	9.80665 m s^{-2}
Alpha particle mass	m_a	6.6×10^{-27} kg
Atomic mass unit	amu	1.66057×10^{-27} kg
Avogadro number	N_A	6.02217×10^{23} mol^{-1}
Bohr magneton	B_e	9.2741×10^{-24} A m^2 (J T^{-1})
Bohr radius	a_o	5.29177×10^{-11} m
Boltzmann constant	K_B	1.3806×10^{-23} m^2 kg s^{-2} K^{-1}
Charge-to-mass ratio for electron	e/m_e	1.75880×10^{11} s A kg^{-1}
Compton wavelength of the electron (h/ m$_3$C)	c	2.42631×10^{-12} m
Electron Lande factor	g_e	2.002
Electron radius	r_e	2.81792×10^{-15} m
Electron rest mass	m_e	9.10955×10^{-31} kg
Elementary charge	e	1.60219×10^{-19} s A
Faraday constant	$F = N_A e$	9.64846×10^4 C mol^{-1}
Gravitational constant	G	6.6732×10^{-11} m^3 kg^{-1} s^{-2}
Hydrogen atom mass	m_H	1.674×10^{-27} kg
Magnetic moment of electron		9.29×10^{-24} J T^{-1}
Magnetic moment of proton		1.41×10^{-26} J T^{-1}
Molar Gas constant	R	8.3143 m^2 kg s^{-2} K^{-1} mol^{-1}
Molar volume	V_{mol}	22.41383 m^3 kmol^{-1}
Molar volume, ideal gas (To = 273.15K, Po = 101.32 kPa)	$Vm = RTo/Po$	0.022414 m^3 mol^{-1}
Nuclear magneton	B_N	5.0505×10^{-27} A m^2 (J T^{-1})
Permeability of a vacuum	u_o	4×10^{-7} m kg s^{-2} A^{-2}
Permitivity of a vacuum	o	8.85418×10^{-12} m^{-3} kg^{-1} s^4 A^2
Planck constant	h	6.6262×10^{-34} m^2 kg s^{-1}
	$h = h/2$	1.0546×10^{-34} m^2 kg s^{-1}
Proton Lande factor	g_H	5.585
Proton magnetogyric ratio	Y_H	2.6752×10^8 kg^{-1} s A
Proton rest mass	M_p	1.67261×10^{-27} kg
Speed of light in a vacuum	c	2.99792×10^8 m s^{-1}
Logarithm (common)	ln(10)	2.30259
Logarithm (natural)	e	2.71828
	l/e	0.36788
Pi	π	3.14159

Data compiled from *Health Physics Handbook,* General Dynamics, Fort Worth Division, OSP-379, 1963. Diem, K. and Lentner, C., Eds., Scientific Tables, Ciba-Geigy, Ltd., Basle, Switzerland, 1970, and *Radiological Health Handbook,* U.S. Department of Health Education and Welfare. Washington, D.C., 1970.

PHYSICAL CONSTANTS AND
CONVERSION FACTORS: TABLE 2
Table of Atomic Mass Units (amu)

Element	^{A}Symbol	Z	Atomic mass units (amu)
Electron	e		0.000549
Neutron	n		1.008665
Proton	p		1.007277
Hydrogen	(^{1}H)	1	1.007825
Deuterium	(^{2}H)	1	2.014102
Tritium	(^{3}H)	1	3.016050
Helium	(^{3}He)	2	3.016030
	(^{4}He)	2	4.002603
	(^{5}He)	2	5.012297
	(^{6}He)	2	6.018893
Carbon	(^{10}C)	6	10.016810
	(^{11}C)	6	11.011432
	(^{12}C)	6	12.000000
	(^{13}C)	6	13.003354
	(^{14}C)	6	14.003242
	(^{15}C)	6	15.010600
Boron	(^{12}B)	5	12.014354
Nitrogen	(^{12}N)	7	12.018641
Oxygen	(^{16}O)	8	15.994915
Phosphorus	(^{32}P)	15	31.973910
Sulfur	(^{32}S)	16	31.972074

From Early, P. J., Razzak, M. A., and Sodee, D. B., *Textbook of Nuclear Medicine Technology,* 3rd ed., C. V. Mosby, St. Louis, 1979. With permission.

PHYSICAL CONSTANTS AND CONVERSION FACTORS: TABLE 3
Fundamental Conversion Factors of Some Important Physical Units

(Length)	km	m	cm	in
1 Kilometer (km)	1	10^3	10^5	3.9370×10^4
1 Meter (m)	10^{-3}	1	100	39.3701
1 Centimeter (cm)	10^{-5}	10^{-2}	1	.3937
1 Inch (in)	2.5400×10^{-5}	2.500×10^{-2}	2.5400	1
1 Foot (ft)	3.0480×10^{-4}	.3048	30.4800	12
1 Yard (yd)	9.1440×10^{-4}	.9144	91.4400	36
1 Mile (mi)	1.6093	1.6093×10^3	1.6093×10^5	6.3360×10^4

(Length)	ft	yds	mi
1 Kilometer (km)	3.2808×10^3	1.0936×10^3	.6214
1 Meter (m)	3.2808	1.0936	6.2137×10^{-4}
1 Centimeter (cm)	3.2808×10^{-2}	1.0936×10^{-2}	6.2137×10^{-6}
1 Inch (in)	8.3333×10^{-2}	2.7778×10^{-2}	1.5783×10^{-5}
1 Foot (ft)	1	.3333	1.8939×10^{-4}
1 Yard (yd)	3	1	5.6817×10^{-4}
1 Mile (mi)	5280	1760	1

(ENERGY)

$$1 \text{ erg} = 1 \text{ dyne-centimeter}$$
$$1 \text{ Joule} = 1 \text{ newton-meter} = 10^7 \text{ ergs}$$
$$1 \text{ Thermochemical calorie} = 4.184 \text{ joules}$$
$$1 \text{ Electronvolt (eV)} = 1.602 \times 10^{-19}$$
$$1 \text{ Atomic mass unit (u)} = 931.478 \text{ MeV}$$
$$\text{Rest mass of the electron } (m_e) = 0.511 \text{ MeV}$$
$$\text{Rest mass of the proton } (m_p) = 938.256 \text{ MeV}$$
$$\text{Rest mass of the neutron } (m_n) = 939.550 \text{ MeV}$$

(Mass)	gm	kg	lb
1 Gram (gm)	1	10^{-3}	2.2046×10^{-3}
1 Kilogram (kg)	10^3	1	2.2046
1 Pound (lb)	453.59	.4536	1

(Time)	Years	Days	Hours	Minutes	Seconds
1 Year	1	365[a]	8.760×10^3	5.256×10^5	3.1536×10^7
1 Day	2.740×10^{-3}	1	24	1.440×10^3	8.640×10^4
1 Hour	1.142×10^{-4}	4.167×10^{-2}	1	60	3.600×10^3
1 Minute	1.903×10^{-6}	6.944×10^{-4}	1.667×10^{-2}	1	60
1 Second	3.171×10^{-8}	1.157×10^{-5}	2.778×10^{-4}	1.667×10^{-2}	1

[a]   For purposes of this table, a year is assumed to be exactly 365 days, instead of its average value of 365.26 days.

(Density)	g/cm³	Pounds/cubic inch	Pounds/cubic foot
g/cm³	1	3.6127292×10^{-2}	62.427961
Pounds/cubic inch	27.679905	1	1728
Pounds/cubic foot	1.6018463×10^{-2}	5.78703×10^{-4}	1

Note: 1 g/ml = 0.999972 g/cm³
   1 g/cm³ = 1.000028 g/ml

PHYSICAL CONSTANTS AND CONVERSION FACTORS: TABLE 3
(continued)
Fundamental Conversion Factors of Some Important Physical Units

(Volume)	Symbol	Relation	Value in SI units
Cubic inch	in^3, cu in	1 in^3 = 1/1728 ft^3	16.387064 × 10^{-6} m^3
Cubic foot	ft^3, cu ft	1 ft^3 = 1/27 yd^3	28.3168 × 10^{-3} m^3
Cubic yard	yd^3, cu yd		0.76555 m^3
Fluid ounce (U.K.)	fl oz (U.K.)	1 fl oz (U.K.) = 1/5 gill (U.K.)	28.4131 × 10^{-6} m^3
Gallon (U.K.)	gal (U.K.)	1 gal (U.K.) = 277.43 in^3	4.54609 × 10^{-3} m^3
Fluid ounce (U.S.)	fl oz (U.S.)	1 fl oz (U.S.) = 1/4 gill (U.S.)	29.5735 × 10^{-6} m^3
Gallon (U.S.)	gal (U.S.)	1 gal (U.S.) = 231 in^3	3.78541 × 10^{-3} m^3
Liter	L (l)	1.000028 dm^3	1.000028 × 10^{-3} m^3

FORCE UNITS

N	kp	Mp	p	dyn
1	0.102	1.02 × 10^{-4}	102	10^5
9.81	1	10^{-3}	10^3	9.81 × 10^5
9.81 × 10^3	10^3	1	10^6	9.81 × 10^6
9.81 × 10^{-3}	10^{-3}	10^{-6}	1	981
10^{-5}	1.02 × 10^{-6}	1.02 × 10^{-9}	1.02 × 10^{-3}	1

ENERGY, WORK UNITS

J	kpm	kWh	kcal	erg	eV
1	0.102	2.78 × 10^{-7}	2.39 × 10^{-4}	10^7	6.24 × 10^{18}
9.81	1	2.72 × 10^{-6}	2.34 × 10^{-3}	9.81 × 10^7	6.12 × 10^{19}
3.6 × 10^6	3.67 × 10^5	860	860	3.6 × 10^{13}	2.25 × 10^{25}
4.19 × 10^3	427	1	1	4.19 × 10^{10}	2.61 × 10^{22}
10^{-7}	1.02 × 10^{-8}	2.39 × 10^{-11}	2.39 × 10^{-11}	1	6.24 × 10^{11}
1.6 × 10^{-19}	1.63 × 10^{-20}	3.83 × 10^{-23}	3.83 × 10^{-23}	1.6 × 10^{-12}	1

POWER UNITS

W	kw	kpm/s	PS	cal/s	kcal/h
1	10^{-3}	0.102	1.36 × 10^{-3}	0.239	0.86
10^3	1	102	1.36	239	860
9.81	9.81 × 10^{-3}	1	1.33 × 10^{-2}	2.34	8.43
736	0.736	75	1	176	632
4.19	4.19 × 10^{-3}	0.427	5.69 × 10^{-3}	1	3.6
1.16	1.16 × 10^{-3}	0.119	1.58 × 10^{-3}	0.278	1

mg % to mEq/L

mg % × valence × 10/atomic wt. = mEqL

In case of gases

vol % × 10/22.4 = mM L

For CO_2, use 22.26 instead of 22.4

PHYSICAL CONSTANTS AND CONVERSION FACTORS: TABLE 3
(continued)
Fundamental Conversion Factors of Some Important Physical Units

At the normal pH of body fluids, 20% of the phosphate radical is combined with one equivalent of base as BH_2PO_4 and 80% with the two equivalents of base as B_2HPO_4. Under these conditions, base equivalence per unit of HPO_4 is therefore $0.2 + (0.8 \times 2) = 1.8$ and the equivalent weight of 53.3 is obtained by dividing the ionic weight by 1.8 instead by 2.

TEMPERATURE CONVERSIONS (CELCIUS TO FAHRENHEIT)

T(°C)	T(°F)	T(°C)	T(°F)	T(°C)	T(°F)	T(°C)	T(°F)
0	32	26	78.8	51	123.8	76	168.8
1	33.8	27	80.6	52	125.6	77	170.6
2	35.6	28	82.4	53	127.4	78	172.4
3	37.4	29	84.2	54	129.2	79	174.2
4	39.2	30	86.0	55	131.0	80	176.0
5	41.0	31	87.8	56	132.8	81	177.8
6	42.8	32	89.6	57	134.6	82	179.6
7	44.6	33	91.4	58	136.4	83	181.4
8	46.4	34	93.2	59	138.2	84	183.2
9	48.2	35	95.0	60	140.0	85	185.0
10	50.0	36	96.8	61	141.8	86	186.8
11	51.8	37	98.6	62	143.6	87	188.6
12	53.6	38	100.4	63	145.4	88	190.4
13	55.4	39	102.2	64	147.2	89	192.2
14	57.2	40	104.0	65	149.0	90	194.0
15	59.0	41	105.8	66	150.8	91	195.8
16	60.8	42	107.6	67	152.6	92	197.6
17	62.6	43	109.4	68	154.4	93	199.4
18	64.4	44	111.2	69	156.2	94	201.2
19	66.2	45	113.0	70	158.0	95	203.0
20	68.0	46	114.8	71	159.8	96	204.8
21	69.8	47	116.6	72	161.6	97	206.6
22	71.6	48	118.4	73	163.4	98	208.4
23	73.4	49	120.2	74	165.2	99	210.2
24	75.2	50	122.0	75	167.0	100	212.0
25	77.0						

PHYSICAL CONSTANTS AND CONVERSION FACTORS:
TABLE 4
Additional Conversion Factors

Energy

1 Electron volt (eV)	$= 1.602 \times 10^{-12}$ erg
1 Kiloelectron volt (keV)	$= 1.602 \times 10^{-9}$ erg
1 Million electron volts (MeV)	$= 1.602 \times 10^{-6}$ erg
1 Joule (J)	$= 10^7$ ergs
1 Watt (W)	$= 10^7$ ergs/s
	$= 1$ J/s
1 Rad	$= 1 \times 10^{-2}$ J/kg
	$= 100$ erg/g
1 Gray (Gy)	$= 100$ rad
	$= 1$ J/kg
1 Sievert (Sv)	$= 100$ rem
	$= 1$ J/kg

PHYSICAL CONSTANTS AND CONVERSION FACTORS:
TABLE 4 (continued)
Additional Conversion Factors

1 Horsepower (HP)	= 746 W
1 Calorie (cal)	= 4.184 J

Charge

1 Electronic charge	= 4.8×10^{-10} electrostatic unit
	= 1.6×10^{-19} C
1 Coulomb (C)	= 6.28×10^{18} charge
1 Ampere (A)	= 1 C/s

Mass and energy

1 Atomic mass unit (amu)	= 1.66×10^{-24} g
	= 1/12 the atomic weight of ^{12}C
	= 931 MeV
1 Electron rest mass	= 0.511 MeV
1 Proton rest mass	= 938.23 MeV
1 Neutron rest mass	= 939.53 MeV
1 Pound	= 453.6 g
1 Kilogram	= 5.6095×10^{29} MeV

Length

1 Micrometer or micron (um)	= 10^{-6} meter
	= 10^{-4} cm
	= 10^{4} Å
1 Nanometer (nm)	= 10^{-9} meter
1 Angstrom (Å)	= 10^{-8} cm
1 Fermi (F)	= 10^{-13} cm

Activity

1 Curie (Ci)	= 3.7×10^{10} disintegrations per second (dps)
	= 2.22×10^{12} disintegrations per minute (dpm)
1 Millicurie (mCi)	= 3.7×10^{7} dps
	= 2.22×10^{9} dpm
1 Microcurie (μCi)	= 3.7×10^{4} dps
	= 2.22×10^{6} dpm
1 Becquerel (Bq)	= 1 dps
	= 2.703×10^{-11} Ci
1 Kilobecquerel (kBq)	= 10^{3} dps
	= 2.703×10^{-8} Ci
1 Megabecquerel (MBq)	= 10^{6} dps
	= 2.703×10^{-5} Ci
1 Gigabecquerel (GBq)	= 10^{9} dps
	= 2.703×10^{-2} Ci
1 Terabecquerel (TBq)	= 10^{12} dps
	= 27.03 Ci

Data compiled from: Weast, R. C., Ed., *CRC Handbook of Chemistry and Physics,* 67th ed. (1986-1987), CRC Press, Boca Raton, FL, 1986. Diem, K. and Lentner, C., Eds., *Scientific Tables,* Ciba-Geigy Ltd., Basle, Switzerland, 1970. *Radiological Health Handbook,* U.S. Department of Health Education and Welfare. Washington, D.C., 1970. *Health Physics Handbook,* General Dynamics, Fort Worth Division, 1963.

PHYSICAL CONSTANTS AND
CONVERSION FACTORS: TABLE 5
Exponential Functions

x	e^{-x}	x	e^{-x}	x	e^{-x}
0.00	1.000	0.38	0.684	1.0	0.368
0.01	0.990	0.39	0.677	1.1	0.333
0.02	0.980	0.40	0.670	1.2	0.301
0.03	0.970	0.41	0.664	1.3	0.273
0.04	0.961	0.42	0.657	1.4	0.247
0.05	0.951	0.43	0.651	1.5	0.223
0.06	0.942	0.44	0.644	1.6	0.202
0.07	0.932	0.45	0.638	1.7	0.183
0.08	0.923	0.46	0.631	1.8	0.165
0.09	0.914	0.47	0.625	1.9	0.150
0.10	0.905	0.48	0.619	2.0	0.135
0.11	0.896	0.49	0.613	2.1	0.122
0.12	0.887	0.50	0.607	2.2	0.111
0.13	0.878	0.52	0.595	2.3	0.100
0.14	0.869	0.54	0.583	2.4	0.0907
0.15	0.861	0.56	0.571	2.5	0.0821
0.16	0.852	0.58	0.560	2.6	0.0743
0.17	0.844	0.60	0.549	2.7	0.0672
0.18	0.835	0.62	0.538	2.8	0.0608
0.19	0.827	0.64	0.527	2.9	0.0550
0.20	0.819	0.66	0.517	3.0	0.0498
0.21	0.811	0.68	0.507	3.2	0.0408
0.22	0.803	0.70	0.497	3.4	0.0334
0.23	0.795	0.72	0.487	3.6	0.0273
0.24	0.787	0.74	0.477	3.8	0.0224
0.25	0.779	0.76	0.468	4.0	0.0183
0.26	0.771	0.78	0.458	4.2	0.0150
0.27	0.763	0.80	0.449	4.4	0.0123
0.28	0.756	0.82	0.440	4.6	0.0101
0.29	0.748	0.84	0.432	4.8	0.0862
0.30	0.741	0.86	0.423	5.0	0.0067
0.31	0.733	0.88	0.415	5.5	0.0041
0.32	0.726	0.90	0.407	6.0	0.0025
0.33	0.719	0.92	0.399	6.5	0.0015
0.34	0.712	0.94	0.391	7.0	0.0009
0.35	0.705	0.96	0.383	7.5	0.0006
0.36	0.698	0.98	0.375	8.0	0.0003
0.37	0.691			8.5	0.0002
				9.0	0.0001

Note: Properties of exponential functions:

$$e^1 = 2.71828 \qquad e^x e^y = e^{x+y} \qquad \ln e^x = x$$

$$e^{-x} = 1/e^x \qquad e^{xy} = (e^x)^y \qquad e^{\ln x} = x$$

$$\exp x = e^x$$

Data compiled from Radioactive decay in *The Radiochemical Manual*, 2nd ed., Amersham, England, 1966, 308 G1, and *Health Physics Handbook*, General Dynamics, Fort Worth Division, 1963.

Miscellaneous

QUALITY ASSURANCE AND QUALITY CONTROL IN NUCLEAR MEDICINE

Quality Assurance (QA) and Quality Control (QC) are two terms which are often confused. QA is the total process, from the initial decision to adopt a particular procedure to the interpretation and recording of the results. In the manufacture of instrumentation and radiopharmaceuticals, it covers the design and development stages through to quality control, and delivery processes to final storage and use by customers.

QC, however, is a fundamental part of the QA process and focuses on the selection, testing, and approval of instruments, radiopharmaceuticals, equipment, and facilities. It cannot be part of the manufacturing function and is set up so that it reports to a higher level within the organization.

Quality cannot be controlled into a product after it is made. It is essential to design in the right qualities, including robustness, at the development phase, so that manufacture, quality control, and use are easy and uncomplicated. The QA process at this time will be directed at both product and regulatory needs and will include the establishment of documented support for product claims, the testing of routinely produced batches stored under normal and stress conditions for setting of specifications, and validation of manufacturing and quality control processes, as well as extensive clinical trial and safety support investigations.

Both the International Atomic Energy Agency (IAEA) and the World Health Organization (WHO) have been active in the field of quality assurance, by formulating advice from international panels of experts and by promoting quality assurance methodology through national seminars and workshops. The IAEA has formed an advisory group on the quality control of nuclear medicine instruments which has published schedules for the various classes of instruments (IAEA 1983). The WHO sponsored a joint meeting in Heidelberg in November 1980, following which it published a guide, *Quality Assurance in Nuclear Medicine*.[21] This contains guidance on the organization of quality assurance programs with reference to the whole field, in addition to defining and tabulating quality control requirements for radiopharmaceuticals and instrumentation.

QUALITY CONTROL TECHNIQUES FOR RADIOPHARMACEUTICALS*

A wide range of modern analytical and control techniques are used to ensure that radiopharmaceuticals are of the highest quality and meet the needs of both users and regulatory authorities. The manufacturing and distribution of the radiopharmaceutical preparations, by assimilation of pharmaceutical preparation, must respond to standards, or in default, to protocols established in agreement with the competent authorities. The standards, which are rendered obligatory, are published in official documents, the pharmacopoeia (French, European, British pharmacopoeia, pharmacopoeia of the U.S.A., etc.)

According to these documents, the establishment of quality control of radiopharmaceutical preparations seems to be relatively easy. In fact, if the general methods of manufacturing, distribution, and control are effectively described, all the radiopharmaceutical preparations are not included in monographs; a homogeneous system of control thus runs through the establishment of internal standards obtained by successive acceptances by the competent authorities. Moreover, as the various pharmacopoeia do not always prescribe the same methods or the same standards, it is necessary to render them compatible. All these facts explain the difficulty to image a control system which takes into consideration the whole international statutory restraints. Some quality control techniques are applicable across the whole product range, whereas others are designed and chosen for individual product application.

---

* From *Amersham Nuclear Medicine Catalogue*, Amersham International, plc., Little Chalfont, England, 1985. With permission.

Study of Radiochemical Purity (RCP)

Radiochemical purity can be defined as the fraction of the radionuclide which is in the correct chemical form. It is an essential quality parameter for all radiopharmaceuticals as well as scanning kits, which are reconstituted with technetium-99m or indium-113m generator eluates before use. The following analytical techniques are routinely used in the determination of RCP:

1.   Thin Layer and Paper Chromatography (TLC/PC)
2.   High Performance Liquid Chromatography (HPLC)
3.   Electrophoresis
4.   Gel Permeation
5.   Solvent Extraction

These techniques and systems are tailored to each product and are designed to separate precursors, known impurities, and decomposition products, as well as to identify the desired product.

1.   **Thin Layer/Paper Chromatography (TLC/PC)** — These methods, which include Reverse Phase Thin Layer Chromatography (RPTLC) and Instant Thin Layer Chromatography (ITLC), have been the main vehicle for the determination of radiochemical purity over many years. They are easy to set up, simple to use, and usually employ mixtures of commonly available solvents and chemicals, but can suffer from the inability of any one system to separate out all the likely impurities. It is the ability to quantify radiochromatograms which has made these techniques the method of choice in the analysis of radiopharmaceuticals. Typically, radiochemical purity is determined by calculating the radioactivity in the desired main peak as a percentage of total radioactivity on the chromatogram. Individual radioactive impurity levels can be similarly calculated. The correct sample positions can be identified by the use of nonradioactive standards which can be easily visualized after development.

2.   **High Performance Liquid Chromatography (HPLC)** — High Performance Liquid Chromatography, formerly known as High Pressure Liquid Chromatography, is increasingly being used for the ultimate purification of radiopharmaceuticals and has found use in their final analyses. Although not so simple to use as TLC/PC, it affords the possibility of separating all known and likely impurities in one analysis and is able to give chemical as well as radiochemical purity information. The conditions of chromatography — flow rate, temperature, particle size of the support or interactive media — together with those factors which affect the kinetic environment, such as multilinear or continuous gradient elution in which pH, ionic concentration, and solvent composition can be varied in a precise way, make it possible for one simple HPLC analysis to be equivalent to an infinite number of PCTLC analyses. The interpretation of chemical purity is more complex than that for radiochemical purity because different chemical entities have different UV absorbing capabilities and the change in solvent composition necessary in continuous gradient elution will also affect UV absorption. Identification of the correct material can be made either through retention time, which is very consistent in such a controlled procedure, or through a nonradioactive marker as used in TLC/PC.

3.   **Electrophoresis** — Electrophoresis utilizes the property of ions to move under the influence of an electric charge. Components of a sample will move at different rates along a strip of paper or gel medium according to their charge and ionic mobility. As such, this technique finds use in a number of applications including the determination of radioactive iodide in iodopharmaceuticals and the measurement of the thallic (^{201}Tl)

ion in Thallous (^{201}Tl) Chloride. The electrophoretograms are measured in the same manner as thin layer and paper chromatograms.

4. **Gel Permeation** —Gel Permeation is used to separate large molecules from small molecules by a sieving effect. Large molecules have difficulty penetrating the pores of gels and are eluted in a column separation procedure more rapidly than small molecules. Quantification can be obtained by passing the eluate through a radioactive counter, but is usually effected by fraction collecting and counting.

5. **Solvent Extraction** — Solvent Extraction is not a particularly convenient technique, but can be useful for some products which are not readily analyzed by other chromatographic techniques. Determination of ion indium (^{111}In) in Indium (^{111}In) Oxine is a case in point where a solvent extraction system with isotonic saline and n-octanol has shown itself to be the only reliable procedure. This technique is also particularly useful in measuring the very low levels of iodide (^{131}I) in iodohippuran (^{131}I) used in effective renal plasma flow investigations.

Study of Radionuclide Purity (RNP)

Radionuclide purity can be defined as the fraction of the total radioactivity in the form of the desired radionuclide. Radionuclidic impurities can arise from extraneous nuclear reactions due to very small levels of impurities in target materials, or from unavoidable nuclear processes, as well as less than optimum separation processes associated with fission and parent-daughter products. These impurities will increase patient radiation dose and may affect imaging processes, so it is important to ensure their accurate and precise measurement, particularly those which are energetic and/or long-lived.

Since all manufacturing processes should be carefully designed and controlled to eliminate or keep these impurities to a very safe level, it is most unusual to find significant levels in any sample submitted for quality control testing. However, methods used in QC to measure RNP include High Resolution Gamma Spectroscopy, Liquid Scintillation Counting, and Chemical Separation (followed by counting).

1. **High Resolution Gamma Spectroscopy** — High Resolution Gamma Spectroscopy utilizing a high purity germanium crystal is a basic tool in the estimation of radionuclidic impurities. It allows many gamma emitting impurities to be resolved, identified, and quantified at very low levels.

2. **Liquid Scintillation Counting** — This technique can be used to estimate beta emitting impurities. It is based on the principle that the energy of photons emitted from an excited phosphor is related to the energy of the radiation which initially excited the phosphor. By suitable electronic gating it is possible to select and measure those photons related to impurities. One use of this technique is found in the determination of indium-114m in indium-111 preparations. This impurity occurs at a very low level due to unavoidable nuclear processes, and although it emits some gamma photons, it is difficult to use high resolution gamma spectroscopy for accurate measurement due to the intensity and similar energies of the indium-111 gamma emissions. However, it has been possible to measure the beta emissions of this very short-lived daughter indium-114 providing that the responses resulting from indium-111 are gated out.

3. **Chemical Separation (Following by Counting)** — This is a well-established method of estimating radionuclidic impurities and improving sensitivity of measurement. One useful variation is to separate out the daughter product of a suspected impurity which itself cannot be separated from the desired or main radionuclide. An example is given by the determination of strontium-90 in strontium-89. Strontium-90 is an impurity produced by neutron irradiation of strontium-89, which is itself produced from neutron irradiation of strontium-88. Both are beta emitters and difficult to separate, but mea-

surement is readily effected by beta counting the yttrium-90 daughter of strontium-90 after separation on an ion exchange column.

Study of Chemical Purity/Identification

Chemical purity can be defined as the fraction of the preparation, labeled or unlabeled, which is in the stated chemical form. This is a particularly important concept for raw chemical starting materials for radiopharmaceutical products which are complex mixtures of buffers, saline, preservatives, stabilizers, chemicals and radiochemicals; chemical purity is usually related to the identification and concentration of excipients and impurities. A variety of techniques are routinely used: (1) Nuclear Magnetic Resonance Spectroscopy, (2) Infra Red Spectroscopy, (3) Ultra Violet/Visible Spectroscopy, (4) Fluorimetry, (5) Emission Spectroscopy, (6) Atomic Absorption Spectroscopy, (7) High Performance Liquid Chromatography, (8) Isotachophoresis, and (9) Microtitration.

1. **Molecular Spectroscopy** — Both Nuclear Magnetic Resonance (NMR) and Infra Red (IF) Spectroscopy are employed in the identification of organic chemical raw materials and final pack excipients, where Ultra Violet/Visible Spectroscopy and Fluorimetry are used as a convenient means of measuring chemical concentrations.

2. **Atomic Spectroscopy** — The wide range and high sensitivity of Emission Spectroscopy makes it an ideal technique for general cationic impurity detection, whereas Atomic Absorption Spectroscopy, both flame and graphite furnace atomization, allows the accurate and specific measurement of low levels of cationic material. Routine procedures are used to screen radiopharmaceutical preparations for "heavy metals", but recent advances in indium-111 labeling of monoclonal antibodies have highlighted the need to use these instruments to measure down to less than one part per million (ppm) of some cations.

3. **High Performance Liquid Chromatography (HPLC)** — The use of HPLC for RCP determinations has already been presented. However, it is also a valuable technique in the separation and quantification of various isometric forms of complex chemicals.

4. **Isotachophoresis** — This technique is based on the ability to separate mixtures of compounds according to their electrophoretic mobility in various media. Identification is confirmed by measuring the output step height, which under defined operating conditions is constant for a given chemical entity. Quantitative estimation of the compound is derived from the output step length, which is related to the time taken for the sample to travel through the UV or conductivity detector cell. Individual samples are assayed by reference to a calibrated curve.

5. **Microtitration** — Most radiopharmaceutical preparations contain exceedingly small levels of chemicals, and any titrimetric or potentiometric assay must, of necessity, be developed so that these low levels, very often less than 1 mg, can be accurately and precisely measured. Examples are found in the estimation of stannous ions in technetium-99m based scanning agents and acid content in Indium (^{111}In) Chloride preparations.

Study of Radioactive Content

Measurement of radioactive concentration is a routine test for all radiopharmaceutical batches as is measurement of radioactive content for all vials and capsules. Ionization Chambers which are reliable and simple to use are selected for this work for most gamma emitters. Low-energy gamma emitters are measured using sodium iodide "well-type" counters and beta emitters are measured using liquid scintillation counters.

Other Quality Control Tests

Whereas some quality control tests are applicable across the whole range of products, such as pH, sterility, apyrogenicity, satisfactory sealing, correct labeling, and freedom from external contamination, other tests can be specific to products or product types.

1. **Biodistribution tests** — Physiological distribution tests are valuable indicators of product performance, and pharmacopeial standards are set for some technetium (^{99m}Tc) radiopharmaceuticals. Such tests, which in some circumstances can be more sensitive and/or specific than physical or chemical testing, are performed as part of the routine batch release testing of all technetium (^{99m}Tc) based scanning agents.
2. **Ion-selective electrode assays** — This is an increasingly important analytical technique used wherever possible to measure concentrations of final pack excipients, such as fluoride and chloride. It is a very sensitive technique and in conjunction with radioactive concentration is useful in the determination of specific activity of "carrier-free" entities, such as iodide ion.
3. **pH** — pH is normally a very simple parameter to measure, but perhaps surprisingly, can cause real difficulties in practice, particularly for those products which are not highly buffered. Experience has shown that pH paper can give misleading values, and measurement by pH meter and electrode is without exception the method of choice. Here, care has to be taken to ensure that the system is correctly set up using standardized pH buffers, and that the electrode is not "poisoned".

Microbiological Control

Microbiological control is of fundamental importance in radiopharmaceutical preparation, and includes essential environmental and equipment control, as well as final pack testing. Experience has shown the need to ensure that facilities such as clean rooms and autoclaves are as firmly controlled as manufacturing procedures and final sterility tests. Since the majority of radiopharmaceuticals are short-lived and of necessity released for use before any sterility testing can be completed, it is of prime importance to control the sterilizing procedure to the most exacting standard.

1. **Environmental control** — Regular testing of preparation areas to ensure that standards of low microbial and particulate contamination are being met is of prime importance in the overall control of radiopharmaceutical preparation. The preparation of vials and closures also demands high quality air and water supplies, and continual monitoring of these is carried out to ensure that safe particulate and microbial levels are being maintained. These tests, combined with the other in-process tests, such as presterilization bioburden and integrity testing of closures, as well as the final sterility and apyrogenicity tests, form a package designed to ensure that only the highest standard radiopharmaceuticals is being prepared.
2. **Autoclave control** — Sterilization by heating in an autoclave is the method of choice for heat-stable aqueous products. Before being accepted into routine use, an autoclave must undergo a rigorous commissioning test involving the use of multipoint recorders with thermocouples distributed throughout the load and chamber. After commissioning, the autoclaves are subjected to a regular sequence of maintenance and revalidation procedures throughout their lifespans.
3. **Pyrogen testing** — Although all processes are designed to limit the bioburden of any product presented to a sterilizing process, it should be noted that the small volumes of radiopharmaceuticals used reduces the patient risk to a minimum. Two tests are in use, the rabbit test and Limulus Amoebocyte Lysate (LAL) test. The LAL test is more sensitive to bacterial endotoxins than the rabbit test and can be made quantitative.

These ease and speeds with which this test can be performed on small volumes of radioactive products means that it is ideally suited for use as an in-process control.

4.   **Sterility test** — The pharmacopoeial sterility tests applied to radiopharmaceuticals are the last in a series of process controls designed to ensure complete safety. Whereas terminally sterilized products are subjected to a high degree of overkill, those products which are produced aseptically have additional related tests, such as integrity testing of final sterilizing filters, to complement the sterility test. Sterility tests may be performed either by direct inoculation of sample into microbial culture media, or by membrane filtration.

QUALITY ASSURANCE OF INSTRUMENTATION*

Quality control of an instrument begins with its selection. The user must decide what facilities and performance are required, and these requirements must be checked against the manufacturer's specification. It should be understood how the performance is to be assessed, and appropriate radionuclide sources, phantoms, and any necessary measuring instruments should be acquired. The supply of spare parts, service manuals, and provision of maintenance should also be considered, and arrangements made for servicing during the proposed lifetime of the equipment.

For many large items of equipment, the siting and installation must be carefully controlled, taking account of such factors as electrical power requirements, background radiation levels, and environmental constraints such as temperature and humidity.

For most instruments it is desirable to define smaller sets of routine tests falling into two categories: operational tests to be undertaken every time the instrument is used, and periodic measurements of performance at appropriate intervals, for example weekly, monthly, or quarterly, depending upon the anticipated reliability.

Dose Calibrators

The dose calibrator (or radionuclide activity meter) is used to measure the quantity of radioactivity administered to the patient. Its response must be calibrated against a source, the activity of which is itself calibrated (to an overall uncertainty of $\pm 5\%$) by a standards laboratory. A sealed long-lived source is required for all stages of quality control; suitable sources are listed below.

SEALED SOURCES FOR CALIBRATION OF ACTIVITY METERS

Radionuclide	Principal photon energies (keV)	Half-life	Activity (MBq)
^{57}Co	122	271 d	40
^{133}Ba	81, 356	10.7 years	10
^{137}Cs	662	30.1 years	4
^{60}Co	1173, 1332	5.3 years	2

Acceptance and reference tests for dose calibrators should include:

1.   Calibration, using standard measurement, geometry, at low and medium gamma-ray energies
2.   Linearity of activity response — up to saturation — using ^{99m}Tc in solution
3.   Measurement of background reading under the most sensitive operating conditions
4.   Calibration for nonstandard measurement geometries (e.g., activity in a syringe)
5.   Test of molybdenum breakthrough option (if applicable)

---

* From Shields, R. A., Quality assurance in nuclear medicine, in McAinsh, T. F., Ed., *Physics in Medicine and Biology Encyclopedia,* Pergamon Press, Oxford, 1986. With permission.

Operational routine tests for dose calibrators include:

1.   Reproducibility using a sealed, medium-energy source of long half-life (not necessarily calibrated)
2.   Measurement of background under normal operating conditions

Periodic routine tests for dose calibrators include:

1.   Calibration against a sealed source
2.   Linearity of activity response
3.   Measurement of background under most sensitive operating conditions

Gamma-Ray Detectors

Three classes of instrument can be considered which share the same scintillation detector technology, and for which basic quality control requirements are similar. These are counters for gamma-emitting samples *in vivo*, probes for uptake measurements *in vivo*, and rectilinear scanners.

For gamma-ray detectors, general acceptance/reference tests should include:

1.   Calibration of the energy response of the pulse-height analyzer (e.g., using the 662 keV emission of ^{137}Cs)
2.   Measurement of linearity of energy response, using radionuclides exhibiting the range of gamma-ray energies
3.   Measurement of sensitivity to relevant radionuclides
4.   Integral background reading (e.g., above 20 keV)
5.   Adjustment of present analyzer peak settings
6.   Measurement of linearity of count-rate response
7.   Measurement of energy resolution (e.g., using ^{137}Cs)
8.   Scaler and/or ratemeter functional verification

Routine tests for all gamma-ray detectors may be summarized as follows:

1.   Operational: checks of mechanical safety, check of analyzer peak setting(s), background measurement and chart recorder or image output function
2.   Periodic: repeat of reference tests

Gamma Cameras

A careful approach to the assessment of performance is essential for effective specification and selection of gamma cameras, and for acceptance and reference testing. Reference testing is particularly important in order to detect and correct long-term slow deterioration in quality. Furthermore, the complexity of the equipment and the nature of the routine clinical investigations demand effective day-to-day control to ensure the validity of the results. There is extensive literature on this subject,[18,19] and there are well-established protocols for performance assessment, notably from the U.S. National Electrical Manufacturers' Association (NEMA)[11,16] and the International Electrotechnical Commission (IEC).[7] These protocols essentially comprise tests by which manufacturers may specify performance parameters. The NEMA system has achieved almost universal acceptance for this purpose. This system concentrates on the intrinsic performance of the detector assembly, whereas the IEC approach is related more to the function of the total system. The various protocols proposed for ongoing quality control have endeavored to marry the desirability of reference to original specifications with practicalities of measurements to be made in hospital departments.

Gamma Cameras: Acceptance/Reference Tests

Unless otherwise stated, these tests should be carried out at count rates less than 10 kcps (kilocounts per second) and with the camera's energy analyzer turned to the photopeak of the relevant gamma radiation with a symmetrical window of $+10\%$.

1. **Analyzer energy settings** — These settings, normally present, must be checked for all radionuclides to be used.

2. **Intrinsic energy resolution** — This parameter, which is fundamental to the performance of the instrument, is difficult to measure in the many modern cameras which employ real-time energy and spatial distortion corrections. The Z pulses, whose amplitudes represent energy absorbed for each detected event, should be taken from the appropriate test point and an amplitude spectrum acquired using a multichannel analyzer, so that there are at least 20 channels within the peak and at least 10 kilocounts are registered in the peak channel. A flood-field source placed on the collimator is suitable; a second radionuclide is needed to calibrate the energy scale. The result is given by the full width at half maximum (FWHM) of the peak, expressed as a percentage of the quoted energy.

3. **Intrinsic spatial resolution** — The spatial resolution of the crystal/photomultiplier tube assembly is a key determinant of system performance. It is usually measured by the line spread function, which is the count-rate profile which would be observed at right angles to the image of an infinitely long and infinitesimally thin line source of activity on the detector face. It is usually quantified in terms of the full width at both half and tenth maximum (FWHM and FWTM).

    Intrinsic resolution may be examined less quantitatively (but much more easily) by producing images using a class of phantoms which comprise patterns of lead placed on the detector face, irradiated by a point source or by a uniform field of activity. Four such phantoms have been used extensively:

    • The quadrant bar phantom, comprising four sets of lead bars mounted in perspex sheet, so that each set is at right angles to those adjacent. Spacing between bars is equal to their width; four values of spacing are chosen so as to indicate the required discrimination of performance.

    • The Anger pie phantom, in which individual sectors of a lead disk each contain a pattern of holes separated by four times the hole diameter. Values of interhole spacing may be chosen between 4 and 10 mm.

    • The orthogonal hole transmission pattern (OHTP), which, in its simplest form, comprises an orthogonal pattern of holes on centers separated by twice the hole diameter. Only one spacing is used over the entire crystal face. For maximum effectiveness, this phantom should be specified to match the camera under test.

    • The Bureau of Radiological Health (BRH) OHTP phantom, a variation in which the interhole spacing changes for each group of six holes in one direction.

4. **System spatial resolution** — This is a measurement of resolution of the detector system including a particular collimator, and may therefore be related directly to the clinical imaging situation. For this reason, a series of measurements is taken with the source at depth (typically 10, 50, 100, 150, and 200 mm) in a scattering medium. The source may be short line of activity, as described in the previous section on intrinsic resolution, or it may be a phantom comprising parallel lines of 0.5 mm bore capillary tubing filled with radioactive solution — an "inverse" of the multiple-slit phantom. As indicated above, the spread of response to the line sources may be expressed in terms of FWHM and FWTM for the particular collimator at the specified depth in scattering medium. Qualitative assessment of system resolution may be carried out by imaging phantoms comprising hot and/or cold "lesions" of different sizes

surrounded by radioactive solution. Two examples are the Williams phantoms and the Shell phantom.[2]

5. **Nonuniformity** — The nonuniformity of sensitivity over the field of view of the camera may be investigated by imaging a structurally rigid flood-field source containing 100-200 MBq of the calibrating radionuclide well mixed throughout the container. This is done with a collimator fitted, in order to give a system measurement. Qualitative images are likely to be affected by inhomogeneities in the display system, and it is desirable to be able to separate out this effect by quantifying the nonuniformity of response of the detector system with a digital computer. A matrix of 64×64 pixels is suitable, within which the useful field of view (UFOV) must be identified. The following parameters may be quoted both for pixels within this area, and also for those within the central field of view (CFOV), defined as falling within a circle of diameter 75% of that of the UFOV:

mean nonuniformity = coefficient of variation of counts

integral nonuniformity (maximum positive) = $(C_{max} - C_m)/C_m \times 100\%$

integral nonuniformity (maximum regative) = $(C_{min} - C_m)/C_m \times 100\%$

where C_{max} and C_{min} are the maximum and minimum pixel counts respectively, and C_m is the mean pixel count.

Also

differential nonuniformity = $(\Delta C/M) \times 100\%$

where ΔC is the maximum difference in counts between two adjacent pixels, and M is the value of the larger of the two counts.

6. **Sensitivity** — The system sensitivity is measured with each collimator by placing a calibrated planar source, 100×100mm, containing approximately 37 MBq of the radionuclide at 100 mm from the collimator surface on its central axis. The result is expressed as the dimensionless quantity counts per second per MBq (or per mCi).

7. **Intrinsic spatial linearity** — Nonuniformity of sensitivity is primarily caused by failure of the detector head positioning circuitry to reproduce faithfully the geometric relationships of points within a source. This spatial nonlinearity, or distortion, is investigated directly by analyzing the image acquired using a multiple slit phantom or a set of perfectly straight line sources on the crystal face. The absolute linearity is given by the maximum displacement of each fitted peak in the image from its ideal position; the differential linearity is the standard deviation of fitted peak positions.[11]

8. **Count rate performance** — This is strongly influenced by measurement conditions because of the effect of scattered radiation on the detector's performance. The IEC protocol attempts to simulate clinical conditions by specifying that the source be placed within a large tank of water on the surface of the collimator. The activity of the source is then increased by known increments until a maximum count rate is obtained, and a graph is plotted of observed count rate against the decay-corrected expected count rate. The observed count rate for 20% loss in relation to the expected count rate, and the maximum count rate, are reported.

9. **Multiple-window spatial registration** — This is a measure of positional deviation of an image acquired at different photon energies, and may conveniently be measured by comparing the images of a ^{67}Ga source acquired at the energy of each of its three emissions.

10. **Shield leakage** — A small 37 MBq source of the radionuclide is used to survey penetration of radiation at several positions around the surface of the detector head, expressing the results as a percentage of on-axis count rate.

11. **Total system performance** — There are dangers inherent in a totally analytical approach to performance assessment[19] and most workers in this field would not be satisfied until their system had produced good images of a known "total performance" phantom, such as the London liver phantom or one of the College of American Pathologists' (CAP) phantoms (WHO 1982).

Gamma Cameras: Routine Tests

It is possible to devise a schedule of routine tests of camera performance to relate to the original NEMA specifications[14] but it is doubtful whether the time taken for such a rigorous approach to quality control would be justified.[1] The following subset of performance tests is suitable for routine quality control:

1. Operational: safety of detector and collimator, analyzer settings uniformity check with ^{99m}Tc or ^{57}Co, display and output verification, and background measurement
2. Weekly: uniformity measurement with ^{99m}Tc, and linearity, sensitivity, and resolution test using an orthogonal hole transmission pattern (OHTP) phantom
3. Periodically: repeat of reference tests

Whole-Body Scanning Attachments

The performance of a whole-body scanning attachment to a gamma camera should be tested daily, to ensure that the collimator axis is perpendicular to the scan plane, and weekly, to verify positioning circuitry by scanning with a flood field fixed to the camera.

Single Photon Emission Tomography

Rotating gamma-camera systems used for emission tomography have special quality control requirements[8,10] which include:

1. Very accurate uniformity correction
2. Assessment of variation of uniformity with rotation
3. Correction for alignment of mechanical and electronic axes of rotation
4. Adjustment of head orientation
5. System uniformity assessment for reconstructed images, and
6. System total performance assessment using a three-dimensional phantom

Computer Systems

Computer systems are often used nowadays for routine clinical analysis, and it is easy to fall into the trap of assuming that "the computer never lies", in spite of the tremendous demands made upon the accuracy, consistency, and speed of the interface circuitry, and of the vulnerability of the processing techniques. There are several tests to be made of computer interface performance which include:

1. Dead-time and count-rate performance
2. Differential and integral linearity of the analog-to-digital converters
3. Accuracy of timing in the list and frame mode acquisitions
4. Accuracy of gated acquisition

An effective routine test is the analysis of a uniformity image acquired with a standardized flood field on the gamma camera. The total counts acquired in a fixed time should be noted, as should the dimensions and position of the image, in addition to the calculation of non-uniformity parameters. Even more information may be derived from the digital image of an orthogonal hole transmission pattern.[19] An alternative scheme whereby a weekly flood field measurement is supplemented by the use of a phantom comprising four point sources set in a square has been proposed by Lancaster et al.[9] The computer analysis gives measurements of system spatial resolution, point source sensitivity, spatial calibration, and spatial distortion.

BIBLIOGRAPHY

1. **Cradduck, T. D., Busemann-Sokole, E.,** Use of NEMA protocols for routine quality assurance, *J. Nucl. Med.,* 26, 95, 1985.
2. Department of Health and Society Security (DHSS), Performance Assessment of Gamma Cameras, Part II, Report No. STB 13, DHSS Scientific and Technical Branch, London, 1982.
3. **Hine, G. J., Paras, P., and Warr, C. P.,** Measurements of the Performance Parameters of Gamma Cameras, Part I, HEW Publication (FDA) 78-8049, Bureau of Radiological Health, U.S. Department of Health, Education and Welfare, Rockville, MD, 1977.
4. **Hine, G. J., Paras, P., Warr, C. P., and Adams, R.,** Measurements of the Performance Parameters of Gamma Cameras, Part II, HEW Publication (FDA) 79-8049. Bureau of Radiological Health, U.S. Department of Health, Education and Welfare, Rockville, MD, 1979.
5. **Horton, P. W., Ed.,** The Theory, Specification and Testing of Anger Type Gamma Cameras, Topic Group Report 27, Hospital Physicists' Association. London, 1978.
6. International Atomic Energy Authority, Quality Control Schedules for Nuclear Medicine Instrumentation, IAEA, Vienna, 1983.
7. International Electrotechnical Commission (IEC), Characteristics and test conditions of radionuclide imaging devices, Draft document 80/22888DC, IEC/BSI, London, 1980.
8. **Jarritt, P. H. and Cullum, I. D.,** Quality control of single photon emission tomographic systems, in Mould, R. F., Ed., *Quality Control of Nuclear Medicine Instrumentation,* Conference Report Series 38, Hospital Physicists' Association, London, 1983, 81.
9. **Lancaster, J. L., Kopp, D. T., Lasher, J. S., and Blumhardt, R.,** Practical gamma camera quality control with a four-point phantom, *J. Nucl. Med.,* 26, 300, 1985.
10. **Mould, R. F., Ed.,** *Quality Control of Nuclear Medicine Instrumentation,* Conference Report Series 38, Hospital Physicists' Association, London, 1983.
11. National Electric Manufacturers' Association (NEMA), Standards for the Performance of Radionuclide Imaging Devices, Publication No. NU-1-1980, Washington, D.C., 1980.
12. Nuclear Medicine — Amersham, Amersham International, plc., Little Chalfont, England, 1985.
13. **Paras, P.,** Quality assurance in nuclear medicine, in *Proc. Int. Symp. Medical Radionuclide Imaging,* Vol. I., IAEA, Vienna, 1977, 3.
14. **Raff, U., Spitzer, V. M., and Hendee, W. R.,** Practicality of NEMA performance specification measurements for user-based acceptance testing and routine quality assurance, *J. Nucl. Med.,* 25, 679, 1984.
15. **Rhodes, B. A., Ed.,** *Quality Control in Nuclear Medicine: Radiopharmaceuticals, Instrumentation and In Vitro Assays,* Mosby, St. Louis, 1977.
16. **Sano, R. M.,** Performance standards: characteristics and test conditions for scintillation cameras, in *Proc. Int. Symp. Medical Radionuclide Imaging,* Vol. II, IAEA, Vienna, 1981, 141.
17. **Shield, R. A.,** Quality assurance, in McAinsh, T. F., Ed., *Nuclear Medicine in Physics in Medicine and Biology Encyclopedia,* Pergamon Press, Oxford, 1986.
18. **Short, M. D., Elliott, A. T., and Barnes, K. J.,** Performance assessment of the Anger camera, in Mould, R. F., Ed., *Quality Control of Nuclear Medicine Instrumentation,* Conference Report Series 38, Hospital Physicists Association, London, 1983, 1.
19. **Todd-Pokropek, A.,** Quality control, detection and display, in Kuhl, D. E., Ed., *Principles of Radionuclide Emission Imaging.* Pergamon, Oxford, 1983, 27
20. **Todd-Pokropek, A.,** Digital quality control of the camera computer interface, in Mould, R. F., Ed., *Quality Control of Nuclear Medicine Instrumentation,* Conference Report Series 38, Hospital Physicists Association, London, 1983, 54.
21. World Health Organization, *Quality Assurance in Nuclear Medicine, A Guide Prepared Following a Workshop in Heidelberg, Federal Republic of Germany,* WHO, Geneva, 1982.

RADIATION PROTECTION SAFETY PRACTICES IN NUCLEAR MEDICINE

1. ORGANIZATIONAL REQUIREMENTS

1.1 General

Good radiation safety practice and the achievement of satisfactory working conditions depend on the effective organization of health physics and safety. The holder of the authority for the use of radioactive material is responsible for the radiological safety of the workers in his employ and that of members of the public liable to exposure as a result of the use of radioactive material.

1.2 Responsible Person

A person with the necessary knowledge and experience must be appointed to accept, on behalf of the holder of the authority, the responsibility for the safe use of all radioactive material under the holder's control and to observe any statutory requirements in connection with the use of radioactive material. An alternate for the responsible person, to whom the duties of the responsible person may be delegated, must also be nominated.

The responsible person's knowledge and experience in the field of radiation protection must be adequate, taking into account the potential radiation hazards attached to the use of the radioactive material under his control. For example, complex procedures involving unsealed sources of relatively high activity will require more knowledge and experience than will the handling of equipment containing sealed sources that form an integral part of the equipment.

Note: it is recommended that the responsible person attend appropriate courses in radiation protection. Whenever necessary, the responsible person should call for advice or assistance from professionally competent persons.

1.3 Duties of the Responsible Person

The responsible person must ensure that

a. New personnel are instructed in safe working practices and in the nature of the biological effects resulting from over-exposure to radiation

b. Operational procedures are so established and maintained that the radiation exposure of each worker is kept as far below the authorized limits as is practicable

c. Each case of excessive or abnormal exposure is investigated to determine its cause and that steps are taken to prevent its recurrence

d. Monitoring devices for personnel are used where required and that records are kept of the results of such monitoring

e. Adequate records are kept of all sources, indicating the locations of these sources or the name of the person to whom they have been assigned

f. Periodic radiation surveys are conducted where required and, if needed, that records of such surveys, including descriptions of corrective measures, are kept

g. All shields, containers and handling equipment are maintained in a satisfactory condition

h. Periodic leak tests of sealed sources are performed

1.4 Classification of Workers

Where persons are employed at institutions or installations where radioactive material is used, it is necessary to distinguish those persons, who as a result of their duties, are potentially liable to exposures in excess of 5 mSv (500 mR) per annum (i.e., one-tenth of the whole body annual dose-equivalent limit for radiation workers). All such persons must be classified as radiation workers; other workers must not be so classified.

It is advisable to limit the number of radiation workers as far as practicable. Measures must be taken to ensure that the exposure of nonradiation workers to radiation sources is kept to a minimum, but in any event the exposure may not exceed the authorized limits. This can be achieved by limiting work with radioactive material to controlled areas to which only radiation workers have access.

1.5 Register

The holder must compile, in respect of all radiation workers, a register that contains at least the following information for each radiation worker:

a.   Results of pre-employment and routine medical examinations
b.   A record of dose equivalents and exposures recorded by personal and pocket dosimeters, respectively
c.   Any other relevant information

1.6 Medical Surveillance

Radiation workers must be medically examined before employment as radiation workers, and then routinely at least once a year or as required by the competent authority. Medical examinations may also be necessary in the event of overexposure or of radiation incidents where the possibility of overexposure exists.

1.7 Register of Sealed Sources

The holder must keep, in respect of all sealed sources, a register that contains at least the following information for each source:

a.   The nuclide, activity and date on which the activity was specified
b.   The date received
c.   The manufacturer's name and the identification number of the source
d.   The purpose for which the source is used
e.   Particulars of leak tests
f.   Particulars of disposal or discarding of the source

1.8 Radiation Warning Signs

Radiation warning signs must be displayed at all entrances to storage places, in areas where radioactive sources are used or installed, and where persons could be exposed to ionizing radiation. A list of the names and telephone numbers of persons who can be telephoned in case of an emergency must be prominently displayed in the locations referred to above.

2. MONITORING AND CALIBRATION
2.1 Monitoring of Persons
2.1.1 General

By the monitoring of persons is meant the routine measurement of the dose equivalents of persons exposed in the course of their work to radiation from external sources and, where applicable, from internally deposited radioactive material. Measurement of the latter will be required only where unsealed sources are used, or where leakage of a sealed source has occurred, and where the possibility of ingestion of radioactive material exists. Unless specifically exempted by the competent authority, all radiation workers must be monitored to determine their dose equivalents due to radiation from external sources, but guidance with regard to the need for internal monitoring must be sought from the competent authority.

2.1.2. Monitoring for External Sources of Radiation

All radiation workers must be issued with personal dosimeters, obtainable from the Radiation Protection Service of the local competent authority. In addition, where working conditions are such that the radiation workers are liable to an exposure from gamma radiation in excess of 185 kBq·kg^{-1} (20 mR) during any one day, direct-reading dosimeters, such as pocket dosimeters, must also be issued to the radiation workers.

Note: The purpose of the pocket dosimeter is for the worker to establish at intervals during the day the rate at which he is exposed to radiation, and to enable him, if necessary, to change working procedures or working conditions to reduce radiation exposures. Pocket dosimeter readings must be recorded at the end of each working day and these recordings filed in the register at the end of each week. This record can be an important source of information when incidents indicated by, or overexposures recorded on personal dosimeters, are investigated at a later date.

2.1.3 Monitoring for Internally Deposited Radioactive Material

Where unsealed sources are used, it may be necessary, in addition to taking personal dosimeter readings, also to monitor for any ingestion of radioactive material. This may be done by whole body counting or by analysis of body excretions, or both. The techniques involved are of a complicated and specialized nature and it is advisable to consult the competent authority in this regard. Whole body counters are available at most of the training hospitals located in the main centers.

2.2 Monitoring of Controlled Areas
2.2.1 General

A systematic program of monitoring of controlled areas must be established to ensure satisfactory working conditions and working procedures, and thereby limit the exposure of persons to radiation. The three types of monitoring involved are

a.   The monitoring of radiation from radioactive sources
b.   The monitoring for surface contamination
c.   The monitoring for air contamination

2.2.2 Monitoring of Direct and Scattered Radiation from Radioactive Sources

All areas around radioactive sources where persons could be exposed to direct or scattered radiation (or both) must be monitored. Adjoining areas or rooms and, when applicable, areas outside buildings must be included as these could also be occupied. Monitoring must be concluded before the start of a project, during its progress, and after significant modifications to existing installations have been made.

Portable ionization chambers, Geiger-Müller counters, and scintillation counters may be used, as applicable. In some cases, thermoluminescent dosimeters or film dosimeters, mounted at strategic places, could also be used.

2.2.3 Monitoring for Surface Contamination (Unsealed Sources)

Every object used for work with unsealed radioactive material is subject to contamination. This includes work surfaces, walls, floors, clothing, and equipment. Contamination by radioactive substances or work surfaces, clothing, and equipment may be a significant hazard to health, and may also interfere with the work being carried out.

All areas where radioactive material has been used and all equipment that has been in contact with radioactive material must be monitored systematically for contamination. Such monitoring must be performed at least when the work has been completed and, if necessary, also at appropriate times during work periods. Whenever they leave the work area, persons (and their clothing) must be monitored so that the spread of contamination is prevented.

TABLE 1
Permitted Levels of Surface Contamination

Source of contamination	Parts of the body, personal clothing, inactive areas	Protective clothing, active areas, glassware, tools/instruments
Alpha emitters	3.7×10^3 Bq $\cdot$ m^{-2} (10^{-1} μCi $\cdot$ m^{-2})	3.7×10^4 Bq $\cdot$ m^{-2} (1 μCi $\cdot$ m^{-2})
Beta emitters	3.7×10^4 Bq $\cdot$ m^{-2} (1 μCi $\cdot$ m^{-2})	3.7×10^5 Bq $\cdot$ m^{-2} (10 μCi $\cdot$ m^{-2})

Monitoring may be performed with the aid of counting instruments and by the taking of smear samples. The instruments used must be suitable for the type of radiation emitted by the radionuclides used, e.g., alpha emitters and soft beta emitters will make the use of alpha scintillation monitors and thin end-window Geiger-Müller counters essential.

The permitted levels of surface contamination, as laid down by the competent authority, are given in Table 1.

2.2.4 Monitoring for Air Contamination

In situations where radioactive gases, aerosols, powders, or dusts are handled or produced, the air must be monitored for contamination.

Where it is possible that, notwithstanding filtration of air exhausted to the atmosphere, the activity released might exceed levels set by the competent authority, a reliable system of air monitoring must be employed.

Note:

a. When aerosols are to be monitored, the airborne substances are caused to be deposited by electrostatic precipitation, impactors, or filtration.
b. Some radioactive gases can be monitored only after collection by chemical or other means.

2.2.5 Suitability of Monitoring Equipment

Monitoring equipment must be carefully selected to ensure that it has an adequate response to the type of radiation to be measured and that the equipment exhibits a minimum of energy dependence over the range of energies concerned. For example, a monitor designed to measure high-energy gamma radiation from, for example, cobalt-60 or iridium-192 sources, may well have a very poor response to lower energy radiation emitted by sources such as americium-241 and iodine-125, and will probably not be capable of detecting beta radiation at all. (Detection of the latter would require thin end-window Geiger-Müller counter or scintillation monitor.)

2.2.6 Recording of Results

Records must be kept of the results of environmental monitoring and of significant events concerning radiation protection. In investigations, such records will usually be the only available sources of data.

2.3 Accidents and Emergencies

Any accidents in which workers have been overexposed to or contaminated with radioactive materials, or in which radioactive material has been spilled, need special action, and special procedures must be followed. Each accident must be reported without delay to the responsible person, who in turn must report it to the competent authority. An incident (i.e., an unplanned event that has taken place and that may lead to a hazardous situation) must be reported immediately to the responsible person.

2.4 Limitation of Exposure to Radiation

All exposure must be kept as low as is reasonably achievable, economic and social factors being taken into consideration. The exposure must therefore be so optimized that a further reduction in exposure would not be justified by the additional cost entailed.

The dose equivalent to individuals must not exceed the dose-equivalent limits laid down by the competent authority. These dose-equivalent limits must be viewed as upper limits, and must not be interpreted as being necessarily allowable. Furthermore, long-continued exposure of a considerable proportion of workers at or near the dose-equivalent limits would be acceptable only if a careful analysis has shown that the resulting higher risk is justified.

It will be possible to achieve the above-mentioned goals only if all levels of contamination of work areas and air concentrations of radionuclides are kept as low as is practicable.

2.5 Calibration of Monitoring Equipment

All equipment, including pocket dosimeters, used for the monitoring of radiation and contamination, must be regularly tested and calibrated by an institution approved for the purpose, as required by the competent authority.

3. SEALED SOURCES
3.1 Choice of sealed sources

A source used to produce a radiation field must be selected on the basis of the criteria given below:

a.   The activity of the source must be as low as possible, consistent with achieving the desired accuracy of measurement.

b.   The energy or penetrating power of the emitted radiation must not be greater than that necessary for accomplishing the task with minimum total exposure.

c.   If possible, the radionuclide in the source must be of low toxicity and in such chemical and physical form as to minimize dispersion and intake and retention in the body, in the event of the encapsulation being broken.

3.2 Working with sealed sources

When working with radioactive sources, the three basic factors of distance, time and shielding must always be kept in mind and so applied that radiation doses are reduced to a minimum.

a.   **Distance** — Distance is an efficient and inexpensive way of protection against exposure from a radioactive source. For gamma radiation the exposure rate decreases with the square of the distance from the source of radiation. (This is true for a point source but can be used as a rule of thumb where the distances are large in comparison with the physical dimensions of the source.) In the case of radiation from a beta emitter, the absorbed dose further decreases with distance because of absorption in the air, while radiation from an alpha emitter has a specific range in air according to the particle energy.

Radioactive sources must never be touched by hand because of the high exposure rates at such small distances. Appropriate tools, e.g., remote handling tongs with a firm grip, must always be used. In some instances it may be necessary to provide more elaborate facilities for the remote manipulation of sources.

The erection of effective barricades to keep persons away from radiation areas is also a way of using distance for protection. Clear warning notices must be displayed at barricades.

b. **Time** — Work with radioactive sources must be so planned that the time in which persons are exposed to these sources is as short as possible. Since the extent of protection provided by the limiting of working time can easily be lost if unexpected difficulties occur in the work, it is advisable that whenever practicable, dummy runs be performed beforehand.

c. **Shielding** — Shielding plays an important role in protection against radiation, and the following facts and recommendations regarding shielding should be considered, when appropriate:

1. External radiation from alpha emitters poses no problem and can easily be shielded.
2. In the case of beta radiation, the skin and eyes must be protected and materials such as acrylic resin, or aluminum of suitable thickness, can be used effectively for this purpose. High-energy beta sources can produce relatively more "bremsstrahlung" (X-rays) in high-density shielding than in low-density shielding. The shielding must be sufficient to reduce the bremsstrahlung to safe levels.
3. The penetrating power of gamma radiation requires the use of dense materials, such as lead and steel, to provide efficient shielding. A general rule is that denser and thicker shielding affords better protection.
4. Neutron sources must be shielded with materials with a high hydrogen or carbon content, such as wood, water, graphite, and paraffin wax. Where gamma rays are also present (e.g., in the case of radium-beryllium sources), additional shielding with dense materials must be provided.
5. In addition to shielding against direct radiation, shielding may be necessary to give adequate protection against backscattering from the floor, the ceiling, and the shielding itself. Air scatter may also be significant in some cases. All materials used for shielding must overlap to prevent penetration of radiation through the joints. In order to achieve maximum economy of design, protective barriers should be positioned as close as possible to the source of radiation. As there are many possibilities for error in calculations of shielding thickness, the adequacy of shielding should always be tested by measurement.

3.3 Source containers

3.3.1 Containers with Permanently Built-In Sources

Containers with permanently built-in sources used, for example, in nuclear instruments, must have the following properties:

a. Where necessary, the normally exposed portion of a sealed source must be protected from damage and abrasion by the provision of an effective covering material.
b. The container must be provided with a lockable shutter that can be operated quickly to avoid undue exposure of the operator and to shut off the useful beam.
c. The maximum exposure rate on the outside of the loaded container must not exceed $1.85\ \mathrm{MBq \cdot kg^{-1} \cdot h^{-1}}$ (200 mR·h^{-1}).
d. The container must have a permanent label fastened to it, giving the following information:
   1. A radiation warning sign
   2. The name or symbol of the radionuclide and its activity and applicable date
   3. The serial number of the source
   4. The serial number of the source container

3.3.2 *Sources not Permanently Built-In*

Sealed sources not permanently built into containers must, when not in use, also be kept in containers that will provide the necessary protection when handled. Every such container must be marked with an identification label that carries the following information in legible and durable marking:

a. A radiation warning sign
b. The names or symbols of the radionuclides and their activities and applicable dates
c. The serial numbers, when available, and any other identification numbers

3.4 *Leak-Testing of Sealed Sources*

Since damage to the encapsulation of a sealed source could result in the leakage and dispersion of the radioactive material, each sealed source must be tested at regular intervals for leakage.

An effective way of testing a source for leakage is to take a smear from the outside surface of the source capsule, using a piece of filter paper or cotton wool wetting with a suitable solvent, and to check the smear for radioactivity, using an instrument sensitive to the type of radiation emitted by the radioactive material. The procedure must be carried out under conditions of adequate protection for the person carrying out the procedure. This can be accomplished by the use of remote handling equipment and radiation shields.

In the case of alpha or low-energy beta emitters, where the radioactive material is usually sealed by a thin protective coating of inactive material, care must be taken not to damage the coating.

A source permanently built into containers must not be removed for leakage-testing, as this will result in unnecessary exposure of the person performing the test. A smear taken from the outside of the container, especially in the region of the shutter activating mechanism, will usually suffice.

If a suitable instrument is not available for the testing of the smear samples, they can be sealed separately in suitable small containers and forwarded to an institution that has the facilities to carry out the tests.

4. UNSEALED SOURCES

4.1 Classified and Design of Laboratories in Which Unsealed Sources Are Used

4.1.1 *General*

The use of unsealed radioactive sources requires special handling and laboratory facilities to

a. Limit external contamination, skin penetration, ingestion and inhalation, in addition to minimizing the usual radiation hazards associated with sealed sources
b. Keep the contamination of apparatus, work surfaces, floors, etc. under control
c. Facilitate cleaning and to avoid difficult and expensive decontamination operations after an accidental spill or the release of radioactive material

4.1.2 *Classification of Laboratories*

The facilities that are required and the precautions to be taken depend on the degree of radiotoxicity and the activity of the radionuclide to be used. Radionuclides are therefore classified according to their relative radiotoxicity per unit activity (Table 2). Each laboratory is classified as Type A, B or C as follows:

a. **Type A** — A laboratory that is specially designed for work with radionuclides having maximum activities in excess of those permitted in a Type B laboratory. Because of

TABLE 2
Classification of Radionuclides According to Relative Radiotoxicity Per Unit Activity

Group 1: High toxicity

^{210}Pb	^{210}Po	^{223}Ra	^{226}Ra	^{228}Ra	^{227}Ac	^{227}Th	^{228}Th	^{230}Th
^{231}Pa	^{230}U	^{232}U	^{233}U	^{234}U	^{237}Np	^{239}Pu	^{238}Pu	^{240}Pu
^{241}Pu	^{242}Pu	^{241}Am	^{243}Am	^{242}Cm	^{243}Cm	^{244}Cm	^{245}Cm	^{246}Cm
^{249}Cf	^{250}Cf	^{252}Cf	^{253}Cf	^{254}Cf	^{253}Es	^{254}Es	^{255}Es	^{256}Fm

Group 2: Medium toxicity upper, Subgroup A

^{22}Ba	^{36}Cl	^{45}Ca	^{46}Sc	^{54}Mn	^{56}Co	^{60}Co	^{89}Sr	^{90}Sr
^{91}Y	^{95}Zr	^{106}Ru	^{110m}Ag	^{115m}Cd	^{114m}In	^{124}Sb	^{125}Sb	^{127m}Te
^{129m}Te	^{125}I	^{126}I	^{131}I	^{133}I	^{134}Cs	^{137}Cs	^{140}Ba	^{144}Ce
^{152}Eu		^{154}Eu	^{160}Tb	^{170}Tm	^{181}Hf	^{182}Ta	^{192}Ir	^{204}Tl
^{207}Bi	^{210}Bi	^{211}At	^{212}Pb	^{224}Ra	^{228}Ac	^{230}Pa	^{234}Th	^{235}U
^{249}Bk	^{254m}Es	^{255}Fm						

Group 3: Medium toxicity lower, Subgroup B

^{7}Be	^{14}C	^{18}F	^{24}Na	^{38}Cl	^{31}Si	^{32}P	^{35}S	^{41}Ar
^{42}K	^{43}K	^{47}Ca	^{47}Sc	^{48}Sc	^{48}V	^{51}Cr	^{52}Mn	^{56}Mn
^{52}Fe	^{55}Fe	^{59}Fe	^{57}Co	^{58}Co	^{63}Ni	^{65}Ni	^{64}Cu	^{65}Zn
^{69m}Zn	^{72}Ga	^{73}As	^{74}As	^{76}As	^{77}As	^{75}Se	^{82}Br	^{85m}Kr
^{87}Kr	^{86}Rb	^{85}Sr	^{91}Sr	^{90}Y	^{92}Y	^{93}Y	^{97}Zr	^{93m}Nb
^{95}Nb	^{99}Mo	^{96}Tc	^{97m}Tc	^{97}Tc	^{99}Tc	^{97}Ru	^{103}Ru	^{105}Ru
^{105}Rh	^{103}Pd	^{109}Pd	^{105}Ag	^{111}Ag	^{109}Cd	^{115}Cd	^{115m}In	^{113}Sn
^{125}Sn	^{122}Sb	^{125m}Te	^{127}Te	^{129}Te	^{131m}Te	^{132}Te	^{130}I	^{132}I
^{134}I	^{135}I	^{135}Xe	^{131}Cs	^{135}Cs	^{131}Ba	^{140}La	^{141}Ce	^{143}Ce
^{142}Pr	^{143}Pr	^{147}Nd	^{149}Nd	^{147}Pm	^{149}Pm	^{151}Sm	^{153}Sm	^{152}Eu
^{155}Eu	^{153}Gd	^{159}Gd	^{165}Dy	^{166}Dy	^{165}Ho	^{169}Er	^{171}Er	
^{171}Tm	^{175}Yb	^{177}Lu	^{181}W	^{185}W	^{187}W	^{183}Re	^{186}Re	^{188}Re
^{185}Os	^{191}Os	^{193}Os	^{190}Ir	^{194}Ir	^{191}Pt	^{193}Pt	^{197}Pt	^{196}Au
^{198}Au	^{199}Au	^{197}Hg	^{197m}Hg	^{203}Hg	^{200}Tl	^{201}Tl	^{202}Tl	^{203}Pb
^{206}Bi	^{212}Bi	^{220}Rn	^{222}Rn	^{231}Th	^{233}Pa	^{239}Np	^{243}Pu	^{244}Pu

Group 4: Low toxicity

^{3}H	^{15}O	^{37}A	^{58m}Co	^{59}Ni	^{69}Zn	^{71}Ge	^{85}Kr	^{85m}Sr
^{87}Rb	^{91m}Y	^{93}Zr	^{97}Nb	^{96m}Tc	^{99m}Tc	^{193}Rh	^{113m}In	^{129}I
^{131m}Xe	^{133}Xe	^{134m}Cs	^{135}Cs	^{147}Sm	^{187}Re	^{191m}Os	^{193m}Pt	^{197m}Pt
^{232}Th	Th-Nat	^{235}U	^{238}U	U-Nat				

the high activities involved, the design of Type A laboratories must be checked by an expert in collaboration with the competent authority, with particular attention being paid to the following:

1. Furniture. The number of items of furniture must be reduced to a minimum and the furniture must be easily washable. Dust-collecting items such as drawers, shelves, and hanging lamps must be reduced to a minimum.
2. Solid-waste receptacles. Each laboratory must be provided with a refuse bin with a foot-operated lid for the collection of solid radioactive waste. The bin must be lined with a removable plastic bag to facilitate the removal of waste without further contamination. All receptables for radioactive waste must be clearly marked with a radiation warning sign.
3. Radiation warning signs. All entrances to a Type A laboratory, as well as any storage facilities and waste receptacles, must be clearly marked with radiation warning signs of an appropriate size.

b.   **Type B** — A laboratory that is specially designed for work with radionuclides and that is suitable for work with unsealed sources of the following categories and maximum activities:

Group 1: up to 3.7×10^8 Bq (10 mCi)
Group 2: up to 3.7×10^9 Bq (100 mCi)
Group 3: up to 3.7×10^{10} Bq (1 Ci)
Group 4: up to 3.7×10^{11} Bq (10 Ci)

c.   **Type C** — A good chemical laboratory that is suitable for work with radionuclides of the following categories and maximum activities:

Group 1: up to 3.7×10^5 Bq (10 µCi)
Group 2: up to 3.7×10^6 Bq (100 µCi)
Group 3: up to 3.7×10^7 Bq (1 mCi)
Group 4: up to 3.7×10^8 Bq (10 mCi)

4.1.3 *The Design of Type B Laboratories*

a.   Floors, walls and work surfaces. The walls and ceiling of a Type B laboratory must be coated with a washable, hard nonporous paint. The floor must be covered with a material such as linoleum or vinyl with sealed joints. The shape of the floor and walls must be rounded in order to facilitate cleaning. Sharp corners, cracks, and rough surfaces must be avoided, and this also applies to all work surfaces. All work surfaces must, in addition, be able to support the mass of any shielding against gamma radiation.

b.   Sinks. The usual type of sink with a smooth white glazed finish, without blemishes, will suffice. It is desirable that two sinks be provided, one of which can be used for radioactive material, while the second one is used for inactive material. A separate wash-hand basin must be provided at the exit. It is desirable to have the sinks connected directly to the main outlet pipe; connections to open channels and to any devices that might accumulate slime must be avoided. The outlet pipe from the sink used for radioactive material must be connected to a liquid storage tank where radioactive fluid can be stored until it has decayed sufficiently to make it safe for disposal into the sewers. Taps must be designed for operation by foot, knee, or elbow rather than by hand.

c.   Fume hoods. A Type B laboratory must be equipped with a well-ventilated fume hood (minimum linear flow 0.5 m·s^{-1}) that has the controls for the water, gas, and electrical supplies fitted on the outside. The inside of the hood and the exhaust ducts must be as easy to clean as is practicable, and the inclusion of an adequate filter on the outlet of the fume hood should be considered. Where multiple hoods are used, they must be so designed that cross-contamination between hoods cannot occur. The operating arrangements of the fume hoods must be clearly indicated.

d.   Lighting and ventilation. A Type B laboratory must be well illuminated and ventilated. Routes of entry and exit for the ventilating air must be clearly defined under all conditions of use, including open and closed positions of doors and windows. The siting of exhaust vents must be such as to prevent recirculation of exhausted air. Lights must preferably be of the recessed type so that they can be mounted flush with the ceiling.

e.   Radiation and contamination monitors. Monitors must be available for measurement of exposures and for routine monitoring of the contamination of work surfaces, etc. Contamination monitors must also be available to enable personnel to monitor their hands, clothes, and shoes every time they leave the laboratory.

f.   Receptacles for contaminated articles. Suitable receptacles must be provided for the storage of contaminated articles, including clothing.

4.2 Tools and Equipment for Safe Working With Unsealed Sources

Special equipment suitable for the type of radiation and level of activity being used must be provided for each kind of operation. The equipment must include handling tools such as tongs, forceps, trays, and mechanical holders. All equipment must be suitably marked and must not be used for work in inactive areas. Long-handled tools provide adequate protection by avoiding proximity to the source when work is done with radionuclides emitting beta particles or gamma photons and having activities of the order of megabecquerels (millicuries). Operations with large amounts of such radioactive material require the use of specially designed, remotely controlled equipment. When the radionuclides concerned are primarily beta emitters, use can be made of transparent plastic shields fitting closely around the equipment to allow good visibility during close work.

Containers for the active material must incorporate the necessary shielding as close to the source as possible. Containers for liquid samples must always be reinforced by an outer, unbreakable container. Manipulations must be carried out over a suitable drip tray. Handling tools and equipment used must be placed in nonporous trays and pans, on absorbent disposable paper that is changed frequently. Equipment must be designed to permit the necessary operations to be carried out expeditiously at considerable distance from the source and, whenever practicable, from behind protective barriers. Operator-source distance, time taken to complete the procedure, and shielding must be carefully controlled to ensure safe working conditions. The use of equipment, containers, glassware, etc., having sharp edges that could cut the hands, must be avoided. Mouth-operated equipment must not be used, and pipettes must be operated by means of suction devices.

4.3 Procedures for Safe Working With Unsealed Sources

4.3.1 General

All operations must be so planned as to limit the spread of radioactive material in the event of spillage. To this end all unnecessary movement of persons or materials must be avoided. Work methods must be studied and procedures adopted that will avoid, as far as possible, the dispersal of radioactive material, in particular through the formation of aerosols, gases, vapors, or dusts. Wet operations must be used in preference to dry ones. Manipulations must be carried out over a suitable drip tray, or with some form of double container that will minimize the effects of breakages or spillage. It is also good practice to cover the work surfaces with absorbent material to soak up minor spills. The absorbent material must be changed when unsuitable for further use, and must be treated as radioactive waste.

Radioactive contamination of the air of the laboratory must be prevented as far as is practicable. All operations likely to produce radioactive contamination of the air through the production of aerosols (in particular the heating of radioactive solutions), smoke, or vapors must be carried out in an airtight enclosure kept below atmospheric pressure (a modified glove box), or in a fume cupboard. Pipettes, stirring rods, and similar equipment must not be placed directly on the work bench or table.

4.3.2 Protective Clothing

Persons working with unsealed radioactive material must wear suitable protective clothing, such as laboratory coats, overalls, overshoes, and gloves. These persons must remove the protective clothing before they leave the area where radioactive contamination could occur. All protective clothing must be monitored before being handed in for laundering. Contaminated clothing must be kept apart from other clothing and laundered separately.

4.3.3 Personal Protective Measures

Unsealed radioactive material must not be manipulated with the unprotected hand. Anyone who has an open skin wound below the wrist (whether protected by a bandage or not) must not work with unsealed radioactive materials without medical approval. All persons must wash their hands thoroughly before leaving a work place. Where the airborne concentration of radioactivity, as laid down by the competent authority, is exceeded, approved respirators, gas masks, or air hoods must be worn by persons working in these laboratories. In this respect the competent authority must be consulted. Such respirators, gas masks or air hoods must be inspected and monitored after each use, and must always be kept clean and in working condition.

4.3.4 Monitoring of a controlled area

Monitoring for surface contamination must be carried out in accordance with permitted levels set in Table 1.

4.3.5 Storage of Volatile Materials

Volatile materials, such as iodine-131 and tritiated water, must be stored in a refrigerator to reduce the production of radioactive vapor.

4.3.6 Prohibited Practices

The following practices are prohibited in a area where radioactive contamination could occur:

a.   Eating, drinking or smoking, and the storing, preparation, or handling of food, medicine, smoking requisites, and cosmetics.
b.   The pipetting by mouth of any liquid that contains radioactive material.

5. RADIOACTIVE WASTE DISPOSAL
5.1 Liquid Waste

Small volumes of liquid of low-level activity may be discharged directly into the sewer in cases where the maximum permissible concentration of the particular radionuclides in water, as laid down by the competent authority, will not be exceeded after dilution. The regulations promulgated by the local authority must also be consulted in this respect. All other liquid waste must be collected in containers of an approved type and discarded in consultation with the competent authority.

5.2 Solid Waste

Solid waste contaminated with radionuclides of short half-life and too active for immediate disposal may be stored in appropriate sealed containers until it has decayed sufficiently to be discarded with nonactive material, in the normal way. All other waste must be collected in approved containers and discarded in consultation with the competent authority. Depleted sealed sources must only be discarded in a manner approved by the competent authority.

6. STORAGE AND TRANSPORTATION OF RADIOACTIVE MATERIAL*
6.1 Storage

When not in use or in transit, sealed and unsealed radioactive sources, or instruments containing radioactive sources, must be stored in a protective enclosure, preferably assigned for this purpose only. The storage place must be adequately shielded, secured to prevent unauthorized access, and so selected or constructed as to minimize risk from fire or flooding. Where a radioactive source is likely to release a radioactive gas, provision must be made

---

*   From SABS 0203 Part 1, The Council of the South African Bureau of Standards, 1985.

to enable the storage place to be ventilated effectively to the open air by mechanical means before any person enters the store.

Underground storage pits must be waterproofed to prevent dampness and the subsequent corrosion of source containers. An inventory must be kept of all radioactive sources in the storage place. Where sources are used by more than one person, a register in which sources are signed in and out must also be kept.

6.2 Transportation
6.2.1 Transportation Inside Premises
No radioactive material must be moved unnecessarily. Radioactive material must be transported in adequately shielded and closed containers. A maximum exposure rate of 1.85 $MBq \cdot kg^{-1} \cdot h^{-1}$ (200 $mR \cdot h^{-1}$) on the outer surface of a transportation container must not be exceeded. A container must be so constructed as to prevent the accidental release of radioactive material in the event of an upset. If radioactive material in liquid, gaseous, powder or other dispersible form is stored in a shatterable container, this container and its contents must be transported in a shatterproof outer container. In the case of a liquid source, the outer container must be lined with absorbent material able to retain all the liquid in the event of breakage.

The transportation container must be clearly marked with warning signs and must bear a transportation tag giving the following information:

a.   The nature and physical condition of the contents
b.   The radionuclide and activity, and the applicable date
c.   The exposure rate on the outer surface of the container and at a distance of 1 m from the container
d.   Any special handling requirements

The outside of a transportation container must be free from contamination.

Any loss of radioactive material during transportation must be reported immediately to the responsible person. Suitably trained workers must be in charge of the transportation of hazardous quantities of radioactive material.

6.2.2 Transportation outside premises
Transportation of radioactive material outside premises must be conducted in accordance with the latest regulations relating to the safe transportation of radioactive materials, issued by the International Atomic Energy Agency.

SAFE HANDLING OF RADIOPHARMACEUTICALS

All radioactive materials emit potentially harmful radiation. Contact with the actual radioactive material may be dangerous and should be kept to a minimum. Radiopharmaceuticals should be handled and used only under the supervision of authorized competent and approved persons. The following procedure should be adhered to in the handling of all radiopharmaceuticals:

Receiving the product:

1.   Check that all documentation (including labels) corresponds to the goods ordered and actually received. If there are any anomalies please notify the supplier as soon as possible.
2.   Notify the local health physicist or other authorized competent person that the package has arrived.

3.   The package should be visually inspected and if any damage is observed (such as wetness and torn packing container) which could possibly result in damage to the product the package must not be opened. It should be made safe and the matter reported immediately to the local competent authority.

4.   If the package is not to be opened immediately a suitable and secure store must be provided. This store should be reserved for radioactive materials only and must be adequately shielded and labeled.

Unpacking the product:

1.   Suitable radiation monitoring instruments should be available to check for contamination and to record dose rates while unpacking radiopharmaceuticals. Measure exposure rates at package surface and at one meter. If exposure rates are more than 14 or 0.7 nC/kg·s (200 or 10 mR/h), respectively, discontinue check-in procedure immediately and notify institution's radiation safety personnel.

2.   The actual products should be unpacked in designated areas by an authorized competent person.

3.   After putting on disposable gloves, open package outer container and remove packing slip. Open inner package to verify content (correct as shipped) and check integrity of final source container (inspect for breakage of seals or vials, loss of liquid, or discoloration of packaging materials). Check also that receipt of shipment does not exceed possession limits.

Inspecting the product:

1.   Care must be taken to restrict personnel dose levels by the use of remote handling implements (e.g., forceps) and suitable shielding. Disposable gloves should be worn whenever radioactive material is handled.

2.   The product should be inspected immediately following removal from the inner container.

3.   Any damage or other causes for concern should be reported to the supplier.

4.   Wipe external surface of final source container with either moistened cotton swab or filter paper held with forceps; assay and record results.

5.   Monitor the packing material and packages for contamination before discarding. Note: If contaminated, treat as radioactive waste. Otherwise, destroy all "radioactive" labeling on package and discard in regular trash.

Using the product:

During preparative procedures in the hospital laboratory, conditions of handling and use must be in accordance with both pharmaceutical and radiological requirements. The various publications listed at the end of this section should be referred to for guidance and advice sought from local regulatory authorities.

Consult the pack leaflet containing information, use, and storage of the product. The decomposition of radiopharmaceutical preparations under the influence of their own radiation is a general phenomenon; in some cases it may shorten the duration of use. It is recommended to maintain the products at a temperature suitable with their physical properties (the particular conditions of storage are notified on the label) as soon as they arrive, and to use them as rapidly as possible.

Disposal of the product:

In general, disposal of unused radiopharmaceuticals does not create significant problems for the hospital. The nuclides tend to have relatively short half-lives — frequently less than 1 week; therefore, they may be disposed of immediately, or stored for a short period to reduce the activity to a level at which disposal is permissible.

Reference should be made to local regulatory authorities for advice on the safe disposal of radioactive material, since requirements may differ in different countries.

Useful publications on the use and safe handling of radiopharmaceuticals:

- IAEA Safety Series.
- No. 1 — Safe Handling of Radionuclides
- No. 9 — Basic Safety Standards for Radiation Protection
- No. 25 — Medical Supervision of Radiation Workers
- No. 38 — Radiation Protection Procedures
- No. 40 — Radioactive Tracers in Industrial Processes
- No. 32 — Planning for Handling Radioactive Accidents
- No. 6 — Regulations for the Safe Transport of Radioactive Materials
- No. 37 — Advisory Material for Application of Transport Regulations
- *Handling, Storage, Use and Disposal of Unsealed Radionuclides in Hospitals and Medical Research Establishments,* ICRP Publication 25.
- *Manual of Radiation Protection in Hospital and General Practice,* 2 volumes, WHO, 1975.
- IAEA publications, many of which are available in English, French, Russian and Spanish, may be obtained from IAEA, Wagramerstrasse 5, P.O. Box 100, A-1400 Vienna, Austria, or from agencies in many countries.

Adapted from *Amersham Nuclear Medicine Catalogue,* Amersham International, plc., Little Chalfont, England, 1985. With permission.

SPECIAL CONSIDERATIONS TO MINIMIZE RADIATION EXPOSURE FROM DIAGNOSTIC NUCLEAR MEDICINE PROCEDURES

PEDIATRIC CONSIDERATIONS

Special care should be taken ideally to keep pediatric doses of radiopharmaceuticals as low as reasonably possible, since the absorbed dose delivered to an infant for a given activity is greater than for adults because of differing body mass relationships and physiological phenomena. A balanced sliding scale must be used to determine the appropriate activity needed to get a statistically valid nuclear medicine examination in a reasonable period of time. Various formulas have been devised for calculating pediatric doses. They are based on age, mass, surface area, or a combination of these. Activities calculated using these various approaches yield similar results, although no method provides for individual variations.

A modified Young's Rule or Webster Rule is one method commonly used — this suggests that the adult dose be multiplied by the following fraction:

$$\frac{\text{child's age in years} + 1}{\text{child's age in years} + 7}$$

Example: The dose for a 3-year old child

$$\frac{3+1}{3+7} = \frac{4}{10} = 40\% \text{ of the adult dose}$$

Clark's Rule is based on the proportionality of child/adult body surface area (using $1.7m^2$ as a normal adult surface area). This suggests that the adult dose be multiplied by the following fraction:

$$\frac{\text{child's surface area in m}^2}{1.7 \text{ m}^2}$$

Example: The dose for a 3-year old child weighing 15 kg, having a surface area of 0.68 m^2

$$\frac{0.68 \text{ m}^2}{1.70 \text{ m}^2} = \frac{4}{10} = 40 \text{ \% of the adult dose}$$

(Nomograms are available in most standard reference sources for determining body surface on the basis of both height and mass.)

EMBRYO, FETUS, AND BREAST-FEEDING INFANT CONSIDERATIONS

Nuclear medicine procedures are generally avoided in pregnant women because of the sensitivity of the fetus to ionizing radiation. However, a nuclear medicine or radiologic study may be the only method of obtaining information of illness during pregnancy. For these cases, special quidelines and recommendations have been implemented.

In 1970 the International Commission on Radiological Protection (ICRP) established the so-called ''10-day rule'', which recommended that less urgent radiologic and radioisotope examinations be confined to the 10 days following the start of menstruation, the time when pregnancy is least probable.

In 1984 the ICRP withdrew its support for this rule, stating: ''During the first 10 days following the onset of a menstrual period there can be no risk to any conceptus, since no conception will have occurred. The risk to a child who has been irradiated *in utero* during the remainder of a four week period following the onset of menstruation is likely to be so small that there need be no special limitation on exposure required within these four weeks.''

In 1985 the National Radiological Protection Board in the United Kingdom issued new guidelines to conform to the ICRP reassessment of the 10-day rule, which had become so cumbersome to implement.

In 1985 the US Food and Drug Administration's Center for Devices and Radiological Health issued a pamphlet, *Embryo, Fetus, Infant: Recommendations to Minimize Diagnostic Nuclear Medicine Exposure.** This is a summary of these recommendations:

1. The patient who is or thinks she might be pregnant, or who is nursing, should be encouraged to give this information to her attending physician when the examination history is taken.
2. The nursing woman should suspend breast feeding for an appropriate period of time following a nuclear medicine examination. The nuclear medicine physician or medical physicist can advise the nursing woman on the length of time that nursing should be suspended.

---

* Copies of the full text of the pamphlet may be obtained from the Center for Devices and Radiological Health, Food and Drug Administration, 5600 Fishers Lane, Rockville, MD, 20857.

Guidelines for Safe Resumption of Breast-Feeding After Radionuclide Administration

Radionuclide	Usual adult dose (MBq)	Breast milk activity at which nursing is considered safe (MBq/ml)	Maximum delay required before resumption of breast-feeding
Technetium (^{99m}Tc) Radiopharmaceuticals	740	30.3×10^{-4}	24 h
Gallium (^{67}Ga) Citrate	111	7.8×10^{-5}	4 weeks
Iodine (^{131}I) Orthoiodohippurate	7.4	6.1×10^{-7}	4.5 d
Iodide	0.185	15.17×10^{-9}	8 weeks
Iodine (^{123}I) Iodide	0.74	4.44×10^{-6}	60 h

From Romney, B. M., Nickoloff, E. L., Esser, P. D. and Alderson, P. O., Radionuclide administration to nursing mothers — mathematically derived guidelines, *Radiology,* 160, 549, 1986.

3. The attending physician can use nuclear medicine consultation request forms in no-nemergency situations to record the pregnancy and nursing status of a woman of childbearing age, and should encourage the patient to elicit this information. If there is a medical emergency, if the nuclear medicine examination will contribute vital information to the diagnosis, and if there are no alternative methods for obtaining this information that would result in lower radiation exposure, then the examination generally should be performed regardless of the patient's pregnancy status, but with particular attention to technical modifications of the procedure that will minimize radiation exposure.

4. The nuclear medicine technologist, in the absence of information about the patient's pregnancy or nursing status, should be encouraged to ask the patient if she is or may be pregnant, or if she is nursing. If the patient replies that she is or may be pregnant or is nursing, the technologist should notify the physician in charge.

5. The nuclear medicine physician should be aware of appropriate alternatives prior to conducting a nuclear medicine procedure on a pregnant or potentially pregnant woman or one who is nursing, and should be prepared to consult with the attending physician on possible alternatives. These alternatives include:

   a. Requesting the use of a radionuclide that delivers a lower radiation dose or one that is less likely to cross the placental barrier than the radionuclide commonly used, if the diagnostic objectives can still be met

   b. In the case of a known pregnancy, assessing the possibility of deferring the examination until the pregnancy is concluded

   c. In the case of a possible but unconfirmed pregnancy, deferring the examination that is not immediately needed until the pregnancy is not confirmed

   d. Cancelling the nonemergency examination once aware that the patient is or may be pregnant

   e. Directing the nursing woman to suspend breast feeding for the period of time that radioactivity is present in the milk

   f. Ascertaining the advisability of using other clinical modalities to diagnose the patient's condition

Other References

- Treves, S. T., *Pediatric Nuclear Medicine,* Springer-Verlag, New York, 1985.
- Alderson, Philip O., Gidlay, David L., and Wagner, Henry H., Jr.: *Atlas of Pediatric Nuclear Medicine,* The C. V. Mosby Company, Saint Louis, Missouri.
- *Pregnancy and Radiation,* Community Education Advisory Committee on Science and Energy, Pennsylvania State University, 1982. (Reviewed and approved by Brent, Robert, Chez, Ronal A., King, Theodore M., and Witzig, Warren F.)

TABLE 3
Effects of Drugs on the Biodistribution of Radiopharmaceuticals

Various drugs induce changes in the biodistribution of radiopharmaceuticals by either enhancing the localization of the radiopharmaceutical in the target organ, or by depressing its uptake. Pharmacological interventions can be used to augment, complement, or differentiate the information obtained from diagnostic nuclear medicine procedures. If the effects are undesirable, it will be useful to know the altered biodistribution while interpreting results from nuclear medicine studies.

Organ (procedure)	Drug	Effects induced by drugs
Thyroid		
Uptake and imaging with Iodine-131, 123 sodium iodide	Lugol, SSKI, cough mixtures,	Decreased uptake
	X-ray contrast agents,	Decreased uptake
	Antithyroid drugs (Tapazole, perchlorate, prophythiouracil),	Decreased uptake
	Thyroid hormones (Thyroxine-Triiodothyronine),	Decreased uptake
	Thyroid stimulating hormone	Increased uptake
Adrenal		
Cortical imaging with Selenium-75 Norcholestenol	Dexamethasone	Suppression of ACTH production
Medullary imaging with Iodine-131, 123-MIBG	Tricyclic antidepressants	Decreased uptake
	Reserpine	Decreased uptake
	Cocaine	Decreased uptake
	Phenylpropanolamine	Decreased uptake
Heart		
Myocardial perfusion imaging with Tallium-201 Chloride	Ergonovine	Decreased myocardial blood flow
	Dipyridamole	Increased myocardial uptake
	Propanolol	Decreased myocardial uptake
	Digitalis	Decreased myocardial uptake
	Furosemide	Increased myocardial uptake
	Isoproterenol	Increased myocardial uptake
Ventricular function imaging with Technetium-99m RBC	Nitroglycerine	Increased left ventricular ejection fraction
	Propanolol	Improves abnormal wall motion
	Calcium channel blockers	Increased left ventricular ejection fraction
Skeleton		
Bone imaging with Technetium-99m phosphate compounds	Corticosteroids	Decreased bone uptake
	Cancer chemotherapeutic drugs	Increased renal activity
		Increased uptake in calvarium
	Melphalan	Increased bone uptake
	Meperidine	Soft tissue uptake
	Aluminum ion	Increased liver uptake
	Dextrose	Increased renal activity
	Phospho-soda	Decreased bone uptake
Liver		
Hepatobiliary imaging with Technetium-99m IDA derivates	Phenobarbital	Increased canalicular bile flow and excretion of bilirubin
	Cholecystokinin, sincalide	Increased gall-bladder contraction
	Atropine	Prolonged gall-bladder activity
	Narcotic analgesics	Prolonged liver to duodenum transit time
RES imaging with Technetium-99m colloids	Aluminum, magnesium	Increased lung activity
	Estrogens	Focal areas of decreased activity in liver
	Androgens	Increased lung activity
	Anesthetics (halothane)	Increased splenic uptake
Spleen		
Splenic imaging with Technetium-99m heat denatured RBCs	Epinephrine	Decrease in spleen volume
Kidneys		
Renogram and imaging with Technetium-99m DTPA	Furosemide	Increased urinary output, diuresis
	Captopril	Decreased renal function in unilateral renal

TABLE 3 (continued)
Effects of Drugs on the Biodistribution of Radiopharmaceuticals

Various drugs induce changes in the biodistribution of radiopharmaceuticals by either enhancing the localization of the radiopharmaceutical in the target organ, or by depressing its uptake. Pharmacological interventions can be used to augment, complement, or differentiate the information obtained from diagnostic nuclear medicine procedures. If the effects are undesirable, it will be useful to know the altered biodistribution while interpreting results from nuclear medicine studies.

Organ (procedure)	Drug	Effects induced by drugs
		artery stenosis
	Cyclosporin A	Decreased renal function
Gastrointestinal		
Gastro-esophageal reflux imaging with Technetium-99m colloid liquid meal	Betanechol	Reduces reflux, increases tone and peristaltic activity of esophagus
		Reduces reflux
	Antacids	Reduces reflux
	Gaviscon	
Gastric emptying imaging with Technetium-99m labeled solid or liquid meals		Accelerates gastric emptying
	Metoclopramide	Accelerates gastric emptying
	Cholinergic agonists	Delays gastric emptying
	Cholinergic antagonists	
Gastrointestinal bleeding imaging with Technetium-99m colloid or labelled RBCs	Glucagon	Inhibits peristalsis, improving imaging of bleeding
	Vasopressin	Produces vasoconstriction reducing bleeding
Meckel's diverticulum imaging with Technetium-99m Pertechnetate	Pentagastrin	Increases localization of Tc-99m Pertechnetate in gastric mucosa
	Cimetidine	Inhibits Tc-99m pertechnetate excretion from gastric mucosa into gastric content, enhances imaging of Meckel's diverticulum
	Glucagon	Increases target-to-background radioactivity ratio
Penis		
Penile blood flow imaging with Technetium-99m Pertechnetate or labeled RBC	Isoxsuprine HCl	Increased blood flow
	Papaverine	Increased blood flow
Tumor and sepsis		
Inflammatory or tumor imaging with Gallium-67 Citrate	Iron dextran	Decreased uptake if given before ^{67}Ga injection
	Iron dextran	Increased uptake if given after ^{67}Ga injection
	Desferoxamine	Decreased uptake if given before ^{67}Ga injection
	Desferoxamine	Increased uptake if given after [67]GA injection
	Chemotherapeutic agents	Increased diffuse lung uptake
	Antibiotics	Increased uptake in colon and kidneys
	Estrogens	Increased uptake in mammary glands
	Anticonvulsants (phenytoin)	Increased lymphoid tissue uptake
	Bleomycin	Increased diffuse lung uptake

TABLE 3 REFERENCES

- **Saha, Gopal B.**, *Fundamentals of Nuclear Pharmacy*, Springer-Verlag, New York, 1986.
- **Spencer, Richard P., Ed.**, *Interventional Nuclear Medicine*, Grune & Stratton, Orlando, FL, 1984.
- **Hadlik, William B., III, Ponto, James A., Lentle, Brian C., and Laven, David L.**, Iatrogenic alterations in the biodistribution of radiotracers as a result of drug therapy, in Hadlik, William B., III, Saha, Gopal B., and Study, Kenneth T., Eds., *Essentials of Nuclear Medicine Science*, Williams & Wilkins, Baltimore, MD, 1987.

TABLE 4
International Airports for Radiopharmaceuticals Distribution

Country/City	Airport	Distance to city		International time + or − Standard GMT
		Miles	km	
North and South America				
Argentina				− 3
Buenos Aires	Ezeiza International	32	51	
Bolivia				− 4
La Paz	El Alto International	9	14	
Brazil				− 3
Rio de Janeiro	Galeao International	13	21	
Sao Paulo	Guarulhos International	16	26	
	Viracopos	60	96	
Canada				
Montreal	Dorval International	15	25	− 5
Toronto	Lester Pearson Int.	17	27	− 5
Vancouver	International	9	15	− 8
Chile				− 4
Santiago	Comodoro Arturo Benitez Merino	13	21	
Colombia				− 5
Bogota	El Dorado International	8	13	
Costa Rica				− 6
San Jose	Juan Santamaria International	11	18	
Ecuador				− 5
Quito	Mariscal Sucre International	5	8	
Guyana				− 3
Georgetown	Timehri	28	44	
Jamaica				− 5
Kingston	Norman Manley International	11	18	
Mexico				− 6
Mexico City	Benito Juarez International	8	13	
Panama				− 5
Panama City	Omar Torrijos Herrera Int.	17	27	
Paraguay				− 4
Asuncion	Silvio Petirosi Int.	10	16	
Peru				− 5
Lima	Jorge Chavez International	10	16	
Puerto Rico				− 5
San Juan	Luis Munoz Marin International	7	11	
Uruguay				− 3
Montevideo	Carrasco International	12	19	
U.S.A.				
Chicago	O'Hare International	21	35	− 6
Los Angeles	International	15	24	− 8
Miami	International	7	11	− 5
New York	J F Kennedy International	14	22	− 5
San Francisco	International	16	26	− 8
Washington	Dulles International	27	43	− 5
Venezuela				− 4
Caracas	Simon Bolivar International	13	22	
Europe and the Soviet Union				
Austria				
Vienna	Schwechat	11	18	+ 1

TABLE 4 (continued)
International Airports for Radiopharmaceuticals Distribution

Country/City	Airport	Distance to city Miles	km	International time + or − Standard GMT
Belgium				+ 1
Brussels	National	8	13	
Cyprus				+ 2
Larnaca	Larnaca	5	8	
Czechoslovakia				+ 1
Prague	Ruzyne	11	18	
Denmark				+ 1
Copenhagen	Copenhagen	6	10	
Finland				+ 2
Helsinki	Helsinki-Vantaa	12	19	
France				+ 1
Paris	Charles de Gaulle	15	24	
	Orly	9	14	
Germany				+ 1
Berlin	Schonefeld	12	19	
	Tegel	5	8	
Frankfurt	Frankfurt International	6	10	
Munich	Riem	7	11	
Greece				+ 2
Athens	Hellinikon	6	10	
Hungary				+ 1
Budapest	Ferihegy	10	16	
Iceland				GMT
Reykjavik	Reykjavik	32	51	
Irish Republic				GMT
Dublin	Dublin	5	8	
Italy				+ 1
Rome	Leonardo da Vinci	22	35	
Milan	Linate	6	10	
Luxembourg	Findel	4	6	+ 1
Malta				+ 1
Valletta	Luqa	4	6	
Netherlands				+ 1
Amsterdam	Schiphol	9	14	
Norway				+ 1
Oslo	Fornebu	5	8	
Poland				+ 1
Warsaw	Okecie	6	10	
Portugal				GMT
Lisbon	Lisbon	5	8	
Romania				+ 2
Bucharest	Otopeni	10	16	
Spain				+ 1
Madrid	Barajas	10	16	
Sweden				+ 1
Stockholm	Arlanda	25	40	
Switzerland				+ 1
Zurich	Zurich	8	13	
Geneva	Geneva	3	5	
Turkey				+ 2
Istanbul	Ataturk	15	24	

TABLE 4 (continued)
International Airports for Radiopharmaceuticals Distribution

Country/City	Airport	Distance to city		International time + or − Standard GMT
		Miles	km	
United Kingdom				GMT
London	Heathrow	15	24	
	Gatwick	28	46	
USSR				+ 3
Moscow	Sheremetyevo	18	29	
Yugoslavia				+ 1
Belgrade	Belgrade	12	19	

Africa

Country/City	Airport	Miles	km	International time + or − Standard GMT
Algeria				GMT
Algiers	Houari Boumediene	12	20	
Egypt				+ 2
Cairo	International	14	22	
Ivory Coast				GMT
Abidjan	Port Bouet	10	16	
Kenya				+ 3
Nairobi	Jomo Kenyatta International	8	13	
Liberia				GMT
Monrovia	Roberts International	36	60	
Morocco				GMT
Casablanca	Mohamed V	19	30	
Mozambique				+ 2
Maputo	Maputo International	5	8	
Nigeria				+ 1
Lagos	Murtala Muhammed	14	22	
South Africa				+ 2
Johannesburg-	Jan Smuts	15	24	
Pretoria		28	45	
Cape Town	D. F. Malan	14	22	
Tunisia				+ 1
Tunis	Carthage	5	8	
Zaire				+ 1
Kinshasa	N'Djili	15	25	
Zambia				+ 2
Lusaka	Lusaka	16	26	
Zimbabwe				+ 2
Harare	Harare	7	12	

Middle East, Asia, and Oceania

Country/City	Airport	Miles	km	International time + or − Standard GMT
Abu Dhabi	International	28	44	+ 4
Australia				
Melbourne	Tullamarine	13	21	+ 10
Sydney	Kingsford Smith	7	11	+ 10
Perth	Perth	13	20	+ 8
Bahrain	Muharraq	4	6	+ 3
China				+ 8
Beijing	Capital	16	26	
Hong Kong	Kai Tak International	3	5	+ 8

TABLE 4 (continued)
International Airports for Radiopharmaceuticals Distribution

Country/City	Airport	Distance to city		International time + or − Standard GMT
		Miles	km	
India				+ 5:30
Bombay	Bombay	18	29	
Delhi	Indira Gandhi International	9	14	
Indonesia				+ 7
Jakarta	Soekarno-Hatta	12	20	
Iran				+ 3:30
Tehran	Mehrabad	3	5	
Iraq				+ 3
Baghdad	Saddam International	11	18	
Israel				+ 2
Tel Aviv	Ben Gurion International	9	14	
Japan				+ 9
Tokyo	Haneda	12	19	
	Narita	40	65	
Jordan				+ 2
Amman	Queen Alia International	20	32	
Korea				+ 9
Seoul	Kimpo International	16	26	
Kuwait				+ 3
Kuwait	International	10	16	
Lebanon				+ 2
Beirut	International	10	16	
Malaysia				+ 8
Kuala Lumpur	Subang International	14	22	
New Zealand				+ 12
Auckland	International	14	22	
Wellington	International	5	8	
Pakistan				+ 5
Karachi	Karachi	8	12	
Philippines				+ 8
Manila	International	5	8	
Republic of China				+ 8
(Taiwan) Taipei	Chiang Kai Shek International	25	40	
Saudi Arabia				+ 3
Jeddah	King Abdulaziz International	11	18	
Singapore	Changi	12	20	+ 8
Thailand				+ 7
Bangkok	International	19	30	
Sri Lanka				+ 5:30
Colombo	Katunayake	20	32	

PATTERNS OF METASTASES*

INTRODUCTION

The management of a cancer patient usually involves a search for metastases at the time of initial diagnosis in order to preclude unnecessary surgery or radiation therapy for cure if distant metastases are found. Searches for metastases are subsequently made if unexplained symptoms occur.

Evidence has shown that early treatment of distant metastases, whether or not specifically identified, can benefit the patient. The clinician needs more than ever to have an accurate knowledge of the propensity of a given cancer to spread to specific organ sites during the evolution of the disease. This describes the results of both clinical examination and autopsy reports of the location and incidence of metastases.

INCIDENCE OF VISCERAL METASTASES

A review of the clinical and autopsy data of the incidence of visceral tumor metastases in liver, lung, bone, and brain is presented in Tables 5 to 9. The distribution of organ involvement by metastatic tumor from a particular primary is not in itself proof of either the anatomic pathway of spread or a predisposition for growth in a particular "soil." The known patterns of spread, however, suggest that the pathway is probably more critical than the "soil."

The presence of cancer in a particular organ at autopsy does not necessarily indicate that screening of that organ at the time of diagnosis would have demonstrated metastases. The data in Tables 5 to 9 are only estimates due to differing degrees of thoroughness of institutional autopsies and procedures. Current clinical screening tests are not accurate for detecting metastases at diagnosis as evidenced, in the tables, by the low incidence of reported visceral involvement at diagnosis. Unless much more sensitive and specific tests are developed, the relative incidence of organ involvement at diagnosis, however, will change very little.

---

*   Adapted from *Patterns of Metastasis*. Courtesy of Adria Laboratories, Columbus, OH, and Farmitalia Carlo Erba, Johannesburg (no date).

TABLE 5
Cancers: Incidence of Metastases, Autopsy Data Only

Site of primary	Bone%	Lung%	Liver%	Brain%
Hepatoma	8	20	N.A.	—
Esophagus	7	25—35	20—32	<1
Stomach	5—10	30	35—50	1—8
Pancreas	5—10	25—40	60—70	1—4

TABLE 6
Pediatric Tumors
Incidence of Metastases at Diagnosis and at Autopsy

Site of Primary	Clinical Status	Bone%	Lung%	Liver%	Brain%
Wilms' Tumor[a]	Diagnosis	<1	20	3—10	0
	Autopsy	1—10	60	30—40	0
Ewing's Sarcoma	Diagnosis	14—28	18—27	0	<5
	Autopsy	59	70	27	5
Neuroblastoma	Diagnosis	<25[b]	<5	25	30[c]
	Autopsy	80	25—30	70	25—50
Rhabdomyosarcoma	Diagnosis	14	21	10	2—4
	Autopsy	70	45—55	44	20
Osteosarcoma	Diagnosis	<5	15	<5	<5
	Autopsy	35—50	75—95	<5	<5

[a] Omentum and mesentery = 25% local and retroperitoneum = 14%.
[b] Only 7% with positive marrow.
[c] Includes mostly epidural extension.

TABLE 7
Genitourinary Tumors:
Incidence of Metastases at Diagnosis and at Autopsy

Site of primary	Clinical status	Bone%	Lung%	Liver%	Brain%
Kidney	Diagnosis[a]	6—10	5—30	13	4
	Autopsy	24—50	50—75	27—40	7—8
Bladder	Diagnosis	<5	5—10	<5	<1
	Autopsy	20—25[b]	25—30	30—50	<1
Prostate	Diagnosis	30—40	5	1	<1
	Autopsy	60—70	63—53	5—13	<2
Testis[c]	Diagnosis	<1	2—12	<1	<1 Seminoma
(germinal)	Autopsy	20—25	70—80	50—80	<10 1%
Penis-urethra	Diagnosis	<1	1	<1	<1
	Autopsy	5	5—10	<10	<1

[a] 40 to 60% off all present with distant disease.
[b] 50% in bone.
[c] Abdominal nodes in 12 to 17%.

TABLE 8
Head and Neck and Colon Cancer:
Incidence of Metastases at Diagnosis and at Autopsy

Site of primary	Clinical status	Bone%	Lung%	Liver%	Brain%
Squamous cell carcinoma of the oral cavity,	Diagnosis	1	2—5	1	1
larynx, pharynx, and salivary gland	Autopsy[a]	5—12	13—23	6—14	5[b]
Colon-rectum[c]	Diagnosis	<1	<5	20—24	1
	Autopsy	5—10	25—40	60—71	<1

[a] At autopsy, the incidence of metastases for cylindroma is 13% bone, 41% lung, and 22% brain. Most metastases from this group originate from primaries in the nasopharynx.
[b] At autopsy, the incidence of brain metastases from squamous cell carcinoma of the nasopharynx is 15%.
[c] At autopsy, the incidence of metastases to the peritoneum from colon/rectal primaries is 71%.

TABLE 9
Gynecologic Cancer:
Incidence of Metastases at Diagnosis and at Autopsy

Site of primary	Clinical status	Bone%	Lung%	Liver%	Brain%
Ovary(Epithelial)	Diagnosis	<1	<5	>5	>1
	Autopsy	2—6	5—10	10—15[a]	<1
Uterus	Diagnosis[b]	<1	<1	<1	<1
	Autopsy[c]	5—12	30—40	10—30	<5
Cervix	Diagnosis	<1	<5	<1	<1
	Autopsy	8—20	20—30	20—35	2—3
Vulva	Diagnosis	<1	<5	<5	<1
	Autopsy	N.A.	15—20	N.A.	N.A.
Choriocarcinoma	In clinical course	5	61	13	13
	Autopsy	2	70—100	40—50	41

[a] Peritoneum into liver 40 to 50%.
[b] 7 to 10% are in nodes outside pelvis.
[c] Peritoneum—30%.

PATHWAYS OF METASTASES

Tumors generally metastasize in an orderly fashion. Metastases, like any living beings cast adrift on an unfriendly sea, have individual preferences for friendly environments. The arterial circulation is a particularly hostile environment for the growth of tumor cell clumps. Tumors rarely invade arteries larger than precapillary arterioles. The lack of arterial dissemination is best exemplified by the rarity (total of less than 10% of all metastases) of muscle, intestinal, kidney, spleen, skin, and heart metastases; the respective percentage of the cardiac arterial output of these organs is 18%, 10%, 22% 10%, 4% and 5% (a total of 69% of the total arterial output). Bone arterial circulation is less than 5% of the cardiac arterial output, yet bone metastases are common and tend to involve the proximal skeleton, which receives only a small proportion of the arterial circulation to bone.

Tumors usually metastasize to major visceral organs (bone, liver, lung) via the venous circulation with or without intervening nodal involvement. Many carcinomas eventually invade visceral organs after passing through one or two lymph node echelons. It is important to be aware that many metastases from some primary cancers that go via lymph nodes are trapped there and treatment of those nodes can produce cure (head and neck, cervix) if the nodal disease is not too extensive.

Intra-abdominal primaries tend to metastasize via the mesenteric lymphatics and portal venous system and into the liver as the initial resting place. From the liver these tumors can metastasize to the lung via the vena cava and pulmonary artery. Liver metastases occur principally as a primary site of drainage of the GI tract, or its serosal are primarily or secondarily involved.

Another mode of metastatic spread relates to tumors of the testicle that metastasize via the lymphatics to nodes of the periarotic area and then enter the venous system to go to the right heart and finally to the lungs. Liver metastases, however, do occur late in the disease course and are frequently present at autopsy.

Ovarian cancer remains confined for long periods of time in the highly favorable environment of the abdominal cavity, especially in the peritoneal surfaces, the posterior gutters, and the diaphragm. These tumors invade the liver only in a small percentage of cases at a very late stage, usually by direct invasion from omental disease or mesenteric venous emboli from omental implants. Lung metastases also occur late in the disease.

Breast cancer metastasizes to the lung via the lymph nodes and superior vena cava and to the bony skeleton via the intercoastal veins, with or without nodal involvement. Liver involvement, although common at autopsy, occurs much later in the course of the disease. Metastasis may arrive there via the pleural lymphatics transdiaphragmatically.

Head and neck cancers metastasize to lymphatics and remain confined in this area. Until recently, it was clinically uncommon for these tumors to metastasize beyond the cervical lymph nodes into their principal visceral target organ, the lungs. As clinicians are effectively able to control local disease, the incidence of clinically obvious visceral metastases late in the disease course will increase in those failing regionally curative therapy. Nasopharynx cancer tends to go to the liver and bone more frequently than other head and neck cancers. The spread to bone is via Batson's plexus in the nasopharynx. Nasopharynx and hypopharynx tumors have a 40% or greater incidence of distant metastases in patients failing treatment.

Lung cancer is the only tumor that has direct access to the arterial circulation and it spreads widely to many organs. Analyses of the pattern of spread of other primary cancers suggest that involvement of the brain, endocrine organs, bones distal to the proximal humerus and femur, and spleen (arterial pattern of spread) usually occur after metastases have first formed in the primary metastatic target organ(s) lung, liver, bone, etc.

Bone metastases to the proximal axial skeleton are usually from direct tumor cell metastases via Batson's paravertebral plexus of veins. Prostate cancer metastases may also travel to the bone via the perineural space. In some cases, bones may be involved by direct extension from local tumor masses in lymph nodes. Cancer clumps from lung, breast, bladder, nasopharynx, prostate, thyroid, and neuroblastoma, etc., that involve the ribs, spinal column, pelvis, skull, shoulder girdles, and proximal femora implant in these bones after traveling in this very leisurely, slow-moving, valveless system of veins. These veins surround the pedicles, lamina, vertebral spines, and spinal cord, and perforate the vertebral bodies as well as enter venous plexi in the pelvis and dural areas. They then join the major cavitary veins (azygos, hemiazygos, and ultimately the vena cava).

Parenchymal brain metastases are truly the end of the metastatic cascade. The brain is secondarily involved following metastasis to the lung for most nonpulmonary malignancies. The lung serves as a primary target organ in these situations, and brain involvement occurs only after pulmonary metastases are present. Lung cancer is the only major cancer in which the brain is the first site of metastasis. In this case it is part of the primary arterial dissemination. At times, the brain will be involved by secondary extension from a bony metastasis in the calvarium, for example, from prostatic cancer, or from secondary extension due to nonbony dural involvement by cancer cells traveling in Batson's plexus. An example is colon cancer which has recurred in the pelvis and invaded the sacrum. The prognosis of these patients is distinctly different from that of patients with arterial-bound parenchymal brain metastases. Epidural spinal cord compression arises from extensions of bony involvement due to Batson's plexus spread.

The unknown adenocarcinoma primary demonstrates the randomness of a primary arterial dissemination pattern. This common entity usually baffles the clinical sleuth even at the time of postmortem examination. The primary site is found in less than 10% of cases premortem. These highly heterogeneous metastatic cells behave more viciously than those from the same primary cancer when it is the presenting phenomenon. Melanoma and kidney appear at times to disseminate also via an arterial pattern. But in greater than 90% of cases, the lung (melanoma of kidney) or liver (melanoma) is involved as well.

TESTING: ACCURACY AND USEFULNESS

Most of the major advances in cancer care today relate to improved disease delineation (staging), but not to improved curability. More tests do not necessarily improve the quality of life, disease curability, or improvement in palliation. Before ordering a test, the physician must decide what information he wants and how a positive or negative result will affect his plans.

The following descriptions of the screening tests are meant to provide a perspective of each test's strengths and weaknesses.

Brain

Radionuclide Scan — This test gives an extremely low yield in a neurologically normal patient, and should not be included in the screening process in asymptomatic patients. Solitary scan abnormalities can be seen in several benign entities (meningioma in a breast cancer patient) or in a primary brain tumor, as well as in a patient with brain metastases. The radionuclide scan is not as sensitive as the CT scan, but in an unusual circumstance it may be positive when the CT is negative.

CT Scan — Few morphological characteristics, such as scan configuration, density, enhancement, etc., are specific for cancer metastases. Benign treatable causes of brain CT scan solitary lesions must be ruled out. The CT scan does detect metastases smaller than those seen on radionuclide scan, but still fails to reveal 40% of all metastases seen on brain autopsy. It should be employed in the asymptomatic patient only in those diseases in which there is effective treatment for early brain metastases (a rare situation). Multiple abnormalities in a neurologically symptomatic patient increase the accuracy and reliability of brain tests.

Nuclear Magnetic Resonance (NMR) — NMR has evolved as a primary imaging modality depicting many intracranial and spinal cord abnormalities. However, it is not possible to distinguish tumor from edema because both entities produce abnormal signals on T1 and T2 weighted images. The use of intravenous paramagnetic contrast agents may soon help us to make the differentiation between neoplastic and inflammatory lesions. Again, the results tend to parallel those seen with iodinated agents in CT.

Lung

Chest Film (AP and Lateral) — Many studies have shown that a well-taken and carefully examined AP and lateral chest film is a good screening exam for most cancers; few patients with lung metastases will be missed. A tomogram will usually reveal more metastatic nodules than seen on the simple roentgenographic chest exam, although a few patients without findings on simple chest film will show metastases by tomography.

CT Scan — CT of the chest will definitely reveal more metastases measuring less than 6 mm than will a tomogram. But half of the lesions less than 6 mm in diameter are benign. Because of the 50% false-positive rate, the CT scan should not be used alone to change decisions. One use for the CT scan would be in a patient in whom the resection of one or more metastases is contemplated. If many more were seen than were demonstrated by the X-ray examination, and if previously unvisualized hilar metastases are seen, resection might be contraindicated.

NMR — NMR appears to be more sensitive in detecting mediastinal masses when compared with CT. Magnetic resonance, however, cannot discriminate between neoplastic and inflammatory lymph node pathology by T1 and T2 relaxation times.

Liver

Radionuclide Scan — Radionuclide scanning to screen for metastatic liver disease in a patient with a normal-size liver (clinically) and negative liver function test is not very productive. It is recommended that screening consist of a clinical examination, an LDH, and an alkaline phosphatase determination. If these tests are negative, fewer than 5 to 10% of primary cancer patients will show lesions with radionuclide scanning (excluding colon, pancreas, and stomach primaries). The usefulness of liver radionuclide scanning is outweighed by the high incidence of false-positive scans (5 to 10%). In some series, the incidence is as high as 40%. There is a high incidence of false-positive scans in alcoholic populations and in patients with fatty livers. Liver cell adenomas, hamartomas, vascular abnormalities, and deviant liver anatomy may foil even those very experienced in interpreting liver scans.

CT Scan — The CT scan is less sensitive but more specific than the radionuclide scan. If the liver radionuclide scan interpretation is equivocal, the patient should be evaluated with a CT scan or a biopsy in order to confirm the presence or absence of metastases, if therapeutic decisions are to be based on this finding.

Ultrasound — This test is very operator-dependent, and should be carefully performed by a highly skilled operator working closely with the clinically astute physician. It is necessary to repeat the test at the same sitting or at future sittings in order to evaluate the findings considered to be abnormal. If used in this setting, the ultrasound can be quite useful, especially in the thin patient. The newer technique of real time ultrasound has made the test more reliable.

NMR — Primary and metastatic neoplasms can be detected with NMR, although optimal pulse sequences in diagnosing intrahepatic metastasis are yet to be determined. The T1 weighted images, as well as heavily T2 weighted images, have improved soft tissue contrast between pathological and normal liver tissue when compared to computed tomography.

Bone

Radionuclide Scan — Bone scans are very nonspecific. Solitary bone scan abnormalities in an asymptomatic cancer patient represent benign entities in as many as 33% of patients. Therefore, interpretation must be done extremely carefully, and therapeutic decisions based on solitary nonarticular abnormalities depend on histologic confirmation or observation over a period of time. In general, scanning is recommended only in patients with an elevated alkaline phosphatase and pain, with the exception of patients with prostate and breast cancer. The scan is not a worthwhile test to screen a Stage I operable breast cancer patient (frequent false-positive and low yield), although breast cancer is known to be a bone seeker, when and if it disseminates. Appropriate bone X-rays are necessary to confirm scan findings especially in the following special circumstances: (1) to better evaluate a patient with pelvic symptoms and a negative scan; (2) in patients with highly destructive tumors such as multiple myeloma; (3) in patients with bone symptomatology and negative scans.

NMR — Although cortical bone is recorded on NMR images as an area of markedly decreased signal, the bone marrow produces an intense signal. Through this process NMR has shown increased sensitivity in detecting skeletal pathology. However, its ability to differentiate neoplastic lesions from inflammatory or traumatic lesions is yet to be confirmed. Both benign and malignant primary osseous tumors, as well as metastatic disease and inflammatory lesions, have shown prolonged T1 and T2 relaxation times.

Chemical Markers

Circulating chemical tumor markers accurately correlate with the volume of metastatic nonendocrine cancer spread to visceral organs in only two instances. The first is the human chorionic gonadotropin titer (HGT), which is a sensitive and specific test for placental cancer and for choriocarcinoma of the genitalia. The second is alpha-fetoprotein (AFP), which is an equally good test for metastatic embryonal yolk sac and testicular cancer. A combination of these two tumor markers is better than either one alone in germinal malignancies.

Carcinoembryonic antigen has not proved clinically useful, but if very high levels are recorded in patients with colon cancer primaries, there appears to be a greater than 50% chance that liver metastases are present. When used to detect early recurrence of colon cancer, this test has not proven to increase the rate of survival in these patients. Most other chemical tests are nonspecific and only variably sensitive. Except in the above circumstances, chemical tumor markers are at best a general guideline and should rarely be used alone for decision making.

SELECTION OF TESTS

Table 10 summarizes which organ(s) should be screened to find visceral spread of a given primary cancer. These organs will be called the primary organs for screening. This may ignore some of the previously discussed pathways of spread because of either weaknesses of clinical screening methods for some of these organs, or the rarity of detecting anything in these organs by conventional methods in spite of their involvement as determined by autopsy studies. The primary metastatic organ(s) indicated will usually be positive if metastases are found elsewhere. A positive test for metastases in the primary organ of spread will alert the clinician to the possibility of visceral involvement. If tests of the primary organs are positive, then the secondary organs may be screened. Screening for visceral metastases in a particular primary tumor is useful, especially in patients with bad prognoses. Screening of secondary organs, however, may be useful if primary screening is positive.

SUMMARY

A well-defined policy of test ordering should be developed which takes into account the following elements:

1. Pathways of tumor spread
2. Incidence of tumor spread based on the overall clinical and autopsy incidence of metastases from a given primary cancer
3. The accuracy of the test (risk-cost benefit ratio)
4. The treatability of the tumor once having spread to that organ

CONCLUSION

The decisions involved in staging and managing the patient with a primary treatable cancer must take into account the natural history of the cancer in the patient being studied. The concept of a primary target organ for metastases sheds light upon the apparent orderliness of venous hematogenous cancer spread and trapping of malignant cells in appropriate viscera. Thus, given (1) the propensity of a particular tumor to develop visceral metastases; (2) a blood-borne pathway for these metastases; (3) a critical therapeutic decision that must be made (i.e., to amputate, to begin chemotherapy, to withhold radiotherapy, etc.); and (4) an accurate test to predict spread, we can rationally order and interpret only those tests which will influence therapy.

A rationale, then, has been presented for the spread and growth of metastases to selected organs from primary malignancies in various sites. Application of the metastatic principles discussed and the tests recommended will yield information that is clinically relevant, thereby protecting the patient from both unnecessary risk and increased expense.

TABLE 10
Organs for Screening in Asymptomatic Patients With a High Risk for Visceral Metastases (Poor Prognostic Factors)

Primary site	Poor prognostic factors	Organs for screening	
		Primary	Secondary
Gynecologic			
Ovary	Teratoma (↑ HCG&AFP)	Chest	Liver
	Stage III		
Uterus	High grade	Chest	Liver
	Ovary extension		
	Deep invasion		
Cervix	Recurrent pelvic cancer	Chest	Bone
	Stage IIIB		Liver?
	Peri-aortic nodes		
Vulva	Deep pelvis nodes	Chest	
Choriocarcinoma	High titers of HCG	Chest	Liver
			Brain
Urologic			
Kidney	Contralateral kidney	Chest	Bone
	Vein involvement		Liver
	Nodes		
	Perinephric spread		
Prostate	Poorly differentiated	Bone	Chest
	Lymph nodes		
	Extracapsular extension		
Testis	High AFP or HCG titer	Chest	Liver
	Multiple nodes in retro peritoneum		
Bladder	High grade	Chest	
	Deep muscle	Bone[a]	
	Positive nodes	Liver[a]	
Pediatric			
Rhabdomyosarcoma	Positive nodes	Liver	
	Nonorbital Primary	Chest	
		Bone	
Neuroblastoma	High grade	Liver	Chest
	High catecholamine titers		Bone
	Not complete resection		
Wilms'	Extracapsular extension	Chest	Liver
	Positive nodes		
	Sarcoma		
Ewing's	All	Bone	Liver
		Chest	
Bone	All	Chest	Bone
Head and neck	Recurrent cancer	Chest	
	Bulky lymph nodes		
Miscellaneous			
Breast	>Four nodes in axilla	Chest	
	Supraclavicular nodes	Bone	Liver
	Primary over 5 cm		
Thyroid	Anaplastic	Chest	Liver
	Extrathyroid extension	Bone	
Melanoma	Skin nodules	Chest	Bone
	Positive nodes	Liver	
Lung	Mediastinal nodes	Bone	Marrow
	Oat cell cancer	Liver	

TABLE 10 (continued)
Organs for Screening in Asymptomatic Patients With a High Risk for Visceral Metastases (Poor Prognostic Factors)

Primary site	Poor prognostic factors	Organs for screening Primary	Secondary
Lymphoma			
Hodgkin's	All	Liver	
		Chest	
		Bone	
		Marrow	
Non-Hodgkin's	All	Liver	Bone
		Chest	
Gastrointestinal			
Pancreas	Nodal involvement		
Stomach	Serosal involvement	Liver	
		Chest	
Colon	Nodal involvement		
	Serosal involvement	Liver	Chest
Rectum	Perirectal involvement	Liver	
	Nodal involvement	Chest	
Sarcoma	High grade	Chest	
	Greater than 5 cm		

ᵃ   Before cystectomy only.

SELECTED JOURNALS PUBLISHING BASIC NUCLEAR MEDICINE SCIENCE AND DIAGNOSTIC MEDICAL IMAGING LITERATURE

Acta Radiologica: Diagnosis
Acta Radiologica: Oncology, Radiation, Physic, Biology
Acta Radiologica Supplementum
Advances in Magnetic Resonance
American Journal of Cardiac Imaging
American Journal of Roentgenology
American Journal of Physiologic Imaging
American Journal of Neuroradiology
Annales de Radiologie
Annals of Nuclear Medicine (Japan)
Annals of Nuclear Medicine (ROC)
Applied Radiation and Isotopes
Applied Radiology
British Journal of Radiology
Cardiovascular and Interventional Radiology
Cardiovascular Ultrasonography
Clinical Nuclear Medicine
Clinical Radiology
Compact News in Nuclear Medicine — NUC
Computerized Radiology
CRC Critical Reviews in Diagnostic Imaging
Diagnostic Imaging
Diagnostic Imaging in Clinical Medicine
European Journal of Nuclear Medicine
Gastrointestinal Radiology
Health Physics
IEEE Transactions — Biomedical Engineering

International Journal of Applied Radiation and Isotopes
International Journal of Nuclear Medicine and Biology
International Journal of Radiation Biology and Related Studies in Physics, Chemistry and Medicine
International Journal of Radiation Oncology, Biology, Physics
Investigative Radiology
Isotope News
Japanese Journal of Magnetic Resonance in Medicine
Journal Belge de Radiologie
Journal de Radiologie
Journal of Clinical Engineering
Journal of Clinical Ultrasound
Journal of Computer Assisted Tomography
Journal of Computerized Tomography
Journal of Magnetic Resonance in Medicine
Journal of Medical Imaging
Journal of Nuclear Medicine
Journal of Nuclear Medicine and Allied Sciences
Journal of Nuclear Medicine Technology
Journal of Physics (E): Scientific Instruments
Journal of Radiation Research
Journal of Ultrasound Medicine
Kaku Igaku
Korean Journal of Nuclear Medicine
Magnetic Resonance Imaging
Magnetic Resonance in Medicine
Magnetic Resonance Quarterly
Medical Physics
Neuroradiology
Noninvasive Medical Imaging
Nuclear Medicine Communications
Nuklearmedizin
Pediatric Radiology
Physics in Medicine and Biology
Physiological Chemistry, Physics and Medical NMR
Polski Przeglad Radiologii i Medycyny Nuklearnej
Progress in Nuclear Medicine
Radiation and Environmental Biophysics
Radiation Medicine
Radiation Research
Radioactive Isotopes in Clinical Medicine
Radiobiologia, Radiotherapia
Radiobiologiia
Radioisotopes
Radiologe
Radiologia Diagnostica
Radiologia Medica
Radiologic Clinics of North America
Radiology
Reviews of Scientific Instruments
ROEFE: Fortschritte auf dem Gebiete der Roentgenstrahlen und der Nuklearmedizin
Recent Advances in Clinical Nuclear Medicine
Recent Advances in Nuclear Medicine
Seminars in Nuclear Medicine
Skeletal Radiology
Urologic Radiology
Vestnik Roentgenologii Radiologii

INDEX TO HANDBOOK

INDEX